# Advances in Immunology

# Advances in Immunology

Edited by **Marcy Ward**

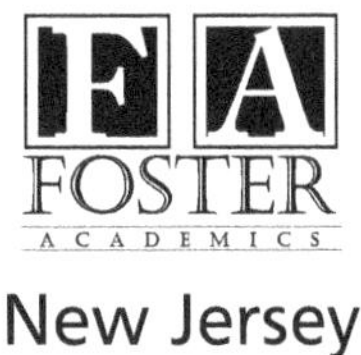


New Jersey

Published by Foster Academics,
61 Van Reypen Street,
Jersey City, NJ 07306, USA
www.fosteracademics.com

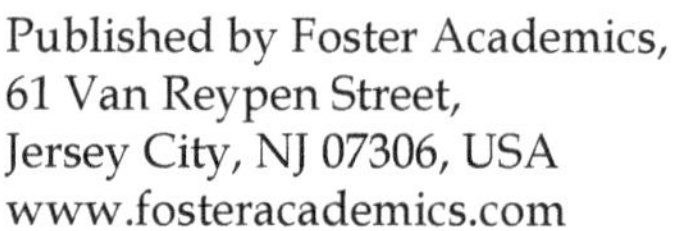

**Advances in Immunology**
Edited by Marcy Ward



International Standard Book Number: 978-1-63242-457-0 (Hardback)



Printed in the United States of America.

# Contents

# Preface

This book discusses the fundamentals as well as modern approaches of immunology. As a branch of bio-medical science, immunology refers to the study of the immune system, its physiological functions, its chemical, physical, biological characteristics and the causes of its malfunction. There are various types of immunological studies like classical immunology, developmental immunology, theoretical immunology, diagnostic immunology, cancer immunology, etc. This text will trace the progress of this field and highlight some of its key concepts and applications. It will attempt to provide a comprehensive understanding of the multiple branches that fall under immunology and their importance. From theories to research to practical applications, case studies related to various topics of relevance to this subject have been included in this book. Students, immunologists, doctors, researchers and all interested in this area will find this book beneficial.

The researches compiled throughout the book are authentic and of high quality, combining several disciplines and from very diverse regions from around the world. Drawing on the contributions of many researchers from diverse countries, the book's objective is to provide the readers with the latest achievements in the area of research. This book will surely be a source of knowledge to all interested and researching the field.

In the end, I would like to express my deep sense of gratitude to all the authors for meeting the set deadlines in completing and submitting their research chapters. I would also like to thank the publisher for the support offered to us throughout the course of the book. Finally, I extend my sincere thanks to my family for being a constant source of inspiration and encouragement.

**Editor**

1

# Lipopolysaccharide Attenuates CD40 Ligand-Induced Regulatory B10 Cell Expansion and IL-10 Production in Mouse Splenocytes

**Mei Lin[1,2], Jiang Lin[1,3], Yuhua Wang[1,4], Nathalie Bonheur[1], Toshihisa Kawai[1], Zuomin Wang[2*], Xiaozhe Han[1*]**

[1]Department of Immunology and Infectious Diseases, The Forsyth Institute, Cambridge, USA
[2]Department of Stomatology, Beijing Chao-Yang Hospital, Capital Medical University, Beijing, China
[3]Department of Stomatology, Fourth Hospital of Harbin Medical University, Harbin, China
[4]Department of Stomatology, Shanghai 9th People's Hospital, Shanghai, China
Email: [*]wzuomin@gmail.com, [*]xhan@forsyth.org

## Abstract

**Toll-like receptors (TLRs) play a key role in B cell-mediated innate and adaptive immunity. It has been shown that interleukin 10 (IL-10)-producing regulatory B cells (B10 cells) can negatively regulate cellular immune responses and inflammation in autoimmune diseases. In this study, we determined the effect of TLR4 signaling on the CD40-activated B10 cell competency. The results demonstrated that LPS and CD40L synergistically stimulated proliferation of mouse splenocytes. The percentage of B10 cells in cultured splenocytes was significantly increased after CD40L stimulation but such increase was diminished by the addition of LPS. Such effects by LPS were only observed in cells from WT but not TLR4$^{-/-}$ mice. IL-10 mRNA expression and protein production in B10 cells from cultured splenocytes were significantly up-regulated by CD40L stimulation but were inhibited after the addition of LPS in a TLR4-dependent manner. This study suggests that LPS-induced TLR4 signaling attenuate CD40L-activated regulatory B10 cell competency.**

## Keywords

**IL10, B10, TLR4, CD40L, LPS**

[*]Corresponding authors.

# 1. Introduction

B cells have been suggested to contribute to the pathogenesis of autoimmune disease through antigen (Ag)-specific autoantibody production [1]. This central role in provoking inflammation in autoimmune diseases has made B cell attractive therapeutic targets through the depletion of these cells [2] [3]. In the past decade, however, data from a number of laboratories have revealed that B cells can also play regulatory roles in the amelioration of inflammation through their interaction with effecter T cells and other innate cells [4]. Recently an IL-10-competent CD1d(high)CD5(+) B cell subset termed B10 cells has been identified in both mice and humans that can play regulatory functions during immune and inflammatory responses [5] [6]. In most autoimmune disease models studied so far, this suppressive or regulatory role of B cells is mediated by the production of IL-10, which inhibits both Th1 and Th2 polarization, Ag presentation and pro-inflammatory cytokine production by myeloid cells [7] [8]. It also has potent activity in limiting DC function in secreting IL-6 and IL-12, and thereby inhibits Th17 cells [9]. B-cell-derived IL-10 is essential for the regulatory function of B cells, as B cells isolated from IL-10 knockout mice failed to mediate the protective function in various autoimmune disease models, such as collagen induced arthritis [10], experimental autoimmune encephalomyelitis [7], non-obese diabetes [11], and inflammatory bowel diseases [12].

CD40 ligation plays a crucial role in B cell activation, T cell-dependent antigen-driven isotype switching and germinal center formation [13]. It has been reported that selective targeting of B cells with agonistic anti-CD40 is an efficacious strategy for the generation of induced regulatory B cells and for the suppression of autoimmune disease [14]. Furthermore, recent studies have shown that B cells express distinct TLRs that determine their ability to respond to microbial patterns, which underlines their direct involvement in the regulatory functions of B cells during autoimmune and infectious diseases [15]. Understanding how B10 cells can be regulated by TLR signaling is of considerable clinical relevance in designing strategies to expand such populations to augment the treatments of autoimmune diseases and overly aggressive inflammatory responses. In this study, we investigated how TLR4 signaling affects CD40-activated B10 cell expansion and IL-10 production.

# 2. Materials and Methods

## 2.1. Mice Strain

Both groups of wild type (WT) and TLR deficient (TLR4$^{-/-}$) mice (n = 10) were of C57BL/6 background and were used for these experiments. TLR4$^{-/-}$ mice backcrossed to the C57BL/6 background were a kind gift from Dr. Toshihisa Kawai (Forsyth Institute, Cambridge, USA). All the mice used in the study (8 - 10 weeks old) were maintained in specific pathogen-free (SPF) units of the Forsyth Institute Animal Facility. The mice were kept on a 12-hour light/dark cycle. The experimental protocols were approved by the Institutional Animal Care and Use Committee of the Forsyth Institute.

## 2.2. Culture of Splenocytes

Mice were euthanized in a $CO_2$ chamber and single-cell suspensions of splenocytes were obtained by dispersing spleen tissues through a 60-gauge stainless steel screen. Erythrocytes were removed by ACK lysing buffer (Lonza, MA). Isolated splenocytes were added into 96-well plates (2.0 × $10^5$/well) in 200 µl RPMI complete medium containing 10% FBS. CD40L (Thermo Scientific) and *E. coli* LPS (strain O55:B5, Sigma-Aldrich) were used as agonist. Splenocytes from WT and TLR4$^{-/-}$ mice were divided into 4 treatment groups: control; *E. coli* LPS (10 µg/ml); CD40L (1 µg/ml); *E. coli* LPS (10 µg/ml) + CD40L (1 µg/ml). Cells were cultured at 37˚C in a humidified incubator with 5% $CO_2$ for 2 days and then were collected for analysis.

## 2.3. Cell Proliferation Analysis

Isolated mouse splenocytes were added into 96-well plates (2 × $10^5$/well ) in 200 µl RPMI complete medium containing 10% FBS and were cultured for 2 days in the presence or absence of *E. coli* LPS (10 µg/ml) and/or CD40L (1 µg/ml). Cell proliferation was evaluated using a MTS reagent CellTiter 96 AQueous Assay (Promega Corp). After 4 hour incubation, the plate was read at OD 490 nm.

## 2.4. Flow Cytometry

At the termination of cell culture, splenocytes in the 96-well plates were washed with PBS followed by incubation with fluorescence conjugated antibodies, including FITC-conjugated anti-mouse CD19, PE-conjugated anti-mouse CD5 and Alexa Fluor 647-conjugated anti-mouse CD1d, using mouse regulatory B cell (B10) flow kit (Biolegend). At least 20,000 cells were counted for analysis and at least 100,000 cells were sorted from each sample for PCR and ELISA.

### 2.5. Reverse Transcription and Quantitative Real Time PCR

Total RNA was extracted from the cells using a Purelink RNA mini kit (Life Technology) following manufacturer's instructions. Isolated mRNA (0.1 μg each) was reverse transcribed into cDNA using the SuperScriptII reverse transcription system in the presence of random primers (Invitrogen). Real-time PCR was carried out in a 20 μl reaction system using SuperScript III Platinum SYBR Green One-Step qRT-PCR Kit (Life Technology) in a Roche LightCycler 480 (Roche Diagnostics, Indianapolis, IN). Each RNA sample was loaded in duplicate into the plate with a template amount of 10 ng. Predesigned primers of GAPDH and IL-10 were from Sigma. The sequences of the primers used were: IL-10: 5'-agcactcccgtctcaaagaa-3' and 5'-tgacgaacatctctggcttg-3' (106 bp); GAPDH: 5'-ccccagcaaggacactgagcaa-3' and 5'-gtgggtgcagcgaactttattgatg-3' (162 bp). The real-time PCR conditions were: 50°C for 3 minutes, 95°C for 10 minutes, followed by 40 cycles of 95°C for 10 seconds, 58°C for 10 seconds, 72°C for 15 seconds. Results were presented as fold changes relative to GAPDH reference.

### 2.6. ELISA

Cell culture supernatant were collected and IL-10 level in the supernatant was detected using a Mouse IL-10 ELISA MAX Standard kit (Biolegend).

### 2.7. Statistical Analysis

All the quantitative data are expressed as means ± standard error. IL-10 gene expression by PCR, IL-10 production by ELISA were evaluated by the Student-Newman-Keuls (SNK) multiple comparison test following one-way analysis of variance (ANOVA). P values of $<0.05$ were considered statistically significant.

## 3. Results

### 3.1. LPS-Induced Proliferation of Mouse Splenocytes Was Enhanced by CD40L

Cultured mouse slpenocytes were treated with *E. coli* LPS and/or CD40L and the overall cell proliferation status was determined. The results demonstrated that *E. coli* LPS significantly promoted proliferation of splenoctes from WT mice but not those from $TLR4^{-/-}$ mice (**Figure 1**). Cell proliferation was not affected when cells were treated with CD40L alone, while LPS-induced cell proliferation was greatly enhanced by the addition of CD40L in WT but not $TLR4^{-/-}$ mice (**Figure 1**). These results suggested that CD40L enhances LPS-induced mouse splenocytes proliferation in a TLR4-dependent manner.

### 3.2. CD40L-Induced B10 Cell Expansion in Mouse Splenocytes Was Inhibited by LPS

After incubation with *E. coli* LPS and/or CD40L for 2 days, $CD19^{+}CD1d^{hi}CD5^{+}$ cells in cultured splenocytes were detected by flow cytometry. The results showed that the percentage of $CD19^{+}CD1d^{hi}CD5^{+}$ cells in cultured splenocytes was unchanged when cells were treated with LPS alone but was significantly increased after CD40L stimulation. Such CD40L-induced expansion of $CD19^{+}CD1d^{hi}CD5^{+}$ cells was diminished when splenocytes were treated with LPS in addition to CD40L (**Figure 2**). However, addition of LPS did not inhibit the CD40L-induced expansion of $CD19^{+}CD1d^{hi}CD5^{+}$ cells in splenocytes from $TLR4^{-/-}$ mice (**Figure 2**), substantiating that such suppressive effect of LPS is TLR4-dependent.

### 3.3. CD40L-Induced IL-10 mRNA Expression by B10 Cells Was Inhibited by LPS

After incubation with *E. coli* LPS and/or CD40L for 2 days, $CD19^{+}CD1d^{hi}CD5^{+}$ cells representing B10 cells in cultured splenocytes were sorted by flow cytometry. After RNA isolation, IL-10 expression levels in sorted B10 cells were detected by real-time PCR. The results showed that IL-10 mRNA level in B10 cells was not affected by LPS treatment but was significantly elevated after CD40L stimulation (**Figure 3**). Such increase was dimi-

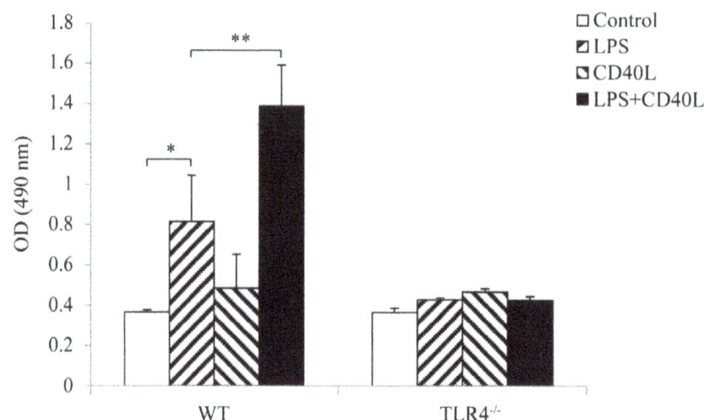


**Figure 1.** Stimulation of mouse splenocytes proliferation by LPS and/or CD40L. Cultured mouse slpenocytes were treated with *E. coli* LPS (10 μg/ml) and/or CD40L (1 μg/ml) for 2 days and the overall cell proliferation status was determined by CellTiter 96 AQueous Assay (Promega Corp). The results are representative of at least six independent experiments in duplicates. Data are presented as mean ± SEM, n = 6. Student t-test, $^{*}P < 0.05$, $^{**}P < 0.01$.

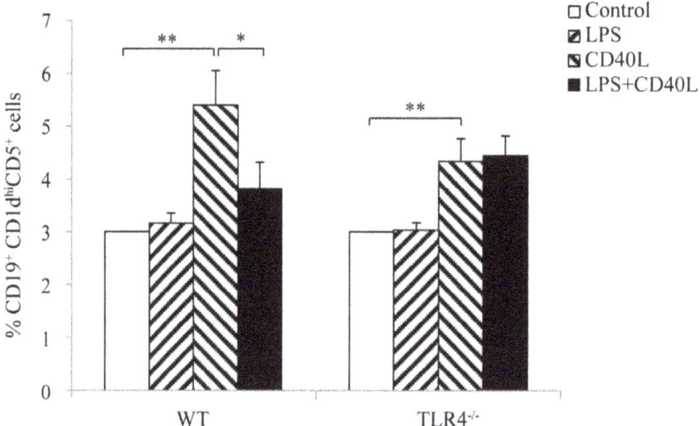


**Figure 2.** B10 cell expansion in mouse splenocytes after LPS and/or CD40L stimulation. Cultured mouse slpenocytes were treated with *E. coli* LPS (10 μg/ml) and/or CD40L (1 μg/ml) for 2 days and $CD19^{+}CD1d^{hi}CD5^{+}$ cells in the cultured splenocytes were detected using flow cytometry. At least 20,000 cells were counted for analysis. Data are presented as mean ± SEM, n = 6. Student t-test, $^{*}P < 0.05$, $^{**}P < 0.01$.

nished when splenocytes were treated with LPS in addition to CD40L (**Figure 3**). However, addition of LPS did not inhibit the CD40L-induced up-regulation of IL-10 expression in B10 cells from $TLR4^{-/-}$ mice (**Figure 3**).

## 3.4. CD40L-Induced IL-10 Protein Production by B10 Cells Was Inhibited by LPS

After incubation with *E. coli* LPS and/or CD40L for 2 days, $CD19^{+}CD1d^{hi}CD5^{+}$ cells in cultured splenocytes were sorted by flow cytometry and IL-10 protein levels in sorted B10 cells were measured by ELISA. The results showed that IL-10 protein level in sorted B10 cells was not affected by LPS treatment but was significantly elevated after CD40L stimulation (**Figure 4**). Such increase was dramatically reduced when splenocytes were treated with both CD40L and LPS (**Figure 4**). However, addition of LPS did not inhibit the CD40L-induced production of IL-10 in cultured splenocytes from $TLR4^{-/-}$ mice (**Figure 4**).

# 4. Discussion

TLR signaling play an important role in bridging innate and adaptive immunity mediated by B cells [16]. Although

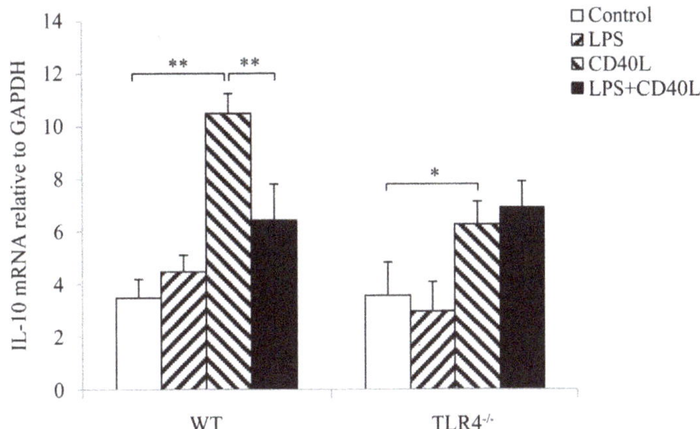


**Figure 3.** IL-10 mRNA expression by B10 cells after LPS and/or CD40L stimulation. Cultured mouse slpenocytes were treated with *E. coli* LPS (10 μg/ml) and/or CD40L (1 μg/ml) for 2 days and $CD19^{+}CD1d^{hi}CD5^{+}$ cells in the cultured splenocytes were sorted out using flow cytometry. Total RNA were isolated from sorted cells using a Purelink RNA mini kit (Life Technology) and IL-10 expression was determined by real time PCR. At least 100,000 cells were sorted from each sample for PCR. Data are presented as mean ± SEM, n = 6. Student t-test, $^{*}P < 0.05$, $^{**}P < 0.01$.

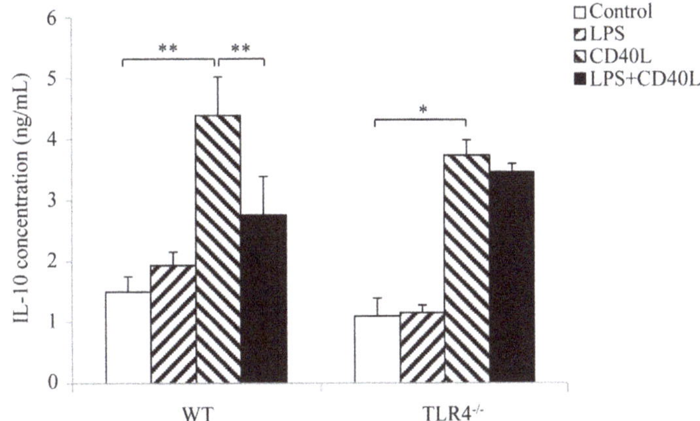


**Figure 4.** IL-10 protein production by B10 cells after LPS and/or CD40L stimulation. Cultured mouse slpenocytes were treated with *E. coli* LPS (10 μg/ml) and/or CD40L (1 μg/ml) for 2 days and $CD19^{+}CD1d^{hi}CD5^{+}$ cells in the cultured splenocytes were sorted out using flow cytometry. Total protein lysate were collected from sorted cells and IL-10 production was determined by ELISA. At least 100,000 cells were sorted from each sample for ELISA. Data are presented as mean ± SEM, n = 6. Student t-test, $^{*}P < 0.05$, $^{**}P < 0.01$.

studies have suggested that agonists for TLR synergized with CD40 stimulation for T cells, little is known about the effects of the CD40 pathway together with TLR-derived stimuli in B cells. Our results suggest that TLR agonists can interact with signals from adaptive immunity to regulate B cell function during host immune response. In particular, activation of TLR4 signaling by LPS together with activation of CD40 pathway by CD40L attenuated regulatory B cell (B10) competency.

It has been demonstrated that TLR agonists synergize with CD40L to induce either proliferation or plasma cell differentiation of mouse B cells [17]. However, how TLR agonists interact with CD40L to modulate the function of regulatory B cells is completely unknown. By performing multi-parametric analysis using CD19, CD5, CD1d antibodies by flow cytometry, we were able to accurately identify low frequency and phenotypically unique regulatory B10 cells and determine their responses to the TLR agonist (LPS) and CD40L. Our results indicated that cell proliferation and regulatory B cell (B10) function are differentially regulated by LPS/CD40L. CD40L synergistically stimulates LPS-induced splenocytes proliferation while LPS antagonize CD40L-induced B10 activations, namely IL-10 production. Previous studies have indicated that TLR-mediated activation of T cells can directly promote the development of autoimmunity and TLR-4-stimulation can activate the antigen presenting cells sufficiently to deliver the signals required to drive the pathogenic function of the T cell [18] [19]. More interestingly, recent data showed that treatment with LPS selectively promoted in the recipient mice the generation of IL-6-producing activated B cells and mediated the differentiation of naive CD4 cells into Th17 phenotypes [20]. Given the pivotal role of regulatory B cells in the control of autoimmunity [7] [8], our findings may provide novel mechanism of autoimmune pathogenesis via LPS-associated suppression of CD40-activated regulatory B cells.

It is noted from our results that the level of IL-10 production detected by PCR and ELISA represent the IL-10 production by B10 cells in the context of cultured splenocytes, not purified B cells as others have demonstrated previously [6]. Yanaba *et al.* clearly showed that LPS as well as CD40 stimulation promotes B10 generation and that LPS, but not CD40, stimulation induces IL-10 secretion in purified B cells *in vitro* [6]. A possible explanation for the discrepancy between these findings and current findings could be that cellular components other than B cells, when responsive to the LPS/CD40L stimulation, are also contributed to the subsequent IL-10 production by B10 cells. B cell responses observed in this study are in the presence of other cellular components in cultured splenocytes, including T cells, dendritic cells and macrophages, which upon LPS/CD40L stimulation, provide potential co-stimulatory or counteractive molecules for the subsequent B cell activation. Therefore, the detected changes in B10 expansion and IL-10 production could be derived from both direct activation of TLR4 and CD40 on B cells and provisions of the co-stimulatory molecules by non-B cells. Studies using purified B cells directly stimulated by LPS/CD40L are warranted to verify if the observed B10 activation and IL-10 regulation in response to LPS/CD40L is solely contributed by and dependent on, intrinsic roles of B cell responses.

## 5. Conclusion

There is an emerging appreciation for the pivotal role played by B cells in several areas of human diseases including autoimmune diseases such as systemic lupus erythematosus (SLE) [21] and Sjögren's syndrome [22]. Established B-cell-directed therapy such as Rituximab has provided a solid foundation for the assessment of the value of other B-cell-based approaches and to survey the range of B-cell involvement in human pathology [23]. The recent research advancement of regulatory B cells in human disease coincides with the vastly accelerated pace of research on the bridging of innate and adaptive immune system [24] [25]. It has been suggested that the *ex vivo* expansion of B10 cells through co-activation of innate and adaptive pathways and reinfusion of autologous B10 cells may provide a novel and effective *in vivo* treatment for severe autoimmune diseases that are resistant to current therapies [26]. Current study and our continued research may provide better understanding of the mechanisms that promote regulatory B10 cell function to counteract exaggerated immune activation in autoimmune as well as non-autoimmune conditions.

## Acknowledgments

This work was supported by NIH Grant DE-021837 and DE-023807 from the National Institute of Dental and Craniofacial Research.

## Disclosure

The authors have no financial conflict of interest.

## References

[1] Lipsky, P.E. (2001) Systemic Lupus Erythematosus: An Autoimmune Disease of B Cell Hyperactivity. *Nature Immunology*, **2**, 764-766. http://dx.doi.org/10.1038/ni0901-764

[2] Dorner, T., *et al.* (2009) Current Status on B-Cell Depletion Therapy in Autoimmune Diseases Other than Rheumatoid Arthritis. *Autoimmunity Reviews*, **9**, 82-89. http://dx.doi.org/10.1016/j.autrev.2009.08.007

[3] Sanz, I., Anolik, J.H. and Looney, R.J. (2007) B Cell Depletion Therapy in Autoimmune Diseases. *Frontiers in Bioscience*, **12**, 2546-2567. http://dx.doi.org/10.2741/2254

[4] Fillatreau, S., Gray, D. and Anderton, S.M. (2008) Not Always the Bad Guys: B Cells as Regulators of Autoimmune Pathology. *Nature Reviews Immunology*, **8**, 391-397. http://dx.doi.org/10.1038/nri2315

[5] Iwata, Y., *et al.* (2011) Characterization of a Rare IL-10-Competent B-Cell Subset in Humans That Parallels Mouse Regulatory B10 Cells. *Blood*, **117**, 530-541. http://dx.doi.org/10.1182/blood-2010-07-294249

[6] Yanaba, K., *et al.* (2009) The Development and Function of Regulatory B Cells Expressing IL-10 (B10 Cells) Requires Antigen Receptor Diversity and TLR Signals. *Journal of Immunology*, **182**, 7459-7472. http://dx.doi.org/10.4049/jimmunol.0900270

[7] Fillatreau, S., *et al.* (2002) B Cells Regulate Autoimmunity by Provision of IL-10. *Nature Immunology*, **3**, 944-950. http://dx.doi.org/10.1038/ni833

[8] Rieger, A. and Bar-Or, A. (2008) B-Cell-Derived Interleukin-10 in Autoimmune Disease: Regulating the Regulators. *Nature Reviews Immunology*, **8**, 486-487. http://dx.doi.org/10.1038/nri2315-c1

[9] Moulin, V., *et al.* (2000) B Lymphocytes Regulate Dendritic Cell (DC) Function *in Vivo*: Increased Interleukin 12 Production by DCs from B Cell-Deficient Mice Results in T Helper Cell Type 1 Deviation. *Journal of Experimental Medicine*, **192**, 475-482. http://dx.doi.org/10.1084/jem.192.4.475

[10] Mauri, C., *et al.* (2003) Prevention of Arthritis by Interleukin 10-Producing B Cells. *Journal of Experimental Medicine*, **197**, 489-501. http://dx.doi.org/10.1084/jem.20021293

[11] Hussain, S. and Delovitch, T.L. (2007) Intravenous Transfusion of BCR-Activated B Cells Protects NOD Mice from Type 1 Diabetes in an IL-10-Dependent Manner. *Journal of Immunology*, **179**, 7225-7232. http://dx.doi.org/10.4049/jimmunol.179.11.7225

[12] Mizoguchi, E., Mizoguchi, A., Preffer, F.I. and Bhan, A.K. (2000) Regulatory Role of Mature B Cells in a Murine Model of Inflammatory Bowel Disease. *International Immunology*, **12**, 597-605. http://dx.doi.org/10.1093/intimm/12.5.597

[13] Castigli, E., Young, F., Carossino, A.M., Alt, F.W. and Geha, R.S. (1996) CD40 Expression and Function in Murine B Cell Ontogeny. *International Immunology*, **8**, 405-411. http://dx.doi.org/10.1093/intimm/8.3.405

[14] Blair, P.A., Chavez-Rueda, K.A., Evans, J.G., Shlomchik, M.J., Eddaoudi, A., Isenberg, D.A., *et al.* (2009) Selective Targeting of B Cells with Agonistic Anti-CD40 Is an Efficacious Strategy for the Generation of Induced Regulatory T2-Like B Cells and for the Suppression of Lupus in MRL/lpr Mice. *Journal of Immunology*, **182**, 3492-3502. http://dx.doi.org/10.4049/jimmunol.0803052

[15] Shen, P., Lampropoulou, V., Stervbo, U., Hilgenberg, E., Ries, S., Mecqinion, A. and Fillatreau, S. (2013) Intrinsic Toll-Like Receptor Signalling Drives Regulatory Function in B Cells. *Frontiers in Bioscience* (*Elite Edition*), **5**, 78-86.

[16] Ren, M., Gao, L. and Wu, X. (2010) TLR4: The Receptor Bridging *Acanthamoeba* Challenge and Intracellular Inflammatory Responses in Human Corneal Cell Lines. *Immunology and Cell Biology*, **88**, 529-536. http://dx.doi.org/10.1038/icb.2010.6

[17] Boeglin, E., Smulski, C.R., Brun, S., Milosevic, S., Schneider, P. and Fournel, S. (2011) Toll-Like Receptor Agonists Synergize with CD40L to Induce Either Proliferation or Plasma Cell Differentiation of Mouse B Cells. *PLoS ONE*, **6**, e25542. http://dx.doi.org/10.1371/journal.pone.0025542

[18] Marsland, B.J., Nembrini, C., Grün, K., Reissmann, R., Kurrer, M., Leipner, C. and Kopf, M. (2007) TLR Ligands Act Directly upon T Cells to Restore Proliferation in the Absence of Protein Kinase C-$\theta$ Signaling and Promote Autoimmune Myocarditis. *Journal of Immunology*, **178**, 3466-3473. http://dx.doi.org/10.4049/jimmunol.178.6.3466

[19] Mellanby, R.J., Cambrook, H., Turner, D.G., O'Connor, R.A., Leech, M.D., Kurschus, F.C., *et al.* (2012) TLR-4 Ligation of Dendritic Cells Is Sufficient to Drive Pathogenic T Cell Function in Experimental Autoimmune Encephalomyelitis. *Journal of Neuroinflammation*, **9**, 248. http://dx.doi.org/10.1186/1742-2094-9-248

[20] Shi, G., Vistica, B.P., Nugent, L.F., Tan, C., Wawrousek, E.F., Klinman, D.M. and Gery, I. (2013) Differential Involvement of Th1 and Th17 in Pathogenic Autoimmune Processes Triggered by Different TLR Ligands. *Journal of Immunology*, **191**, 415-423. http://dx.doi.org/10.4049/jimmunol.1201732

[21] Dolff, S., Abdulahad, W., Bijl, M. and Kallenberg, C. (2009) Regulators of B-Cell Activity in SLE: A Better Target for Treatment than B-Cell Depletion? *Lupus*, **18**, 575-580. http://dx.doi.org/10.1177/0961203309102296

[22] Abdulahad, W.H., Meijer, J.M., Kroese, F.G.M., Meiners, P.M., Vissink, A., Spijkervet, F.K.L., Kallenberg, C.G.M. and Bootsma, H. (2011) B Cell Reconstitution and T Helper Cell Balance after Rituximab Treatment of Active Primary Sjogren's Syndrome: A Double-Blind, Placebo-Controlled Study. *Arthritis & Rheumatism*, **63**, 1116-1123. http://dx.doi.org/10.1002/art.30236

[23] Herrera, D., Rojas, O.L., Duarte-Rey, C., Mantilla, R.D., Ángel, J. and Franco, M.A. (2014) Simultaneous Assessment of Rotavirus-Specific Memory B Cells and Serological Memory after B Cell Depletion Therapy with Rituximab. *PLoS ONE*, **9**, e97087. http://dx.doi.org/10.1371/journal.pone.0097087

[24] Marcenaro, E., Carlomagno, S., Pesce, S., Moretta, A. and Sivori, S. (2011) Bridging Innate NK Cell Functions with Adaptive Immunity. *Advances in Experimental Medicine and Biology*, **780**, 45-55. http://dx.doi.org/10.1007/978-1-4419-5632-3_5

[25] Scotet, E., Nedellec, S., Devilder, M.C., Allain, S. and Bonneville, M. (2008) Bridging Innate and Adaptive Immunity through $\gamma\delta$ T-Dendritic Cell Crosstalk. *Frontiers in Bioscience*, **13**, 6872-6885. http://dx.doi.org/10.2741/3195

[26] Yoshizaki, A., Miyagaki, T., DiLillo, D.J., Matsushita, T., Horikawa, M., Kountikov, E.I., *et al.* (2012) Regulatory B Cells Control T-Cell Autoimmunity through IL-21-Dependent Cognate Interactions. *Nature*, **491**, 264-268. http://dx.doi.org/10.1038/nature11501

## Abbreviations

TLR: toll-like receptor;
LPS: lipopolysaccharide;
CD40L: CD40 ligand;
IL10: interleukin 10;
ELISA: enzyme-linked immunosorbent assay.

# 2

# Plant Digestive Supplement Designed by Lactobacillus Regulated Leukocyte Subsets through Activation of Complement Components and Implication for Use against Tumor Bearing Host against Infection

**Kohji Ohtubo[1], Nobuo Yamaguchi[1,2*], Nurmuhamamt Amat[3], Dilxat Yimit[3], Parida Hoxur[4] Hiroshi Ushijima[2] and Yousuke Watanabe[2]**

[1]Ishikawa Natural Medicinal Products Research Center, Ishikawa, Japan
[2]Department of Fundament Research for CAM, Kanazawa Medical University, Ishikawa, Japan
[3]Traditional Uighur Medicine Department, Xinjiang Medical University, Urumqi, China
[4]Traditional Chinese Medicine Hospital, Xinjiang Medical University, Urumqi, China
Email: *serumaya@kanazawa-med.ac.jp

## Abstract

**A plant material consisted by Family Poaceae was fermented by Yeast and *Lactobaccilli* (U-164). This material was proved by as safe in animal safety experiment for oral administration. In order to prove the effect of U-164 against physiological function, the animal and human trials were set up to look into mainly leukocyte functions. In animal experiment, anti-oxidative effect and anti-body response in immune-compromised host and diabetes meritus were made up. For human use, peripheral lymphocyte in number and subset ratio were followed up to one month after adminis-tration. In order to understand its effect, human complement component analysis was made by immune-electrophoresis. Our results showed that U-164 augmented the level of lymphocytes, while U-164 down regulated the level of granulocytes. In our clinical study with 19 healthy volun-teers, granulocyte and lymphocyte ratio was obtained as neutral in peripheral blood being in-creased significantly 30 days after the ingestion of U-164. In experimental animal study, the com-promised host as well as normal animal was administered with cancer chemotherapeutic agent (Mytomycin-C). Our observations showed against antibody producing cell, this material recovered the antibody production in the host compromising the immure responsiveness. We also proposed an idea that U-164 exhibited tonic effects via activating complement components. Moreover, we tried to access further to the anti-oxidative activities of this U-164. This modification brought to**

*Corresponding author.

**the significant lifted up for anti-oxidative activity for phagocytic cell.**

## Keywords

**Family Poaceae, Fermentation, Yeast, Lactobacillus, Cancer Chemotherapeutic Agent, Compromised Host, Complement, C3b Fragment, Anti-Oxidant, Diabetes, Blood Sugar**

## 1. Introduction

In recent years, complementary and alternative medicines (CAM) have achieved more and more attentions since they are able to treat many chronic illnesses, such as fatigue syndrome that plagues the industrialized world. The present team has reported that typical styles of CAM, preparing special molecule for both digestive and easy to activated human complement component regulate functions of leukocytes in human immune system [1] [2]. Dietary and fermented formula holds promise as strong inducers of acquired immunity. While the immune system is working against the local infection of pathogens, cytokine and immuno-competent cells react throughout the body in close connection to the brain, the endocrine and immune system [3]. In this study, we hypothesize that U-164 may influence immuno-competent cells qualitatively and quantitatively U-164 targeting lymphocytes based on the constitution dependent manner. U-164 has been employed as tonic agent and the implication has little been made on the characteristics of the levels of leukocyte subset, such as granulocytes and lymphocytes. In this report, we seek to focus on the identity of U-164 formula, comparing to another herbal medicine. The influence of U-164 on leukocyte and/or lymphocyte subpopulations in human peripheral blood is also discussed. Moreover, some preliminary trials for the new processing of herbal formulae by degradation of acidophilic bacteria and yeast fungus [4].

## 2. Materials and Methods

### 2.1. Animal Study

#### 2.1.1. Single and Multiple Dose Toxicity Study

Nine female seven-week-old ddY mice, were used for the acute oral toxicity study. The tests were carried out according to Ethics of the Organization for Economic Co-operation and Development (OECD) Test Guideline 401. The mice were housed at 24˚C ± 1˚C, 50% relative humidity. Both conventional and charged water were suspended in sterile and administered to mice in free supplemental system, calculating daily consumption. Mice were weighted at 0 - 7 days after administration, and clinical observations were made once a day. Necropsy was performed on all mice seven days after administration.

#### 2.1.2. Schematic Diagram for Bone Marrow Suppressed Immune-Compromised Mice

In the animal model of immuno-competency reduction, male C57BL/6J mice, aged 8 - 9 weeks, were injected with Mitomycin-C (MMC) (5 mg/kg) to inhibit the bone marrow. Then, U-164 extracts was administered orally at a dosage of 1 g/kg/day for five consecutive days. Normal animals were chosen as controls [5] (**Figure 1**).

### 2.2. Preparation of U-164

U-164 was prepared using method of Ohtubo, *et al.* A plant material, sugarcane, consisted by Family Poaceae were fermented by Yeast and Lactobaccilli (U-164). After the incaution for five years, liquid materials were served for U-164 (COSMOS Co. Ltd. Kurume, Fukuoka, Japan).

### 2.3. Recovery of Immuno-Competence

#### 2.3.1. Recovery off White Blood Cells by U-164

The bone marrow-suppressed mice were administered herbal decoction U-164 1 g/kg dairy for 5 days and after 1 week later, their blood were withdrawn from their tail vain. Then, the number of leukocytes was counted in Bürker-Türk solution.

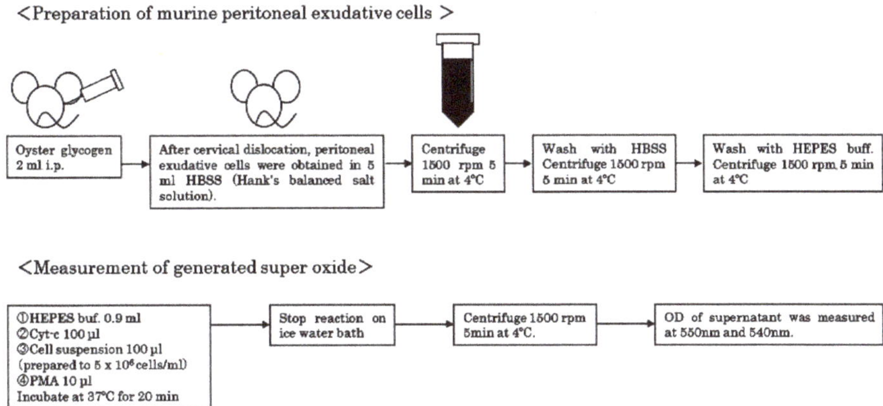


**Figure 1.** Experimental design for this report. The bone marrow suppressed mice were administered fermented decoction of U-164 (1 g/kg/day) for 5 days. One week later, mice were immunized with sheep red blood cells, ($2 \times 10^8$/mouse) intraperitoneally. Five days later, their spleen cells were collected. Plague-forming cells (PFC) were developed, and the ability of IgM and IgG antibody production was tested U-164 by the method reported in the text.

### 2.3.2. Regulatory Effect of Leukocyte Subsets

Bone marrow-suppressed mice were administered with herbal decoction of U-164 (1000 mg/kg) for 10 days. One week later, the blood from their tail vain was withdrawn. Then the granulocyte and lymphocyte subsets were counted in Bürker-Türk solution.

### 2.3.3. Recovery of Macrophage Activity, Migration

Cells from peritoneal exudates were collect from the peritoneal cavity of bone marrow-suppressed mice. Phagocytes were purified using adherent technique to get cell suspensions which contained more than 95% of phagocytes. The purified cells were loaded to the upper room of Boyden chamber to test migration ability at a concentration of $1 \times 10^4$ cell/ml. Human serum treated at 56°C for 30 min was for the chemo tactic agent of mouse phagocyte [6].

### 2.3.4. Recovery of Macrophage Activity, Phagocytosis

The same cells suspension was purified by adherent technique for phagocyte, which produces cells contained more than 95% of phagocytes. The purified cells were adjusted to $1 \times 10^4$ cell/cm$^2$ and mixed with latex beads that are 5um in granule wit U-164 luorescence isochianate. After 90 min of incubation, remained granule were washed out from the glass slide. Number of phagocytic cell and their ability to catch up the latex beads were automatically measured by ACAS system, which outputs the result in a digital form (Adherent cell activity evaluating system; Shimazu, Kyoto, Japan).

### 2.3.5. Augmentation of Lymphocyte Activity, Antibody Secreting Cell

The bone marrow suppressed mice were administered herbal decoction of U-164 (1 g/kg/day) for 5 days. One week later, mice were immunized with sheep red blood cells, ($2 \times 10^8$/mouse) intraperitoneally. Five days later, their spleen cells were collected. Plague-forming cells (PFC) were developed, and the ability of IgM and IgG antibody production was tested U-164he method reported by Jerne and Nordin [7] [8].

### 2.3.6. Effect for CD Positive Lymphocyte Distribution by U-164 against Different Constitution

Whole blood obtained from the subjects was washed twice with PBS. One hundred micro-liters of the suspensions were stained with 20 µl of fluorescent monoclonal antibodies (anti-human CD2$^+$, CD4$^+$, CD8$^+$, CD11b$^+$, CD14$^+$, CD16$^+$, CD19$^+$ and CD56$^+$ antibodies). Ten thousands stained cells were re-suspended in PBS to detect surface markers by flow cytometry (FACS Calibur; Becton Dickinson Immnocytometry Systems, CA, USA).

### 2.3.7. Recovery of Cytokine Producing Lymphocytes in Different Constitution

The blood cell suspensions were cultured with PMA (phorbol 12-myristate 13-acetate), ionomycin and BSA (bovine serum albumin) for 4 - 5 hours at 37˚C. After that, the cell suspensions were stained using the monoclonal antibodies of PE-IL-4, FITC-IFN-$\gamma$and FITC-IL-1$\beta$. Then they were analyzed U-164he FACScan (Becton Dickinson Co. Ltd. USA). The antibodies and reagents used in the test were purchased from Becton Dickinson Immunocytometry System (USA).

#### 2.3.8. Evaluation of Macrophage Activity, Phagocytosis

The peritoneal exudates cells were collect from the peritoneal cavity of bone marrow-suppressed mice. Cell suspensions were purified by adherent technique for phagocyte, getting a suspension which contained over 95% of phagocytes. The purified cells were adjusted to 1 × $10^4$ cell/ml and loaded at the upper chamber of Boyden chamber for test migration. Human serum with treated at 56˚C for 30 min was for the chemotactic agent for mouse phagocyte.

Phagocytic activity and antibody production of macrophages were analyzed using a classical test that could test the total activity of the immune system by examine chemotaxis, phagocytosis and intracellular degradation of macrophage. For identifying antibody-forming cells, plaque-forming cells were detected using heterogeneous erythrocyte; sheep erythrocyte was a target antigen. Peritoneal macrophages were collected and purified in fetal calf serum (FCS)-coated petri-dishes. The cell population was approximately 97% uniform in function and morphology. These cells were applied to the nuclepore-membrane (pore size: 5 μm; Neuro Probe Co. Ltd., Cabin John MD, USA) with a chemotaxis chamber (Neuro Probe Co. Ltd.). After 90 minutes' incubation, the membrane was vigorously washed with saline (37˚C), fixed, and then stained with methylene blue dye. After counting under a microscope for the total field of the membrane, the average number of migrating cells was expressed as cell counts/$mm^2$.

The same cells suspension was purified by adherent technique for phagocyte, which contained over 95% of phagocytes. The purified cells were adjusted to 1 × $10^4$ cell/$cm^2$ and mixed with latex beads that were 5um in granule wit U-164 luorescence isochianate. After 90 min of incubation, the remained granule were washed out from the glass slide and counting automatically by ACAS system, which outputs digital presentation, for evaluating phagocytes in number and in their ability to catch up the latex beads (ACAS: adeherent cell activity analyzing system, Shimazu, Kyoto, Japan). Latex beads in 5 μm with fluorescence were used to test phagocytic activity and *Candida albicans* was cell killing activity. A macrophage-target cell ratio of 1:10 was considered to be optimum. Ten minutes after incubating phagocytes and target cells, intracellular Candida cells were cultured on an agar dish with conventional medium 1640 until the next day to perform the colony forming assay. In this way, the phagocytic ability of the macrophages was monitored. To document intracellular killing activity, the same procedures were performed excepting that the incubation time was changed to 90 minutes.

#### 2.3.9. Antibody Forming Cell Study by U-164

Sheep erythrocyte (SRBC), a T-dependent antigen, was used for antibody formation cell study. Ten days after tumor transplantation, each antigen was intra-peritoneally injected. After four and six days, the antibody-forming cells were detected using localized hemolysis in an agar gel. Plaque-forming cells were developed U-164he method of Jerne and Nordin [7] [8].

### 2.4. Anti-Oxidative Evaluation of U-164 by Phagocytic Cell

#### 2.4.1. Animals for This Test

Eight week-old female C57BL/6 were purchased from Sankyo Laboratory Service Corporation (Shizuoka, Japan). All mice were kept under specific pathogen-free conditions. Mice food and distilled water were freely accessible for each mouse. Housing temperature and humidity were controlled 25˚C ± 1˚C and 60%.

#### 2.4.2. Reagents for This Measurment

As for the basic medium, HEPES buffer (HEPES 17mM, NaCl 120mM, Glucose 5mM, KCl 5mM, $CaCl_2$ 1mM, $MgCl_2$ 1mM) was prepared and sterilized by filtration. Phorbol 12-myristate 13-acetate (PMA, Sigma, USA) was diluted to $10^{-6}$ M by dimethyl sulfoxide DMSO, Sigma, USA) and used as a stimulant for super oxide anion generation for murine peritoneal exudates cells. Cytochrome-c (Sigma, USA) was diluted to 1mM by HEPES buffer. Since cytochrome-c reduced by super oxide showed maximum absorbance at 550 nm, we used cytochrome-c to measure the amount of super oxide anion generation through spectro-photometrical technique. Oyster glycogen (type Ⅱ, Sigma, USA) was diluted in the purified water (10% w/v, Wako, Japan) and autoclaved at 120C for 20min. This solution was used for intraperitoneal injection to mice in order to induce peripheral neutrophils into the abdominal cavity.

#### 2.4.3. Estimating the Amount of Super Oxide Anion Generated by Murine Peritoneal Exudates Cells

Each remedy was orally administered to mice (500 mg/kg) for one week. Two milliliters of 10% Oyster glycogen was injected intraperitoneally 10 hours before the assay. Sufficient murine peritoneal exudative cells were induced ten hours after the stimulation. Mice were euthanized by cervical dislocation, murine peritoneal exudates cells (PEC) suspension was centrifuged twice for 5 minutes at 1500 rpm at 4°C. Then PEC was prepared to $1 \times 10^6$ cells/ml of HEPES buffer. One hundred microliters of cytochrome-c and 10 μl of PMA were added to the cell suspension and this was incubated for 20 minutes at 37°C. The reaction mixture was then centrifuged for 10 minutes at 1500 rpm, 4°C. An OD of supernatant was measured at both 550 nm and 540 nm, the amount of generated super oxide anion was shown in the formula; increased absorbance at 550 nm $(\Delta A_{50\text{-}540})/19.1 \times 10^3$ (mmol/ml). In order to ensure if we really measured the amount of generated super oxide anion or not, we tried to add super oxide anion dismutase (SOD), an enzyme for its anti-oxidative effect, into our experimental system. The result was as expected that the reduction of cytochrome-c was inhibited after the addition of SOD. This showed us that our experimental system could be used properly for measuring the amount of generated super oxide anion.

### 2.5. Statistical Analysis

Data are expressed as means ± standard deviations. The differences between U-164-treated and non-treated conditions were compared using a one-tailed analysis of variance. A $P$ value $< 0.05$ was considered to be statistically significant.

## 3. Clinical Findings by U-164

### 3.1. Volunteers and Assessing QOL for U-164

Twenty healthy volunteers aged from 21 to 70 years for both sex were recruited and were administered U-164 for 30 days. Fifteen milliliters of blood were drawn from the forearm vein one hour before the first administration of U-164 and 30 days after the last U-164 administration (day 30). All volunteers provided informed consent prior to participation for this trial. This study was approved by Ethics Committee of Kanazawa Medical University.

### 3.2. Leukocyte Counts Test for U-164

The assessments including a total number of leukocytes was ordered to count with blood chemical test for the medical diagnosis of public institution (Ishikawa Preventive Medicine Association, Ishikawa, Japan). In the differential counting, 200 cells were counted on a May-Grünewald-Gimsa stained slide, and percentages of lymphocytes and granulocytes were determined.

### 3.3. Leukocyte Subset Analyses for U-164

The assessments including a total number of leukocytes was ordered to count with blood chemical test for the medical diagnosis of public institution (Ishikawa Preventive Medicine Association, Ishikawa, Japan). In the differential counting, 200 cells were counted on a May-Grunewald-Gimsa stained slide, and percentages of lymphocytes and granulocytes were determined [8].

## 4. Results for U-164

### 4.1. Animal Experiment

#### 4.1.1. One Shot and Multiple Shots Toxicity Study of Conventional Sugarcane and Fermented Sugarcane (U-164)

No deaths or abnormalities of body weight, water and food consumption, or coat condition were observed in the treated mice. Necropsy evaluation of the mice did not reveal any significant differences in thymus, liver, spleen, kidney, adrenal gland and testicle weights between the control group and both conventional sugarcane and fermented sugarcane groups, or between males and females.

#### 4.1.2. Recovery of Whole Body Weight by U-164

The body weight and thymus weight reduced in bone marrow-suppressed mice, resulting in the reduction of peripheral blood leukocyte to around 40%. After administered each herbal decoction 1 g/kg dairy for 5 days and after 1 week later, their blood were recovered to around 90% of normal value (**Figure 2**).

#### 4.1.3. Recovery of Thymus Weight by U-164

The bone marrow-suppressed mice were administered U-164 1 g/kg dairy for 5 days, and one week later, their blood was withdrawn from their tail vein. The cell count of the peripheral blood is showed in **Figure 4**, **Table 1**. shows that the thymus weight decreased to half of normal control after 5 mg/kg of MMC was injected. However, all the three U-164s recovered thymus weight to about 70% of the control.

#### 4.1.4. Augmentation of CD⁺ Cells and Cytokine Producing Cells by U-164

CD3, CD4 and CD19 cells of MMC treated mice were recovered to almost normal values after the administration of U-164s. As for the functional recovery, IFN-$\gamma$ and IL-4 producing cells were also recovered U-164. The all three decoction, including U-164 and a functionally depressive agent of TCM. In cytokine producing cells, IFN-$r$ and IL-4 producing cell were recovered with U-164. In all these sugarcanes derivatives tested, cytokine producing cells were recovered with U-164 was the most and even conventional sugarcane formulae.

#### 4.1.5. Sorting Subjects into Two Groups, G-Type and L-Type by Granulocyte and Lymphocyte Proportion by U-164

The volunteers were healthy subject, with no drastic change for the total number of leukocytes. However, we tried to check the regulative effect of herbal formulae for two different constitution, G-rich type and L-rich type. Analysis that mixed both groups together showed no significant differences in total leukocyte number except that for FBT; in G-type group, total number of leukocytes was down regulated by BT derivatives. This was a results of the down regulation of major group of leukocyte, granulocyte.

As for the L-type, no significant changes were found after the treatment of both FBTs. In the L-type group, on the other hand, increased the tonal leukocyte and granulocyte in number, on the contrary to the down regulation for lymphocytes. To further clarify the influence of hemopoietic formula, we divided the subjects into two groups: the G-type group, who had a granulocyte count over 60%, and the L-type group, who had a lymphocyte count over 40%. In the L-type group, lymphocyte counts tended to decrease on day 10, accompanied by an increase in granulocyte numbers by U-164 but not by conventional sugarcane. On the contrary, the granulocyte counts of G-type group tended to decrease on day 10. The decrease of granulocyte count was raised by U-163, but not by conventional sugarcane on day 10 (**Table 2**, **Table 3**).

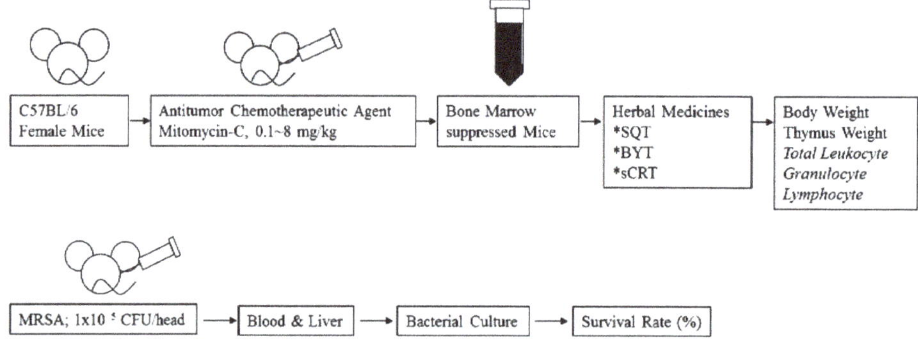


**Figure 2.** Twenty-four hours change of total peripheral leukocyte count on the basis of each constitution/condition. We tried to express the effect of peripheral total leukocyte number by individual level of change and plot in the x-axis as in each age. Variations in leukocyte subpopulations in the peripheral blood before and after U-164 therapy.

### 4.1.6. Augmentation of Lymphocyte Activity, Antibody Secreting Cell

The bone marrow-suppressed mice were administered herbal decoction U-164 for five days. One week later,

**Table 1.** Constitution Dependent Regulation of Leukocyte Subset by U-164.

| | G-type individual | | L-type individual | |
|---|---|---|---|---|
| | *Original Sugarcane* | | *Fermented Sugarcane* | |
| | **Before** | **After** | **Before** | **After** |
| Total WBC ($\times 10^3$ µl) | 6.56 | 5.78 | 4.97 | 6.88 |
| Lymphocyte (%) | 25.8 | 27.6 | 45.8 | 47.2 |
| Granulocyte (%) | 69.7 | 69.7 | 60.2 | 65.6 |
| Neutrophil (%) | 65.8 | 62.4 | 49.6 | 51.4 |
| Eosinophil (%) | 2.9 | 2.5 | 2.4 | 3.9 |
| Basophil (%) | 0.6 | 0.7 | 0.8 | 0.8 |

**Table 2.** Constitution dependent regulation of leukocyte by U-164.

| | G-type individual | | L-type individual | |
|---|---|---|---|---|
| | *Original Sugarcane* | | *Fermented Sugarcane* | |
| | **Before** | **After** | **Before** | **After** |
| Total WBC ($\times 10^3$µl) | 6.11 | 5.98 | 5.62 | 6.88 |
| Lymphocyte (%) | 24.7 | 26.8 | 41.3 | 44.5 |
| Granulocyte (%) | 66.6 | 67.6 | 52.6 | 58.9 |
| Neutrophil (%) | 63.5 | 62.6 | 51.0 | 53.2 |
| Eosinophil (%) | 1.5 | 2.1 | 2.3 | 3.8 |
| Basophil (%) | 0.5 | 0.9 | 0.6 | 0.8 |

**Table 3.** Constitution dependent regulation of lymphocyte by Sugarcane Derivatives.

| CD | G-type individual | | L-type individual | |
|---|---|---|---|---|
| | *Original Sugarcane* | | *Fermented Sugarcane* | |
| | **Before (%)** | **After (%)** | **Before (%)** | **After (%)** |
| CD2 | 61.45 | 73.34 | 62.46 | 71.46 |
| CD4 | 18.44 | 29.78 | 33.43 | 47.66 |
| CD8 | 37.56 | 42.54 | 29.69 | 28673 |
| CD11 | 73.56 | 73.56 | 65.63 | 73.74 |
| CD14 | 0.05 | 0.05 | 0.06 | 0.07 |
| CD16 | 65.79 | 57.35 | 55.54 | 47.54 |
| CD19 | 8.67 | 8.46 | 8.21 | 7.99 |
| CD56 | 1.03 | 1.96 | 2.06 | 2.75 |

mice were immunized with sheep red blood cells, (2 × $10^8$/mouse) intraperitoneally. Four and six days later, their plague-forming cells (PFC) were developed. The ability of IgM and IgG antibody production was tested U-164 he method reported by Jerne and Nordin [7]. In this mouse model, MMC did not reduce the antibody forming cells significantly but the tendency was the same as shown in the former section. In this test, B was the most effective than that of A. U-164 was the strongest material to augment antibody secreting cell among the four formulae.

#### 4.1.7. Macrophage Phagocytic Activity by U-164

So as to detect the supportive effect and important immunological stimulation U-164onic agent, Bu-Ji, we traced the augmentation pattern of each remedy. As results of this trial, the phagocytic patterns U-164onic agents, Bu-Ji, were clearly different from MMC-treated mice. Moreover, augmentation of phagocytes were different between each sugarcane derivatives. U-164 was prominent in activating phagocytes quantitatively and qualitatively compared to conventional sugarcane. We showed the diversity in the recovery pattern of U-164. Famous tonic remedies in Japan, U-164, strongly recovered phagocytic activity in compromised hosts, but the recovery by fermented sugarecane/U-164 was much less than that by original sugarcane (**Table 4**).

### 4.2. The Level of Generated Super Oxide Anion Controlled by U-164

The amount of generated super oxide anion was calculated in the formula shown above. The generated super oxide anion after one week administration of *Agaricus* and *Chlorella* were 2.64 and 1.95 $\times 10^{-5}$ mmol/ml, respecttively, whereas that was 2.85 × $10^{-5}$ mmol/ml in control group. The generated super oxide anion after one week administration of conventional turmeric, fermented formulae, were 1.24, 1.25 and 2.88 × $10^{-5}$ mmol/ml, respectively. The generated super oxide anion after one week administration of Propolis was 2.55 × $10^{-5}$ mmol/ml. All these drugs, except for U-164, decreased super oxide anion generation after administration for one week in mice.

#### The Estimation of Generated Super Oxide Anion between the Fermented and Not Fermented Sugarcane/U-164

Since the antioxidative effects of herbal medicine were demonstrated, we investigated the way to reinforce this effect. The fermentation is one of the possibilities. Since the fermentation is preceded by bacterial digestion and degradation, less efficient constituents would be lost than commonly used extraction by hot water. Therefore, we decided to ferment the herbal medicine by yeast (*Saccharomyces cerevisiae*), expecting the enhancement of its antioxidative effects. The generated super oxide anion after one week administration of fermented U-164. All the fermented herbal medicine decreased super oxide anion generation in compare with their corresponding unfermented ones (**Table 5**).

## 5. Clinical Findings

### 5.1. Regulation in Cell Number of Total Leukocyte and Subsets

Leukocyte numbers have been counted one hour before and 15 days after the treatment of hemopoitic formula.

**Table 4.** Relative activities of macrophage phagocytosis.

| | Phagocytosis | |
|---|---|---|
| | Positive Cells/$10^6$ cells | |
| | Law active (%) | High active (%) |
| Normal | 52 (100) | 45 (100) |
| MMC | 34 (65) | 5 (11) |
| MMC + *C. Sugarcane* | 108 (207) | 59 (131) |
| MMC + *F. Sugarcane* | 187 (326) | 89 (199) |

**Table 5.** Anti-oxidative Activity of Peritoneal Macrophages treated by U-164.

| Materials | Generated $O_2^-$ ($\times10^5$ mmol/ml) |
|---|---|
| *Agaricus burazei* | 2.79 |
| *Conv. Sugarcane* | 1.94 |
| *F. Sugarcane/U*-164 | 1.63 |
| Propolis | 2.55 |
| Control | 2.99 |

The cell number measured one hour before the administration was set as 100%. Relative percentage of cell number on the 15th day was calculated. No significant changes were observed in G-group after the administration of U-164. However, significant change was found in L-type group.

### 5.2. Dividing Subjects into Two Groups, G-Type and L-Type by the Ratio to Granulocyte and Lymphocyte

The volunteers were healthy subject, with no drastic change for the total number of leukocytes. However, we tried to check the regulative effect of herbal formulae for two different constitution, G-rich type and L-rich type. Analysis that mixed both groups together showed no significant differences in total leukocyte number except that for U-164; in G-type group, total number of leukocytes was down regulated by U-164. This was a results of the down regulation of major group of leukocyte, granulocyte.

As for the L-type, no significant changes were found after the treatment of both U-164. In the L-type group, on the other hand, increased the tonal leukocyte and granulocyte in number, on the contrary to the down regulation for lymphocytes. To further clarify the influence of hemopoietic formula, we divided the subjects into two groups: the G-type group, who had a granulocyte count over 60%, and the L-type group, who had a lymphocytecount over 40%. In the L type group, lymphocyte counts tended to decrease on day 15, accompanied by an increase in granulocyte numbers by conventional sugarcane but not by U-164. On the contrary, the granulocyte counts of G-type group tended to decrease on day 15. The decrease of granulocyte count was raised by U-164, but not by conventional sugarcane on day 10.

### 5.3. Lymphocyte Subsets Reveal Significant Variation by U-164

After U-164 treatment, cell counts of $CD2^+$, $CD4^+$, $CD8^+$, $CD11b^+$, $CD16^+$, $CD19^+$ and $CD56^+$ were tested to evaluate variations in T cells, B cells, macrophages and NK cells. These values were measured one hour before hemopoietic formula and 15 days thereafter. Our results showed that CD2 and CD4 cells were increased by both U-164 and SQT. $CD11b^+$ and $CD14^+$ cell counts, which are closely associated with macrophage activity, increased by U-164 in the L-type subjects. In particular, there was a remarkable increase in $CD11b^+$ cell number on day 15. T cell subsets that are closely associated with activity of immature T cells, ($CD2^+$, $CD4^+$ and $CD8^+$), the $CD2^+$ ($P < 0.05$) showed an increase with the treatment of U-164 15 days after administration. The number of $CD19^+$ cells, which is closely associated with B cell activity, was not changed by both U-164 throughout the trial, neither were the numbers of $CD16^+$ and $CD56^+$ cells (**Table 6**).

## 6. Products of Complement Activation Combining the Biological Activity

Activation of either the alternative or the classical pathway results in the generation of many important peptides involved in inflammatory responses. The anaphylaxis increase of vascular permeability Degradation of mast cells and basophils with release of histamine Degradation of eosinophils Aggregation of platelets opsonization of particles and solubilization of immune complexes with subsequent facilitation of phagocytosis Release of neutrophils from bone marrow resulting in leukocytosis Smooth muscle contraction Increase of vascular permeability Smooth muscle contraction Increase of vascular permeability Degradation of mast cells and basophils with release of histamine Degradation Degranulation of eosinophils Aggregation of platelets Chemotaxis of basophils, eosinophils, neutrophils, and monocytes Release of hydrolytic enzymes from neutrophils Chemotaxis of neutrophils Release of hydrolytic enzymes from neutrophils Inhibition of migration and insulation of spreading

**Table 6.** Constitution dependent regulation of $CD^+$ lymphocyte by U-164.

| CD | G-type individual | | L-type individual | |
|---|---|---|---|---|
| | *Original Sugarcane* | | *Fermented Sugarcane* | |
| | Before (%) | After (%) | Before (%) | After (%) |
| CD2 | 66.56 | 73.65 | 62.43 | 74.98 |
| CD4 | 18.43 | 29.54 | 32.55 | 4532 |
| CD8 | 34.33 | 43.45 | 27.66 | 26853 |
| CD11 | 74.54 | 72.65 | 62.68 | 7253 |
| CD14 | 0.03 | 0.06 | 0.07 | 0.07 |
| CD16 | 65.54 | 55.87 | 57.43 | 46.73 |
| CD19 | 8.65 | 8.21 | 8.36 | 8.54 |
| CD56 | 1.30 | 1.87 | 1.93 | 2.47 |

of monocytes and macrophages anaphylatoxins C3a, C4a, and C5a are derived from the enzymatic cleavage of C3, C4, and C5 respectively. Historically, C3a and C5a were defined as factors derived from activated serum possessing spasmogenic activity. The anaphylatoxins are now recognized as having many additional biologic functions. Both C3a and C5a are known to induce the release of histamine from mast cells and basophils (chapter 20A). As shown in **Figure 4** both anaphylatoxins cause smooth muscle contraction and induce the release of vasoactive amines, which cause an increase in vascular permeability.

The effect of C5a anaphylatoxin on neutrophils is of considerable importance in the inflaammatory response. Not only can C5a induce neutrophil aggregation, but this anaphylatoxin appears to be the main chemotactic peptide generated by activation of either complement pathway. In vitro, nanomolar concentrations of C5a will induce the unidirectional movement of neutrophils. Other inflammatory cells, such as monocytes, eosinophils, basophils, and macrophages, have also been shown to exhibit a chemotactic response to C5a. The removal of the carboxy-terminal arginine from C5a by serum carboxy peptidase N, generating C5a-des-arg, inactivates the spasmogen, yet restoration of full chemotactic activity of C5a-des-are may occur in the presence of serum. Therefore, C5a-desarg may also be responsible for in vivo neutrophil chemotactic activity.

As described earlier, the cleavage of C3 by either the alternative or the classical C3 convertases results in the production of two major split products, the C3a anaphylatoxin and cab. The larger C3b fragment can serve as an opsonin (promoter of phagocytosis) by binding to a target through the thioester mechanism. This renders the particle or cell immediately susceptible to ingestion by a variety of phagocytic cells that carry specific receptors for C3b.

Many recent observations point to additional roles for complement fragments in regulating the activity 9f cells of the immune system. These observations include the presence of receptors on lymphocytes for various complement proteins, including C3 split products and Factor H, affecting B and T cell function. This is an important area for future research with this concept, we tried to demonstrate visually by the immune-electrophoresis. The human serum was prepared after administrating f-Black Turmeric together with the sample with before fermentation. Immuno-electrophoresis was setting up for 90 mins, followed by incubating with anti-human whole serum and specific for C3 and Bf component. These specifi anti complement component serum were kindly supplied by Dr Syunnosuke SAKAI, Cancer Research Institute of Kanazawa University, Japan (**Figure 3**, **Figure 4**).

## 7. Discussion

Our investigation clarified how U-164 influenced the immune system (e.g. leukocyte, granulocyte and lymphocyte subsets in particular). We quantified CD positive cell counts as indicators of T cells, B cells, macrophages and NK cells. For qualitative and quantitative evaluation, we examined the cytokine expression levels, and directly measured the expression levels of cytokine-containing cells in peripheral blood, eliminating possible artificial factors that could arise from culturing in test tubes or changes in net value by catalyzation. To avoid any possible influence from the circadian rhythm, we obtained the whole blood from all donors at the same time. In

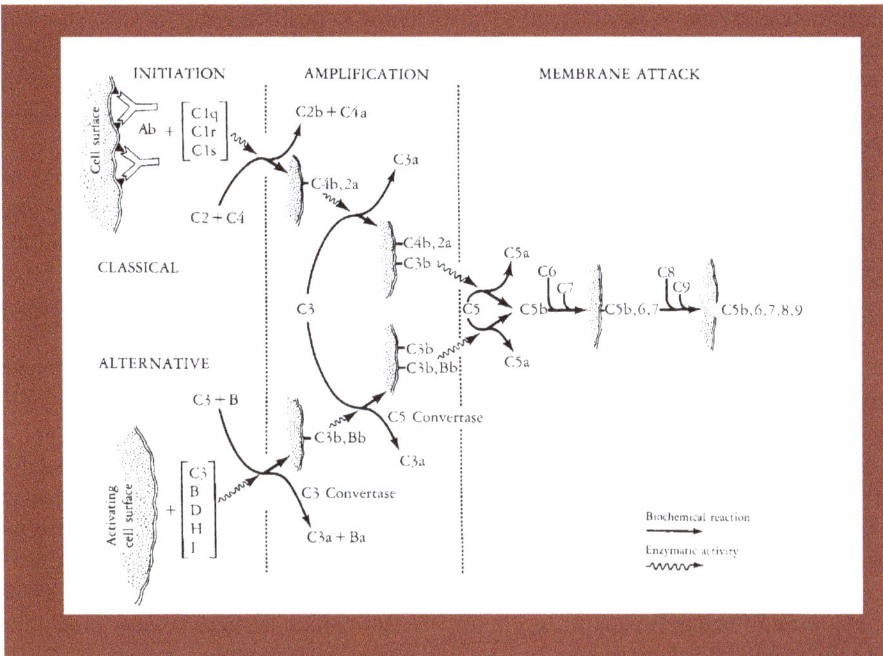


**Figure 3.** Diagrammatical representation of complement component in vertebrate. The analysis of CD positive cells by FCM was measured by gating in the lymphocytes region on the scattered gram. Figure shows an example analysis. Nonspecific reaction of the PE fluorescence was found in the isotype control.

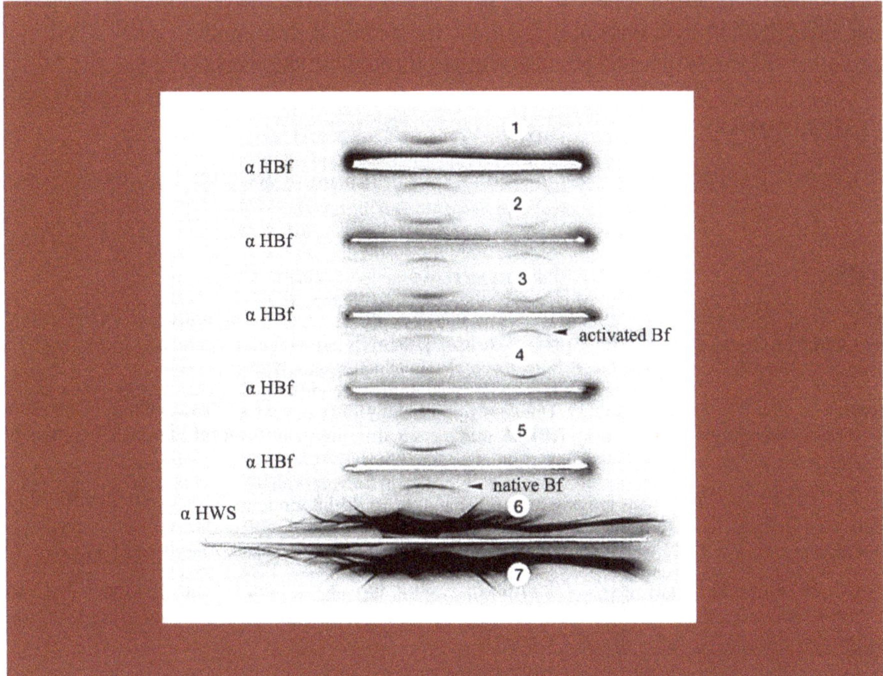


**Figure 4.** Immunoe; ectrophoretic demonstration of activated human Complement.

this investigation, we confirmed that U-164 quantitatively and qualitatively regulated leukocytes, granulocytes, lymphocytes and their subsets. The increase of $CD2^+$, $CD4^+$, $CD8^+$, $CD11b^+$, $CD16^+$, $CD19^+$ and $CD56^+$ cell counts as well as the levels of IL-1$\beta$, IL-4 and IFN-$\gamma$ in blood cells suggested that hemopoitic formula might enhance the activities of humoral and cellular immunities, as well as NK cells. We also observed that levels of cytokine producing cells, in particular, increased rather than CD-positive lymphocytes, showing that U-164 augmented lymphocyte production qualitatively than quantitatively. Moreover, U-164 activated both CD11b cells and IL-1$\beta$ producing cells, suggesting the activation of phagocyte cells both in number and in function. Consequently, these data further demonstrated that U-164 acted in macrophages in the same manner as *Mycobacterium tuberculosis* that had cell walls constructed of waxy substances [9]-[19].

In previous reports about hot-spring hydrotherapy and acupuncture, we had proposed that immune system regulation was an important factor for evaluating CAM. Since other substances, such as endotoxin and waxy substances from *Mycobacterium tuberculosis*, similar to proplis, were known for augmenting host immune responses. This time, we decided to focus solely on propolis. A possible explanation for immune enhancement could be the activation of the circular system and/or autonomic nervous system, although the details of the mechanism remained unclear. Further research regarding to the mechanism was necessary.

Abo *et al.* reported that granulocyte count was increased U-164he excitation of the sympathetic nervous system, while lymphocyte count was increased by excitation of parasympathetic nervous system [20]-[28]. Our data also showed that granulocyte count was decreased in subjects with a high granulocyte count, while lymphocyte count was increased in the same subjects. The lymphocyte count, however, was decreased in subjects with a high lymphocyte level, while granulocyte count was increased in the same subjects. In other words, the subjects dominated U-164he sympathetic nerve could release stress, whereas the sympathetic activity of subjects who were dominated U-164he parasympathetic nerve might be excited by hemopoietic formula. This way, the cell counts appeared to converge at appropriate levels after hemopoietic formula. Finally, in order to determine whether the elevation of leukocyte counts resulted from an infection triggered by hemopoitic formula or not, the subjects were followed up for 8 days after the last administration of hemopoitic formula. During that period, we could not observe any infectious signs such as pyodermitis, fever, or enhancement of C-reactive protein (CRP). The value of CRP was 0.57 g/dl to 1.23 g/dl in our subjects, suggesting very mild inflammatory responses, which showed that hemopoitic formula did not cause infection. Since the meridian may influenced cells through out the body and might pass through every organ system, hemopoitic formula stimulation might provide maximum benefits without dangerous side effects [28] [29]. As an immune-enhancer, fermented sugarcane, U-164 merits further investigation as a possible treatment for acquired immunodeficiency syndrome, chronic fatigue syndrome and other disorders that had been concerned throughout the world.

## Acknowledgements

This project was partly supported by the Committee of Promotion of Acupuncture and Moxibustion Therapies in Japan.

## References

[1] Kitada, Y., Wan, W., Matsui, K., Shimizu, S. and Yamaguchi, N. (2000) Regulation of Peripheral White Blood Cells in Numbers and Functions through Hot-Spring Bathing During a Short Term—Studies in Control Experiments. *Journal of Japanese Society Balneology Climatology Physiological Medicine*, **63**, 151-164.

[2] Yamaguchi, N., Takahashi, T., Sugita, T., Ichikawa, K., Sakaihara, S., Tsugiyasu Kanda T., Arai, M. and Kawakita, K. (2007) Acupuncture Regulates Leukocyte Subpopulations in Human Peripheral Blood. *Evidence-Based Complementary and Alternative medicine*, **4**, 447-453.

[3] Suzuki, S., Toyabe, S., Moroda, T., Tada, T., Tsukahara, A. and Iiai, T. (1997) Circadian Rhythm of Leukocytes and Lym-Phocytes Subsets and Its Possible Correlation with the Function of the Autonomic Nervous System. *Clinical Experimental Immunology*, **110**, 500-508. http://dx.doi.org/10.1046/j.1365-2249.1997.4411460.x

[4] Yamaguchi, N., Kawada, N., Ja, X.-S., Okamoto, K., Okuzumi, K., Chen, R. and Takahashi, T. (2014) Overall Estimation of Anti-Oxidant Activity by Mammal Macrophage, *Open Journal of Rheumatology and Autoimmune Diseases*, **4**, 13-21. http://dx.doi.org/10.4236/ojra.2014.41002

[5] Hamada, M. and Yamaguchi, N. (1988) Effect of Kanpo Medicine, Zyuzentaihoto, on the Immune Reactivity of Tumor-Bearing Mice. *Journal of Ethnopharmacology*, **24**, 311-320. http://dx.doi.org/10.1016/0378-8741(88)90160-2

[6] Tu, C.C., Li, C.S., Liu, C.M. and Liu, C.C. (2011) Comparative Use of Biomedicine and Chinese Medicine in Taiwan: Using the NHI Research Database. *Journal of Alternative and Complementary Medicine*, **17**, 339-346. http://dx.doi.org/10.1089/acm.2010.0200

[7] Jerne, N.K. and Nordin, A.A. (1963) Plaque Formation in Agar by Single Antibody Producing Cells. *Science*, **140**, 405-408. http://dx.doi.org/10.1126/science.140.3565.405

[8] Yamaguchi, N., Ueyama, T., Amat, N., Yimit, D., Hoxur, P., Sakamoto, D., Katoh, Y., Watanabe, I. and Su, S.-Y. (2015) Bi-Directional Regulation by Chinese Herbal Formulae to Host and Parasite for Multi-Drug Resistant *Staphylococcus aureus* in Humans and Rodents. *Open Journal of Immunology*, **4**, 18-32. http://dx.doi.org/10.4236/oji.2015.51003

[9] Jong, M.S., Hwang, S.J., Chen, Y.C., Chen, T.J., Chen, F.J. and Chen, T.P. (2010) Prescriptions of Chinese Herbal Medicine for Constipation under the National Health Insurance in Taiwan. *Journal of the Chinese Medical Association*, **73**, 375-383. http://dx.doi.org/10.1016/S1726-4901(10)70081-2

[10] Navo, M.A. and Phan Vaughan, J.C. (2004) An Assessment of the Utilization of Complementary and Alternative Medication in Women with Gynecologic or Breast Malignancies. *Journal of Clinical Oncology*, **22**, 671-677. http://dx.doi.org/10.1200/JCO.2004.04.162

[11] Liu, J.P., Yang, H., Xia, Y. and Cardini, F. (2009) Herbal Preparations for Uterine Fibroids. *Cochrane Database of Systematic Reviews*, No. 2, CD005292. http://dx.doi.org/10.1002/14651858.cd005292.pub2

[12] Murayama, T., Yamaguchi, N., Iwamoto, K. and Eizuru, Y. (2006) Inhibition of Ganciclovir-Resistant Human Cytomegalovirus Replication by Kampo (Japanese Herbal Medicine). *Antiviral Chemistry & Chemotherapy*, **17**, 11-16. http://dx.doi.org/10.1177/095632020601700102

[13] Abo, T., Kawate, T., Itoh, K. and Kumagai, K. (1981) Studies on the Bioperiodicity of the Immune Response. 1. Circadian Rhythms of Human T, B and K Cell Traffic in the Peripheral Blood. *Journal of. Immunology*, **126**, 1360-1363.

[14] Abo, T. and Kumagai, K. (1978) Studies of Surface Immunoglobulins on Human B Lymphocytes. Physiological Variations of $Sig^+$ Cells in Peripheral Blood. *Clinical Experimental Immunology*, **33**, 441-452.

[15] Landmann, R.M., Muller, F.B., Perini, C., Wesp, M., Erne, P. and Buhler, R. (1984) Changes of Immunoregulatory Cells Induced by Psychological and Physical Stress: Relationship to Plasma Catecholamines. *Clinical Experimental Immunology*, **58**,127-135.

[16] Iio, A., Ohguchi, K., Naruyama, H., Tazawa, S., Araki, Y., Ichihara, K., Nozawa, Y. and Ito, M. (2012) Ethanolic Extract of Brazilian Red Propolis ABCA1 Expression and Promote Cholesterol Effulux from THP-1 Macrophage. *Phytomedicine*, **19**, 383-388. http://dx.doi.org/10.1016/j.phymed.2011.10.007

[17] Kitada, Y., Okamoto, K., Takei, T., Jia, X.F., Chen, R., Yamaguchi, N., Tsubokawa, M., Wu, W.H., Murayama, T. and Kawakita, K. (2013) Hot Spring Hydro Therapy Regulate Peripheral Leukocyte Together with Emotional Hormone and Receptor Positive Lymphocytes According to Each Constitution/Condition. *Open Journal of Rheumatology and Autoimmune Diseases*, **3**, 140-153. http://dx.doi.org/10.4236/ojra.2013.33022

[18] Kitada, Y., Wan, W., Matsui, K. Matsui, K., Shimizu, S. and Yamaguchi, N. (2000) Regulation of Peripheral White Blood Cells in Numbers and Functions through Hot-Spring Bathing During a Short Term—Studies in Control Experiments. *Journal of Japanese Society Balneology Climatology Physiological Medicine*, **63**, 151-164.

[19] Jerne, N.K. and Nordin, A.A. (1963) Plaque Formation in Agar by Single Antibody Producing Cells. *Science*, **140**,405-408. http://dx.doi.org/10.1126/science.140.3565.405

[20] Jerne, N.K., Nordin, A.A. and Henry, C. (1963) The Agar Technique for Recognizing Antibody Producing Cells. In: Amons, B. and Kaprowski, H., Eds., *Cell-Bound Antibodies*, Wistar Institute Press, Philadelphia, 109-125.

[21] Hamada, M. and Yamaguchi, N. (1988) Effect of Kanpo Medicine, Zyuzentaihoto, on the Immune Reactivity of Tumor-Bearing Mice. *Journal of Ethnopharmacology*, **24**, 311-320. http://dx.doi.org/10.1016/0378-8741(88)90160-2

[22] Jyumonji, N. and Fujii, Y. (1993) A New Assay for Delayed-Type Hypersensitivity *in Vitro* Detection F-CHLORELLA. The Macrophage Migration by Boyden Chamber. *The Journal of Kanazawa Medical University*, **18**, 198-203.

[23] Yamaguchi, N., Shimizu, S. and Izumi, H. (2004) Hydrotherapy Can Modulate Peripheral Leukocytes: An Approach to Alternative Medicine. *Advances in Experimental Medicine and Biology*, **546**, 239-251. http://dx.doi.org/10.1007/978-1-4757-4820-8_18

[24] Murayama, T., Yamaguchi, N., Matsuno, H. and Eizuru, Y. (2004) *In Vitro* Anti-Cytomegalovirus Activity of Kampo (Japanese Herbal) Medicine. *Evidence-Based Complementary and Alternative Medicine*, **1**, 285-289.

[25] Abe, S., Yamaguchi, N., Tansho, S. and Yamaguchi, H. (2005) Preventive Effects of Juzen-taiho-to on Infectious Disease, Juzen-taiho-to (Shi-Quan-Da-Bu-Tang) Scientific Evaluation and Clinical Applications. In: Yamada, H. and Saiki, I., Eds., *Traditional Herbal Medicines for Modern Times*, CRC Press, Boca Raton.

[26] Nakano, S., Noguchi, T., Takekoshi, H., Suzuki, G. and Nakano, M. (2005) Maternal-Fetal Distribution and Transfer of Dioxins in Pregnant Women in Japan, and Attempts to Reduce Maternal Transfer with Chlorella (*Chlorella pyrenoidosa*) Supplements. *Chemosphere*, **61**, 1244-1255. http://dx.doi.org/10.1016/j.chemosphere.2005.03.080

[27] Yamaguchi, N., Shimizu, S. and Izumi, H. (2004) Hydrotherapy Can Modulate Peripheral Leukocytes: An Approach to Alternative Medicine, Complementary and Alternative Approaches to Biomedicine. Kluwer Academic/Plenum Publishers, New York, 239-251. http://dx.doi.org/10.1007/978-1-4757-4820-8_18

[28] Shimizu, S., Kitada, H., Yokota, H., Yamakawa, J., Murayama, T., Sugiyama, K., Izumi, H. and Yamaguchi, N. (2002)

Activation of the Alternative Complement Pathway by *Agaricus blazei* Murill. *Phytomedicine*, **9**, 536-545. http://dx.doi.org/10.1078/09447110260573047

[29] Yamaguchi, N., Araai, M. and Murayama, T. (2015) Aspect of QOL Assessment and Proposed New Scale for Evaluation. *Open Journal of Immunology*, **4**, in press.

## Abbreviations

Conventional Sugarcane. Normal Sugarcane, Family Poaceae, befor fermentation.

CAM: Complementary and alternative medicine, beside the western medicine, there are many traditional medicine and/or health promoting menu all over the world.

CD: Cluster of differentiation. Each lymphocyte has name that expressed CD number, for example CD2, CD4, etc.

DM: Diabetes mellitus.

FCM: Flow Cytometry.

Fermented Sugarcane: Fermented Sugarcane by Lactobacili, abbreviate U-154 in the text.

G-rich type: The individual that exhibit over 60% of granulocyte in peripheral blood, finding many in young gentleman.

L-rich type: The individual that exhibit over 40% of lymphocyte in peripheral blood, finding lot in ladies and senile.

U-164: Fermented sugarcane, Family Poaceae, that degradated by Lactobacilli.

# 3

# Region Specific Effects of Maternal Immune Activation on Offspring Neuroimmune Function

**Heping Zhou**

Department of Biological Sciences, Seton Hall University, New Jersey, USA
Email: heping.zhou@shu.edu

## Abstract

**Growing evidence suggests that maternal immune activation has a significant impact on the immuno-competence of the offspring. The present study aimed to characterize region-specific effects of maternal immune activation on the offspring's neuroimmune function. The offspring born to dams treated with saline or lipopolysaccharide (LPS) at gestational day 18 was stimulated with saline or LPS at postnatal day 21, and the mRNA expression of various inflammatory genes in different brain regions of the offspring was analyzed. The offspring born to saline-treated dams exhibited a typical neuroimmune response with elevated levels of cytokines and chemokines following LPS stimulation in all four brain regions examined. In contrast, the offspring born to LPS-treated dams exhibited significantly reduced mRNA induction of cytokines and chemokines following LPS stimulation in the prefrontal cortex but not in the brainstem when compared with pups born to saline-treated dams. Furthermore, the mRNA expression of LPS-induced I-κBζ was significantly attenuated in the prefrontal cortex when compared with pups born to saline-treated dams. These results suggest that maternal LPS may have differential effects on the neuroimmune function in different regions of the offspring brain, and highlight the importance of maternal milieu in the development of neuroimmune function in the offspring.**

## Keywords

**Maternal Immune Activation, Lipopolysaccharide, Neuroimmune, Cytokine, Chemokine**

## 1. Introduction

A well-organized neuroimmune response is critical for the first-line defense against invading microorganisms and restoring homeostasis in the central nervous system (CNS). The pattern recognition receptors such as Toll-like receptors (TLRs) widely expressed in the CNS play an important role in the initiation of a neuroimmune response. Lipopolysaccharide (LPS), a main component of the Gram-negative cell wall, binds to CD14, an LPS co-receptor, and TLR-4, which triggers the activation of MyD88-dependent and independent signaling pathways, leading to the activation of transcription factors such as nuclear factor kappa-light-chain-enhancer of activated B cells (NF-κB), and thereby increasing the expression of cytokines and chemokines [1].

NF-κB consists of a family of transcription factors including p65 and p50. The transcriptional activity of NF-κB is regulated by canonical inhibitors of κB (I-κBs), such as I-κB$\alpha$, which sequester NF-κBs in the cytosol and thereby prevent them from binding to κB target DNA sequences in the promoter region of inflammatory genes such as interleukin (IL)-6 and tumor necrosis factor (TNF)-$\alpha$ [2], as well as by non-classical I-κBs such as I-κB$\zeta$ in the nucleus. Studies have shown that I-κB$\zeta$ increases the expression of such NF-κB target genes as IL-6 and monocyte chemoattractant protein (MCP)-1 by forming a complex with NF-κB p50 homodimers or facilitating transcription-enhancing nucleosome remodeling in the nucleus of immune cells [3]-[5]. Furthermore, the duration and strength of NF-κB transcriptional activity may also be affected by posttranslational modifications such as ubiquitination, acetylation, methylation, phosphorylation, oxidation/reduction, and prolyl isomerization [6].

There is accumulating evidence that maternal immune activation affects the developing immune and nervous system in the offspring. For example, the offspring born to polyriboinosinic-polyribocytidilic acid (poly I:C)-treated pregnant rats exhibits neural, behavioral, and pharmacological changes relevant to schizophrenia [7]. The cord blood monocytes isolated from neonatal preterm lambs following maternal exposure to LPS exhibit decreased production of IL-6 in response to LPS stimulation when compared with monocytes from preterm control animals [8]. Consistently, the offspring born to LPS-treated pregnant rats exhibits diminished immune response to LPS challenge as compared to the pups born to vehicle-treated rats [9] [10]. These studies suggest that maternal immune stimulation may suppress the offspring's immune response to infections.

Maternal treatment with LPS has also been found to have region-specific effects on offspring brain. For example, intraperitoneal (i.p.) injection of LPS at 70% gestation significantly increases the level of cell death in the cortex but not in the periventricular white matter of the fetus compared to those injected with vehicles [11]. Maternal immune activation induces region-specific changes in the expression of cytokines in the offspring mouse brain [12]. Previously, we reported that maternal exposure to LPS has a significant impact on offspring neuroinflammation [10]. However, how maternal LPS stimulation affects the offspring's neuroimmune function in different brain regions is still largely unknown.

This study aimed to examine the regional pattern of the effects that maternal immune activation has on the offspring's neuroimmune function. Pregnant rats were treated with 500 μg/kg LPS via i.p. injection on gestational day 18 to induce immune activation. The offspring was allowed to develop up to the time of weaning at postnatal day 21 (P 21). The expression of cytokines, chemokines, and other mediators of the TLR-4 signaling pathway in the prefrontal cortex, hippocampus, cerebellum, and brainstem of the offspring at 2 h following stimulation with saline or 250 μg/kg LPS was examined.

## 2. Materials and Methods

### 2.1. Animals

Adult male and female Sprague-Dawley® rats were purchased from Harlan Inc. (Indianapolis, IN), maintained in a temperature- and humidity-controlled facility with a 12-h light/dark cycle, and fed a standard rat diet and water *ad libitum*. Animals were allowed to acclimate to the animal facility for at least 7 days prior to beginning the experiments. Animal studies including animal breeding were conducted with the approval of the Institutional Animal Care and Use Committee (IACUC) at Seton Hall University.

Each male rat (250 - 300 g) was housed with three female rats (200 - 230 g) at night, and the female rats were visually inspected for the presence of a vaginal plug the next morning. The female rat with a vaginal plug was moved to a separate cage under above-mentioned conditions and the day with a vaginal plug found was defined as gestational day 0. On gestational day 18, the pregnant dams were randomly assigned to receive 500 μg/kg LPS (*Salmonella enterica* serovar Typhimurium; Sigma, St. Louis, MO) or saline via intraperitoneal (i.p.) injection. Following injection with LPS or saline, the dams continued to be housed in above-mentioned conditions. After birth, the litter size was culled to 10 wherever applicable, and the offspring was allowed to develop up to the time of weaning at postnatal day (P) 21 when they were randomly assigned to receive one i.p. injection of saline or 250 μg/kg LPS and sacrificed 2 h later. Different brain regions were then dissected and stored at −80˚C for further analyses.

## 2.2. Total RNA Extraction

Total RNA from dissected brain tissues was isolated using the TRIzol reagent (Invitrogen, Grand Island, NY) according to manufacturer's instructions. The prepared RNA samples were dissolved in RNase-free water and stored at −80˚C.

## 2.3. Semi-Quantitative Reverse Transcriptase-Polymerase Chain Reaction (RT-PCR) Assay

cDNA was synthesized from 2 μg of total RNA using oligo $(dT)_{12-18}$ primer and Moloney Murine Leukemia Virus (M-MLV) reverse transcriptase (Promega, Madison, WI). After cDNA synthesis, PCR amplification was carried out using appropriate sense and antisense primers specific for rat $\beta$-actin (a house-keeping gene), IL-1$\beta$, IL-6, Mob-1, KC, CD14, TLR-4, Myd88, NF-κB, I-κB$\alpha$, and I-κB$\zeta$ synthesized by Eurofins Genomics (Huntville, AL) in a final volume of 20 μl containing 1 μl of cDNA, 1X PCR buffer, 0.2 μM of each sense and antisense primer, 0.2 mM of dNTPs, and 0.5 unit of Taq DNA polymerase (Applied Biosystems, Foster City, CA) [10] [13]. The reaction was heated to 94˚C for 5 min, followed by appropriate cycles of denaturation at 94˚C for 30 s, annealing at 57˚C for 30 s, and extension at 72˚C for 30 s. After the final cycle, a 7-min extension step at 72˚C was included. PCR products were then run on a 2.0% agarose gel and the gel image was recorded using a UVP GelDoc-It™ imaging system (UVP, Upland, CA). The band intensities of genes of interest were digitized using VisionWorks™ LS software (UVP, Upland, CA) and normalized against the intensity of $\beta$-actin in the same sample.

## 2.4. Statistical Analysis

All data were presented as means ± SD. Two-way analysis of variance (ANOVA) was used to analyze the data with maternal LPS treatment and postnatal LPS stimulation as between-subject factors. Bonferroni post-tests were performed if the overall treatment effects were significant. Results with $p < 0.05$ were considered statistically significant.

# 3. Results

## 3.1. Expression of Cytokines in Different Regions of Offspring Brain Following LPS Stimulation

To evaluate region-specific effects of maternal LPS on the neuroimmune response in the offspring brain, dams were treated with one dose of saline or 500 μg/kg LPS on gestational day 18 via i.p. injection, and the pups were subsequently stimulated with one i.p. injection of saline or 250 μg/kg LPS at P 21. At two hours after the injection, the pups were sacrificed, and prefrontal cortex, cerebellum, hippocampus, and brainstem were dissected. Total RNA was extracted from these tissues and the relative mRNA levels of cytokines were measured using semi-quantitative RT-PCR.

The basal level of mRNA expression of IL-1$\beta$ in the cerebellum (**Figure 1(a)**), hippocampus (**Figure 1(b)**), brainstem (**Figure 1(c)**), and prefrontal cortex (**Figure 1(d)**) of pups born to dams treated with LPS on gestational day 18 (L/S) trended higher than that in pups born to dams treated with saline (S/S) although the difference was not statistically significant. LPS stimulation significantly elevated the mRNA level of IL-1$\beta$ in the cerebellum, hippocampus, brainstem, and prefrontal cortex of P 21 pups born to dams treated with saline (S/L) and LPS (L/L) as compared to S/S and L/S pups respectively (**Figure 1**). Furthermore, the mRNA expression of IL-1$\beta$ was significantly lower in the prefrontal cortex of L/L than S/L pups. Although not statistically significant, the mRNA expression of IL-1$\beta$ was dramatically lower in the cerebellum and hippocampus of L/L than S/L pups while IL-1$\beta$ expression in the brainstem of L/L pups appeared to be comparable to that in S/L pups (**Figure 1**).

The mRNA expression of IL-6 in different brain regions of P 21 pups was also examined. The basal mRNA level of IL-6 was very low in all brain regions of S/S and L/S pups. IL-6 mRNA expression was significantly higher in the cerebellum (**Figure 2(a)**), hippocampus (**Figure 2(b)**), brainstem (**Figure 2(c)**), and prefrontal

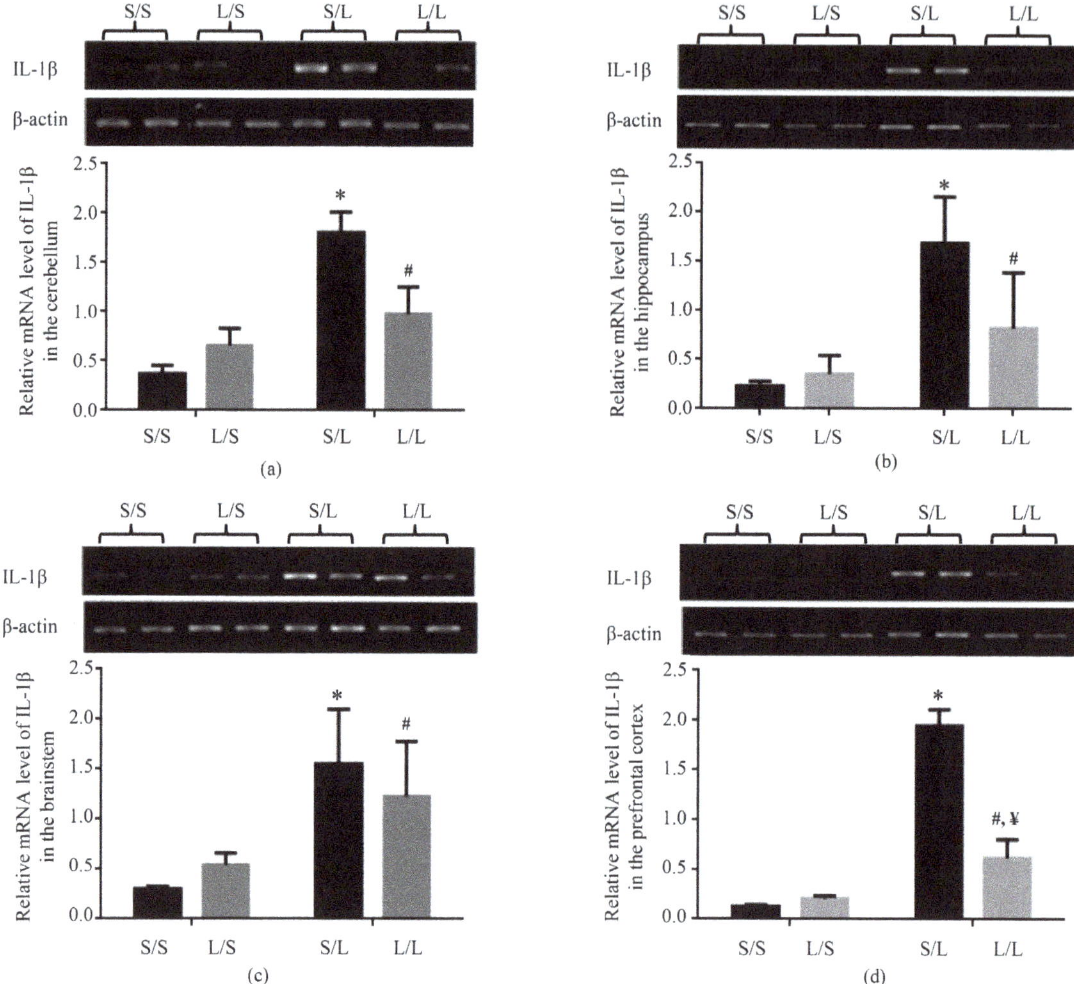


**Figure 1.** Relative mRNA expression of IL-1*β* in the cerebellum (a), hippocampus (b), brainstem (c), and prefrontal cortex (d) of P 21 pups born to saline or LPS-treated dams at 2 h following stimulation with saline or 250 μg/kg LPS as measured by semi-quantitative RT-PCR. *, vs. S/S; #, vs. L/S; ¥, vs. S/L.

cortex (**Figure 2(d)**) of S/L than S/S pups. IL-6 mRNA expression was also dramatically higher in all four brain regions of L/L than L/S pups even though the difference in the hippocampus and brainstem did not pass the threshold of statistical significance. Furthermore, the mRNA expression of IL-6 was significantly attenuated in the cerebellum and prefrontal cortex and trended lower in the hippocampus of L/L than S/L pups while it was comparable in the brainstem of S/L and L/L pups (**Figure 2**).

## 3.2. Expression of Chemokines in Different Regions of Offspring Brain Following LPS Stimulation

The expression of chemokines, key soluble factors involved in recruiting immune cells to the brain parenchyma, was then examined. The basal mRNA expression of KC in the cerebellum (**Figure 3(a)**), hippocampus (**Figure 3(b)**), brainstem (**Figure 3(c)**), and prefrontal cortex (**Figure 3(d)**) of L/S pups appeared to be comparable to that in S/S pups. The mRNA level of KC was significantly higher in the cerebellum, hippocampus, brainstem, and prefrontal cortex of S/L and L/L pups than S/S and L/S pups respectively. Furthermore, the mRNA expression of KC was significantly reduced in the cerebellum and prefrontal cortex, and trended lower in the hippocampus and brainstem of L/L than S/L pups (**Figure 3**).

The basal level of Mob-1 mRNA expression was very low in the cerebellum (**Figure 4(a)**), hippocampus (**Figure 4(b)**), brainstem (**Figure 4(c)**), and prefrontal cortex (**Figure 4(d)**) of S/S and L/S pups. LPS stimula-

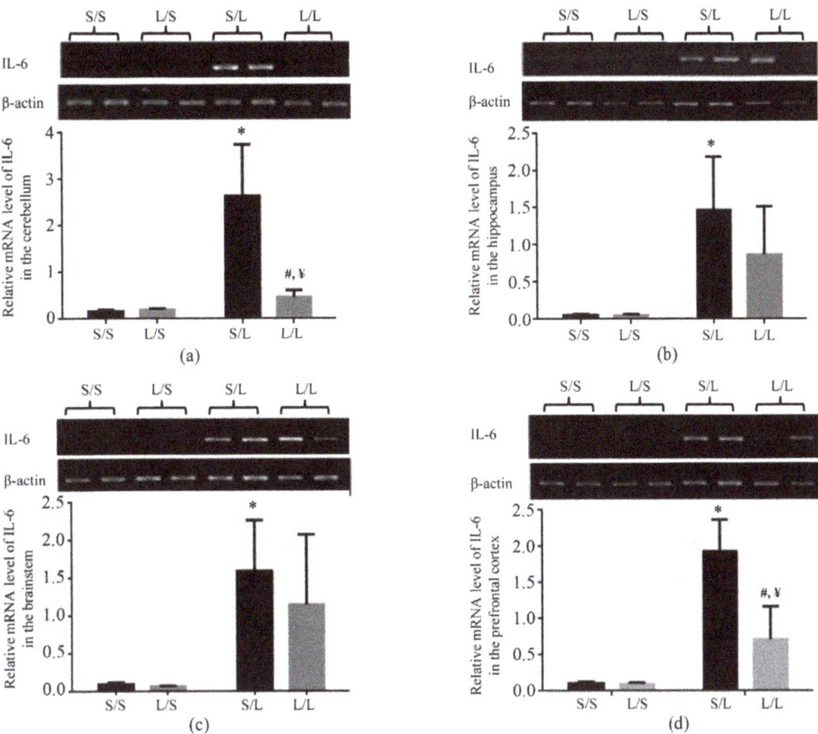


**Figure 2.** Relative mRNA expression of IL-6 in the cerebellum (a), hippocampus (b), brainstem (c), and prefrontal cortex (d) of P 21 pups born to saline or LPS-treated dams at 2 h following stimulation with saline or 250 μg/kg LPS as measured by semi-quantitative RT-PCR. *, vs. S/S; #, vs. L/S; ¥, vs. S/L.

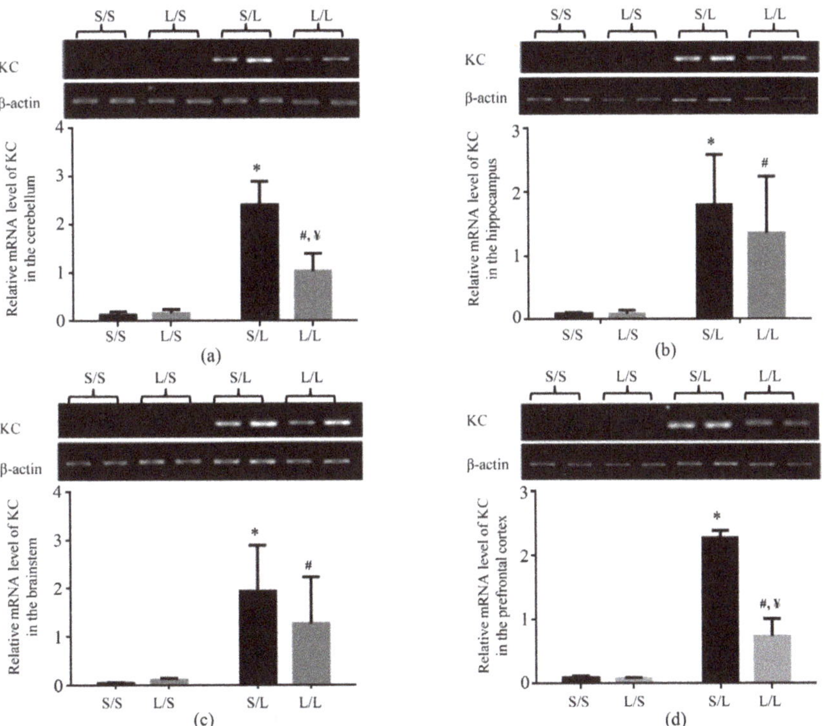


**Figure 3.** Relative mRNA expression of KC in the cerebellum (a), hippocampus (b), brainstem (c), and prefrontal cortex (d) of P 21 pups born to saline or LPS-treated dams at 2 h following stimulation with saline or 250 μg/kg LPS as measured by semi-quantitative RT-PCR. *, vs. S/S; #, vs. L/S; ¥, vs. S/L.

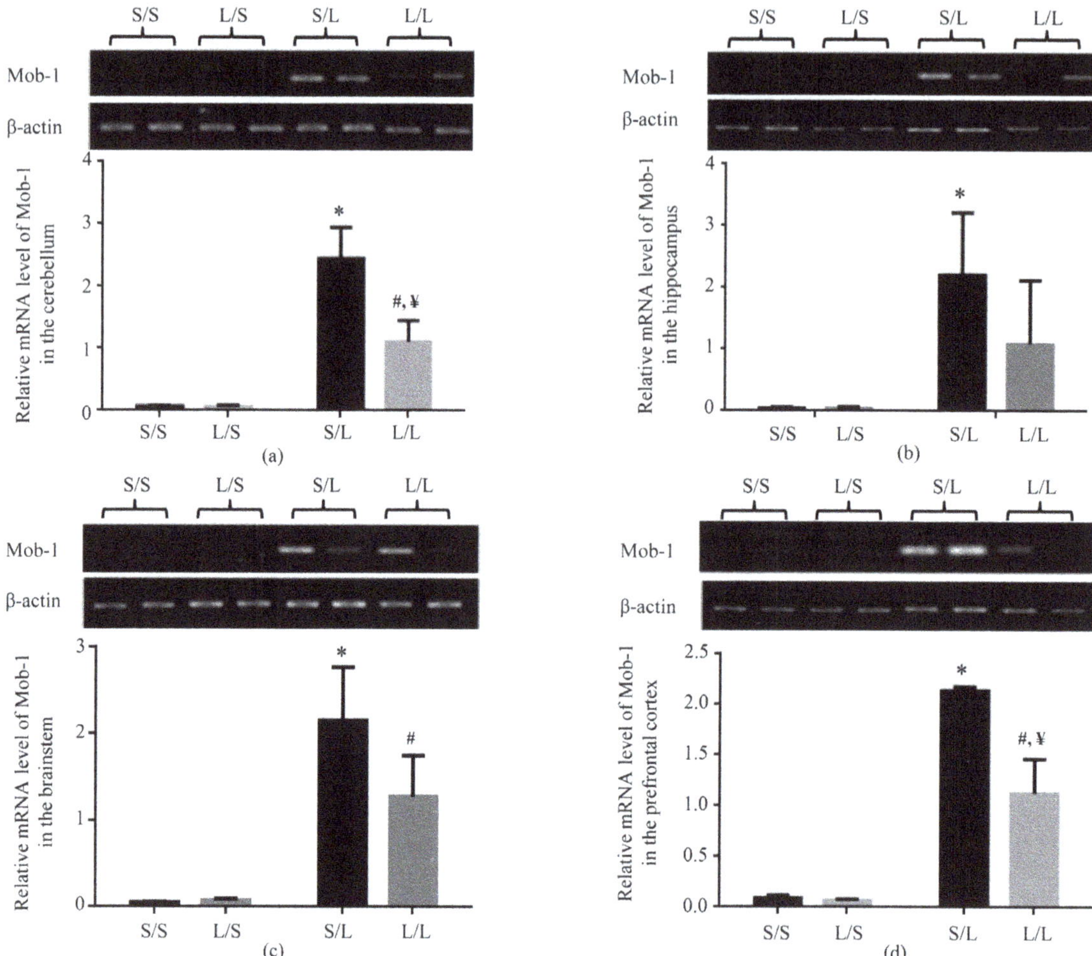


**Figure 4.** Relative mRNA expression of Mob-1 in the cerebellum (a), hippocampus (b), brainstem (c), and prefrontal cortex (d) of P 21 pups born to saline or LPS-treated dams at 2 h following stimulation with saline or 250 μg/kg LPS as measured by semi-quantitative RT-PCR. *, vs. S/S; #, vs. L/S; ¥, vs. S/L.

tion significantly elevated the mRNA expression of Mob-1 in all four brain regions of S/L pups as compared to that in S/S pups. The mRNA expression of Mob-1 was also significantly elevated in the cerebellum, brainstem, and prefrontal cortex, and trended higher in the hippocampus of L/L when compared with L/S pups. Furthermore, the mRNA expression of Mob-1 was significantly attenuated in the cerebellum and prefrontal cortex, and trended lower in the hippocampus and brainstem of L/L when compared with S/L pups (**Figure 4**).

### 3.3. Expression of Upstream Mediators of TLR-4 Signaling Pathway in Different Regions of Offspring Brain Following LPS Stimulation

The mRNA expression of upstream mediators of TLR-4 signaling pathway, namely Myd88, CD14 and TLR-4, in different brain regions of the offspring was then examined. Neither maternal nor postnatal LPS significantly changed the mRNA expression of Myd88 in the cerebellum (**Figure 5(a)**), hippocampus (**Figure 5(b)**), brainstem (**Figure 5(c)**), and prefrontal cortex (**Figure 5(d)**) of the offspring. The mRNA expression of TLR-4 in the cerebellum (**Figure 6(a)**), hippocampus (**Figure 6(b)**), brainstem (**Figure 6(c)**), and prefrontal cortex (**Figure 6(d)**) was not significantly affected by maternal or postnatal LPS treatment either.

The mRNA expression of CD14 in the cerebellum (**Figure 7(a)**), hippocampus (**Figure 7(b)**), and prefrontal cortex (**Figure 7(d)**) of S/S pups was not significantly different from that in L/S pups while it trended higher in the brainstem (**Figure 7(c)**) of L/S than S/S pups. CD14 mRNA expression appeared to be elevated in all four brain regions of S/L when compared with S/S pups, but only the increase in prefrontal cortex was statistically

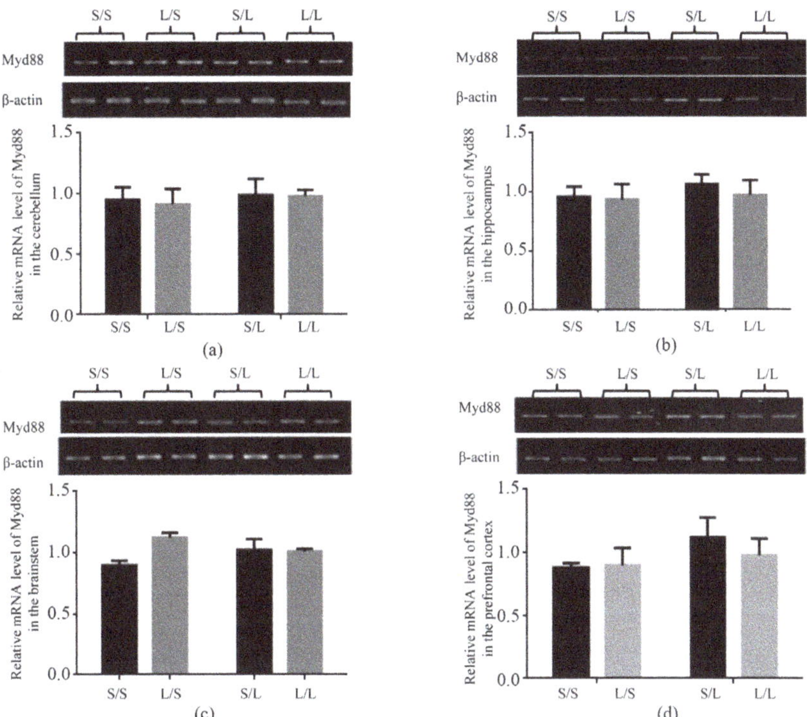


**Figure 5.** Relative mRNA expression of Myd88 in the cerebellum (a), hippocampus (b), brainstem (c), and prefrontal cortex (d) of P 21 pups born to saline or LPS-treated dams at 2 h following stimulation with saline or 250 μg/kg LPS as measured by semi-quantitative RT-PCR.

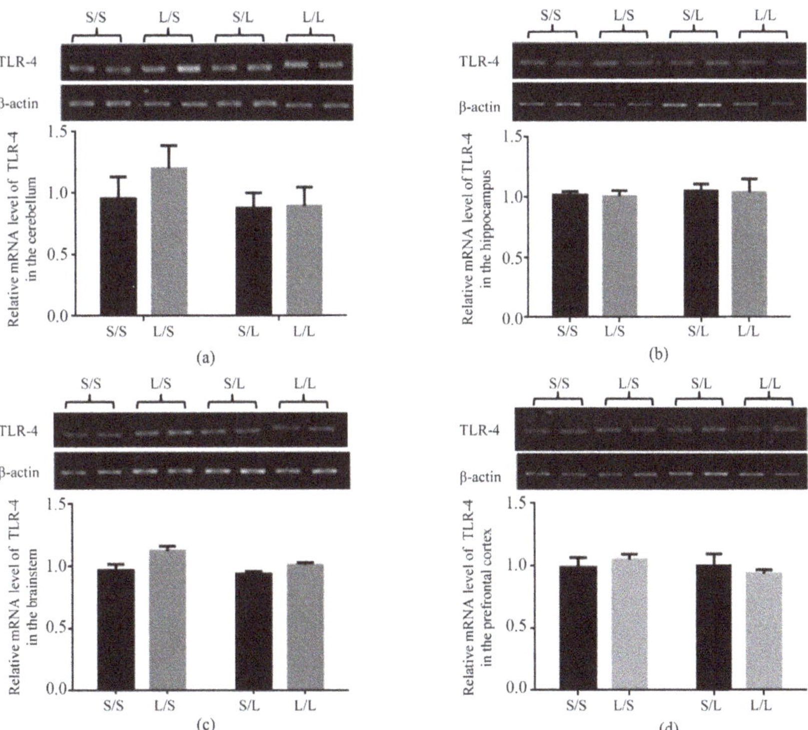


**Figure 6.** Relative mRNA expression of TLR-4 in the cerebellum (a), hippocampus (b), brainstem (c), and prefrontal cortex (d) of P 21 pups born to saline or LPS-treated dams at 2 h following stimulation with saline or 250 μg/kg LPS as measured by semi-quantitative RT-PCR.

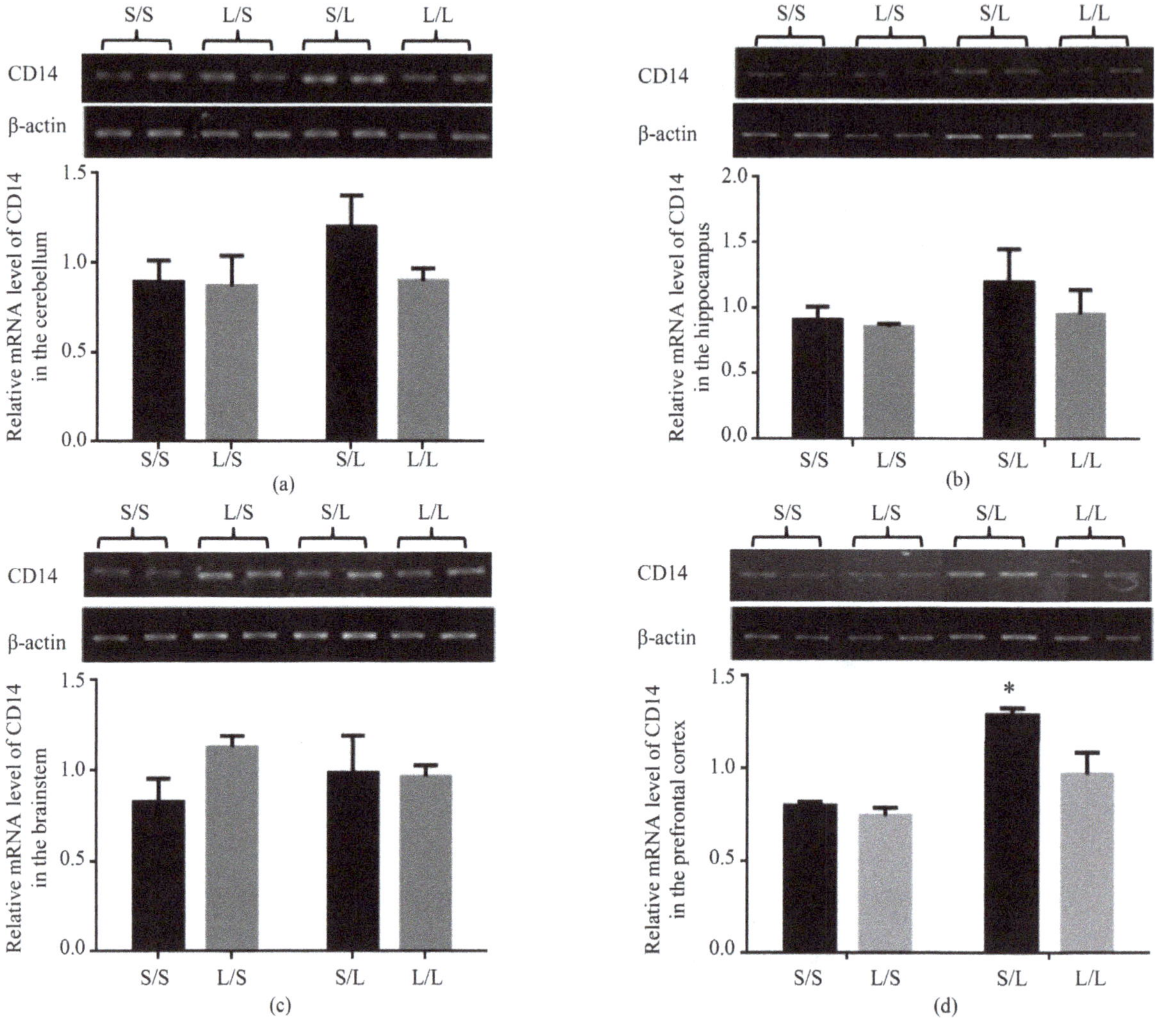


**Figure 7.** Relative mRNA expression of CD14 in the cerebellum (a), hippocampus (b), brainstem (c), and prefrontal cortex (d) of P 21 pups born to saline or LPS-treated dams at 2 h following stimulation with saline or 250 μg/kg LPS as measured by semi-quantitative RT-PCR. *, vs. S/S.

significant. The mRNA expression of CD14 trended higher in the prefrontal cortex of L/L when compared with L/S pups, and was comparable in the cerebellum, hippocampus, and brainstem of L/L pups and L/S pups. Additionally, the mRNA expression of CD14 was lower in the cerebellum, hippocampus, and prefrontal cortex of L/L pups than that in S/L pups, although the difference was not statistically significant (**Figure 7**).

## 3.4. Expression of Transcription Regulators in Different Regions of Offspring Brain Following LPS Stimulation

We then examined the mRNA expression of NF-κB p65 and its regulators in different brain regions of the offspring. The mRNA expression of NF-κB p65 in the cerebellum (**Figure 8(a)**), hippocampus (**Figure 8(b)**), brainstem (**Figure 8(c)**), and prefrontal cortex (**Figure 8(d)**) of S/S pups was not significantly affected by maternal or postnatal treatment with LPS. The mRNA expression of I-κB$\alpha$ in all four brain regions was comparable in S/S and L/S pups, and elevated to equivalent degrees at 2 h following LPS stimulation in S/L and L/L pups (**Figure 9**).

The mRNA expression of I-κB$\zeta$ in the cerebellum (**Figure 10(a)**), hippocampus (**Figure 10(b)**), brainstem (**Figure 10(c)**), and prefrontal cortex (**Figure 10(d)**) of S/S pups was comparable to that in L/S pups. LPS stimulation significantly elevated the mRNA level of I-κB$\zeta$ in all four brain regions of S/L and L/L pups. Further-

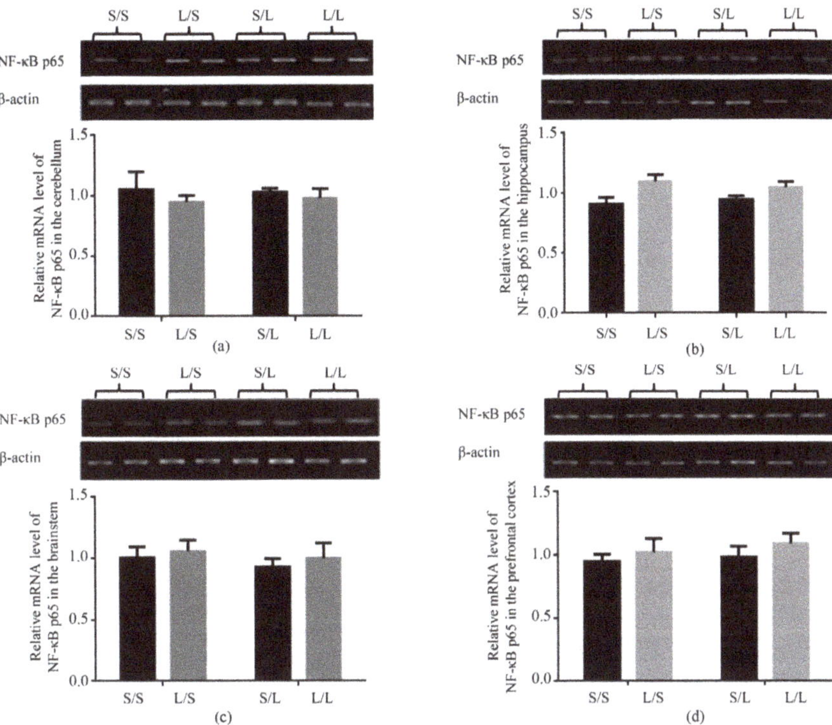


**Figure 8.** Relative mRNA expression of NF-κB p65 in the cerebellum (a), hippocampus (b), brainstem (c), and prefrontal cortex (d) of P 21 pups born to saline or LPS-treated dams at 2 h following stimulation with saline or 250 μg/kg LPS as measured by semi-quantitative RT-PCR.

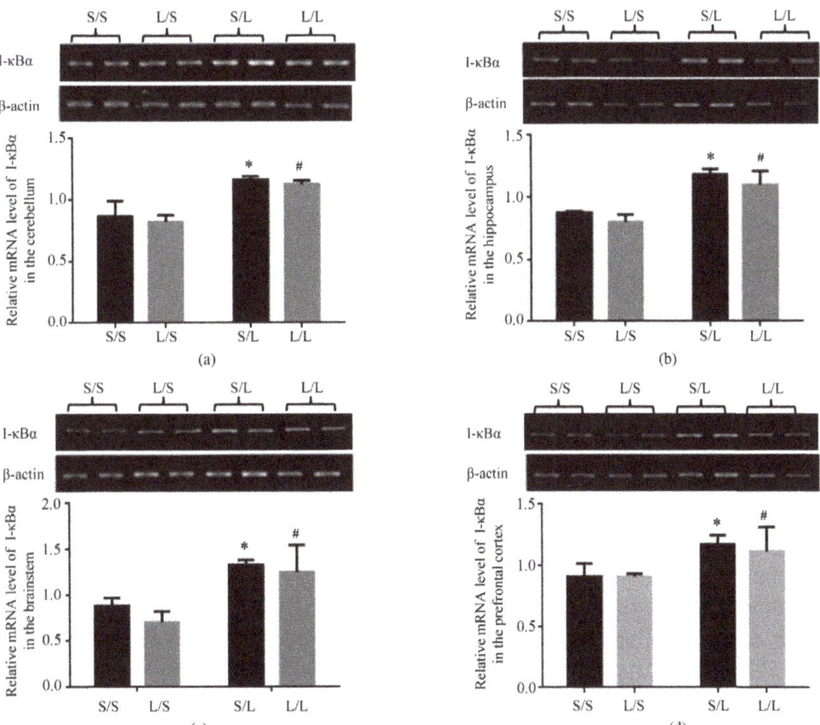


**Figure 9.** Relative mRNA expression of I-κBα in the cerebellum (a), hippocampus (b), brainstem (c), and prefrontal cortex (d) of P 21 pups born to saline or LPS-treated dams at 2 h following stimulation with saline or 250 μg/kg LPS as measured by semi-quantitative RT-PCR. *, vs. S/S; #, vs. L/S.

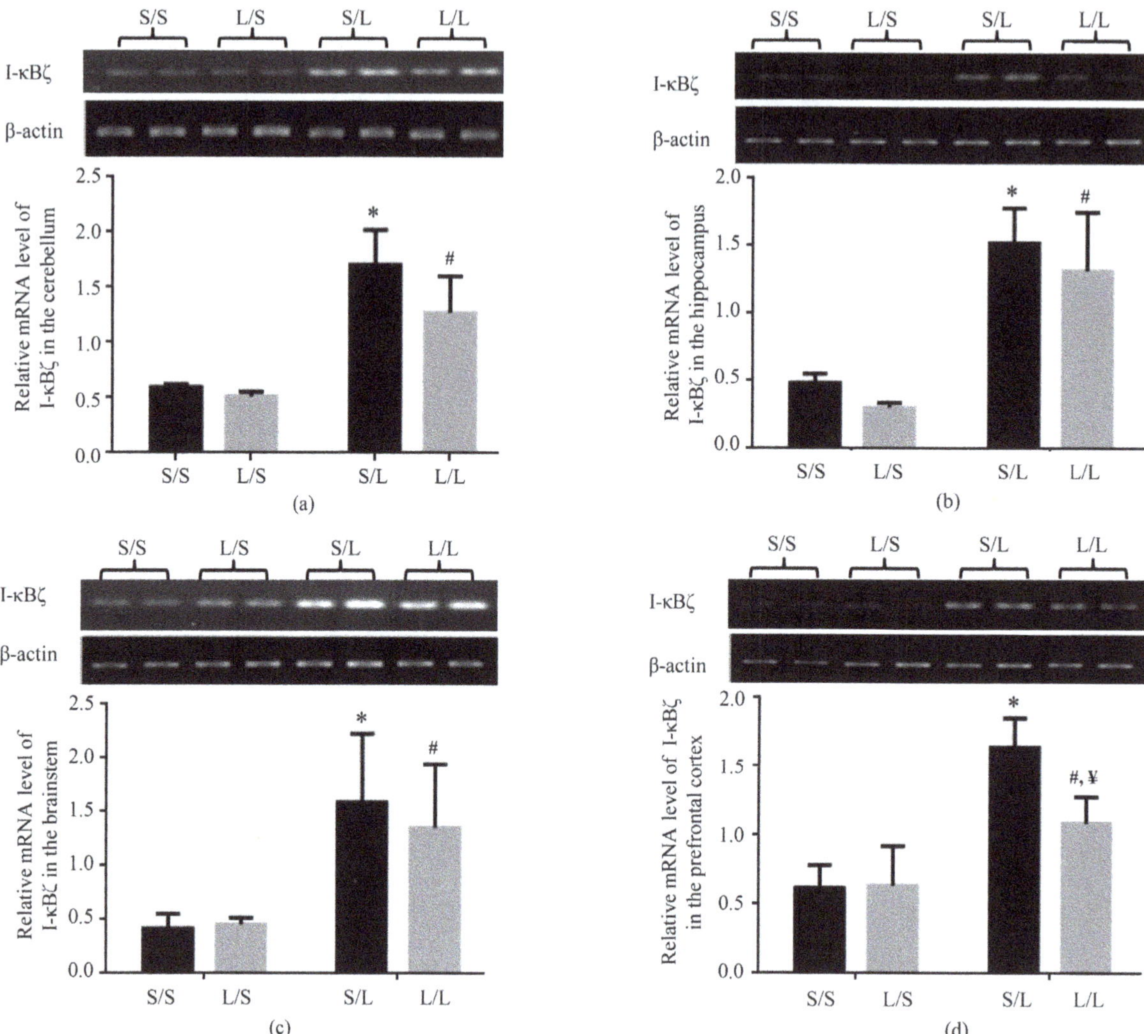


**Figure 10.** Relative mRNA expression of I-κBζ in the cerebellum (a), hippocampus (b), brainstem (c), and prefrontal cortex (d) of P 21 pups born to saline or LPS-treated dams at 2 h following stimulation with saline or 250 μg/kg LPS as measured by semi-quantitative RT-PCR. *, vs. S/S; #, vs. L/S; ¥, vs. S/L.

more, while the mRNA expression of I-κBζ was comparable in the hippocampus and brainstem of S/L and L/L pups, it trended lower in the cerebellum of L/L than S/L pups, and was significantly reduced in the prefrontal cortex of L/L when compared with S/L pups (**Figure 10**).

## 4. Discussion

Neuroimmune function plays a key role in combating infections, removing debris, promoting repairs, and maintaining homeostasis in the brain. Previous studies have shown that maternal immune activation affects immune as well as neuroimmune responses in the offspring [7] [9] [10]. In this study, we investigated the relationship between maternal immune activation and the neuroimmune function in different regions of the offspring brain. The prefrontal cortex and cerebellum of L/L pups exhibited attenuated mRNA induction of cytokines, namely IL-1$\beta$ and IL-6, and chemokines, namely KC and Mob-1, when compared with S/L pups at 2 h following LPS stimulation even though the difference in IL-1$\beta$ was not statistically significant in the cerebellum. Furthermore, mRNA expression of these cytokines and chemokines in the hippocampus of L/L pups trended lower than that in S/L pups while the mRNA expression of these cytokines and chemokines was not dramatically different in the brainstem of L/L and S/L pups. These findings suggest that the neuroimmune function in four different brain regions of the offspring was susceptible to maternal immune activation to different degrees with prefrontal cortex and cerebellum being the most vulnerable and brainstem the least while the hippocampus was somewhat affected.

In association with reduced mRNA levels of cytokines and chemokines in the prefrontal cortex and cerebellum, the mRNA expression of CD14 in the prefrontal cortex and cerebellum of L/L pups also trended lower than that in S/L pups. Additionally, the mRNA expression of I-κB$\zeta$ was significantly reduced in the prefrontal cortex and trended lower in the cerebellum of L/L when compared with S/L pups. Studies have shown that I-κB$\zeta$ is a positive regulator of a subset of NF-κB target genes such as IL-6 [3] [14], which suggests that the reduced induction of I-κB$\zeta$ in the prefrontal cortex of L/L may have contributed to the attenuated mRNA induction of cytokines and chemokines when compared with S/L pups. Further studies on the protein levels of NF-κB and I-κB$\zeta$ as well as posttranslational modifications of NF-κB would help to better understand how NF-κB regulation contributes to the observed effects of maternal immune activation on offspring neuroimmune function in our animal model.

While the transcriptional activity of NF-κB is regulated by I-κBs, the expression of I-κB$\zeta$ is, in turn, transcriptionally regulated by NF-κB as part of a feed back loop [15] [16]. Consistently, LPS has been reported to induce the expression of I-κB$\zeta$ in mouse embryonic NIH-3T3 fibroblast cells [16], human myelomonocytic U937 cells [17], and mouse RAW264 macrophages [18], and in the spleen, lymph node, and lung of mice [14]. Our study also show that LPS stimulation significantly elevated the mRNA expression of I-κB$\zeta$ in all brain regions of the offspring compared to the saline controls.

A well-organized neuroimmune response is essential for appropriate tissue maintenance and immune surveillance of the CNS, to defend the CNS against pathogens, and to help it recover from stress and injury [19]-[22]. Neuroinflammation has generally been regarded as a double-edged sword that can cause injury to or protect the CNS. There is evidence that neuroinflammation is a risk factor for neurodegenerative disorders, such as Alzheimer's [23] and Parkinson's diseases [20] [24]. On the other hand, insufficient neuroinflammation and microglial dysfunction could lead to insufficient clearance of $\beta$-amyloid plaques and have been proposed as a possible pathway in the pathogenesis of Alzheimer's disease [25] [26]. Additionally, a neuroimmune-based mechanism has been posited for the etiology of schizophrenia and autism [27]-[30]. Graciarena *et al.* reported that subcutaneous injections of LPS into pregnant rats every other day from gestational days 14 to 20 leads to persistent microglial activation specifically in the hippocampus of adult offspring animals [31]. The present study did examine the mRNA induction of cytokines and chemokines in L/S and S/S pups and found that the mRNA expression of IL-1$\beta$ trended higher in all four brain regions of L/S than S/S pups while the basal level of IL-6, KC, and Mob-1 expression was barely detectable in L/S and S/S pups under the experimental conditions. While it is of interest to further examine the status of neuroinflammation of the offspring at the basal level, the results in this study suggest that the offspring's neuroimmune response to an immune insult may be impacted to different degrees depending on the brain regions. Considering that neuroinflammation involves finely regulated expression of pro-inflammatory and anti-inflammatory mediators [20]-[22], profiling of neuroinflammatory mediators at different time points following LPS stimulation would help to further delineate the effects of maternal immune activation on the neuroimmune function of the offspring pups and provide a better understanding of the interplay between disturbances in maternal environment and development of neuropathologies in the offspring later in life.

## 5. Conclusion

In summary, this study demonstrated that the prefrontal cortex and cerebellum of L/L pups exhibited attenuated mRNA induction of cytokines, namely IL-1$\beta$ and IL-6, and chemokines, namely KC and Mob-1, when compared with S/L pups at 2 h following LPS stimulation even though the difference in IL-1$\beta$ was not statistically significant in the cerebellum. Furthermore, mRNA expression of these cytokines and chemokines in the hippocampus of L/L pups trended lower than that in S/L pups while the mRNA expression of these cytokines and chemokines was not dramatically different in the brainstem of L/L and S/L pups. In association with reduced mRNA levels of cytokines and chemokines in the prefrontal cortex and cerebellum, the mRNA expression of CD14 in the prefrontal cortex and cerebellum of L/L pups also trended lower than that in S/L pups. Additionally, the mRNA expression of I-κB$\zeta$ was significantly reduced in the prefrontal cortex and trended lower in the cerebellum of L/L when compared with S/L pups. These findings suggest that the neuroimmune function in four distinct brain regions of the offspring was susceptible to maternal immune activation to different degrees with prefrontal cortex and cerebellum being the most vulnerable and brainstem the least while the hippocampus was somewhat affected, and help to delineate the effects of maternal immune activation on the development of neuropathologies in the offspring later in life.

## Acknowledgements

This work was supported in part by the National Institute of Health Grant R15-HD065643 to H.Z.

## Conflict of Interest

The author declares that there is no conflict of interests regarding the publication of this paper.

## References

[1] Hanke, M.L. and Kielian, T. (2011) Toll-Like Receptors in Health and Disease in the Brain: Mechanisms and Therapeutic Potential. *Clinical Science* (Lond), **121**, 367-387. http://dx.doi.org/10.1042/CS20110164

[2] Cutolo, M., Soldano, S., Contini, P., Sulli, A., Seriolo, B., Montagna, P. and Brizzolara, R. (2013) Intracellular NF-kB-Decrease and IKBalpha Increase in Human Macrophages Following CTLA4-Ig Treatment. *Clinical and Experimental Rheumatology*, **31**, 943-946.

[3] Trinh, D.V., Zhu, N., Farhang, G., Kim, B.J. and Huxford, T. (2008) The Nuclear IkappaB Protein IkappaB Zeta Specifically Binds NF-kappaB p50 Homodimers and Forms a Ternary Complex on kappaB DNA. *Journal of Molecular Biology*, **379**, 122-135. http://dx.doi.org/10.1016/j.jmb.2008.03.060

[4] Kayama, H., Ramirez-Carrozzi, V.R., Yamamoto, M., Mizutani, T., Kuwata, H., Iba, H., Matsumoto, M., Honda, K., Smale, S.T. and Takeda, K. (2008) Class-Specific Regulation of Pro-Inflammatory Genes by MyD88 Pathways and IkappaBzeta. *Journal of Biological Chemistry*, **283**, 12468-12477. http://dx.doi.org/10.1074/jbc.M709965200

[5] Hildebrand, D.G., Alexander, E., Horber, S., Lehle, S., Obermayer, K., Munck, N.A., Rothfuss, O., Frick, J.S., Morimatsu, M., Schmitz, I., Roth, J., Ehrchen, J.M., Essmann, F. and Schulze-Osthoff, K. (2013) IkappaBzeta Is a Transcriptional Key Regulator of CCL2/MCP-1. *Journal of Immunology*, **190**, 4812-4820.

[6] Huang, B., Yang, X.D., Lamb, A. and Chen, L.F. (2010) Posttranslational Modifications of NF-kappaB: Another Layer of Regulation for NF-kappaB Signaling Pathway. *Cell Signal*, **22**, 1282-1290. http://dx.doi.org/10.1016/j.cellsig.2010.03.017

[7] Zuckerman, L. and Weiner, I. (2005) Maternal Immune Activation Leads to Behavioral and Pharmacological Changes in the Adult Offspring. *Journal of Psychiatric Research*, **39**, 311-323. http://dx.doi.org/10.1016/j.jpsychires.2004.08.008

[8] Kramer, B.W., Ikegami, M., Moss, T.J., Nitsos, I., Newnham, J.P. and Jobe, A.H. (2005) Endotoxin-Induced Chorioamnionitis Modulates Innate Immunity of Monocytes in Preterm Sheep. *American Journal of Respiratory and Critical Care Medicine*, **171**, 73-77. http://dx.doi.org/10.1164/rccm.200406-745OC

[9] Hodyl, N.A., Krivanek, K.M., Lawrence, E., Clifton, V.L. and Hodgson, D.M. (2007) Prenatal Exposure to a Pro-Inflammatory Stimulus Causes Delays in the Development of the Innate Immune Response to LPS in the Offspring. *Journal of Neuroimmunology*, **190**, 61-71. http://dx.doi.org/10.1016/j.jneuroim.2007.07.021

[10] Lasala, N. and Zhou, H. (2007) Effects of Maternal Exposure to LPS on the Inflammatory Response in the Offspring. *Journal of Neuroimmunology*, **189**, 95-101. http://dx.doi.org/10.1016/j.jneuroim.2007.07.010

[11] Harnett, E.L., Dickinson, M.A. and Smith, G.N. (2007) Dose-Dependent Lipopolysaccharide-Induced Fetal Brain Injury in the Guinea Pig. *American Journal of Obstetrics and Gynecology*, **197**, 179. e1-179. e7. http://dx.doi.org/10.1016/j.ajog.2007.03.047

[12] Garay, P.A., Hsiao, E.Y., Patterson, P.H. and McAllister, A.K. (2013) Maternal Immune Activation Causes Age- and Region-Specific Changes in Brain cytokines in Offspring throughout Development. *Brain, Behavior, and Immunity*, **31**, 54-68. http://dx.doi.org/10.1016/j.bbi.2012.07.008

[13] Ortega, A., Jadeja, V. and Zhou, H.P. (2011) Postnatal Development of Lipopolysaccharide-induced Inflammatory Response in the Brain. *Inflammation Research*, **60**, 175-185. http://dx.doi.org/10.1007/s00011-010-0252-y

[14] Kitamura, H., Kanehira, K., Okita, K., Morimatsu, M. and Saito, M. (2000) MAIL, a Novel Nuclear IκB Protein That Potentiates LPS-Induced IL-6 Production. *FEBS Letters*, **485**, 53-56. http://dx.doi.org/10.1016/S0014-5793(00)02185-2

[15] Sun, S.C., Ganchi, P.A., Ballard, D.W. and Greene, W.C. (1993) NF-κB Controls Expression of Inhibitor IκB Alpha: Evidence for an Inducible Autoregulatory Pathway. *Science*, **259**, 1912-1915. http://dx.doi.org/10.1126/science.8096091

[16] Yamazaki, S., Muta, T., Matsuo, S. and Takeshige, K. (2005) Stimulus-Specific Induction of a Novel Nuclear Factor-κB Regulator, IκB-Zeta, via Toll/Interleukin-1 Receptor Is Mediated by mRNA Stabilization. *Journal of Biological Chemistry*, **280**, 1678-1687. http://dx.doi.org/10.1074/jbc.M409983200

[17] Kitamura, H., Kanehira, K., Shiina, T., Morimatsu, M., Jung, B.D., Akashi, S. and Saito, M. (2002) Bacterial Lipopolysaccharide Induces mRNA Expression of an IκB MAIL through Toll-Like Receptor 4. *Journal of Veterinary Medical Science*, **64**, 419-422. http://dx.doi.org/10.1292/jvms.64.419

[18] Ito, T., Morimatsu, M., Oonuma, T., Shiina, T., Kitamura, H. and Syuto, B. (2004) Transcriptional Regulation of the MAIL Gene in LPS-Stimulated RAW264 Mouse Macrophages. *Gene*, **342**, 137-143. http://dx.doi.org/10.1016/j.gene.2004.07.032

[19] Lehnardt, S. (2010) Innate Immunity and Neuroinflammation in the CNS: The Role of Microglia in Toll-Like Receptor-Mediated Neuronal Injury. *Glia*, **58**, 253-263.

[20] Skaper, S.D. (2007) The Brain as a Target for Inflammatory Processes and Neuroprotective Strategies. *Annals of the New York Academy of Sciences*, **1122**, 23-34. http://dx.doi.org/10.1196/annals.1403.002

[21] Jean-Baptiste, E. (2007) Cellular Mechanisms in Sepsis. *Journal of Intensive Care Medicine*, **22**, 63-72. http://dx.doi.org/10.1177/0885066606297123

[22] Bosshart, H. and Heinzelmann, M. (2007) Targeting Bacterial Endotoxin: Two Sides of a Coin. *Annals of the New York Academy of Sciences*, **1096**, 1-17. http://dx.doi.org/10.1196/annals.1397.064

[23] Blasko, I., Stampfer-Kountchev, M., Robatscher, P., Veerhuis, R., Eikelenboom, P. and Grubeck-Loebenstein, B. (2004) How Chronic Inflammation Can Affect the Brain and Support the Development of Alzheimer's Disease in Old Age: The Role of Microglia and Astrocytes. *Aging Cell*, **3**, 169-176. http://dx.doi.org/10.1111/j.1474-9728.2004.00101.x

[24] Sekiyama, K., Sugama, S., Fujita, M., Sekigawa, A., Takamatsu, Y., Waragai, M., Takenouchi, T. and Hashimoto, M. (2012) Neuroinflammation in Parkinson's Disease and Related Disorders: A Lesson from Genetically Manipulated Mouse Models of Alpha-Synucleinopathies. *Parkinson's Disease*, **2012**, Article ID: 271732. http://dx.doi.org/10.1155/2012/271732

[25] Napoli, I. and Neumann, H. (2009) Microglial Clearance Function in Health and Disease. *Neuroscience*, **158**, 1030-1038. http://dx.doi.org/10.1016/j.neuroscience.2008.06.046

[26] Streit, W.J., Conde, J.R., Fendrick, S.E., Flanary, B.E. and Mariani, C.L. (2005) Role of Microglia in the Central Nervous System's Immune Response. *Neurological Research*, **27**, 685-691.

[27] Meyer, U. (2013) Developmental Neuroinflammation and Schizophrenia. *Progress in Neuro-Psychopharmacology and Biological Psychiatry*, **42**, 20-34. http://dx.doi.org/10.1016/j.pnpbp.2011.11.003

[28] Zhou, H.P. (2012) Maternal Infection and Neurodevelopmental Disorders in the Offspring. *American Journal of Immunology*, **8**, 10-17. http://dx.doi.org/10.3844/ajisp.2012.10.17

[29] Boksa, P. (2008) Maternal Infection during Pregnancy and Schizophrenia. *Journal of Psychiatry & Neuroscience*, **33**, 183-185.

[30] Buehler, M.R. (2011) A Proposed Mechanism for Autism: An Aberrant Neuroimmune Response Manifested as a Psychiatric Disorder. *Medical Hypotheses*, **76**, 863-870. http://dx.doi.org/10.1016/j.mehy.2011.02.038

[31] Graciarena, M., Depino, A.M. and Pitossi, F.J. (2010) Prenatal Inflammation Impairs Adult Neurogenesis and Memory Related Behavior through Persistent Hippocampal TGF$\beta_1$ Downregulation. *Brain, Behavior, and Immunity*, **24**, 1301-1309. http://dx.doi.org/10.1016/j.bbi.2010.06.005

4

# Multiple Comparisons of Traditional Acupuncture Therapies of Japan, Korea and China—A Preliminary Report of Three Countries' Acupuncture (TCA) Project

**Kenji Kawakita[1*], Yong-Suk Kim[2], Nobuo Yamaguchi[3], Xiao-Pin Lin[4], Matsuo Arai[4], Naomi Takazawa[4], Shan-Yu Su[5]**

[1]Department of Physiology, Meiji University of Integrative Medicine, Kyoto, Japan
[2]Department of Acupuncture & Moxibustion, (Brain & Neurological Disorders and Pain), Kangnam Korean Hospital, Kyung Hee University, Seoul, Korea
[3]Kanazawa Medical University, Ishikawa, Japan
[4]Ishikawa Natural Medicinal Products Research Center, Kanazawa, Japan
[5]School of Post-Baccalaureate Chinese Medicine, College of Chinese Medicine, China Medical University, Taichung, Taiwan
Email: [*]k_kawakita@meiji-u.ac.jp

## Abstract

**Acupuncture therapy had established in China and it distributed among Asian countries and developed in each country as traditional medicine. In this project we compared the procedures and effects of traditional acupuncture therapies in China, Korea and Japan by using 10 healthy young male volunteers with written informed consent. Total white cell counts, leukocyte subsets and noradrenalin contents were used as outcomes. Three well trained traditional acupuncture therapists were chosen and they treated the same subjects at random order with intervals of at least two months. Each acupuncturist made his diagnosis and points selection for potentiate vital conditions. Clearly different procedures and point selections were used among three traditional acupuncture therapies on the same subject and the obtained changes of outcome measures also differed. Although variations of data were quite large, these results clearly demonstrated that acupuncture therapies have developed among three countries in unique manner.**

## Keywords

**Acupuncture, Total Leukocyte, Leukocyte Subset, Emotional Hormone, QOL, Comparison Among**

[*]Corresponding author.

**Chinese, Korean and Japanese Traditional Acupuncture**

## 1. Introduction

It is widely accepted that acupuncture and moxibustion therapies are originated from China, and it has grown and established its own system as traditional medicine, then it distributes to worldwide as traditional Chinese Medicine (TCM). The diagnosis and procedure of TCM have been well established and recently various re-evaluation of TCM has been conducted [1]-[4]. The majority of practitioners have learned acupuncture therapy in China or Chinese doctors in the different countries, so TCM way of acupuncture therapy may be considered as only one acupuncture therapy in the world.

During the process of development and worldwide distribution, it has modified in different countries with their nature, social customs, foods and other things. Thereafter the term "acupuncture and moxibustion therapies" includes several different procedures of diagnosis and treatment in them, although existence of the differences has not been hardly noticed the researcher of clinical trials of acupuncture in the Western world.

In Korea and Japan, acupuncture therapy has developed as one of traditional therapies with different characteristics from that of TCM. Korean acupuncture has developed on the basis of "Sasang" constitutional medicine, and Saam acupuncture has established as Korean particular way of diagnosis and treatment procedures of acupuncture [5] [6]. Sasang constitutional medicine is characterized as holistic tailored medicine [7], and its reliability of a questionnaire for the diagnosis is confirmed recently [8].

In Japan, acupuncture therapy has long been used as the main stream medicine until Edo era (the middle of 19 century), and it is usually characterized by its use of needling tube with fine needles and gentle manipulation without de-qi sensation [9]-[11]. In our previous multi-center trial, gentle manipulation to the specific point at the throat is used as acupuncture for prevention of the symptoms of common cold [12]. In practical situation, wide variation of diagnosis and needling techniques are used such as meridian, reaction point, trigger point, skin impedance, anatomy-physiology, and so on. These variations of Japanese acupuncture may due to its position of the medical systems in Japan. It has developed for the requirement of the patients. Recently, more modernized acupuncture based on physiology and anatomy of the body has been developed to cooperate with Western medical doctors.

On the other hand, recent clinical trials of acupuncture have provided an important evidence of efficacy and safety of acupuncture treatment, and the majority of acupuncture interventions used in the trials is based on TCM theory of acupuncture points selection and manipulations [13]. The mega trials conducted in German clearly demonstrate that real TCM style acupuncture has a statistically superior effect compared with conventional and/or standardized Western therapies [14]. The economic analysis also demonstrates the cost-benefit of acupuncture therapy in German acupuncture trials [15].

The major issues to be considered now is that there is no statistically significant difference between real TCM acupuncture group and those of sham acupuncture (minimal acupuncture) group, that is no specific effect of acupuncture therapy was proven by high quality RCTs conducted in German. In the trials, minimal acupuncture is characterized by shallow needling to non-acupuncture points without de-qi sensation. As the majority of researchers of clinical trials of acupuncture in the Western world have learned and trained TCM as standard acupuncture therapy, so the location of acupuncture points and provocation of particular de-qi sensation is considered to be essentially important. So the German trials choose the minimal acupuncture as sham intervention might be reasonable.

However, the shallow needling without de-qi used in minimal acupuncture have been widely used in Japan and selection of acupuncture points tended to be based on careful palpation of the skin and/or deep tissues not restricted at the precise location in textbook [16]. In other words, the minimal acupuncture is not adequate intervention as inert sham intervention because it has been used in Japan as one of the procedure of real acupuncture manipulation.

Therefore it is important to know the existence of different procedures of acupuncture except for TCM acupuncture therapy, however, no clinical researches comparing various traditional acupuncture therapies have been conducted in evidence based manner so far.

Our previous study clearly demonstrated that one session of acupuncture treatment by Japanese acupuncture, called Tai-chi (太極) therapy, one of traditional acupuncture therapies could induced remarkable effects on immune system [17]. Then Prof. Yamaguchi proposed a project called "鍼三国師 (TCA: three countries' acupuncture) project" to investigate the different therapeutic properties of traditional acupuncture in Japan, Korea and China. The protocol of the present project conducted was determined through several meetings and discussions among the researcher in China, Korea and Japan.

The purpose of TCA project is to clarify the different characteristics of traditional acupuncture procedures in three countries and it may help to understanding and development of potential roles of acupuncture therapy in the future CAM.

## 2. Methods

### 2.1. Subjects and Practitioners

Subjects were healthy young subjects with informed consent (male, average 21 years, 20 - 25, $n = 10$). They had no experience of acupuncture treatment. The experimental design used was cross-over and each subject was randomly allocated to Chinese, Korean and Japanese acupuncture in order of their registration. One subject received three different treatments. The experiments were conducted in April, June and August in 2009 at Kanazawa.

Acupuncture practitioners were well-experienced traditional acupuncture therapists in Japan, Korea and China (their clinical experiences were over 20 years). The practitioners were asked to make diagnosis on each subject by their own methodology and selected best acupuncture points for individualized treatments in each subject to improve their conditions based on their diagnosis. The purpose of the treatment was to enhance self-defense system and to make better health condition in each subject. The concrete procedures of diagnosis and treatment were recorded on the chart in detail, and the processes of diagnosis and treatment were recorded by video camera with permission of the subjects and practitioners.

The subjects were treated by three practitioners in three different styles of acupuncture treatments at intervals of about 2 months or more. The experiments usually started in a clinic at 19:00 in each time to avoid the circadian changes in adrenalin contents and white blood cells [18]. The experiments were conducted on April, June and August. An additive experiment by Chinese acupuncture treatment was performed on January 2010 as the initial Chinese practitioner was accidentally exchanged and the first three subjects data collected in April was replaced by the new samples. Three beds were prepared and each practitioner treated three subjects in each experimental session. The average treatment time was about 30 mins. The procedures of diagnosis and treatments were recorded by three video cameras with permission of the subjects and practitioners.

The written informed consents were obtained, and the protocol of this project was approved by the Ethics Committee of Kanazawa Medical School.

### 2.2. Measurement of White Blood Cell Composition and Adrenalin Contents

Blood samples were collected by nurse before acupuncture treatment and 24 hours after the treatment. The blood samples were analyzed conventional procedures and measured the total leukocytes (WBC: white blood cell) number and ratio of granulocytes and lymphocytes. The catecholamine content (adrenalin) was also measured by ELISA (Enzyme-Linked Immuno Sorbent Assay).

### 2.3. Statistical Analysis

The data were expressed as mean+/− standard deviation. The WBC is number of cells, granulocytes and lymphocytes were shown as % of total leukocytes and adrenalin content was expressed by pg (pikogram/ml). Group comparison of data was performed by ANOVA and post hoc multiple test. Difference of point selection between two countries was analyzed by chi-square test (Statview, 5.0, SAS). The correlation between baseline data and ratio of each WBC composition and adrenalin were also calculated.

## 3. Results

### 3.1. Diagnosis and Treatment of Three Countries

Subjects included in this pilot project were ten healthy young male university students, and they were diagnosed by three traditional acupuncturists in each treatment session and point selections were performed by individualized manner. Korean acupuncturist clearly classified based on Sasang constitution theory, a traditional Korean medical theory. Nine subjects were classified into Soeum-in type ($n = 4$), Soyang-in type ($n = 1$), Taeum-in type ($n = 3$) and Tayang-in type ($n = 0$) by Sasang constitutional medicine, and deficiency of responsible meridians were pointed out. The point selection was conducted by base on the Saam acupuncture theory, and the points located in the periphery were frequently used. Supplement or drain technique on the selected points were restrictedly performed.

Chinese acupuncturist used pulse and tongue diagnosis then selected the points. No TCM diagnosis of condition was performed as the subjects were basically healthy young students. The relatively thick acupuncture needles were used and inserted deep in tissues and de-qi sensation frequently provoked by the needle manipulation.

Japanese acupuncturist did careful palpation of the skin and deep tissues to detect reaction points, no pulse diagnosis was used. The needling procedure was gentle manipulation without any subjective sensation called de-qi. He chose the points regardless of the precise location of acupuncture points so no information regarding selection of the acupuncture points used was available but rough location of needling points was recorded. The extremely different characteristic of the Japanese style acupuncture from that of C and K treatment is apparent.

All practitioners used the single-use disposable acupuncture needle in sterile package.

### 3.2. Point Selection of Korean and Chinese Acupuncturists

**Table 1** summarizes the acupuncture points selected by Korean and Chinese practitioner in all subjects of this study. The total numbers of acupuncture points used were similar but the actual points used were quite different between C and K treatments. Total number of acupuncture points used in C and K treatment were 83 (4 - 17, mean of 9.2/subject) and 75 (6 - 9, mean of 8.3/subject), and less and regular number of points selection were observed in K treatment.

The acupuncture points used in C and K treatments were obviously different, and only 5 acupuncture points (ST36, V12, LI11, LR3, SP2) were used in both K and C treatment, although the subjects were the same and a total of 44 acupuncture points were used in K and C treatment. The major points used in C and K treatments were listed in **Table 2**.

## 4. WBC Number

The total WBC number, lymphocyte (%), granulocyte (%), serum adrenalin content (pg/ml) were measured before treatment as baseline. The baseline data of nine subjects who complete three acupuncture therapies received were listed in **Table 3**.

One subject was dropout for his personal reason. There was no significant difference among three groups (China, Korea and Japan) in their baseline data although individual variations tended to be large.

### WBC Counts

The effects of C, K and J acupuncture treatment on the total number of WBC counts were summarized in **Figure 1** and **Figure 2**. Relative changes in percentage compared with the baseline (before treatment) were indicated as

**Table 1.** Point selection by K and C practitioners.

| | points | range | mean |
|---|---|---|---|
| China | 83 | 6-9 | 9.22 |
| Korea | 75 | 4-17 | 8.33 |

**Table 2.** Rank of the acupuncture points frequently used in K and C treatments.

| Points | 1 | 2 | 3 | 4 | 5 | 6 | 7 |
|---|---|---|---|---|---|---|---|
| China | BL23 | ST36 | SP6 | CV4 | KI3 | GV4 | CV12 |
| Korea | SP3 | CV12 | ST36 | LI4 | SI2 | HT7 | SI3 |

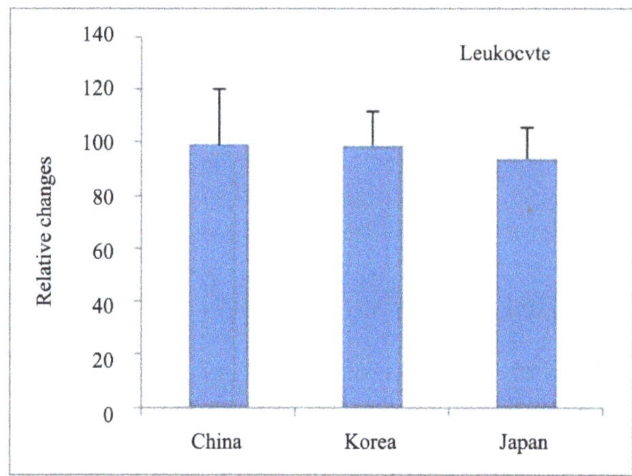


**Figure 1.** Changes of WBC numbers (% of baseline) after one acupuncture session.

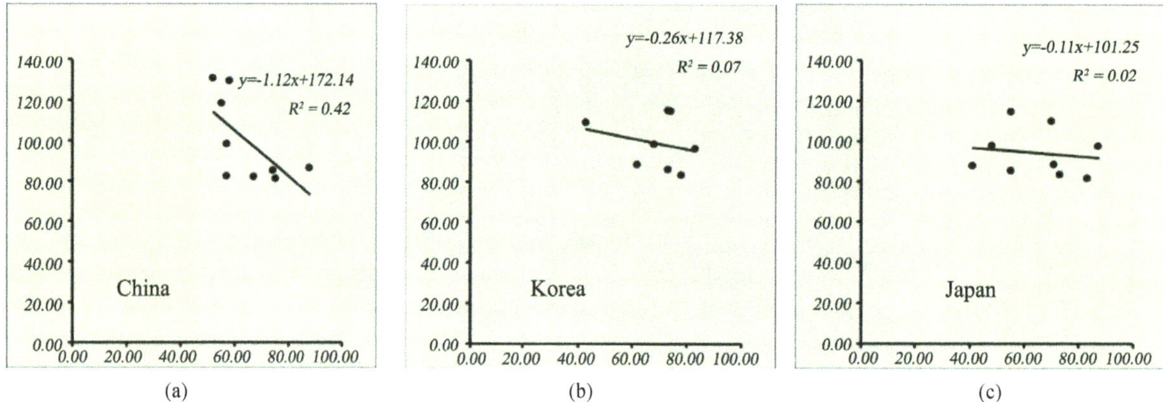


**Figure 2.** (a)-(c) Relations between the baseline data and percent change after acupuncture treatments. Vertical scale: relative changes in leukocyte number 24 hrs after treatment. Horizontal scale: baseline data of leukocyte number (×100/mm$^3$).

**Table 3.** Baseline data of leukocytes (number *100), lymphocytes (%), Lymphocytes(%) and serum adrenalin (pg/ml).

| | mean | SD | *n* |
|---|---|---|---|
| **Leukocytes** | | | |
| China | 64.78 | 12.04 | 9 |
| Korea | 69.25 | 12.30 | 8 |
| Japan | 64.78 | 15.80 | 9 |
| **Lymphocytes** | | | |
| China | 39.91 | 9.49 | 9 |
| Korea | 31.21 | 7.23 | 8 |
| Japan | 37.12 | 10.03 | 9 |
| **Granulocytes** | | | |
| China | 55.54 | 9.61 | 9 |
| Korea | 64.76 | 8.29 | 8 |
| Japan | 58.98 | 11.26 | 9 |
| **Adrenalin** | | | |
| China | 51.67 | 21.05 | 9 |
| Korea | 57.00 | 16.21 | 8 |
| Japan | 61.78 | 29.04 | 9 |

columns and vertical bars (mean and SD) in **Figure 1**.

Total WBC counts did not change after the treatment and slight decrease in J treatment is observed. The largest SD in C treatment indicates the strong influence of C treatment on WBC counts. No significant differences were observed (ANOVA, $p = 0.749$). **Figures 2(a)-(c)** summarizes the relations between the baseline data and degrees of changes in percentages after three treatments. All subject's data were plotted and regression lines in three treatments was shown in each figures. In C treatment, negative slope of regression line indicates the higher baseline WBC subjects tended to be reduced by the treatment. In K and J treatments, no such tendencies could be observed, although the individual variations tend to be large (small coefficients of determination).

## 5. Lymphocyte Ratio

The effects of C, K and J treatments on the lymphocytes were summarized in **Figure 3** and **Figure 4** Influences of acupuncture treatments on lymphocytes differ among the countries. In C treatment tended to decrease the relative value to 91.1%, whereas K and J treatments increase to 109.5 and 108.6%, although no statistical significance observed (one way ANOVA, $P = 0.0784$).The variation of SD among the countries is similar.

**Figure 4** summarizes the relation between the baseline data and degree of changes in percentages of lymphocytes ratios after the treatment. In C and J treatments, negative regression lines, whereas K treatment produce slight positive regression.

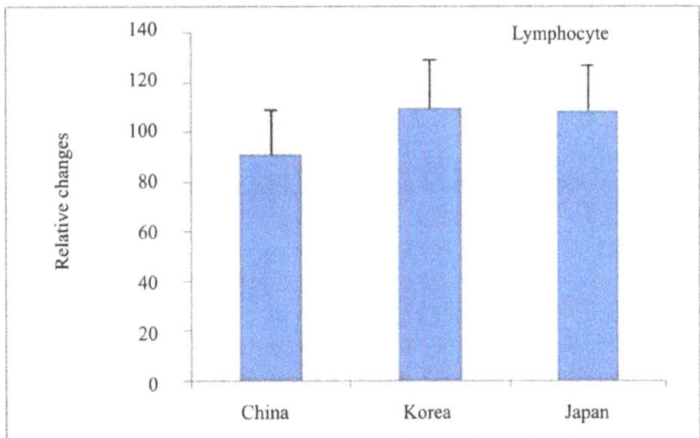


**Figure 3.** Changes of Lymphocyte ratios (% of baseline) after acupuncture session.

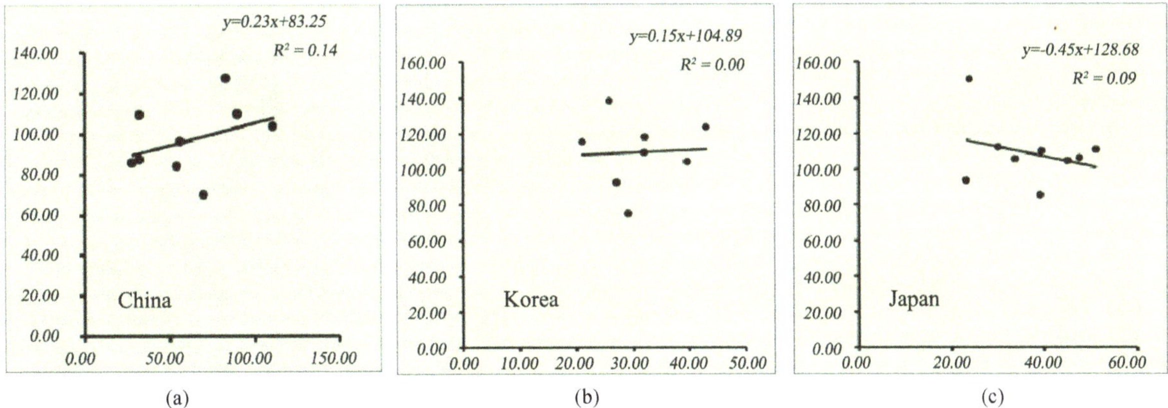


**Figure 4.** (a)-(c) Relations between the baseline data and percent change after acupuncture treatments. Vertical scale: relative changes in lymphocytes number 24 hrs after treatment. Horizontal scale: baseline data of ratios of lymphocytes (%).

### Granulocyte Ratio

The effects of C, K and J treatment on the ratio of lymphocytes were summarized in **Figure 5** and **Figure 6**. Effects of acupuncture treatments on granulocytes ratios are shown in **Figure 5**.

On granulocytes ratios are basically opposite pattern of those of lymphocyte. Only C treatment increased to 108.8% and K and J treatments reduced to 95.1 and 95.5, respectively. There are significant difference among the countries (ANOVA, $p = 0.026$).

The negative slope of regression lines was observed in C treatments and positive slopes were obtained in K and J treatments.

## 6. Changes in Adrenaline Contents

Relative changes in adrenalin contents are shown in **Figure 7** and **Figure 8**. Regarding adrenalin contents, three treatments have different influences. In C treatment, increase of the contents with large variation in C treatment whereas slight reduction with small variation in J treatment. K treatment has no changes as the mean value although its variation is large,

Relative changes of adrenalin contents after acupuncture treatments are shown as a regression lines in **Figure 8**. The negative slopes of regression lines in C and K treatments are observed whereas a positive line in J treatment is detected. These patterns of regression lines are different from those observed WBC and their subclasses (granulocytes and lymphocytes).

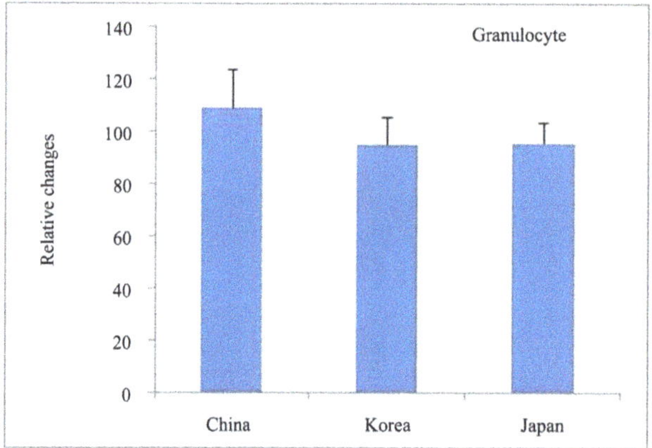


**Figure 5.** Changes of Granulocyte ratios (% of baseline) after one acupuncture session.

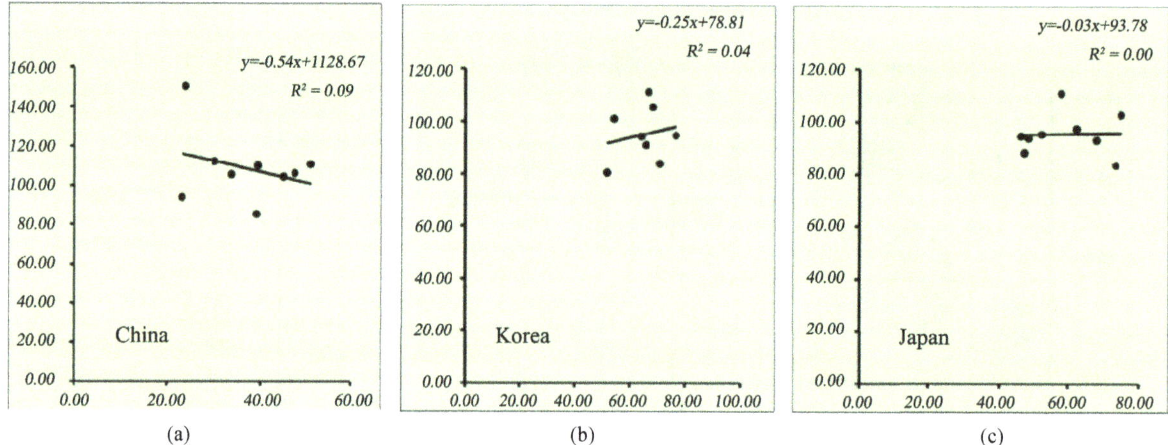


**Figure 6.** (a)-(c) Relations between the baseline data and percent change after acupuncture treatments. Vertical scale: relative changes in leukocyte number 24 hrs after treatment. Horizontal scale: baseline data of ratios of granulocytes (%).

## 7. Discussion

In the present pilot study, we compared the effects of three different individualized diagnoses and treatments of

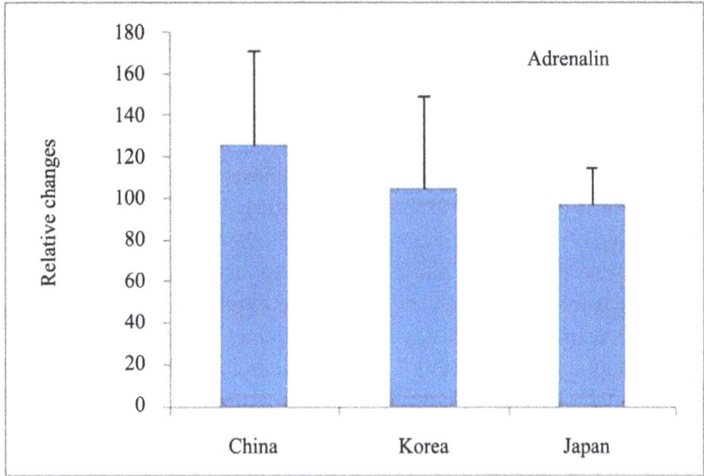


**Figure 7.** Changes of Adrenalin contents (% of baseline) after one acupuncture session.

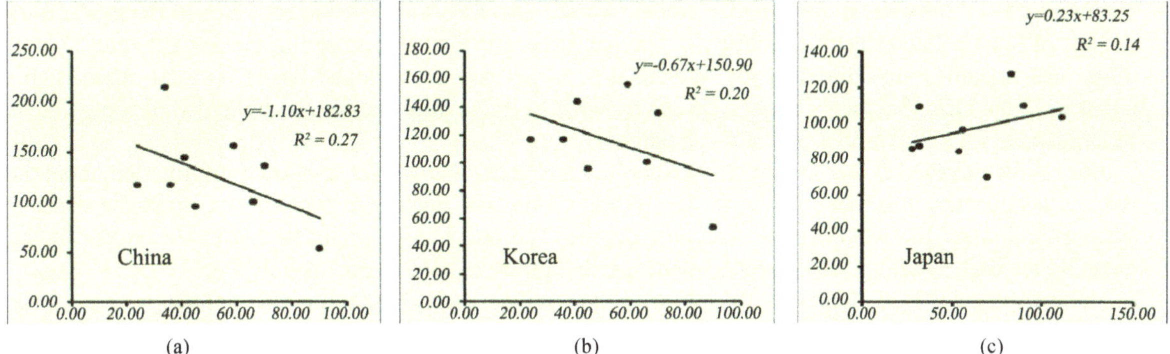


**Figure 8.** (a)-(c) Relations between the baseline data and percent change after acupuncture treatments. Vertical scale: relative changes in leukocyte number 24 hrs after treatment. Horizontal scale: baseline data of serum adrenalin contents (pg/ml).

traditional ways of Chinese, Korean and Japanese acupuncture on the WBC composition and adrenalin in the same subject. The apparently clear differences of point selection and procedure of acupuncture manipulations among the countries were observed. A total of 44 acupuncture points was selected but only 5 points were common in K and C treatments. Three different acupuncture treatments also induced different tendencies in modification of the WBC counts and lymphocyte and granulocyte ratios and serum adrenalin although no statistically significant as obvious individual variations also observed.

The facts that multi-directional changes in the outcome measures could be produced by three different acupuncture treatments suggested the importance of procedures of acupuncture needling. In this study, Chinese acupuncture produced de-qi sensation, and Korean acupuncture frequently used the acupuncture points in the hand. On the contrary, Japanese acupuncture provoked almost no subjective sensation but the practitioner detected slight changes in respiratory movement during his needling technique. These three acupuncture treatments undoubtedly induced several modifications on the immune and autonomic nervous systems in different manner.

The immune system was strongly influenced by various factors. Psychological state such as depression and mental stress suppressed the immune activities [19] Acupuncture and moxibustion treatment could improve and modify the immune activity by measuring cytotoxicity of lymphocytes and NK cell count [20]-[22]. On the contrary, lack of effect of acupuncture on the immune modulatory effects was also reported [23].

Recently analysis of gene by using cDNA microarray analysis demonstrated participation of several genes which related to the up-regulation of NK cell activity by electro-acupuncture (EA) [24]. Down-regulation of proinflammatory cytokine such as IL-I beta mRNA by EA was also shown [25].

In mice, EA activated the spleen NK cells and IFN-gamma level also increased, and EA also increased beta endorphin level and its effects were antagonized by naloxone [26]-[29].

Anti-inflammatory effect of acupuncture was suggested to be mediated by vagal nerve stimulation and deactivation of macrophages [21], and the fact that existence of acetylcholine receptors on the lymphocytes [30] suggested the importance of tune of autonomic nervous system on the immune activity.

Our previous study clearly demonstrated that one of Japanese-style acupuncture treatment induces prolonged increases of cytokines and shift of ratios of granular cells and lymphocytes depending on the previous condition of the subjects. The increases of IFN-gamma and IL-I6 and other leukocytes with various CD marker including NK cells were observed. These promoting influences of acupuncture on the immune systems and reciprocal effects on lymphocytes and granulocytes might be a possible explanation of bio-regulatory function of acupuncture [18] [30] [31]. Then measurement of ratios of the lymphocytes and granulocytes proposed as a useful outcome measures in complementary and alternative (CAM) medicine [17].

In the present study no such changes in lymphocytes and granulocyte was observed in the subgroup analysis of G-type and L-type subjects, although the same acupuncture practitioner with the previous study participated in this project.

The large variation of baseline data in small sample size might be a possible cause of the discrepancy of results. Health conditions of the subjects, young university students, varied during the relatively long periods (4 months) accompanied with seasonal changes of circumstances, so the present data could not be assumed as the simple results of J treatment. The similar problems were also found in the characteristics of the modulating potentials of K and C acupuncture treatments. Another issue was the subject used in the present study. The traditional acupuncture procedures and its theoretical concepts might developed based on their subjects in each country, so the facts that the subjects in this study were Japanese young students might also be a possible cause of large variation of the results in K and C treatments.

The results obtained in the present study were not conclusive but we got important information about the variety of acupuncture treatments in Japan, Korea and China, and they have potentials to modulate the immune systems and stress level in different way with degree. The information might be useful for understanding the meaning the each system of traditional acupuncture therapy developed in each country.

The present study also offers a useful information regarding issues of specific effect of acupuncture. Recently a society of researchers of acupuncture (Society of Acupuncture Research: SAR) reported a white paper on future acupuncture research in the next decade [32]. One of the important issues of the SAR white paper is to explain the results obtained by well-designed acupuncture clinical trials conducted in USA [33]. The purpose of the RCT was to clarify the specific effect of acupuncture and significance of individualized TCM point selection. The obtained results indicated no statistically significant differences among the individualized TCM treatment, standardized TCM treatment and simulated acupuncture treatment (the skin was stimulated by tooth pick), although they were significantly more effective than Western standard therapy [33].

One simple explanation is to assume these acupuncture treatments are strong placebo effects, and no specific effect exists. The comparison of TCM acupuncture and simulated acupuncture with tooth pick seems to be reasonable protocol to clarify the specific effect of acupuncture, however the present study clearly demonstrated that TCM acupuncture is one of acupuncture procedures and other procedures developed in Japan and Korea also have modulatory effects on bio-regulatory systems. So simulated acupuncture, it might be included as real acupuncture technique in Japan, could not assume an inert sham intervention. So it is keenly required to develop inert sham acupuncture device or technique to clarify the existence of specific effects of acupuncture.

It should be noted that this project had several limitations. The major issue is the choice of subjects. The initial protocol was planned to select the subjects from three countries, but the time schedule of practitioners could not allow the selection from three countries, and small number of Japanese young male students who have no experience of acupuncture could be prepared. The selection of subjects in three countries might be one important issue in the future project. The selection of traditional acupuncture practitioners was also important issue. In Japan a practitioner who participated in the previous study [17] was adopted as key member of this project. In Korea, members of the Korean Acupuncture and Moxibustion Society (KAMS) discussed and recommended the practitioner in this study. In Chinese acupuncture, one Chinese acupuncturist who has acupuncture clinic in Japan was adopted. The individual variation of diagnosis of TCM doctors was pointed out [3], so it is important to prepare several practitioners in each country for obtaining sufficient and representative results of each country.

The feature of the present study was to examine three different traditional acupuncture treatments by applying to the same subjects. So crossover design was used. However the remarkable variation of baseline data and lack of control subjects, who received no acupuncture treatments, made it difficult to analyze and discuss the data sufficiently.

This clinical study of JCK traditional acupuncture was the first attempt in the world and it offered important information to establish the role of acupuncture therapy in CAM as an individualized therapy, and also offer interesting information for the future researches.

## References

[1] Anastasi, J.K., Currie, L.M. and Kim, G.H. (2009) Understanding Diagnostic Reasoning in TCM Practice: Tongue Diagnosis. *Alternative Therapies in Health and Medicine*, **15**, 18-28.

[2] Coyle, M. and Smith, C. (2005) A Survey Comparing TCM Diagnosis, Health Status and Medical Diagnosis in Women Undergoing Assisted Reproduction. *Acupuncture Medicine*, **23**, 62-69. http://dx.doi.org/10.1136/aim.23.2.62

[3] Hogeboom, C.J., Sherman, K.J. and Cherkin, D.C. (2001) Variation in Diagnosis and Treatment of Chronic Low Back Pain by Traditional Chinese Medicine Acupuncturists. *Complementary Therapies in Medicine*, **9**, 154-166. http://dx.doi.org/10.1054/ctim.2001.0457

[4] Zhang, G.G., Lee, W., Bausell, B., Lao, L., Handwerger, B. and Berman, B. (2005) Variability in the Traditional Chinese medicine (TCM) diagnoses and herbal prescriptions provided by three TCM practitioners for 40 patients with rheumatoid Arthritis. *Journal of Alternative and Complementary Medicine*, **11**, 415-421. http://dx.doi.org/10.1089/acm.2005.11.415

[5] Lee, S.W., Jang, E.S., Lee, J. and Kim, J.Y. (2006) Current Researches on the Methods of Diagnosing Sasang Constitution: An Overview. *Evidence-Based Complementary and Alternative Medicine*, **6**, 43-49. http://dx.doi.org/10.1093/ecam/nep092

[6] Kim, Y.S., Jun, H., Chae, Y., Park, H.J., Kim, B.H., Chang, I.M., *et al.* (2005) The Practice of Korean Medichine: An Overview of Clinical Trials in Acupuncture. *Evidence-Based Complementary and Alternative Medicine*, **2**, 325-352. http://dx.doi.org/10.1093/ecam/neh102

[7] Kim, J.Y. and Pham, D.D. (2009) Sasang Constitutional Medicine as a Holistic Tailored Medicine. *Evidence-Based Complementary and Alternative Medicine*, **6**, 11-19. http://dx.doi.org/10.1093/ecam/nep100

[8] Yoo, J.H., Kim, J.W., Kim, K.K., Kim, J.Y., Koh, B.H. and Lee, E.J. (2007) Sasangin Diagnosis Questionnaire: Test of Reliability. *Journal of Alternative and Complementary Medicine*, **13**, 111-122. http://dx.doi.org/10.1089/acm.2006.5293

[9] Kobayashi, A., Uefuji, M. and Yasumo, W. (2010) History and Progress of Japanese Acupuncture. *Evidence-Based Complementary and Alternative Medicine*, **7**, 359-365. http://dx.doi.org/10.1093/ecam/nem155

[10] Kawakita, K., Shichidou, T., Inoue, E., Nabeta, T., Kitakoji, H., Aizawa, S., *et al.* (2008) Do Japanese Style Acupuncture and Moxibustion Reduce Symptoms of the Common Cold? *Evidence-Based Complementary and Alternative Medicine*, **5**, 481-489. http://dx.doi.org/10.1093/ecam/nem055

[11] Birch, S. and Jamison, R.N. (1998) Controlled Trial of Japanese Acupuncture for Chronic Myofascial Neck Pain: Assessment of Specific and Nonspecific Effects of Treatment. *The Clinical Journal of Pain*, **14**, 248-255. http://dx.doi.org/10.1097/00002508-199809000-00012

[12] Kawakita, K., Shichidou, T., Inoue, E., Nabeta, T., Kitakouji, H., Aizawa, S., *et al.* (2004) Preventive and Curative Effects of Acupuncture on the Common Cold. A Multicentre Randomized Controlled Trial in Japan. *Complementary Therapies in Medicine*, **12**, 181-188. http://dx.doi.org/10.1016/j.ctim.2004.10.004

[13] Witt, C., Brinkhaus, B., Jena, S., Linde, K., Streng, A., Wagenpfeil, S., *et al.* (2005) Acupuncture in Patients with Osteoarthritis of the Knee: A Randomised Trial. *Lancet*, **366**, 136-143. http://dx.doi.org/10.1016/S0140-6736(05)66871-7

[14] Cummings, M. (2009) Modellvorhaben Akupunktur—A Summary of the ART, ARC and GERAC Trials. *Acupuncture in Medicine*, **27**, 26-30. http://dx.doi.org/10.1136/aim.2008.000281

[15] Witt, C.M. and Brinkhaus, B. (2010) Efficacy, Effectiveness and Cost-Effectiveness of Acupuncture for Allergic Rhinitis—An Overview about Previous and Ongoing Studies. *Autonomic Neuroscience*, **157**, 42-45. http://dx.doi.org/10.1016/j.autneu.2010.06.006

[16] WHO (2008) WHO Standard Acupuncture Point Locations in the Western Pacific Region. WPRO Nonserial Publication, Acpuncture Point Location.

[17] Yamaguchi, N., Takahashi, T., Sakuma, M., Sugita, T., Uchikawa, K., Sakaihara, S., *et al.* (2007) Acupuncture Regulates Leukocyte Subpopulations in Human Peripheral Blood. *Evidence-Based Complementary and Alternative Medicine*, **4**, 447-453. http://dx.doi.org/10.1093/ecam/nel107

[18] Abo, T., Kawate, T., Itoh, K. and Kumagai, K. (1988) Studies on the Bioperiodicity of the Immune Response. I. Circadian Rhythms of Human T, B and K Cell Traffic in the Peripheral Blood. *The Journal of Immunology*, **126**, 1360-1363.

[19] Evans, D.L., Pedersen, C.A. and Folds, J.D. (1988) Major Depression and Immunity-Preliminary Evidence of Decreased Natural Killer Cell Populations. *Progress in Neuro-Psychopharmacology and Biological Psychiatry*, **12**, 739-748. http://dx.doi.org/10.1016/0278-5846(88)90019-X

[20] Arranz, L., Guayerbas, N., Siboni, L. and De la Fuente, M. (2007) Effect of Acupuncture Treatment on the Immune Function Impairment Found in Anxious Women. *The American Journal of Chinese Medicine*, **35**, 35-51. http://dx.doi.org/10.1142/S0192415X07004606

[21] Kavoussi, B. and Ross, B.E. (2007) The Neuroimmune Basis of Anti-Inflammatory Acupuncture. *Integrative Cancer Therapies*, **6**, 251-257. http://dx.doi.org/10.1177/1534735407305892

[22] Yamashita, H., Ichiman, Y. and Tanno, Y. (2001) Changes in Peripheral Lymphocyte Subpopulations after Direct Moxibustion. *The American Journal of Chinese Medicine*, **29**, 227-235. http://dx.doi.org/10.1142/S0192415X01000265

[23] Kho, H.G., Van Egmond, J., Eijk, R.J. and Kapteyns, W.M. (1991) Lack of Influence of Acupuncture and Transcutaneous Stimulation on the Immunoglobulin Levels and Leukocyte Counts Following Upper-Abdominal Surgery. *European Journal of Anaesthesiology*, **8**, 39-45.

[24] Kim, C.K., Choi, G.S., Oh, S.D., Han, J.B., Kim, S.K., Ahn, H.J., *et al.* (2005) Identification of Genes Altering Their Expressions in Electroacupuncture Induced Up-Regulation of Natural Killer Cell Activity. *Journal of Neuroimmunology*, **168**, 144-153.

[25] Wang, J., Zhao, H., Mao-Ying, Q.L., Cao, X.D., Wang, Y.Q. and Wu, G.C. (2009) Electroacupuncture Downregulates TLR2/4 and Pro-Inflammatory Cytokine Expression after Surgical Trauma Stress without Adrenal Glands Involvement. *Brain Research Bulletin*, **80**, 89-94. http://dx.doi.org/10.1016/j.brainresbull.2009.04.020

[26] Yu, Y., Kasahara, T., Sato, T., Guo, S.Y., Liu, Y., Asano, K., *et al.* (1997) Enhancement of Splenic Interferon-Gamma, Interleukin-2, and NK Cytotoxicity by S36 Acupoint Acupuncture in F344 Rats. *The Japanese Journal of Physiology*, **47**, 173-178. http://dx.doi.org/10.2170/jjphysiol.47.173

[27] Yu, Y., Kasahara, T., Sato, T., Asano, K., Yu, G., Fang, J., *et al.* (1998) Role of Endogenous Interferon-Gamma on the Enhancement of Splenic NK Cell Activity by Electroacupuncture Stimulation in Mice. *Journal of Neuroimmunology*, **90**, 176-186. http://dx.doi.org/10.1016/S0165-5728(98)00143-X

[28] Sato, T., Yu, Y., Guo, S.Y., Kasahara, T. and Hisamitsu, T. (1996) Acupuncture Stimulation Enhances Splenic Natural Killer Cell Cytotoxicity in Rats. *The Japanese Journal of Physiology*, **46**, 131-136. http://dx.doi.org/10.2170/jjphysiol.46.131

[29] Ma, Z., Wang, Y. and Fan, Q. (1992) The Influence of Acupuncture on Interleukin 2 Interferon-Natural Killer Cell Regulatory Network of Kidney-Deficiency Mice. *In Contact with Professor Kawakita K.*, **17**, 139-142.

[30] Toyabe, S., Iiai, T., Fukuda, M., Kawamura, T., Suzuki, S., Uchiyama, M., *et al.* (1997) Identification of Nicotinic Acetylcholine Receptors on Lymphocytes in the Periphery as Well as Thymus in Mice. *Immunology*, **92**, 201-205. http://dx.doi.org/10.1046/j.1365-2567.1997.00323.x

[31] Abo, T. (2003) Immune Revolution. Kohdansha International Publisher, Tokyo. (in Japanese)

[32] Langevin, H.M., Wayne, P.M., Macpherson, H., Schnyer, R., Milley, R.M., Napadow, V., *et al.* (2011) Paradoxes in Acupuncture Research: Strategies for Moving Forward. *Evidence-Based Complementary and Alternative Medicine*, **2011**, Article ID: 180805. http://dx.doi.org/10.1155/2011/180805

[33] Cherkin, D.C., Sherman, K.J., Avins, A.L., Erro, J.H., Ichikawa, L., Barlow, W.E., *et al.* (2009) A Randomized Trial Comparing Acupuncture, Simulated Acupuncture, and Usual Care for Chronic Low Back Pain. *Archives of Internal Medicine*, **169**, 858-866. http://dx.doi.org/10.1001/archinternmed.2009.65

# 5

# Single Cellular Algae Digestive Supplement Designed by Yeast & Lactobacillus Rearranged Leukocyte Subsets through Activation of Complement Components

**Hitoshi Kubota[1,2*], Nurmuhamamt Amat[3], Dilxat Yimit[3], Parida Hoxur[4], Nobuo Yamaguchi[1,2]**

[1]Ishikawa Natural Medicinal Products Research Center, Ishikawa, Japan
[2]Department of Fundament Research for CAM, Kanazawa Medical University, Ishikawa, Japan
[3]Traditional Uighur Medicine Department, Xinjiang Medical University, Urumqi, China
[4]Traditional Chinese Medicine Hospital, Xinjiang Medical University, Urumqi, China
Email: [*]serumaya@kanazawa-med.ac.jp

## Abstract

**A plant fermentation was carried out by Yeast and Lactobacilli against single cellular algae (*f-Chlorella*). These materials were proved by as safe in animal safety experiment. We sought to look into changes of immune-competent cells that commonly utilized *f-Chlorella* including after administration of immno-suppressed animals. The effects by *f-Chlorella* on the reguratіonal effect to the host were measured. Our results showed that *f-Chlorella* regulated the level of lymphocytes, while *conventional-Chlorella* worked to adjust the level of granulocytes. In our clinical study with 20 healthy volunteers, granulocyte and lymphocyte ratio was obtained as neutral in the peripheral blood. In rodents, immune-compromised host as well as normal animal were prepared with cancer chemotherapeutic agent (Mytomycin-C), and then tried to rescue the immune-competent rebel. Our observations showed that both *Chlorella* derivatives regulated in number and functions. The effect was more prominent in *f-Chlorella* than that of conventional one. We discussed the significance and mechanism of *f-Chlorella* on the level of leukocyte subsets in number and function. These effects were considered to bring the potential elevation of antibody secreting cell by the localized heamolysis in gel method. We also proposed an idea that exhibited tonic effects were brought via activating the complement components in the serum. Moreover, we tried to access further to the anti-oxidative activities of this *f-Chlorella*. This modification brought to the significant lifted up for immune competent cells and anti-oxidative activity for phagocytic cells.**

[*]Corresponding author.

## Keywords

**Family Poaceae, *Chlorella pyrenoidosa*, Fermentation, Yeast, Lactobacillus, Cancer Chemotherapeutic Agent, Compromised Host, Lipidosis, Cardiovascular Disease, Diabetes Meritus, Immune Augmentation**

## 1. Introduction

In recent years, complementary and alternative medicines (CAM) have achieved more and more attentions since they are able to treat many chronic illnesses, such as fatigue syndrome that plagues the industrialized world. The present team has reported that typical styles of CAM, preparing special molecule for both digestive and easy to activated human complement component.

Beside the complement activation, we have been reported as immune-regulatory menu by hot spring hydrotherapy and acupuncture [1] [2]. About the dietary system, here we report Chlorella derivatives Dietary and fermented formula as strong inducers of acquired immunity. While the immune system is working against the local infection of pathogens, cytokine and immuno-competent cells react throughout the body in close connection to the brain, the endocrine and immune system [3]. In this study, we hypothesize that *f-Chlorella* may influence immuno-competent cells qualitatively and quantitatively *f-Chlorella* targeting lymphocytes based on the constitution dependent manner. *f-Chlorella* has been employed as tonic agent and the implication has little been made on the characteristics of the levels of leukocyte subset, such as granulocytes and lymphocytes. In this report, we seek to focus on the identity of *f-Chlorella* formula, comparing to another herbal medicine. The influence of *f-Chlorella* on leukocyte and/or lymphocyte subpopulations in human peripheral blood is also discussed. Moreover, some preliminary trial that concerns the new processing of *Chlorella* cells by degradation of acidophilic bacteria and yeast fungus [4]-[10] (**Figure 1**).

## 2. Experimental Animal

### 2.1. Toxicity Test by Single and Multiple Administration

Ten female seven-week-old ddY mice, were used for the acute oral toxicity study. The tests were carried out

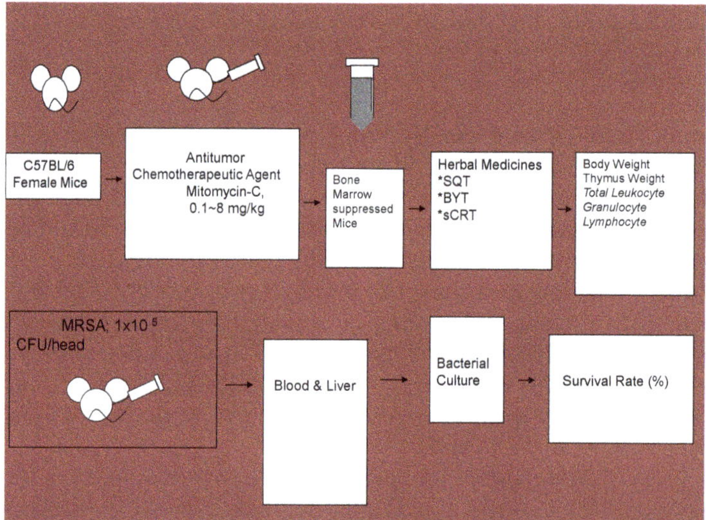


**Figure 1.** Experimental procedure for this animal experiments. We sampled peripheral blood from the 12 volunteers before and after hot hydro therapy, at the same time on each day, in accordance with the consideration of circadian rhythm of leukocyte. The spring quality is a weak sodium chloride with sodium carbohydrate of the water temperature 41˚C ± 1˚C. During the night and in the morning of the next day, they had a bath in the hot spring two or three times, for 20 - 30 minutes each time. Time interval of blood sampling between before and after hot-spring hydrotherapy was approximately 24 hours. The total and differential leukocyte counts were measured Control waterhe automated hematology analyzer.

according to Ethics of the Organization for Economic Co-operation and Development (OECD) Test Guideline 401. The mice were housed at 24˚C ± 1˚C, 50% relative humidity. Both conventional and charged water were suspended in sterile and administered to mice in free supplemental system, calculating daily consumption. Mice were weighted at 0 - 7 days after administration, and clinical observations were made once a day. Necropsy was performed on all mice seven days after administration.

## 2.2. Experimental Design for Bone Marrow Suppressed Immune-Compromised Mice

In the animal model of immuno-competency reduction, male C57BL/6J mice, aged 8 - 9 weeks, were injected with Mitomycin-C (MMC) (5 mg/kg) to inhibit the bone marrow. Then, *f-Chlorella* extracts was administered orally at a dosage of 1 g/kg/day for five consecutive days *f-Chlorella* and conventional *Chlorella* was chosen as controls [11].

### 2.2.1. Recovery of Total Leukocytes and Subsets of Leukocytes

The bone marrow-suppressed mice were administered herbal decoction *f-Chlorella* 1 g/kg dairy for 5 days and after 1 week later, their blood were withdrawn from their tail vain. Then, the number of leukocytes was counted in Bürker-Türk solution.

### 2.2.2. A Recovery of Leukocyte Subsets by *f-Chlorella*

Bone marrow-suppressed mice were administered with herbal decoction of *f-Chlorella* (1 g/kg/day) for five days. One week later, the blood from their tail vain was withdrawn. Then the granulocyte and lymphocyte subsets were counted in Bürker-Türk solution.

### 2.2.3. A Recovery of Macrophage Activity, Migration

Cells from peritoneal exudates were collect from the peritoneal cavity of bone marrow-suppressed mice. Phagocytes were purified using adherent technique to get cell suspensions which contained more than 95% of phagocytes. The purified cells were loaded to the upper room of Boyden chamber to test migration ability at a concentration of $1 \times 10^4$ cell/ml. Human serum treated at 56˚C for 30 min was for the chemo tactic agent of mouse phagocyte [12].

### 2.2.4. Recovery of Macrophage Activity, Phagocytosis

The same cells suspension was purified by adherent technique for phagocyte, which produces cells contained more than 95% of phagocytes. The purified cells were adjusted to $1 \times 10^4$ cell/cm$^2$ and mixed with latex beads that are 5 μm in *f-Chlorella*, fluorescence isochianate. After 90 min of incubation, remained granule were washed out from the glass slide. Number of phagocytic cell and their ability to catch up the latex beads were automatically measured by ACAS system, which outputs the result in a digital form (Adherent cell activity evaluating system; Shimazu, Kyoto, Japan).

### 2.2.5. Recovery of Macrophage Activity, Target Cell Killing

The same phagocyte suspension, which contained over 95% of phagocytes, was produced by adherent technique for phagocyte. The purified cells were adjusted to $1 \times 10^5$ cell/ml to examine the macrophage activity of killing, the nitro blue tetrazolium (NBT) reduction test [13] [14].

### 2.2.6. A Recovery of Lymphocyte Activity, Antibody Secreting Cell

The bone marrow suppressed mice were administered herbal decoction of *f-Chlorella* (1 g/kg/day) for 5 days. One week later, mice were immunized with sheep red blood cells, ($2 \times 10^8$/mouse) intraperitoneally. Five days later, their spleen cells were collected. Plague-forming cells (PFC) were developed, and the ability of IgM and IgG antibody production was tested *f-Chlorella* he method reported by Jerne and Nordin [15].

### 2.2.7. CD Positive Lymphocyte Distribution by *f-Chlorella* against Different Constitution

Whole blood obtained from the subjects was washed twice with PBS. One hundred micro-liters of the suspensions were stained with 20 μl of fluorescent monoclonal antibodies (anti-human $CD2^+$, $CD4^+$, $CD8^+$, $CD11b^+$, $CD14^+$, $CD16^+$, $CD19^+$ and $CD56^+$ antibodies). Ten thousands stained cells were re-suspended in PBS to detect surface markers by flow cytometry (FACS Calibur; Becton Dickinson Immnocytometry Systems, CA, USA).

#### 2.2.8. Distribution of Cytokine Producing Lymphocytes in Different Constitution

The blood cell suspensions were cultured with PMA (phorbol 12-myristate 13-acetate), ionomycin and BSA (bovine serum albumin) for 4 - 5 hours at 37˚C. After that, the cell suspensions were stained using the monoclonal antibodies of PE-IL-4, FITC-IFN-$\gamma$ and FITC-IL-1$\beta$. Then they were analyzed *f-Chlorella* FACScan (Becton Dickinson Co. Ltd. USA). The antibodies and reagents used in the test were purchased from Becton Dickinson Immunocytometry System (USA).

The peritoneal exudates cells were collect from the peritoneal cavity of bone marrow-suppressed mice. Cell suspensions were purified by adherent technique for phagocyte, getting a suspension which contained over 95% of phagocytes. The purified cells were adjusted to $1 \times 10^4$ cell/ml and loaded at the upper chamber of Boyden chamber for test migration. Human serum with treated at 56˚C for 30 min was for the chemotactic agent for mouse phagocyte.

Phagocytic activity and antibody production of macrophages were analyzed using a classical test that could test the total activity of the immune system by examine chemotaxis, phagocytosis and intracellular degradation of macrophage. For identifying antibody-forming cells, plaque-forming cells were detected using heterogeneous erythrocyte; sheep erythrocyte was a target antigen. Peritoneal macrophages were collected and purified in fetal calf serum (FCS)-coated petri-dishes. The cell population was approximately 97% uniform in function and morphology. These cells were applied to the nuclepore-membrane (pore size: 5 μm; Neuro Probe Co. Ltd., Cabin John MD, USA) with a chemotaxis chamber (Neuro Probe Co. Ltd.). After 90 minutes' incubation, the membrane was vigorously washed with saline (37˚C), fixed, and then stained with methylene blue dye. After counting under a microscope for the total field of the membrane, the average number of migrating cells was expressed as cell counts/mm$^2$.

The same cells suspension was purified by adherent technique for phagocyte, which contained over 95% of phagocytes. The purified cells were adjusted to $1 \times 10^4$ cell/cm$^2$ and mixed with latex beads that were 5 um in granule with *f-Chlorella* fluorescence isochianate. After 90 min of incubation, the remained granule were washed out from the glass slide and counting automatically by ACAS system, which outputs digital presentation, for evaluating phagocytes in number and in their ability to catch up the latex beads (Adherent cell activity evaluating system, Shimazu, Kyoto, Japan). Latex beads in 5 μm with fluorescence were used to test phagocytic activity and *Candida albicans* was cell killing activity. A macrophage-target cell ratio of 1:10 was considered to be optimum. Ten minutes after incubating phagocytes and target cells, intracellular *Candida* cells were cultured on an agar dish with conventional medium 1640 until the next day to perform the colony forming assay. In this way, the phagocytic ability of the macrophages was monitored. To document intracellular killing activity, the same procedures were performed excepting that the incubation time was changed to 90 minutes.

### 2.3. Antibody Forming Cell Study

Sheep erythrocyte (SRBC), a T-dependent antigen, was used for antibody formation cell study. Ten days after tumor transplantation, each antigen was intra-peritoneally injected. After four and six days, the antibody-forming cells were detected using localized hemolysis in an agar gel. Plaque-forming cells were developed *f-Chlorella* the method of Jerne and Nordin [15].

### 2.4. Anti-Oxidative Effect Evaluation

#### 2.4.1. Animal

Eight week-old female C57BL/6 were purchased from Sankyo Laboratory Service Corporation (Shizuoka, Japan). All mice were kept under specific pathogen-free conditions. Mice food and distilled water were freely accessible for each mouse. Housing temperature and humidity were controlled 25˚C ± 1˚C and 60%.

#### 2.4.2. Reagents

As for the basic medium, HEPES buffer (HEPES 17 mM, NaCl 120 mM, Glucose 5 mM, KCl 5 mM, $CaCl_2$ 1 mM, $MgCl_2$ 1 mM) was prepared and sterilized by filtration. Phorbol 12-myristate 13-acetate (PMA, Sigma, USA) was diluted to $10^{-6}$ M by dimethyl sulfoxide DMSO, Sigma, USA) and used as a stimulant for super oxide anion generation for murine peritoneal exudates cells. Cytochrome-c (Sigma, USA) was diluted to 1 mM by HEPES buffer. Since cytochrome-c reduced by super oxide showed maximum absorbance at 550 nm, we used cytochrome-c to measure the amount of super oxide anion generation through spectro-photometrical technique. Oyster glycogen (type, Sigma, USA) was diluted in the purified water (10% w/v, Wako, Japan) and autoclaved at 120˚C for 20 min. This solution was used for intraperitoneal injection to mice in order to induce peripheral neutrophils into the abdominal cavity.

#### 2.4.3. The Measuring the Amount of Super Oxide Anion Generated by Murine Peritoneal Exudates Cells

*Fermented Chlorella* and *Conventional Chlorella* were orally administered to mice (500 mg/kg) for one week. Two milliliters of 10% Oyster glycogen was injected intraperitoneally 10 hours before the assay. Sufficient murine peritoneal exudative cells were induced ten hours after the stimulation. Mice were euthanized by cervical dislocation, murine peritoneal exudates cells (PEC) suspension was centrifuged twice for 5 minutes at 1500 rpm at 4˚C. Then PEC was prepared to $1 \times 10^6$ cells / ml of HEPES buffer. One hundred micro liters of cytochrome-c and 10 μl of PMA were added to the cell suspension and this was incubated for 20 minutes at 37˚C. The reaction mixture was then centrifuged for 10 minutes at 1500 rpm, 4˚C. An OD of supernatant was measured at both 550 nm and 540 nm, the amount of generated super oxide anion was shown in the formula; increased absorbance at 550 nm ($\triangle A_{550\text{-}540}$)/$19.1 \times 10^3$ (mmol/ml). In order to ensure if we really measured the amount of generated super oxide anion or not, we tried to add super oxide anion dismutase (SOD), an enzyme for its anti-oxidative effect, into our experimental system. The result was as expected that the reduction of cytochrome-c was inhibited after the addition of SOD. This showed us that our experimental system could be used properly for measuring the amount of generated super oxide anion [4].

## 3. Clinical Findings

### 3.1. Volunteers and Evaluation Methods

Twenty healthy volunteers aged from 21 to 70 years for both sex were recruited and were administered *f-Chlorella* for 30 days. Fifteen milliliters of blood were drawn from the forearm vein one hour before the first administration of *f-Chlorella* and 30 days after the last *f-Chlorella* administration (day 30). All volunteers provided informed consent prior to participation for this trial. This study was approved by Ethics Committee of Kanazawa Medical University (**Table 1**).

### 3.2. *Chlorella* Derivatives and Assessment for Host Immune Factor

Dried formula of *conventional Chlorella.* and *f-Chlorella* in granules were chosen as representatives of *f-Chlorella* [12] and were chosen as controls. A dose of 5.25 g dried powder of each formula (SUN *Chlorella* Co. Ltd., KYOTO, Japan) was administered two times per day for 30 days. Physiological functions were checked and possible side effects of the drug were inquired for all the subjects to ensure the safety of the trial.

### 3.3. Leukocyte Counts

The assessments including a total number of leukocytes was ordered to count with blood chemical test for the medical diagnosis of public institution (Ishikawa Preventive Medicine Association, Ishikawa, Japan). In the differential counting, 200 cells were counted on a May-Grünewald-Gimsa stained slide, and percentages of lymphocytes and granulocytes were determined.

### 3.4. Leukocyte Subset Analyses

The assessments including a total number of leukocytes was ordered to count with blood chemical test for the medical diagnosis of public institution (Ishikawa Preventive Medicine Association, Ishikawa, Japan). In the differential counting, 200 cells were counted on a May-Grunewald-Gimsa stained slide, and percentages of lymphocytes and granulocytes were determined [14].

The whole blood obtained from the subjects was washed twice in phosphate buffered saline (PBS). One hundred micro-liters of the suspensions were stained with 20 μl of fluorescent monoclonal antibodies (anti-human

**Table 1.** Constitution dependent regulation of lymphocyte by *Chlorella* Derivatives.

| CD | G-type individual | | L-type individual | |
|---|---|---|---|---|
| | *Conv. Chlorella* | | *f-Chlorella* | |
| | Before (%) | After (%) | Before (%) | After (%) |
| CD2 | 63.95 | 76.91 | 60.25 | 77.79 |
| CD4 | 19.75 | 28.53 | 31.05 | 45.14 |
| CD8 | 38.44 | 40.37 | 26.52 | 28.03 |
| CD11 | 73.54 | 70.36 | 63.37 | 70.78 |
| CD14 | 0.03 | 0.05 | 0.08 | 0.01 |
| CD16 | 66.93 | 58.02 | 54.00 | 41.23 |
| CD19 | 8.33 | 8.00 | 8.39 | 7.26 |
| CD56 | 1.68 | 1.74 | 1.96 | 2.41 |

$CD2^+$, $CD4^+$, $CD8^+$, $CD11b^+$, $CD14^+$, $CD16^+$, $CD19^+$ and $CD56^+$ antibodies). About 10,000 stained cells were re-suspended in PBS, then surface markers were detected by flow cytometry (FACS Calibur; Becton Dickinson Immnocytometry Systems, CA, USA).

### 3.5. Measurement of Cytokine Expression Levels in Blood Cells

To test whether *f-Chlorella* affected the functional maturation of immunocytes within a short period of time, we examined the number of cytokine containing cells using FACS analysis. This method reveals cytokine producing cell by peering off the surface of lymphocyte, enable to assess the cells in a festival evening, compare than serum cytokine level that correspond to paper tips of post festival [14].

Blood cell suspensions were cultured in phorbol 12-myristate 13-acetate (PMA), ionomycin and bovine serum albumin (BSA) (Sigma CO. Ltd., Mo, USA) for 4 - 5 hrs at 37˚C. Subsequently, the cell suspensions were stained with monoclonal antibodies (Percp-CD3, Percp-CD45, FITC-interferon (IFN)-$\gamma$, PE-interleukin (IL)-4, FITC- IL-1$\beta$) and analyzed by flow cytometry. All antibodies used in this study were purchased from Becton Dickinson Immunocytometry System (CA, USA).

## 4. Results

### 4.1. Animal Test

#### 4.1.1. Single and Multiple Dose Toxicity Study of *Conventional Chlorella* and *Fermented Chlorella*

No deaths or abnormalities of body weight, water and food consumption, or coat condition were observed in the treated mice. Necropsy evaluation of the mice did not reveal any significant differences in thymus, liver, spleen, kidney, adrenal gland and testicle weights between the control group and both *conventional Chlorella* and *f-Chlorella* treatment groups, or between males and females.

#### 4.1.2. Immuno-Compromized Host by Mytomicin-C Treated Mice

In theanimal model, theimmuno-competencywas reduced in C57BL/6J mice, aged 8-9 weeks,by injecting with Mitomycin-C (MMC) (5mg/kg) to inhibit the bone marrow. Then, *Chloreralla* samples were administered orally at a dosage of 1g/kg/day for five consecutive days.

#### 4.1.3. Recovery of Whole Body Weight

The body weight and thymus weight reduced in bone marrow-suppressed mice, resulting in the reduction of peripheral blood leukocyte to around 40%. After administered each herbal decoction 1 g/kg dairy for 5 days and after 1 week later, their blood were recovered to around 90% of normal value.

#### 4.1.4. Recovery of Thymus Weight

The bone marrow-suppressed mice were administered *f-Chlorella*1g/kg dairy for 5 days, and one week later, their blood was withdrawn from their tail vein. The cell count of the peripheral blood is showed in **Figure 4**. **Table 5** shows that the thymus weight decreased to half of normal control after 5 mg/kg of MMC was injected. However, all the three *f-Chlorella* recovered thymus weight to about 70% of the control.

#### 4.1.5. Recovery of CD+ Cells and Cytokine Producing Cells

CD3, CD4 and CD19 cells of MMC treated mice were recovered to almost normal values after the administration of *f-Chlorella* As for the functional recovery, IFN-$\gamma$ and IL-4 producing cells were also recovered the all three decoction, including *f-Chlorella* and a functionally depressive agent of TCM. In cytokine producing cells, IFN-*r* and IL-4 producing cell were recovered with *f-Chlorella* in all the three *f-Chlorella* tested, cytokine producing cells were recovered with *f-Chlorella* and even conventional *Chlorella* (**Table 2**).

#### 4.1.6. Recovery of Macrophage Activity, Phagocytosis

We show that MMC clearly suppressed the phagocytic activity of mice both in number and function. After the treatment of *f*-Chlorella, the mice recovered their phagocytic activity to normal range. With a precise observation, the recovery activity was different between *f-Chlorella* and *f-Chlorella* was the strongest *f-Chlorella* among the four formulae to augment in number and function of phagocytes. On the other hand, the augmentation by *f-Chlorella* was less than that by *Chlorella* (**Table 3**, **Figures 2-5**).

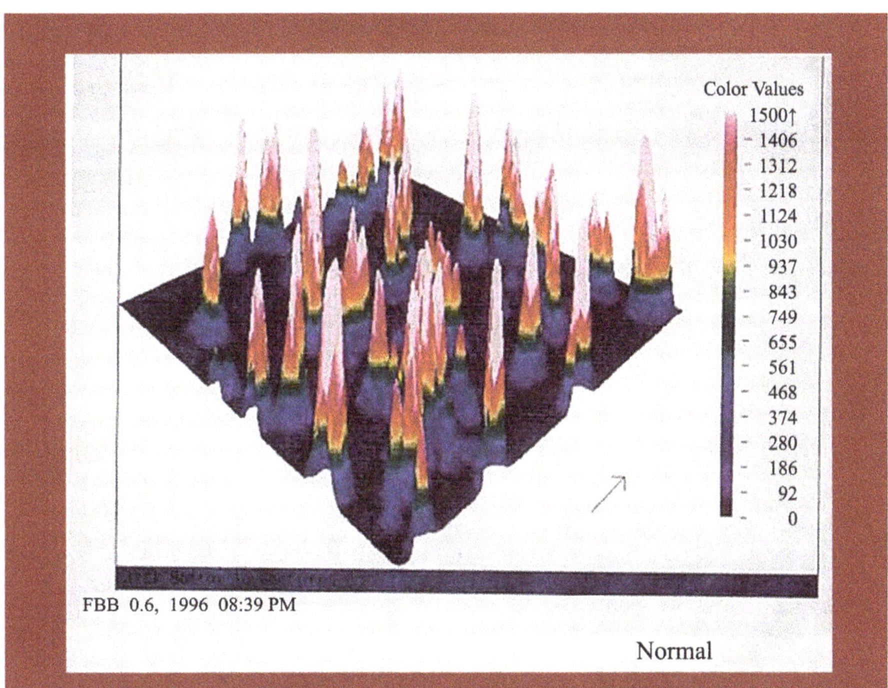


**Figure 2.** Macrophage pahgocytosis accessed by ACAS system targeting florescent activated latex beads in normal mice We tried to express the effect of peripheral total leukocyte number by individual level of change and plot in the x-axis as in each age. Variations in leukocyte subpopulations in the peripheral blood before and after hot spring hydrotherapy.

**Table 2.** Plaque forming/antibody secreting cell Supported by *Chlorella* Derivatives.

| Group Number | PFC/$10^6$ Spleen ells |
|---|---|
| 1 Normal Mice | 556 ± 21 |
| 2 MMC Control | 128 ± 64 |
| 3 MMC + *C. Chlorella* | 386 ± 55$^*$ |
| 4 MMC + *f-Chlorella* | 789 ± 54$^{**}$ |

$^*$p < 0.01 comparing to MMC control. $^{**}$p < 0.05 comparing to non-fermented formulae.

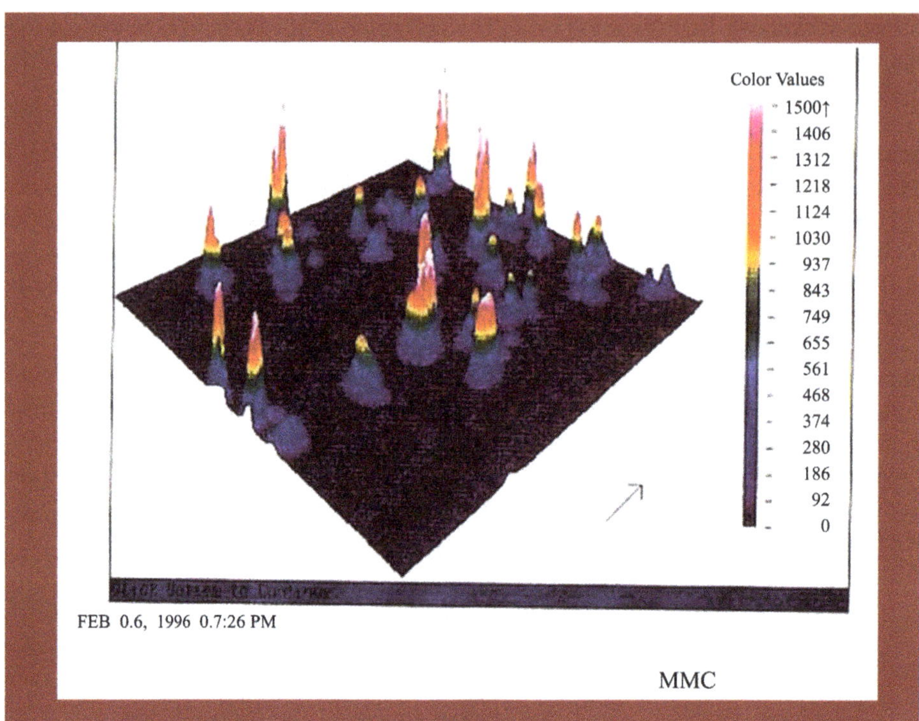


**Figure 3.** Macrophage pahgocytosis accessed by ACAS system targeting florescent activated latex beads in Mytomicin-C treated mice. We sampled peripheral blood from the 12 volunteers before and after hot spring hydrotherapy, at the same time on each day, in accordance with the consideration of circadian rhythm of leukocyte In this figure, we tried to show the date simply pooled and make mean, then compared.

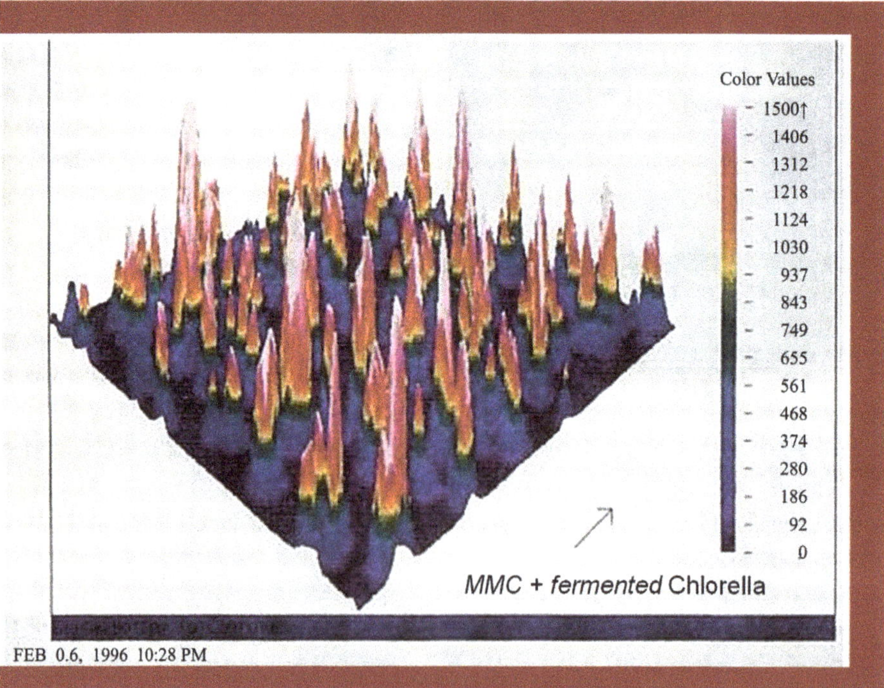


**Figure 4.** Macrophage pahgocytosis accessed by ACAS system targeting florescent activated latex beads in MMC+ *f-Chlorella*. Each spot were obtained from the calculation comparing relative value from before and after levels in the serum, Catecholamines levels in the peripheral blood. The constitution dependent analysis, the detail change and vector of each change could find from individual data, showing higher value volunteer down regulated much more than lower leveled one.

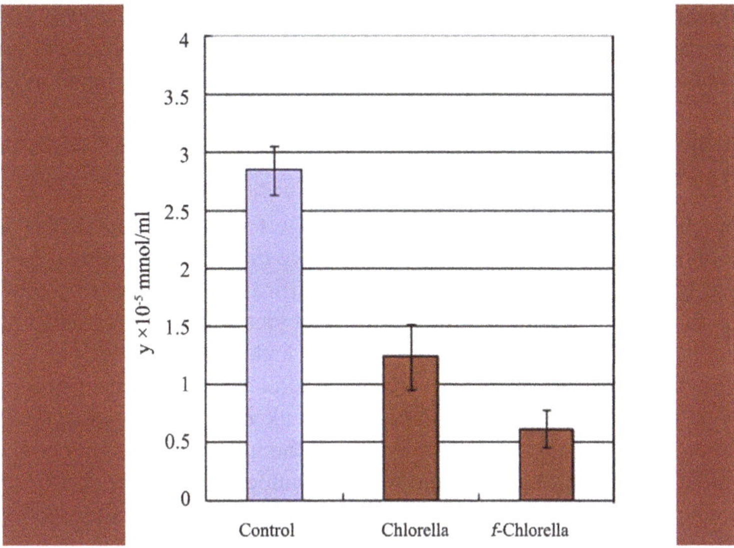


**Figure 5.** Anti-oxidative effect by *Chlorella* Derivatives. The analysis of CD positive cells by FCM was measured by gating in the lymphocytes region on the scattered gram. Fig. shows an example analysis. Nonspecific reaction of the PE fluorescence was found in the isotype control.

**Table 3.** Relative activities of macrophage phagocytosis supported by *Chlorella* Derivatives.

| | Phagocytosis | |
|---|---|---|
| | Positive Cells/10$^6$ cells | |
| | Law active (%) | High active (%) |
| Normal | 52 (100) | 45 (100) |
| MMC | 34 (65) | 5 (11) |
| MMC + *C.Chlorella* | 108 (207) | 59 (131) |
| MMC + *f-Chlorella* | 187 (326) | 89 (199) |

### 4.1.7. Recovery of Lymphocyte Activity, Antibody Secreting Cell

The bone marrow-suppressed mice were administered herbal decoction *f-Chlorella* for five days. One week later, mice were immunized with sheep red blood cells, (2 × 10$^8$ cells/mouse) intraperitoneally. Four and six days later, their plague-forming cells (PFC) were developed. The ability of IgM and IgG antibody production was tested method reported by Jerne and Nordin [15]. In this mouse model, MMC did not reduce the antibody forming cells significantly but the tendency was the same as shown in the former section. In this test, B was the most effective than that of A. *f-Chlorella* was the strongest material to augment antibody secreting cell among the four formulae.

### 4.1.8. The amount of Generated Super Oxide Anion

The amount of generated super oxide anion was calculated in the formula shown above. The generated super oxide anion after one week administration of *Agaricus* and *Chlorella* were 2.64 and 1.95 × 10$^{-5}$ mmol/ml, respectively, whereas that was 2.85 × 10$^{-5}$ mmol/ml in control group. The generated super oxide anion after one week administration of herbal medicine, *Chlorella* were 1.24, 1.25 and 2.88 × 10$^{-5}$ mmol/ml, respectively. The generated super oxide anion after one week administration of Propolis was 2.55 × 10$^{-5}$ mmol/ml. All these drugs, except for *Chlorella* decreased super oxide anion generation after administration for one week in mice.

## 5. Clinical Findings

### 5.1. Regulation in Cell Number of Total Leukocyte and Its Subsets

Leukocyte numbers have been counted one hour before and 15 days after the treatment of hemopoitic formula.

The cell number measured one hour before the administration was set as 100%. Relative percentage of cell number on the 15th day was calculated. No significant changes were observed in G-group after the administration of both types of *Chlorella* derivatives. However, significant change was found in L-type group (**Table 4**).

## 5.2. Dividing Subjects into Two Groups, G-Type and L-Type by Granulocyte and Lymphocyte Proportion

The volunteers were healthy subject, with no drastic change for the total number of leukocytes. However, we tried to check the regulative effect of herbal formulae for two different constitution, G-rich type and L-rich type. Analysis that mixed both groups together showed no significant differences in total leukocyte number except that for *f-Chlorella*. In G-type group, total number of leukocytes was down regulated by both style of *Chlorella*. This was a results of the down regulation of major group of leukocyte, granulocyte.

As for the L-type, no significant changes were found after the treatment of both *f-Chlorella* In the L-type group, *f-Chlorella*, on the other hand, increased the tonal leukocyte and granulocyte in number, on the contrary to the down regulation for lymphocytes. To further clarify the influence of hemopoietic formula, we divided the subjects into two groups: the G-type group, who had a granulocyte count over 60%, and the L-type group, who had a lymphocyte count over 40%. In the L-type group, lymphocyte counts tended to decrease on day 15, accompanied by an increase in granulocyte numbers by conventional *Chlorella* but not by *f-Chlorella*. On the contrary, the granulocyte counts of G-type group tended to decrease on day 15. The decrease of granulocyte count was raised by *f-Chlorella* on day 15 (**Table 5**).

**Table 4.** Constitution dependent regulatory effect by *f-Chlorella*.

| | G-type individual | | L-type individual | |
|---|---|---|---|---|
| | *Conv. Chlorella* | | *f-Chlorella* | |
| | Before | After | Before | After |
| Total WBC (x $10^3$µl) | 6.66 | 5.95 | 5.82 | 7.04 |
| Lymphocyte (%) | 24.6 | 265.4 | 34.3 | 43.2 |
| Granulocyte (%) | 66.5 | 66.4 | 49.8 | 56.8 |
| Neutrophil (%) | 65.8 | 62.6 | 48.3 | 53.4 |
| Eosinophil (%) | 1.8 | 2.7 | 2.4 | 4.8 |
| Basophil (%) | 0.9 | 0.8 | 0.6 | 0.9 |

**Table 5.** Constitution dependent regulation of lymphocyte by Chlorella Derivatives.

| CD | G-type individual | | L-type individual | |
|---|---|---|---|---|
| | *Conv. Chlorella* | | *f-Chlorella* | |
| | Before (%) | After (%) | Before (%) | After (%) |
| CD2 | 632.93 | 77.93 | 64.25 | 78.88 |
| CD4 | 18.76 | 29.52 | 32.15 | 44.15 |
| CD8 | 37.43 | 43.07 | 27.52 | 29.13 |
| CD11 | 72.55 | 71.23 | 65.23 | 71.55 |
| CD14 | 0.04 | 0.04 | 0.08 | 0.09 |
| CD16 | 63.99 | 58.42 | 53.11 | 49.45 |
| CD19 | 8.44 | 8.23 | 8.44 | 7.97 |
| CD56 | 1.25 | 1.88 | 1.78 | 2.56 |

## 5.3. Lymphocyte Subsets Showed Significant Variation and Regulation

After *f-Chlorella* treatment, cell counts of $CD2^+$, $CD4^+$, $CD8^+$, $CD11b^+$, $CD16^+$, $CD19^+$ and $CD56^+$ were tested to evaluate variations in T cells, B cells, macrophages and NK cells. These values were measured one hour before hemopoietic formula and 15 days thereafter. Our results showed that CD2 and CD4 cells were increased by both *f-Chlorella* and SQT. $CD11b^+$ and $CD14^+$ cell counts, which are closely associated with macrophage activity, increased by *f-Chlorella* in the L-type subjects. In particular, there was a remarkable increase in $CD11b^+$ cell number on day 15. T cell subsets that are closely associated with activity of immature T cells, ($CD2^+$, $CD4^+$ and $CD8^+$), the $CD2^+$ ($P < 0.05$) showed an increase with the treatment of *f-Chlorella* 15 days after administration. The number of $CD19^+$ cells, which is closely associated with B cell activity, was not changed by both *f-Chlorella* throughout the trial, neither were the numbers of $CD16^+$ and $CD56^+$ cells.

## 5.4. Cytokine Producing Cells

To test whether herbal decoction affected the functional maturation of immunocytes in a short time, we investigated the number of cytokine producing/containing cells by FACS analysis. This method reveals cytokine producing cell number by peering off the surface of lymphocyte, enable to express the number of cells in festival evening, compare than serum cytokine level that correspond to the paper tips of post festival. To determine whether *f-Chlorella* influences functional maturation of immuno-competent cells, levels of IL-1$\beta$-, IL-4- and IFN-$\gamma$-expressed T cells were further examined using fluorescence-activated cell sorter analyses. There was a significant increase in the levels of IFN-$\gamma$ and IL-4 containing cells after administration of SQT. The result revealed that IFN-$\gamma$ expression, which increased highly on the 15th day after treatment, was different from the expression of IL-1$\beta$ and IL-4, those on the other hand, exponentially increased on day 15 after the administration of SQT. The augmentation of cytokine expression was confirmed by a classical method in the lymphoid organ, *i.e.* antibody-forming cells and plaque-forming cells. Both *f-Chlorella* down-regulated IL-1$\beta$ producing cells in both G-type and L-type groups (**Table 6**).

# 6. The Complement System-Another Stage for Focusing by Fragmented Polysaccharide

We would like to focus on the another important factor of immunological component, complement. These protein are compose of at least 9 components. These protein are famous for its defensive activity against infections organisms as in the defense immunity. However, we had found that the complement had worked when we introduced fragmented /fermented polysaccharide as complement activator, so called alternative pathway conjunct to Alternative Medicine. So in this chapter, we would like to show the nature of complement and activated mechanism that lead to the activation of all the physical activities through the augmentation of complement receptor positive structure cells. Activation of the complement system results in a cascade of interactions of these proteins, leading to the generation of products that have important biologic activities and that constitute an important humoral mediator system involved in inflammatory reactions. First, coating of particles, such as bacteria or immune complexes, with certain components of complement facilitates the ingestion of the particle by phagocytic cells (opsonic function of complement). Second, the activation event generates many fission products of complement proteins for which specific receptors exist on a variety of inflammatory cells, such as granulocytes, lymphocytes, and other cells. Binding of these complement-derived products to such receptors results in biologic activities such as chemotaxis and hormone-like activation of cellular functions (inflammatory function of complement).

**Table 6.** Constitution dependent regulation of cytokine producing cell by *Chlorella* Derivatives.

| Cytokine | G-type individual | | L-type individual | |
|---|---|---|---|---|
| | *Conv. Chlorella* | | *f-Chlorella* | |
| | Before (%) | After (%) | Before (%) | After (%) |
| IFN-$\gamma$ | 6.66 | 5.67 | 3.45 | 5.56 |
| IL-4 | 1.5 | 2.5 | 2.9 | 4.8 |
| IL-1$\beta$ | 0.7 | 0.9 | 0.7 | 0.8 |

## 6.1. Pathways of Complement Activation and Complement Components

Activation of complement can occur by two separate pathways: the classical and the alternative pathways. Both pathways lead to a common terminal pathway referred to as the pathway of membrane attack. Twenty plasma proteins, are now known to be constituents of these pathways. These proteins can be divided into functional proteins, which represent the elements of the various pathways, and regulatory proteins, which exhibit control function. The concentration of the proteins in normal human plasma covers a broad range. They are synthesized in the liver but also by cells of the lympho-reticular system, such as lymphocytes and monocytes. Both the classical and the alternative complement pathways can be organized into various operational units: initiation, amplification, and membrane attack. Following an initial recognition event, which leads to initiation of the pathway, an amplification phase takes place that involves the action of proteases and the recruitment of additional molecules; this is followed by a terminal phase of membrane attack during which the cell dies. The recognition unit for the classical pathway, C1, is composed of three separate proteins, Clq, Clr, and Cls. The initiation of this pathway of complement typically involves the reaction of antibody with antigen, which may be soluble or on the surface of a target cell. This antigen-antibody reaction allows the binding of Clq to two or more Fc regions of certain IgG subclasses (IgG1, IgG2, IgG,) or IgM. Activators of the classical pathway. The ultra structure of Clq has been demonstrated by electron microscopy to consist of six subunits similar to a bouquet of six flowers. The central stalks of Clq resemble collagen in primary and secondary structure. Upon binding of one Clq molecule to the Fc regions of two or more antigen-bound antibody molecules, Clr proenzymes are activated. The chemical basis of this activation is the cleavage of a peptide bond by an autocatalytic mechanism, leading to the formation of activated Clr, a protease that subsequently cleaves the proenzyme Cls. Thus, the binding of Clq to an immunoglobulin in complex with the antigen represents the recognition event of the classical pathway, resulting in the activation of Clr and Cls. The final result is the generation of an enzymatically active component, Cls, which will cleave and thereby activate the next proteins in the cascade, leading to amplification of the recognition event.

The enzyme Cls has two physiologic substrates, C4 and C2. C4 is cleaved by Cls into C4a, one of the three anaphylatoxins (molecules that promote increased vascular permeability and smooth muscle contraction), and C4b, which binds to the target cell surface. Cls also cleaves C2 when C2 is in complex with C4b. Cleavage of C2 generates C2b, which is released, and C2a, which remains bound to C4b. The bimolecular complex C4b, 2a is a protease that cleaves C3 and therefore is called C3 convertase. Cleavage of C3 by the C3 convertase generates two important biologically active peptides, C3a (another anaphylatoxin) and cab, which attaches to target cell surfaces and can bind to C5. C5, when in complex with C3b, can be cleaved by the C3 convertase (then referred to as C5 convertase). The C5 convertase hydrolyzes C5, which generates the C5a anaphylatoxin and C5b. C5b is the nucleus for the formation of the membrane attack complex. Immediately following their generation, C3b and C4b exhibit a unique transient ability to covalently bind to target cells ("metastable binding site"). This property has reentry been shown to be due to an intramolecular thioester bond that is present between the sulfhydryl group of a cysteine residue and the gamma carbonyl group of a glutamine residue on C3 and C4. Upon activation of C3 or C4, this thioester becomes highly reactive and can react with a cell surface hydroxyl or amino group. This results in the covalent attachment of C3b or C4b to the target cell. An additional function of the thioester bond is its hydrolysis by water, occurring during activation of the alternative pathway as described below.

The alternative pathway can be activated when a molecule of C3b is bound to a target cell. This C3b molecule combines with the plasma protein Factor B, which is a zymogen, and which, when bound to C3b, can be activated by the plasma protein Factor D by cleavage into two fragments, Ba and Bb. The Bb fragment, which contains the active enzymatic site, remains bound to C3b, as C3b, Bb. This complex, like C4b, 2a in the classical pathway, is a C3 convertase (C3b; Bb); it is stabilized by the binding of another plasma protein, properdin. Thus, the alternative pathway used to be called the properdin pathway. The presence of a single molecule of C3b generates many molecules of C3b, Bb, resulting in a tremendous amplification. The C3 convertase (C3b, Bb) cleaves C3, thereby generating more molecules of C3b, which can combine with other molecules of factor B to give more molecules of cab, Bb, which can, in turn, cleave more molecules of C3. Therefore, the central feature of the alternative pathway is a positive feedback loop that amplifies the original recognition event. As in the classical pathway, attachment of many C3b molecules to the target cell -will allow binding of C5 and its cleavage into C5a and C5b by the enzyme C3b, Bb, now referred to as C5 convertase.

Owing to the potential of this positive feedback loop to rapidly use up Factor B and C3, the positive feedback must be carefully regulated. There are two important regulatory proteins in plasma. The first protein, Factor H (formerly referred to as PIH), competes with Factor B for binding to C3b and also dissociates C3b, Bb into C3b and Bb. The second control protein, Factor I (formerly referred to as C3b in activator), cleaves C3b that is bound to Factor H or to a similar protein found on the surface of the host cell. The resulting cleaved C3b, termed iC3b, can no longer form a C3 convertase. The action of these two control proteins prevents the consumption of Factor B and C3 in plasma; in addition, these two proteins in activate C3b, Bb on host cell surfaces. In contrast, surfaces of many target cells, such as bacteria and other microorganisms, protect C3b, Bb from in activation by Factors H and I. This protection allows the positive feedback loop to proceed on the surface of the target cell, leading to the activation of the pathway and subsequent cell death. In other words, the alternative pathway is activated by those substances that prevent the inactivation of the positive feedback loop enzyme C3b, Bb. A substance is therefore treated as "foreign" if it restricts the action of Factors H and I and allows the positive feedback loop to continue.

The chemical structures on surfaces of particles and cells responsible for activation or non-activation of the alternative pathway have not been identified. There is some evidence that carbohydrate moieties are involved, particularly sialic acid. The alternative pathway protein(s) responsible for the recognition of these structures also remains to be determined. As pointed out earlier, the activation of the alternative pathway requires a C3b molecule bound to the surface of a target cell. An intriguing question is, "Where does the critical first cab molecule come from?". Although it can be provided by the C3 convertase of the classical pathway or by cleavage of C3 by plasmin and certain bacterial and other cellular proteases, the alternative pathway can generate this first C3b molecule without these proteases. The intramolecular thioester, which is highly reactive in nascent C3b and is responsible for the covalent attachment to targets, is also accessible in native C3 to water molecules. Thus, spontaneous hydrolysis of the thioester bond occurs constantly in plasma at a low rate. The C3 molecules in which the thioester bond has been hydrolyzed behave like C3b, although the C3a domain has not been removed. C3 with a hydrolyzed thioester is called C3 (H20) or C3b-like C3. It can bind Factor B and allow Factor D to activated Factor B, which results in formation of a fluid-phase C3 convertase, C3, Bb. This enzyme is continuously formed and produces C3b molecules that can randomly attach to cells. Although these C3b molecules will be rapidly inactivated on host cells by Factors H and I, they will start the positive feedback loop on foreign surfaces, as outlined previously. In other words, the alternative pathway is constantly activated at a low rate, but amplification with subsequent cell death occurs only on foreign particles.

## 6.2. Activated Products of Complement and Their Biological Activity

Activation of either the alternative or the classical pathway results in the generation of many important peptides involved in inflammatory responses. The anaphylaxis increase of vascular permeability degranulation of mast cells and basophils with release of histamine Degranulation of eosinophils Aggregation of platelets opsonization of particles and solubilization of immune complexes with subsequent facilitation of phagocytosis Release of neutrophils from bone marrow resulting in leukocytosis Smooth muscle contraction Increase of vascular permeability Smooth muscle contraction Increase of vascular permeability Degranulation of mast cells and basophils with release of histamine Degranulation of eosinophils Aggregation of platelets Chemotaxis of basophils, eosino phils, neutrophils, and monocytes Release of hydrolytic enzymes from neutrophils Chemotaxis of neutrophils Release of hydrolytic enzymes from neutrophils Inhibition of migration and indulation of spreading of monocytes and macrophages latoxinsna C3a, C4a, and C5a are derived from the enzymatic cleavage of C3, C4, and C5 respectively. Historically, C3a and C5a were defined as factors derived from activated serum possessing spasmogenic activity. The anaphylatoxins are now recognized as having many additional biologic functions. Both C3a and C5a are known to induce the release of histamine from mast cells and basophils (chapter 20A). As shown in **Figure 6** both anaphylatoxins cause smooth muscle contraction and induce the release of vasoactive amines, which cause an increase in vascular permeability.

The effect of C5a anaphylatoxin on neutrophils is of considerable importance in the inaammatory response. Not only can C5a induce neutrophil aggregation, but this anaphylatoxin appears to be the main chemotactic peptide generated by activation of either complement pathway. In vitro, nanomolar concentrations of C5a will induce the unidirectional movement of neutrophils. Other inflammatory cells, such as monocytes, eosinophils, basophils, and macrophages, have also been shown to exhibit a chemotactic response to C5a. The removal of the

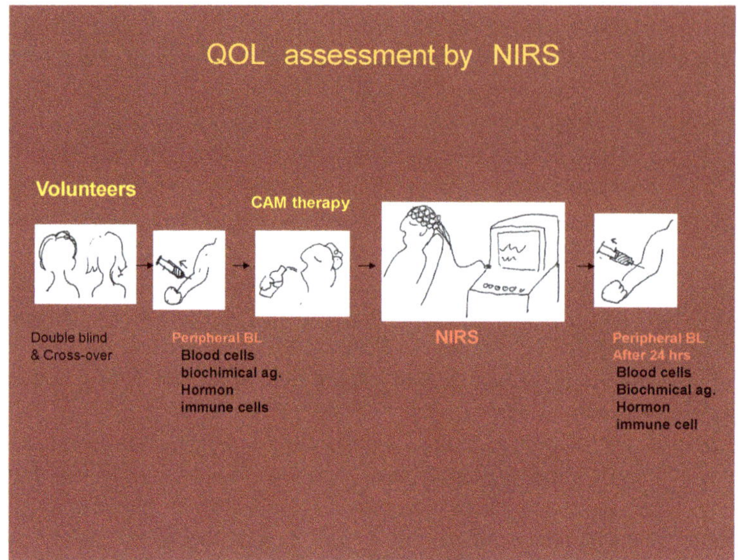


**Figure 6.** Experimental Design for Assessing CAM Therapy. The analysis of $\beta_2$-AR expressing cells and CD positive cells by FCM was measured by gating in the lymphocytes region on the scattered gram. Figure shows an example analysis.

carboxy-terminal arginine from C5a by serum carboxy peptidase N, generating C5a-des-arg, inactivates the spasmogen, yet restoration of full chemotactic activity of C5a-des-are may occur in the presence of serum. Therefore, C5a-desarg may also be responsible for in vivo neutrophil chemotactic activity.

As described earlier, the cleavage of C3 by either the alternative or the classical C3 convertases results in the production of two major split products, the C3a anaphylatoxin and cab. The larger C3b fragment can serve as an opsonin (promoter of phagocytosis) by binding to a target through the thioester mechanism. This renders the particle or cell immediately susceptible to ingestion by a variety of phagocytic cells that carry specific receptors for C3b.

Many recent observations point to additional roles for complement fragments in regulating the activity 9f cells of the immune system. These observations include the presence of receptors on lymphocytes for various complement proteins, including C3 split products and Factor H, affecting B and T cell function. This is an important area for future research (**Figures 7-9**).

## 7. Cardio-Vascular Disease

Daily consumption of the *Chlorella* extract of *Chlorella. Pyrenoidosa* significantly reduces the serum levels of total cholesterol, LDL-C, and triglyceride (TG) and oxidative stress in hyper lipidemic patients. Therefore, this extract could be considered as a potential agent for treatment of dyslipidemia and prevention of atherosclerosis development.

## 8. Discussion

Our investigation clarified how hemopoitic formula, also known as tonic agent and Bu-Ji, influenced the immune system (e.g. leukocyte, granulocyte and lymphocyte subsets in particular).

We quantified CD positive cell counts as indicators of T cells, B cells, macrophages and NK cells. For qualitative and quantitative evaluation, we examined the cytokine expression levels, and directly measured the expression levels of cytokine-containing cells in peripheral blood, eliminating possible artificial factors that could arise from culturing in test tubes or changes in net value by cartelization. To avoid any possible influence from the circadian rhythm, we obtained the whole blood from all donors at the same time.

In this investigation, we confirmed that *f-Chlorella* quantitatively and qualitatively regulated leukocytes, granulocytes, lymphocytes and their subsets. The increase of $CD2^+$, $CD4^+$, $CD8^+$, $CD11b^+$, $CD16^+$, $CD19^+$ and

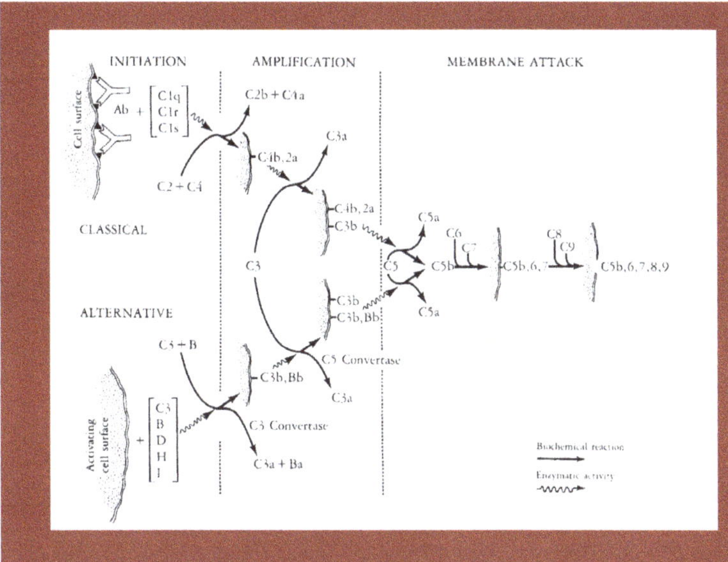


**Figure 7.** Complement Cascade from Start to the Final. An East and Lactobacilli can degradate the macromolecular substances to low molecular one to get their energy. This procedure had been so called fermentation, This process is good for storage and finding new taste for human being as well as other creatures. This product was to find to get through intestinal barrier and activated the complement component that was succeeded to augment receptor positive physiological cell scattered around the each organ including immunological competent organ.

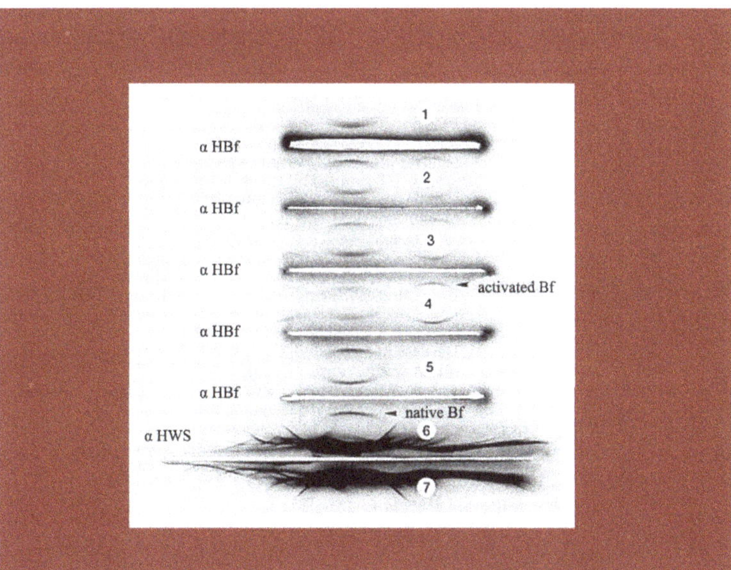


**Figure 8.** An Immuno Electrophoresis to Show Direct Evidence of Activated Complement Fragment Administrating *f-Chlorella*. The analysis of $\beta_2$-AR receptor expressing cells and CD positive cells by FCM was measured by gating in the lymphocytes region on the scattered gram. Figure shows an example analysis.

$CD56^+$ cell counts as well as the levels of IL-1$\beta$, IL-4 and IFN-$\gamma$ in blood cells suggested that hemopoitic formula might enhance the activities of humoral and cellular immunities, as well as NK cells. We also observed that levels of cytokine producing cells, in particular, increased rather than CD-positive lymphocytes, showing

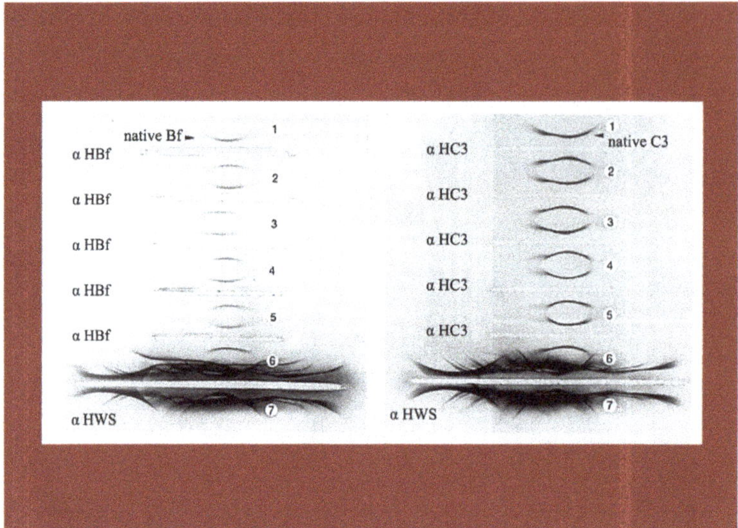


**Figure 9.** An Immuno Electrophoresis to Show Direct Evidence of Activated Complement Fragment Administrating *f-Chlorella*. Time interval of blood sampling between before and after hot-spring hydrotherapy was approximately 24 hours. Measurements of the total and differential leukocyte counts and 3 catecholamines levels in the peripheral blood.

that *f-Chlorella* augmented lymphocyte production qualitatively than quantitatively. Moreover, *f-Chlorella* activated both CD11b cells and IL-1$\beta$ producing cells, suggesting the activation of phagocyte cells both in number and in function. Consequently, these data further demonstrated that *f-Chlorella* acted in macrophages in the same manner as *Mycobacterium tuberculosis* that has cell walls constructed of waxy substances [13].

In previous reports about hot-spring hydrotherapy and acupuncture, we had proposed that immune system regulation was an important factor for evaluating CAM. Since other substances, such as endotoxin and waxy substances from *Mycobacterium tuberculosis*, similar to proplis, were known for augmenting host immune responses. This time, we decided to focus solely on propolis. A possible explanation for immune enhancement could be the activation of the circular system and/or autonomic nervous system, although the details of the mechanism remain unclear. Further research regarding to the mechanism was necessary.

Abo *et al.* reported that granulocyte count was increased *f-Chlorella* the excitation of the sympathetic nervous system, while lymphocyte count was increased by excitation of parasympathetic nervous system [11] [12]. Our data also showed that granulocyte count was decreased in subjects with a high granulocyte count, while lymphocyte count was increased in the same subjects [16]-[20]. The lymphocyte count, however, was decreased in subjects with a high lymphocyte level, while granulocyte count was increase in the same subjects. In other words, the subjects dominated *f-Chlorella* the sympathetic nerve could release stress, whereas the sympathetic activity of subjects who were dominated parasympathetic nerve might be excited by hemopoietic formula. This way, the cell counts appeared to converge at appropriate levels after hemopoietic formula. Finally, in order to determine whether the elevation of leukocyte counts resulted from an infection triggered by hemopoitic formula or not, the subjects were followed up for 8 days after the last administration of hemopoitic formula [21]-[30]. During that period, we could not observe any infectious signs such as pyodermitis, fever, or enhancement of C-Reactive Protein (CRP). The value of CRP was 0.57 g/dl to 1.23 g/dl in our subjects, suggesting very mild inflammatory responses, which showed that hemopoitic formula did not cause infection. Since the meridian might influence cells throughout the body and might pass through every organ system, hemopoitic formula stimulation might provide maximum benefits without dangerous side effects. As an immune-augmentation system, hemopoietin formulae merit health investigation as a possible treatment for acquired immune-deficiency system. The other failure especially for the senile required throughout the world [31]-[39].

## References

[1] Kitada, Y., Wan, W., Matsui, K., Matsui, K., Shimizu, S. and Yamaguchi, N. (2000) Regulation of Peripheral White

Blood Cells in Numbers and Functions through Hot-Spring Bathing during a Short Term—Studies in Control Experiments. *Journal of Japanese Society Balneology Climatology Physiological Medicine*, **63**, 151-164.

[2] Yamaguchi, N., Takahashi, T., Sugita, T., Ichikawa, K., Sakaihara, S., Kanda, T., Arai, M. and Kawakita, K. (2007) Acupuncture Regulates Leukocyte Subpopulations in Human Peripheral Blood. *Evidence-Based Complementary and Alternative Medicine*, **4**, 447-453. http://dx.doi.org/10.1093/ecam/nel107

[3] Suzuki, S., Toyabe, S., Moroda, T., Tada, T., Tsukahara, A. and Iiai, T. (1997) Circadian Rhythm of Leukocytes and Lymphocytes Subsets and Its Possible Correlation with the Function of the Autonomic Nervous System. *Clinical Experimental Immunology*, **110**, 500-508. http://dx.doi.org/10.1046/j.1365-2249.1997.4411460.x

[4] Yamaguchi, N., Kawada, N., Ja, X.S., Okamoto, K., Okuzumi, K., Chen, R. and Takahashi, T. (2014) Overall Estimation of Anti-Oxidant Activity by Mammal Macrophage. *Open Journal of Rheumatology and Autoimmune Diseases*, **4**, 13-21. http://dx.doi.org/10.4236/ojra.2014.41002

[5] Hamada, M. and Yamaguchi, N. (1988) Effect of Kanpo Medicine, Zyuzentaihoto, on the Immune Reactivity of Tumor-Bearing Mice. *Journal of Ethnopharmacology*, **24**, 311-320. http://dx.doi.org/10.1016/0378-8741(88)90160-2

[6] Tu, C.C., Li, C.S., Liu, C.M. and Liu, C.C. (2011) Comparative Use of Biomedicine and Chinese Medicine in Taiwan: Using the NHI Research Database. *Journal of Alternative and Complementary Medicine*, **17**, 339-346. http://dx.doi.org/10.1089/acm.2010.0200

[7] Yamaguchi, N., Chen, R., Okamoto, K., Takei, T., Tsubokawa, M., Sakamoto, D., Jia, X.S., Wenhan, W.W. and Murayama, T. (2013) Quantitative Regulation of Peripheral Leukocyte by Light Exercise and Tailored Scale for Assessment. *Open Journal of Immunology*, **3**, 175-183. http://dx.doi.org/10.4236/oji.2013.34022

[8] Yamaguchi, N., Wenhan, N., Wan, W., Sakamoto, D., Nurmuhammad, A., Matsumoto, K., Takei, T., Okuzumi, K., Murayama, T. and Takahashi, T. (2013) Regulative Effect for Natural Killer Cell by Hot Spring Hydrotherapy—Quantitative and Qualitative Discussion. *Open Journal of Immunology*, **3**, 201-209. http://dx.doi.org/10.4236/oji.2013.34025

[9] Navo, M.A., Phan, J. and Vaughan, C. (2004) An Assessment of the Utilization of Complementary and Alternative Medication in Women with Gynecologic or Breast Malignancies. *Journal of Clinical Oncology*, **22**, 671-677. http://dx.doi.org/10.1200/JCO.2004.04.162

[10] Murayama, T., Yamaguchi, N., Iwamoto, K. and Eizuru, Y. (2006) Inhibition of Ganciclovir-Resistant Human Cytomegalovirus Replication by Kampo (Japanese Herbal Medicine). *Antiviral Chemistry & Chemotherapy*, **17**, 11-16. http://dx.doi.org/10.1177/095632020601700102

[11] Abo, T., Kawate, T., Itoh, K. and Kumagai, K. (1981) Studies on the Bioperiodicity of the Immune Response. I. Circadian Rhythms of Human T, B and K Cell Traffic in the Peripheral Blood. *Journal of Immunology*, **126**, 1360-1363.

[12] Abo, T. and Kumagai, T. (1978) Studies of Surface Immunoglobulins on Human B Lymphocytes. Physiological Variations of Sig+ Cells in Peripheral Blood. *Clinical Experimental Immunology*, **33**, 441-452.

[13] Landmann, R.M.A., Muller, F.B., Perini, C., Wesp, M., Erne, P. and Buhler, F.R. (1984) Changes of Immunoregulatory Cells Induced by Psychological and Physical Stress: Relationship to Plasma Catecholamines. *Clinical Experimental Immunology*, **58**, 127-135.

[14] Iio, A., Ohguchi, K., Naruyama, H., Tazawa, S., Araki, Y., Ichihara, K., Nozawa, Y. and Ito, M. (2012) Ethanolic Extract of Brazilian Red Propolis ABCA1 Expression and Promote Cholesterol Effulux from THP-1 Macrophage. *Phytomedicine*, **19**, 383-388. http://dx.doi.org/10.1016/j.phymed.2011.10.007

[15] Jerne, N.K. and Nordin, A.A. (1963) Plaque Formation in Agar by Single Antibody Producing Cells. *Science*, **140**, 405-408. http://dx.doi.org/10.1126/science.140.3565.405

[16] Jyumonji, N. and Fujii, Y. (1993) A New Assay for Delayed-Type Hypersensitivity *in Vitro* Detection F-CHLORELLA. The Macrophage Migration by Boyden Chamber. *The Journal of Kanazawa Medical University*, **18**, 198-203.

[17] Yamaguchi, N., Shimizu, S. and Izumi, H. (2004) Hydrotherapy Can Modulate Peripheral Leukocytes: An Approach to Alternative Medicine. *Advances in Experimental Medicine and Biology*, **546**, 239-251. http://dx.doi.org/10.1007/978-1-4757-4820-8_18

[18] Murayama, T., Yamaguchi, N., Matsuno, H. and Eizuru, Y. (2004) *In Vitro* Anti-Cytomegalovirus Activity of Kampo (Japanese Herbal) Medicine. *Evidence-Based Complementary and Alternative Medicine*, **1**, 285-289.

[19] Abe, S., Yamaguchi, N., Tansho, S. and Yamaguchi, H. (2005) Preventive Effects of Juzen-taiho-to on Infectious Disease. In: Haruki, Y. and Isao, S., Eds., *Juzen-taiho-to* (*Shi-Quan-Da-Bu-Tang*): *Scientific Evaluation and Clinical Applications*, Traditional Herbal Medicines for Modern Times, CRC Press, Boca Raton.

[20] Nakano, S., Noguchi, T., Takekoshi, H., Suzuki, G. and Nakano, M. (2005) Maternal-Fetal Distribution and Transfer of Dioxins in Pregnant Women in Japan, and Attempts to Reduce Maternal Transfer with *Chlorella* (*Chlorella pyrenoidosa*) Supplements. *Chemosphere*, **61**, 1244-1255. http://dx.doi.org/10.1016/j.chemosphere.2005.03.080

[21] Otsuki, T., Shimizu, K., Iemitsu, M. and Kono, I. (2011) Salivary Secretory Immunoglobulin a Secretion Increases after 4-Weeks Ingestion of Chlorella-Derived Multicomponent Supplement in Humans: A Randomized cross over Study. *Nutrition Journal*, **10**, 91. http://dx.doi.org/10.1186/1475-2891-10-91

[22] Otsuki, T., Shimizu, K., Iemitsu, M. and Kono, I. (2012) Chlorella Intake Attenuates Reduced Salivary SIgA Secretion in Kendo Training Camp Participants. *Nutrition Journal*, **11**, 103.

[23] Hasegawa, T., Ito, K., Ueno, S., Kumamoto, S., Ando, Y., Yamada, A., Nomoto, K. and Yasunobu, Y. (1999) Oral Administration of Hot Water Extracts of *Chlorella vulgaris* Reduces IgE Production against Milk Casein in Mice. *International Journal of Immunopharmacology*, **21**, 311-323. http://dx.doi.org/10.1016/S0192-0561(99)00013-2

[24] Hsu, H.Y., Jeyashoke, N., Yeh, C.H., Song, Y.J., Hua, K.F. and Chao, L.K. (2010) Immunostimulatory Bioactivity of Algal Polysaccharides from *Chlorella pyrenoidosa* Activates Macrophages via Toll-Like Receptor 4. *Journal of Agricultural and Food Chemistry*, **58**, 927-936. http://dx.doi.org/10.1021/jf902952z

[25] Nakano, S., Takekoshi, H. and Nakano, M. (2010) *Chlorella pyrenoidosa* Supplementation Reduces the Risk of Anemia, Proteinuria and Edema in Pregnant Women. *Plant Foods for Human Nutrition*, **65**, 25-30. http://dx.doi.org/10.1007/s11130-009-0145-9

[26] Soontornchaiboon, W., Joo, S.S. and Kim, S.M. (2012) Anti-Inflammatory Effects of Violaxanthin Isolated from Microalga *Chlorella ellipsoidea* in RAW 264.7 Macrophages. *Biological and Pharmaceutical Bulletin*, **35**, 1137-1144. http://dx.doi.org/10.1248/bpb.b12-00187

[27] Vecina, J.F., Oliveira, A.G., Araujo, T.G., Baggio, S.R., Torello, C.O., Saad, M.J. and Queiroz, M. (2014) *Chlorella* Modulates Insulin Signaling Pathway and Prevents High-Fat Diet-Induced Insulin Resistance in Mice. *Life Sciences*, **95**, 45-52. http://dx.doi.org/10.1016/j.lfs.2013.11.020

[28] Cherng, J.Y. and Shih, M.F. (2005) Preventing Dyslipidemia by *Chlorella pyrenoidosa* in Rats and Hamsters after Chronic High Fat Diet Treatment. *Life Sciences*, **76**, 3001-3013. http://dx.doi.org/10.1016/j.lfs.2004.10.055

[29] Ryu, N.H., Lim, Y., Park, J.E., Kim, J., Kim, J.Y., Kwon, S.W. and Kwon, O. (2014) Impact of Daily *Chlorella* Consumption on Serum Lipid and Carotenoid Profiles in Mildly Hypercholesterolemic Adults: A Double-Blinded, Randomized, Placebo-Controlled Study. *Nutrition Journal*, **13**, 57. http://dx.doi.org/10.1186/1475-2891-13-57

[30] Mizoguchi, T., Takehara, I., Masuzawa, T., Saito, T. and Naoki, Y. (2008) Nutrigenomic Studies of Effects of *Chlorella* on Subjects with High-Risk Factors for Lifestyle-Related Disease. *Journal of Medicinal Food*, **11**, 395-404. http://dx.doi.org/10.1089/jmf.2006.0180

[31] Jong, Y.C. and Mei, F.S. (2005) Potential Hypoglycemic Effects of *Chlorella* in Streptozotocin-Induced Diabetic Mice. *Life Sciences*, **77**, 980-990. http://dx.doi.org/10.1016/j.lfs.2004.12.036

[32] Dauchet, L., Amouyel, P., Hercberg, S. and Dallonggeville, J. (2006) Fruit and Vegetable Consumption and Risk of Coronary Heart Disease: A Meta-Analysis of Cohort Studies. *The Journal of Nutrition*, **136**, 2588-2593.

[33] Shimbo, M., Kawagishi, H. and Yokogoshi, H. (2005) Erinacine A Increases Catecholamine and Nerve Growth Factor Content in the Central Nervous System of Rats. *Nutrition Research*, **25**, 617-623. http://dx.doi.org/10.1016/j.nutres.2005.06.001

[34] Kawagishi, H. and Zhuang, C. (2008) Compounds for Dementia from *Hericium erinaceum*. *Drug of the Future*, **33**, 149-155. http://dx.doi.org/10.1358/dof.2008.033.02.1173290

[35] Mizuno, M., Morimoto, M., Minato, K. and Tsuchida, H. (1998) Polysaccharides from *Agaricus blazei* Stimulate Lymphocyte T-Cell Subsets in Mice. *Bioscience, Biotechnology, and Biochemistry*, **62**, 434-437. http://dx.doi.org/10.1271/bbb.62.434

[36] Nakamura, T., Matsugo, S., Uzuka, Y., Matsuo, S. and Kawagishi, H. (2004) Fractionation and Anti-Tumor Activity of the Mycelia of Liquid-Cultured *Phellinus linteus*. *Bioscience, Biotechnology, and Biochemistry*, **68**, 868-872. http://dx.doi.org/10.1271/bbb.68.868

[37] Lindequist, U., Niedermeyer, T.H.J. and Jülish, W.D. (2005) The Pharmacological Potential of Mushrooms. *Evidence-Based Complementary and Alternative Medicine*, **2**, 285-299. http://dx.doi.org/10.1093/ecam/neh107

[38] Yamaguchi, N., Ueyama, T., Amat, N., Yimit, D., Hoxur, P., Sakamoto, D., Katoh, Y., Watanabe, I. and Su, S.Y. (2015) Bi-Directional Regulation by Chinese Herbal Formulae to Host and Parasite for Multi-Drug Resistant *Staphylococcus aureus* in Humans and Rodents. *Open Journal of Immunology*, **4**, 18-32. http://dx.doi.org/10.4236/oji.2015.51003

[39] Shimizu, S., Kitada, H., Yokota, H., Yamakawa, J., Murayama, T., Sugiyama, K., Izumi, H. and Yamaguchi, N. (2002) Activation of the Alternative Complement Pathway by *Agaricus blazei* Murill. *Phytomedicine*, **9**, 536-545. http://dx.doi.org/10.1078/09447110260573047

6

# Bi-Directional Regulation by Chinese Herbal Formulae to Host and Parasite for Multi-Drug Resistant *Staphylococcus aureus* in Humans and Rodents

**Nobuo Yamaguchi[1,2], Takanao Ueyama[3], Nurmuhamamt Amat[4], Dilxat Yimit[4], Parida Hoxur[5], Daisuke Sakamoto[6], Yuma Katoh[2,7], Ikkan Watanabe[2], Shan-Yu Su[8,9]**

[1]Department of Fundamental Research for CAM, Kanazawa Medical University, Uchinada, Japan
[2]Ishikawa Natural Medicinal Products Research Center, Kanazawa, Japan
[3]Department of Medicine II, Kansai Medical University, Osaka, Japan
[4]Traditional Uighur Medicine Department, Xinjiang Medical University, Urumqi, China
[5]Traditional Chinese Medicine Hospital, Xinjiang Medical University, Urumqi, China
[6]Department of Chest Surgery, Kanazawa Medical University, Himi Citizen Hospital, Himi, Japan
[7]Department of Respiratory Medicine, Tohkai Central Hospital, Gifu, Japan
[8]Department of Chinese Medicine, China Medical University Hospital, Taichung City, Taiwan
[9]School of Post-Baccalaureate Chinese Medicine, College of Chinese Medicine, China Medical University, Taichung City, Taiwan
Email: serumaya@kanazawa-med.ac.jp

## Abstract

**A decline in the immunopotential of the host plays acritical factor(s) in the occurrence of infections with methicillin-resistant *Staphylococcus aureus* (MRSA) or microorganisms by opportunistic infection. In such an infection, no way out for therapeutic concept, therefore bi-directional trial was the final choice. So we selected aformula, Dang Gui Liu Huang Tang (dLHT), which could both augmentimmune factorsin host and exert bacteriostatic effect. We sought to break through the epidemic by MRSA especially in elderly patient, by the fundamental and clinical trial by employing minor TCM, characterizing bidirectional ability of the decoction by western methods. Animal Experiment: Mitomycin-C (MMC)-treated mice with or without the infection of MRSA were made. The experimental design was made up to examine the bacteriostatic action as well as the immunopotentiating bias of the promising Chinese herbal medicine, dLHT, which was first proved for its immune potentiating activities as well as their sensitivity to antibiotics, but not direct aseptic effect was clear for MRSA. Both basic and clinical data showed that this formula was effective on re-**

**pelling from the infectious focus after the treatment of MRSA infection. After the administration of dLHT, the number of white blood cells in MMC-treated mice recovered to 80% of the normal level. In addition, the phagocytic activity of macrophages increased to 70% in the dLHT-treated group, while that of the non-treated group was only 20%. The bactericidal activity also recovered to the level close to the normal value by dLHT. The ratio of neutrophils in the dLHT-administered group increased to 2.2% (normal mice, 2.6%), whereas that in the non-terated group was only 0.5%. The bacterial count in the liver of MRSA-challenged mice reached the peak at six hours after the challenge in both dLHT-treated and non-treated mice. However, the number of bacteria in dLHT group was much greater than that in the non-treated group. The bacterial count in the blood showed an increase 12 and 24 hours after the challenge. Even 24 hours after the challenge, a significant number of bacteria existed in the blood of dLHT-administered group, whereas only a small number of bacteria detectable 6 hours after the challenge and the number gradually decreased thereafter in the dLHT-administered group. MRSA-challenged MMC-treated mice were treated by dLHT, vancomycin, or dLHT and vancomycin. All of non-treated mice died 8 days after the MRSA challenge, whereas the survival rates were 60% after dLHT treatment, 40% after vancomycin treatment, and 80% after dLHT and vancomycin treatment. All of MMC-treated mice, to which the phagocytic cells prepared from MMC-treated mice with dLHT administration had adoptively been transferred, survived from MRSA challenge. On the other hand, the survival rate of MMC-treated mice, to which the lymphocytes prepared from the same mice had adoptively been transferred, was 40%. Clinical Trial: All cases with dLHT treatment showed negative culture results for MRSA after the dLHT administration. The culture generally became negative less than 50 days after the initial administration, whereas one control case needed more than 100 days and the other was dead of the infection. One representative case, who was a 78-year-old woman suffering from hypertension, atrial fibrillation, and cerebral bleeding in the right occipital lobe, infected with MRSA during the antibiotic therapy for *Streptococcus pneumoniae*. The antibiotic therapy was halted and the dLHT administration started. Three weeks later, the culture result became negative. In addition, serum protein and albumin values also returned to the level that they had had before the infection of MRSA.**

## Keywords

**Drug Sensitivity, Multiple Resistance, Dang Gui Liu Huang Tang, MRSA, Nosocomical Infection, Host Immunity**

## 1. Introduction

The decline in the immunopotential of the host plays an essential role in the occurrence of infections even by low pathogenic bacteria, methicilline-resistant *Staphylococcus aureus* (MRSA) or *pseudomonas*. There are two primary systems, innate immunity and adaptive immunity. Despite these defense systems, the overwhelming problems of possessing these dual systems, the innate and adaptive does not seem to guard or even prevent the development of one internal threat to survival. However, every individual exposes to the list of immunodeficiency in daily life with both internal and externals [1]-[10]. The factors that influence the acquired immune activity are systemic metabolic disorders such as diabetes, malnutrition, extreme exhaustion, extensive stress, aging and medical side effects [1]-[10]. So we have to select appropriate menu to regulate immune function through leukocyte storage. The menu had been summarized and listed as CAM: complementary and alternative medicine [11]-[18]. The use of the menu in conjunction with exercise recipe is in a quandary due to the lack of information concerning these cross-interactions among general public and a lack in information among the health professionals with a potentially significant health scale.

In other words, there are no tentative scales for evaluating the intense of exercise for each patient. A propose of this study is to suggest the best tailored scale for evaluating the intense of menu. For this purpose, we sought to set up a mouse model in which mice were infected with MRSA and treated with mitomycin-C (MMC) to examine the bacteriostatic and anti-inflammatory actions as well as the immuno-competent actions of the promising Chinese herbal medicine, Dang Gui Liu Huang Tang (dLHT). dLHT was also administered to patients who were infected with MRSA. Both animal and clinical experiments compared dLHT with standard hemopoietic herbal decoction in the MRSA infection system.

## 2. Experimental Design

### 2.1. Experimental Mice

Eight-week-old male C57BL/6J mice (Sankyo Animal Laboratory Inc.) were kept at clear animal housing at specific pathogen free condition (SPF) with a room temperature of 24˚C ± 1˚C and a humidity of 60%. The water and mice food were freely accessed.

### 2.2. Experimental Animal Model

In the animal model of immuno-competency reduction, mice were injected with MMC (5 mg/kg) to inhibit the bone marrow. An extract of dLHT, which was freezed and dried, was administered orally at a dosage of 1 g/kg/day for five consecutive days. The white cell count, the ability of the macrophages to migrate, and phagocytosis of MRSA clinical were examined. The bacteria count in the liver reached the peak six hours after the injection. In the combined treatment group with dLHT + antibiotics, the number of bacteria decreased markedly. Moreover, in the joint treatment group, the blood bacteria number increase 6 hours and 12 hours after treatment, and a great number of bacteria lasted after 24 hours. On the other hand, there was no increasing in bacteria count in the treatment group. After introducing MMC, dLHT was administered orally for five days. Two days after the last administration, spleen cells were removed, and phagocytic cells and lymphocytes were passively transferred into recipient mice whose bone marrows were inhibited. MRSA was injected into the peritoneal cavity of the mice thereafter, and the survival rate was observed. After two weeks, all the mice which were injected with phagocytes survived longer, but the survival rate in the group that were injected with lymphocytes was only 40% (**Figure 1**).

#### 2.2.1. Survey of White Blood Cell after dLHT Administration

The bone marrow suppressed mice were administered herbal decoction dLHT 1 g/kg dairy for 5 times and after 2 weeks later, their blood were withdrawn from their tail vain. Then, leukocytes were counted the using Bürker-Türk solution.

#### 2.2.2. Survey of Leukocyte Subsets after dLHT Administration

The bone marrow suppressed mice were administered herbal decoction dLHT 1 g/kg dairy for 5 days, and after 2 weeks, their blood was withdrawn from their tail vain. Then, granulocytes and lymphocytes were counted using Bürker-Türk solution.

#### 2.2.3. Survey of Macrophage Activity, Migration after dLHT Administration

Cells of peritoneal exudates were collect from the peritoneal cavity of bone marrow. The cell suspension was purified by adherent technique for phagocyte, which resulted in over 95% of cells being phagocytes. The purified cells were adjusted to $1 \times 10^4$ cell/ml and loaded at the upper chamber of Boyden chamber for test migration. Human serum was incubated at 56˚C for 30 min for the chemotactic agent for mouse phagocyte [19]-[22].

#### 2.2.4. Macrophage Activity, Phagocytosis

The same cells suspension was purified by adherent technique for phagocyte, which resulted in over 95% of cells being phagocytes. The purified cells were adjusted to $1 \times 10^4$ cell/cm$^2$ and mixed with latex beads which are 5 μm in granule with fluorescence isochianate. After 90 min of incubation, the remained granules were washed out from the glass slide and counting was done automatically by ACAS system, which made digital presentation, to evaluate phagocytic cell in number and their ability to catch up the latex beads (Adherent Cell Activity Evaluating System, Shimazu, Kyoto, Japan).

#### 2.2.5. Recovery of Macrophage Activity, Target Cell Killing

The same phagocytes suspension was purified by adherent technique for phagocyte, which resulted in over 95%

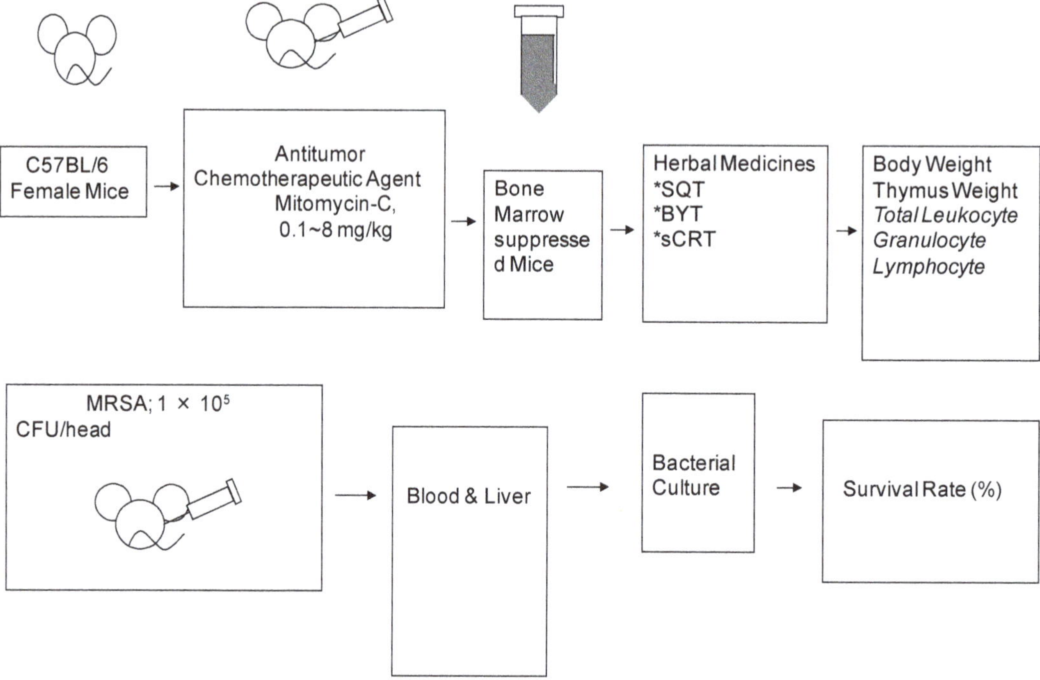


**Figure 1.** Experimental design was dialoged in the figure. 8-week-old C57BL/6 female mice were prepared as experimentally bone marrow suppressed animals. Herbal decoctions dLHT (500 mg/kg/day) were administered just after MMC injection. After one month later of TCM administration, each group of mice were server for each experiment. For the infectious experiment, the mice were challenged with $1 \times 10^6$ of MRSA via peritoneal. Then the number of MRSA in the organ and survival rate were followed up to two weeks.

of cells being phagocytes. The purified cells were adjusted to $1 \times 10^5$ cell/ml and the macrophage migration, the phagocytic activity, and the bactericidal activity were examined by the Boyden chamber method, by the phagocytosis of sheep blood cells, and by the nitroblue tetrazolium (NBT) reduction test [23]-[27].

## 2.3. Recovery of Lymphocyte Activity, Antibody Secreting Cell

The bone marrow suppressed mice were administered herbal decoction dLHT and BYT 8 g/kg dairy for 10 times. After 2 weeks, mice were immunized with sheep red blood cells, ($2 \times 10^8$/mouse) intraperitoneally. Five days later, their spleen cells were collected and plague-forming cells (PFC) were develop and tested the ability of IgM and IgG antibody production using the method reported by Jerne and Nordin [28] [29].

## 2.4. Effects on Drug Sensitivity

So as to test the effect of herbal decoction dLHT on the drug sensitivities of multi-drug-resistant bacteria, dLHT were directory co-cultured with the each bacterium. The strains of clinical origin were *H. influluenzae* I-105, *H. influluenzae* I-147, *E. coli* ML 4901/Rms212, *E. coli* ML 4901/Rms213, *E. coli* ML 4901/Rte16, *E. coli* ML. 4901/Rms149, and *P. aeruginosa* PAO0214/pMG26. Each bacterium was co-cultured with either 3 mg/ml or 30 mg/ml of dLHT. The bacteria were co-cultured with or without dLHT and amino benzylpenicillin. After 120 min of culture at 37°C, remained ABPC were estimated.

## 2.5. Experimental Infection by MRSA

Eight-week-old male C57BL/6J mice were injected with MMC at a dosage of 5 mg/kg to inhibit the bone marrow, thus creating a mouse model with the reduced immunopotential. The decoction of dLHT was administered orally at a dosage of 1 g/kg/day for five consecutive days, with or without a intraperitoneal injection of vancomycin (10 mg/kg) per day in the combined group for herbal medicine and antibiotics. For the infection of MRSA, $5 \times 10^8$ CFU were injected intraperitoneally, and their survival were followed up for 4 weeks.

#### 2.5.1. Kinetics of Intra-Organ Number of Bacteria

Eight-week-old male C57BL/6J mice were injected with MMC at a dosage of 5 mg/kg to inhibit the bone marrow, thus creating a mouse model with the reduced immunopotential. The decoction of dLHT was administered orally at a dosage of 500 mg/kg/day for five consecutive days, and 10 mg/kg of vancomycin was injected intraperitoneally once a day in the combined-treatment group for herbal medicine and antibiotics. To induce the infection of MRSA, $1 \times 10^9$ or $5 \times 10^8$ cells were injected intraperitoneally. Each 5 days, mice were sacrificed to check the intra-bacterial number/bacterial clearance. Their blood and liver were harvested to test the number of bacteria. For this experiment, their liver was homogenized by Teflon homogenizer at 100 rpm/one minute in the ice chilled basket. Then cultured by agar plate made by BHI medium (Nissui Co Ltd., Tokyo).

#### 2.5.2. Kinetics of Survival Curb in Mice

After preparing reduced immunopotential mice model, the decoction of dLHT was administered orally at a dosage of 500 mg/kg/day for five consecutive days, and 10 days later their phagocyte and lymphocyte were separated. Then they were intraperitoneally challenged with $5 \times 10^8$ cells of MRSA. The survival was followed up for 4 weeks.

#### 2.5.3. Adoptive Transfer Experiment for Identify the Critical Cell for Augment against MRSA Infection

The immune-suppressed C57BL/6J mice were administered the extract of dLHT orally at a dosage of 500 mg/kg/day for five consecutive days. Ten days later their phagocyte and lymphocyte were separated. Then the mice were adoptively injected either phagocyte or lymphocyte ($1 \times 10^5$ cell/ head). Then they were challenged with MRSA, $5 \times 10^8$ cells intraperitoneally, and their survival was followed up to 4 weeks.

### 2.6. Statistical Analysis

Data are expressed as means ± standard deviations. The association between the baseline and changes after the treatment of hemopoitic formula were analyzed in each individual using a one-tailed analysis of variance. A $P$ value less than 0.05 was considered to be statistically significant.

### 2.7. Clinical Trial in Infection Control Bed Side

Six elderly MRSA-infected patients, whose age ranged from 78 to 91 years, were selected and provided written informed consent. This clinical trial was approved by ethics committee in Kanazawa Medical University. Four patients were administered orally with an extract of dLHT at a dosage of 5.25 g/day. The clinical findings and laboratory results were observed continuously. Blood test and bacterial check were routine for inpatients in Kanazawa Medical University Hospital.

## 3. Results

### 3.1. Recovery of White Blood Cell by dLHT

The peripheral blood leukocytes were reduced to 20% in bone marrow-suppressed mice two weeks after MMC injection. The leukocyte count recovered to 57.1% of baseline in the dLHT group, 14 days after administration of the herbal decoction of dLHT at a dose of 1 g/kg/day for 5 days (**Figure 2**).

### 3.2. Recovery of Leukocyte Subsets

The bone marrow-suppressed mice were administered herbal decoction dLHT 1 g/kg/day for 10 days. One week later, levels of lymphocyte, granulocyte, and monocyte in the peripheral blood from the tail vein were counted using flow cytometry. MMC, at a dosage of 5 mg/kg, decreased the level of granulocyte. However, administered herbal decoction dLHT recover the leukocyte proportion almost to the level of normal control (**Table 1**).

#### 3.2.1. Recovery of Macrophage Activity, Migration

The bone marrow-suppressed mice were administered herbal decoction of dLHT at 1 g/kg/day for 5 days, and 1 week later, cells in peritoneal exudates were collected from peritoneal cavity. The cell suspension was purified

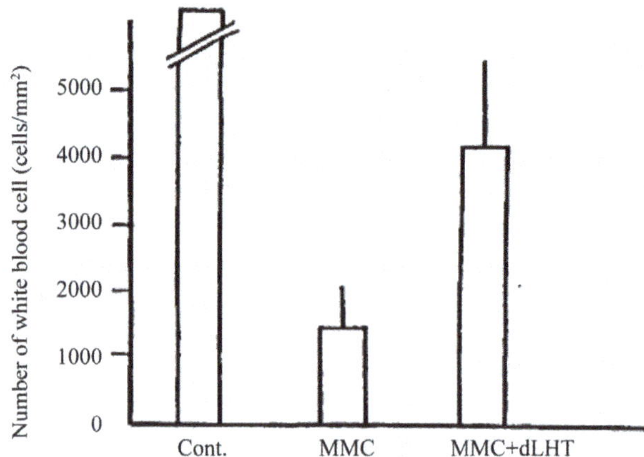


**Figure 2.** The capacity of dLHT on total white blood cell recovery. After the dLHT administration for 2 weeks. the peripheral blood were collected from the tail vain and counted by Bűrkel-Tűrk counter. Data are expressed as the means ± SE. $^*P < 0.01$, MMC versus MMC + dLHT group.

**Table 1.** Flow cytometric analysis of white blood cell subsets in mice.

| | Control[a] | MMC[b] | MMC + dLHT[C] |
|---|---|---|---|
| Lymphocyte | 58.9 | 65.0 | 54.5 |
| Granulocyte | 2.6 | 0.5 | 2.2 |
| Monocyte | 4.9 | 6.4 | 5.8(%) |

[a]Normal mice; [b]MitomycinC (MMC)-treated mice; [c]MMC-treated mice with dLHT administration.

by adherent technique for phagocyte, which resulted in over 95% of cells being phagocytes. The purified cells were adjusted to $1 \times 10^6$ cell/ml and loaded at the upper chamber of Boyden chamber for test migration. Human serum that has been treated at 56°C for 30 min was used as the chemotactic agent for mouse phagocytes. MMC treatment brought depression of migration activity ($P < 0.05$), while dLHT administration increase their migration to 90% as compared to the normal control (**Figure 3**).

### 3.2.2. Recovery of Macrophage Activity, Phagocytosis by dLHT

The cell suspension was purified by adherent technique for phagocyte, which resulted in over 95% of cells being phagocytes. The purified cells were adjusted to $1 \times 10^4$ cell/cm$^2$ and mixed with latex beads 5um in granule with fluorescence isocyanate. After incubated for 90 minutes, remained granule were washed out from the glass slide and counting automatically by ACAS system. The phagocytic activity of MMC-treated mice was clearly depressed both in number and function (**Figures 4(a)-(d)**).

### 3.2.3. Recovery of Macrophage Activity, Killing

The bone marrow suppressed mice were administered herbal decoction dLHT 1 g/kg/day for 10 days. One week later, cells in peritoneal exudates were collected from the peritoneal cavity. The cell suspension was purified by adherent technique for phagocyte, which resulted in over 95% of cells being phagocytes. The purified cells were adjusted to $1 \times 10^6$ cell/ml to perform the nitroblue tetrazolium (NBT) reduction test. Activity of macrophage was decreased significantly in MMC-treated mice, whereas, dHLT treatment recovered their activity to normal level (**Figure 5**).

## 3.3. Recovery of Lymphocyte Activity, Antibody Secreting Cell

The bone marrow suppressed mice were administered herbal decoction dLHT and BYT 8 g/kg/day for 10 days

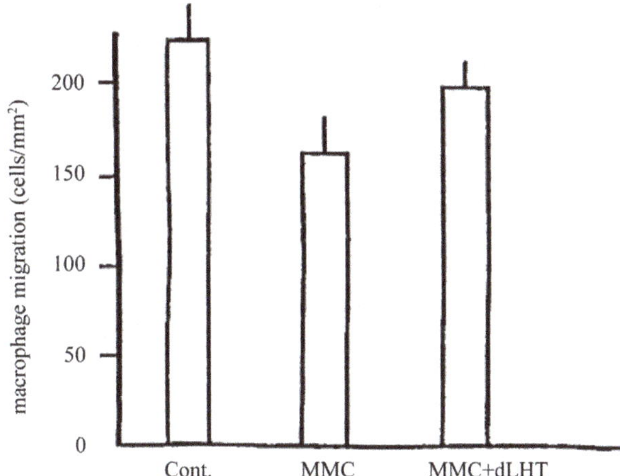


**Figure 3.** The effect on macrophage migration by dLHT after administrating MMC. The procedure of treatment was the same as in **Figure 2**. The macrophage migration capacity was detected by millipore membrane method separated by 0.25 μm in diameter. Data are expressed as the means ± SE. $^*P < 0.05$, MMC versus MMC + dLHT group.

as positive control. Two weeks later, mice were immunized with sheep red blood cells ($2 \times 10^8$/mouse) intraperitoneally. Four and six days later, their plague-forming cells (PFC) were developed and antibody producing ability for IgM and IgG was tested by the method reported by Jerne and Nordin [28] [29]. In this mice system, MMC did not reduced the antibody forming cell in statically significant level. The tendency was the same as shown in the former section (**Figure 6**).

## 3.4. Effects on Drug Sensitivity

So as to test the effect of herbal decoction dHLT on the drug sensitivities of multidrug-sensitive bacteria MRSA, dHLT were directory co-cultured with the bacteria. The strains of clinical origin were *H. influluenzae* I-105, *H. influluenzae* I-147, *E. coli* ML 4901/Rms212, *E. coli* ML 4901/Rms213, *E. coli* ML 4901/Rte16, *E. coli* ML 4901/Rms149, *P. aeruginosa* PAO0214/pMG26. Each bacterium was co-cultured with either 3 mg/ml or 30 mg/ml with dLHT in the presence of amino benzyl penicillin. After the co-culture with herbal decoction, and multi-resistant bacterial strains turned to sensitive at least for amino benzyle penicillin. Moreover, the relative inhibition was dose-dependent to the concentration of dLHT (**Table 2**).

### 3.4.1. Effects of dLHT on Survival Rate in MRSA-Infected Mice

The infection experiment was designed to integrate with the above results, exhibiting the augmentation of each component of host defense factors. Eight-week-old male C57BL/6J mice were injected with MMC at a dosage of 5 mg/kg to inhibit the bone marrow, thus a mouse model with the reduced immunopotential was created. The decoction of dLHT were administered orally at a dosage of 1g/kg/day for five consecutive days, and 10 mg/kg of vancomycin was injected intraperitoneally once a day for the combined-treatment group of herbal medicine and antibiotics. For the infection of MRSA, $1 \times 10^9$ or $5 \times 10^8$ bacteria were injected intraperitoneally, and their survival were followed up to 4 weeks. **Figure 7** shows that the antibiotics plus dLHT group survived much longer than groups of dLHT alone and antibiotics alone.

### 3.4.2. Adoptive Transfer Experiment for Identify the Critical Point for Augment against MRSA Infection

The total estimation of host augmentation, adoptive transfer experiment was performed to identify the factor of activated site by dLHT. Eight-week-old male C57BL/6J mice were injected with MMC at a dosage of 5 mg/kg to inhibit the bone marrow, to create a mouse model of reduced immunopotential. An extract of dLHT in powder form was administered orally at a dosage of 500 mg/kg/day for five consecutive days. Ten days later their

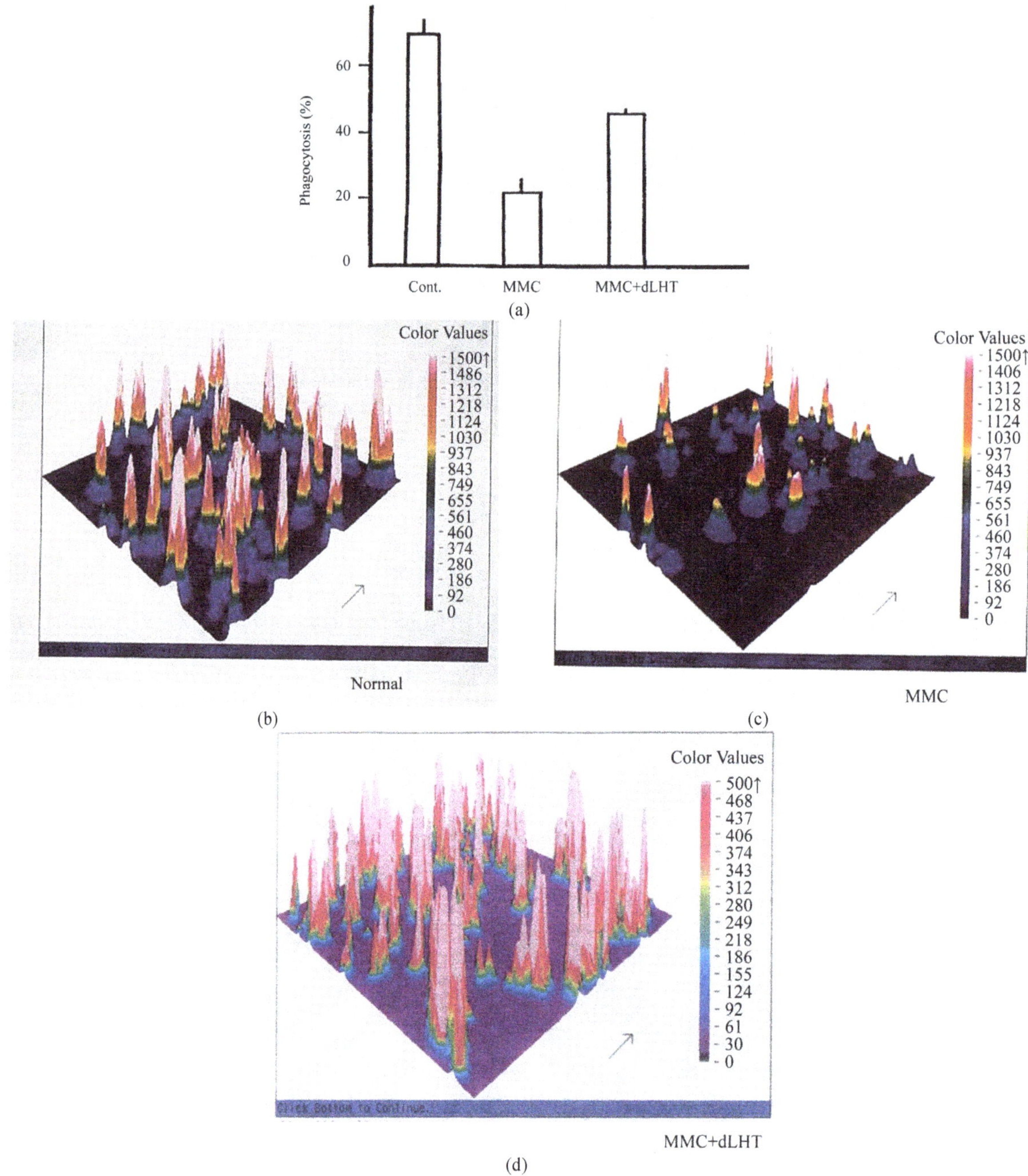


**Figure 4.** (a) A classical presentation of macrophagephagocytosis agaist microorganism by dLHT after administrating MMC. The procedure of treatment was the same in **Figure 2**. The macrophage migration capacity in Normal control was detected by computer analysis, ACAS. Data are expressed as the means ± SE. $^{*}P < 0.01$, MMC versus MMC + dLHT group; (b) CG presentation for the effect on macrophage phagocytosis against latex beads by normal mice. Cells from peritoneal exudates were collect from the peritoneal cavity. The cell suspension was purified by adherent technique for phagocyte, which resulted in over 95% of cells being phagocytes. The purified cells were adjusted to $1 \times 10^4$ cell/ml in the slass slide. The procedure of treatment was the same in **Figure 2**. The macrophage phagocytosis capacity after MMC administration was detected by computer analysis, by ACAS; (c) CG presentation for the effect on macrophage phagocytosis against latex beads after administrating MMC. The procedure of treatment was the same in **Figure 2**. The macrophage migration capacity was detected by computer analysis, ACAS. The data was shown from MMC-treated mice; (d) CG presentation for the effect on macrophage phagocytosis against latex beads by dHLT after administrating MMC. The procedure of treatment was the same in **Figure 2**. The macrophage migration capacity was detected by computer analysis, ACAS. The data was shown from MMC-treated and dLHLT rescued mice.

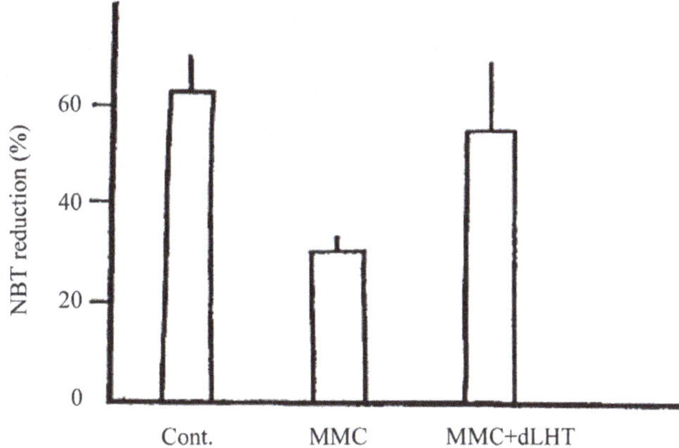


**Figure 5.** The effect on macrophage killing activity revealed with NBT reduction test by dHLT after administrating MMC. The procedur of treatment was the same in **Figure 2**, except that the killing activity was detected by Nitro-blue Tetrazolium. Data are expressed as the means ± SE. $^{*}P < 0.001$, MMC versus MMC + dLHT group.

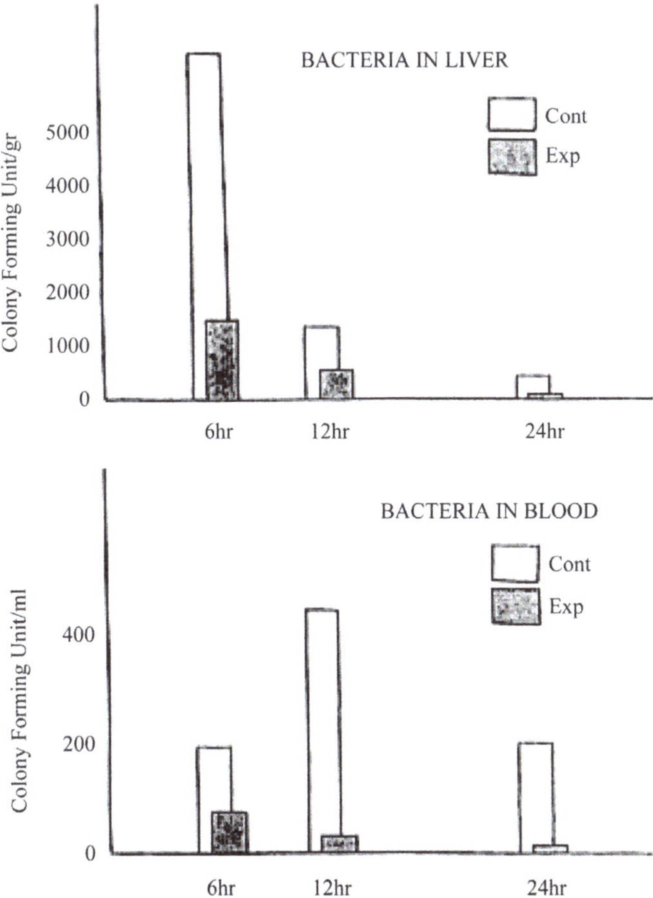


**Figure 6.** The infection test was tried to express number of micro organisms in each lymphoid organ. The number of MRSA counting in the organ that experimentally infected by $5 \times 10^6$ of microorganisms. Data are expressed as the means ± SE. $^{*}P < 0.001$, MMC versus MMC + dLHT group.

**Table 2.** Effect on drug sensitivity by dHLT to multi & high dose resistant clinical strain of bacteria.

| Enzyme | Class | % Inhibition of penicillinase | | | | | |
|---|---|---|---|---|---|---|---|
| | | dHLT (mg/ml) | | SQT (mg/ml) | | BYT (mg/ml) | |
| | | 30 | 3 | 30 | 3 | 30 | 3 |
| *H. influenza* I -105 | * | 83.5 ± 11.3** | 3.9 ± 1.6 | 94.7 ± 5.7 | 1.5 ± 1.4 | 20.1 ± 3.2 | - |
| *H. influenza* I -147 | * | 24.9 ± 5.4 | -*** | 57.7 ± 7.4 | - | - | - |
| *E. coil* ML4901/Rms212 | Type I | 30 ± 12 | 11 ± 6 | 107 ± 9 | 13 ± 3 | 29 ± 8 | 11 ± 4 |
| *E. coil* ML4901/Rms213 | Type II | 85 ± 7 | - | 100 ± 24 | 31 ± 10 | 104 ± 8 | - |
| *E. coil* ML4901/Rte16 | Type III | 73 ± 9 | 5 ± 3 | 97 ± 27 | 34 ± 9 | 100 ± 9 | 4 ± 3 |
| *E. coil* ML4901/Rms149 | Type IV | 40 ± 9 | - | 94 ± 32 | - | 59 ± 13 | - |
| *P. aeruginosa* PAO2142RP$^r$/Pmg26 | * | 104 ± 3 | 13 ± 3 | 103 ± 12 | 47 ± 5 | 103 ± 18 | 5 ± 4 |

*Not classified; **Results are an arithmetic mean from three determinations ± standard deviation; ***Not inhibited.

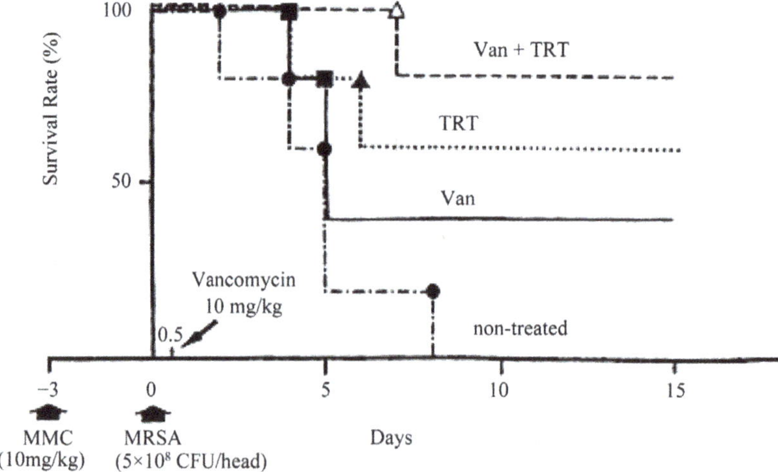


**Figure 7.** The experimental infection test. The test were performed by the mice divided into 4 group. The groups were consisted by normal, MMC-treated, MMC-treated + dHLT, MMC-treated + dLHT plus chemotherapeutic agency vancomycin. Each survival was followed up to six week.

phagocyte and lymphocyte were separated. Then the mice were adoptively injected either phagocyte or lymphocyte ($1 \times 10^5$ cell/ head). Then they were challenged intraperitoneally with $5 \times 10^8$ cells of MRSA. Their survival was followed up until the fourth week. The survival rate of the group that was transferred with phagocytic cell was kept 100% during the two weeks after MRSA challenge. After the administration of dLHT, the number of white blood cells in MMC-treated mice was increase to 80% of that of the control group. In addition, the relative phagocytic activity of macrophages increased to 50% of that of the control group, while that of non-treated group was only 20% (**Figure 8**). The bactericidal activity also recovered to the level close to the normal value The ratio in neutrophils in dLHT administered MMC-treated group increased to 2.2% (normal mice, 2.6%), whereas that in MMC-treated group was only 0.5%. The bacteria count in the liver of MRSA-challenged mice with and without dLHT administration peaked six hours after the challenge. However, the number of bacteria in the group with dLHT administration was much greater than that of the group without dLHT administration. The bacteria count in the blood showed an increase at the 12th and 24th hours after the challenge. Even 24 hours after MRSA challenge, a significant number of bacteria remained in the blood of the group without dLHT administration, whereas only a small number of cells were detected 6 hours after the challenge, and the bacterial number was gradually decreased thereafter in the group of dLHT administration (**Figure 8**). MRSA-challenged MMC-treated mice were treated by dLHT, vancomycin, or dLHT combined with vancomycin. All of the non-treated mice died eight days after the MRSA challenge, whereas the survival rates in the dLHT group was 60%,

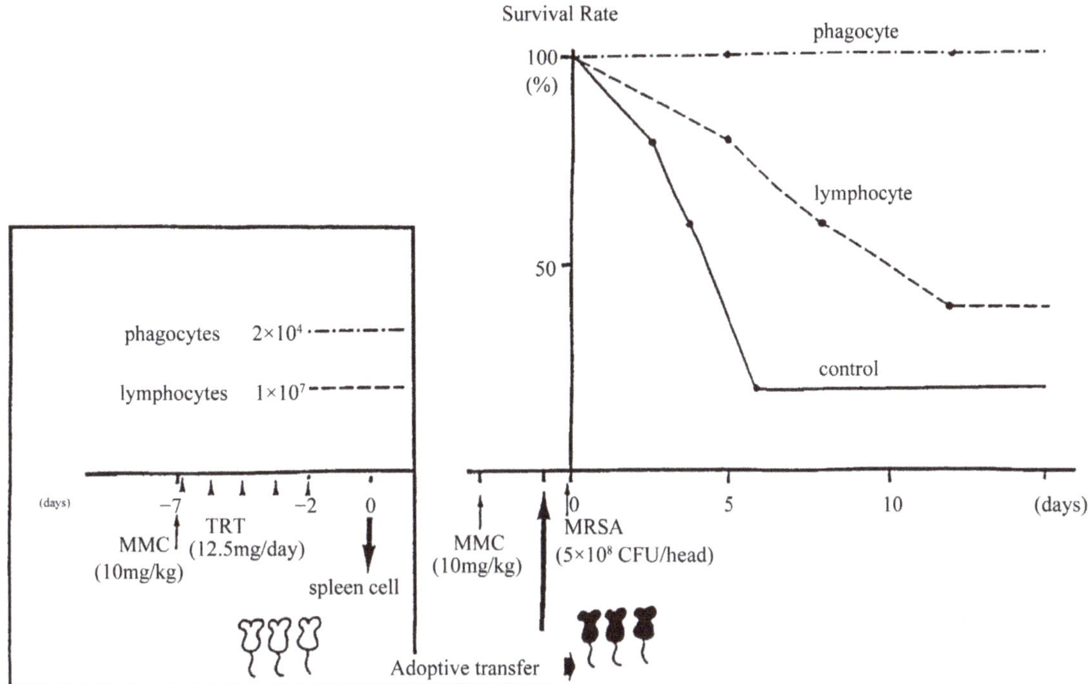


**Figure 8.** The adoptive transfer of leukocyte sublet. The leukocyte from MMC treated and dLHT administered mice were separated granulocyte and lymphocyte. One week later, 5 × $10^5$ MRSA were challenged and followed up their survival rate.

that of vancomycin group was 40%, and that of dLHT and vancomycin-combined group was 80% (**Figure 8**). All of dLHT administered MMC-treated mice, to which the phagocytic cells prepared from MMC-treated mice with dLHT administration had adoptively been transferred, survived after the MRSA challenge. On the other hand, the survival rate of MMC-treated mice, to which the lymphocytes prepared from the same mice had adoptively been transferred, was 40% (**Figure 8**).

## 4. Clinical Trial in Infection Control in Bed Side

Six patients were recruited for this trial. They were inpatient in substantially infection control bed from outpatient for their nosocomial infection by MRSA. The original focuses were atrial attack and cerebral bleeding by hypertension and low value of serum albumin. Two of the same type of patients attended as control for the disagreement by their family. There were no new antibiotics in the commercial base for hospital, selecting the augmentation of host defense immunity. We selected four candidate herbalmedicines that augment blood cells in number and functions in previous studies. Based on the research in the MMC-generated immunocompromised host, dHLT is the best herbal medicine for both augmentation of host immune factors and increased sensitivity of MRSA to antibiotics. All four cases with dLHT treatment showed culture results of MRSA negative after the dLHT administration. The MRSA culture became negative within 50 days after the initial administration in four of the six subjects (**Figure 9**). In the control group, one case needed more than 100 days to become MRSA-negative and another died from the infection (**Figure 10**). One representative case is a 78-year-old woman suffering from hypertension, atrial fibrillation, and cerebral bleeding in the right occipital lobe. During the antibiotic therapy for *Streptococcus pneumoniae*, MRSA appeared. The antibiotic therapy was halted and the dLHT administration started. The culture result became negative in three weeks after the dLHT treatment. In addition, serum protein and albumin values also returned to the values that they had had before the infection of MRSA (**Figure 9** and **Figure 10**).

## 5. Discussion

When dLHT was administered orally in mouse models whose immunopotential had been inhibited, the herbal

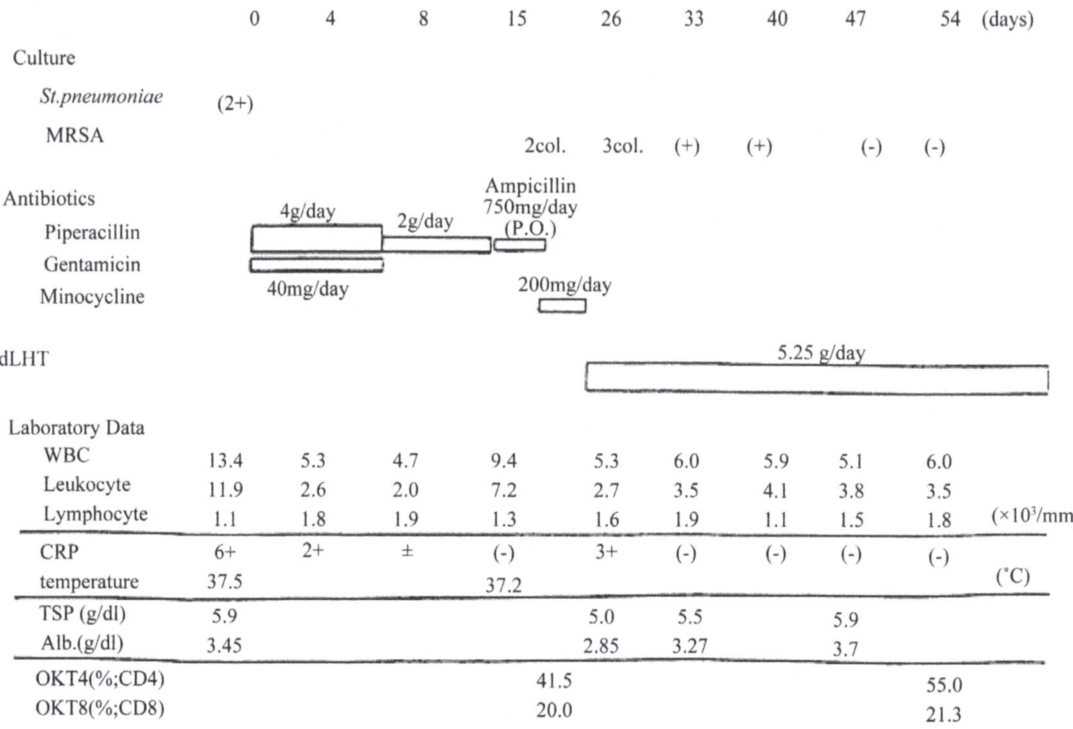

0 4 8 15 26 33 40 47 54 (days)
Culture
St.pneumoniae (2+)
MRSA 2col. 3col. (+) (+) (-) (-)
Antibiotics
Piperacillin 4g/day 2g/day
Ampicillin 750mg/day (P.O.)
Gentamicin 40mg/day
Minocycline 200mg/day
dLHT 5.25 g/day
Laboratory Data
WBC 13.4 5.3 4.7 9.4 5.3 6.0 5.9 5.1 6.0
Leukocyte 11.9 2.6 2.0 7.2 2.7 3.5 4.1 3.8 3.5
Lymphocyte 1.1 1.8 1.9 1.3 1.6 1.9 1.1 1.5 1.8 (×10³/mm)
CRP 6+ 2+ ± (-) 3+ (-) (-) (-) (-)
temperature 37.5 37.2 (°C)
TSP (g/dl) 5.9 5.0 5.5 5.9
Alb.(g/dl) 3.45 2.85 3.27 3.7
OKT4(%;CD4) 41.5 55.0
OKT8(%;CD8) 20.0 21.3


**Figure 9.** Human bed side test. The trial was done for stroke and/or heart infarction patient after informed and consented. Trial schedule and chemical data were show in the figure. The herbal decoction, 8 g/head of dLHT was administered daily for at least one month. Then MRSA were chased by collecting sputa from the patient. The blood chemical data were shown in the figure.

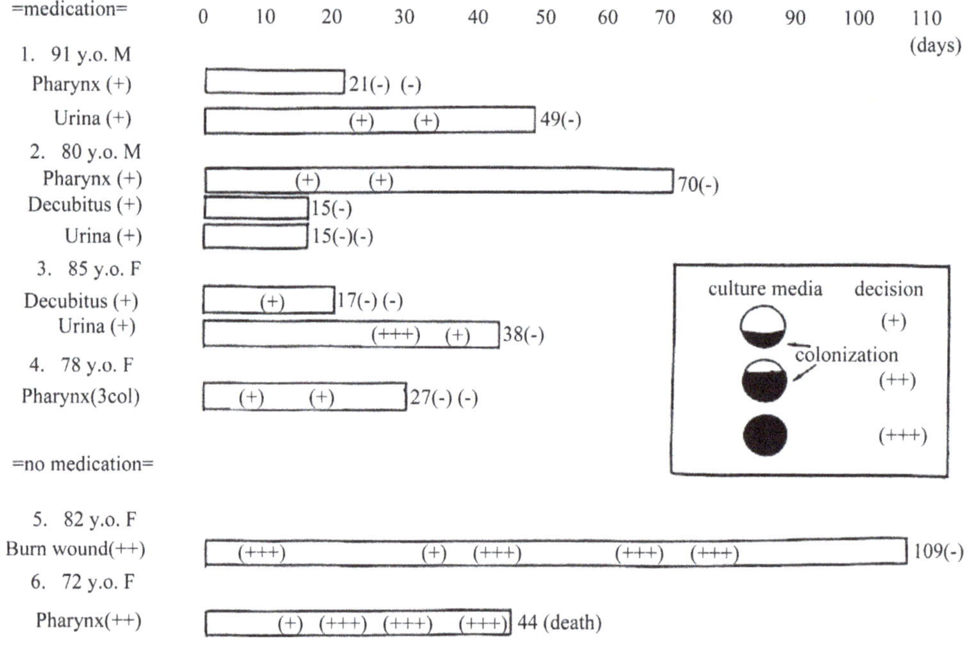


**Figure 10.** Time course presentation of MRSA from the sanple of patient. Human bed side test was done for the patient who were suffering heat infarction positive with administrating dLHT. The herbal decoction, 8 g/head of dLHT was administered daily for at least one month. Then MRSA were chased by collecting sputa from the patient. The MRSA containing from the patient sample were shown in the figure.

medicine activated the phagocytes both quantitatively and qualitatively, indicating dLHT to be an effective interstitial medicine [29]-[34]. In addition, based on the data from both the animal models and the clinical trial, no side effects were observed, confirming the complete efficacy of the drug. Of late, as we move towards a society with a high percentage of elderly people, the authors speculate that this Chinese herbal medicine which activates the immunopotential would be very helpful in the treatment of opportunistic infections that are commonly seen among the elder patients in the developed countries [35]-[40].

At the time of this clinical trial, vancomycin was not commercially available, so there were no suitable antibiotics for MRSA patients. Thereafter, vancomysin was purchased from markets with governmental approval. However, bacteria which are resistant against new drug might emerge after several years' use. So the trial to host immune defense enhanced by herbal decoction is important for infections of microorganisms.

This study selected dLHT because this formula was composed of several single herbs, which possessed the effects of augmentation of blood cell number and function. In a famous China textbook for herbal formulae in Qin Dynasty, the only descriptive is found stating that dLHT is effective for fever. Therefore, this formula is minor, not listed up in Japanese authorized herbal formulae for government.

From a pharmaceutical stand point of view, dLHT is composed with several anti-septic harbs, supposing the effect of dLHT for infection came from anti-septic effect. So we tried to compare dLHT, BYT and SDT against clinical derived MRSA *in vitro* agar plate. However, dLHT was not significantly effective for direct anti-septic effect for MRSA. So we conclude our result that, dLHT affects host immune activity especially for macrophage phagocytosis for this MRSA infection system.

In a simultaneous report, we tried to identify some herbal formulae which could augment blood cells in number and function in Shi-Quan-Da-Bu-Tang and Bu-Zong-Ye-Qi-Tang. dLHT exhibited has a similar character with Shi-Quan-Da-Bu-Tang, which also augments granulocyte/phagocyte.

Abo pointed out that he could differentiate granulocyte rich type from lymphocyte rich type according to the constitution. He reported that gentleman sorted out for G-rich type; on the other hand, ladies are lymphocyte rich type in the same. Within the gentleman G-rich type turned to L-rich-type at the senile. So in general, young people are recommended to employ Bu-Zong-Ye-Qi-Tang. On the other hand, senile is good for Shi-Quan-Da-Bu-Tang [36]-[41].

## References


[1] Kurashige, S., Yoshida, T. and Mitsuhashi, S. (1980) Immune Responsein Sarcoma 10-Bearing Mice. *Annual Report of Gunnma University*, **1**, 36-44.

[2] Miyazaki, S. (1977) Immunodificiency in Clinical Origin. *Clinical Pediatrics*, 1001-1006.

[3] Kishida, K., Miyazaku, S., Take, H., Fujimoto, T., Shi, H., Sasaki, K. and Goya, N. (1978) Granial Irradiation and Lymphocyte Subpopulation in Acute Lymphatic Leukemia. *Journal of Pediatrics*, **92**, 785-786. http://dx.doi.org/10.1016/S0022-3476(78)80155-3

[4] Yamaguchi, N., Takei, T., Chen, R., Wushuer, P. and Wu, W.H. (2013) Maternal Bias of Immunity to Her Offspring: Possibility of an Autoimmunity Twist out from Maternal Immunity to Her Young. *Open Journal of Rheumatology and Autoimmune Diseases*, **3**, 40-55. http://dx.doi.org/10.4236/ojra.2013.31008

[5] Murgita, R.A. and Tomasi Jr., T.B. (1975) Suppression of the Immune Response by Alpha-Fetoprotein. *The Journal of Experimental Medicine*, **141**, 269-286. http://dx.doi.org/10.1084/jem.141.2.269

[6] Paul, G., Margaret, S., Liew, Y.F. and Allan, M.M. (1995) CD4+ but Not CD8+ T Cells Are Required for the Induction of Oral Tolerance. *International Immunology*, **7**, 501-504. http://dx.doi.org/10.1093/intimm/7.3.501

[7] Koshimo, H., Miyazawa, H.Y., Shimizu, Y. and Yamaguchi, N. (1989) Maternal Antigenic Stimulation Actively Produces Suppressor Activity in Offspring. *Developmental & Comparative Immunology*, **13**, 79-85. http://dx.doi.org/10.1016/0145-305X(89)90020-7

[8] Zoeller, M. (1988) Tolerization during Pregnancy: Impact on the Development of Antigen-Specific Help and Suppression. *European Journal of Immunology*, **18**, 1937-1943. http://dx.doi.org/10.1002/eji.1830181211

[9] Shinka, S., Dohi, Y., Komatsu, T., Natarajan, R. and Amano, T. (1974) Immunological Unresponsiveness in Mice. I. Immunological Unresponsiveness Induced in Embryonic Mice by Maternofetal Transfer of Human-Globulin. *Biken Journal*, **17**, 59-72.

[10] Aase, J.M., Noren, G.R., D.V. Reddy, and Geme Jr., J.W. (1972) Mumps-Virus Infection in Pregnant Women and the Immunologic Response of Their Offspring. *The New England Journal of Medicine*, **286**, 1379-1382. http://dx.doi.org/10.1056/NEJM197206292862603

[11] Wang, X.X., Kitada, Y., Matsui, K., Ohkawa, S., Sugiyama, T., Kohno, H., Shimizu, S., Lai, J.E., Matsuno, H. and Yamaguchi, N. (1999) Variation of Cell Populations Taking Charge of Immunity in Human Peripheral Blood Following Hot Spring Hydrotherapy Quantitative Discussion. *The Journal of Japanese Association of Physical Medicine, Balneology and Climatology*, **62**, 129-134.

[12] Matsuno, H., Wang, X.X., Wan, W., Matsui, K., Okawa, S., Sugiyama, T., Kohno, H., Shimizu, S., Lai, J.E. and Yamaguchi, N. (1999) Variation of Cell Populations Taking Charge of Immunity in Human Peripheral Blood Following Hot Spring Hydrotherapy Qualitative Discussion. *The Journal of Japanese Association of Physical Medicine, Balneology and Climatology*, **62**, 135-140.

[13] Yamaguchi, N., Hashimoto, H., Arai, M., Takada, S., Kawada, N., Taru, A., Li, A.L., Izumi, H. and Sugiyama, K. (2002) Effect of Acupuncture on Leukocyte and Lymphocyte Subpopulation in Human Peripheral Blood-Quantitative Discussion. *The Journal of Japanese Association of Physical Medicine, Balneology and Climatology*, **65**, 199-206.

[14] Wan, W., Li, A.L., Izumi, H., Kawada, N., Arai, M., Takada, A., Taru, A., Hashimoto, H. and Yamaguchi, N. (2002) Effect of Acupuncture on Leukocyte and Lymphocyte Subpopulation in Human Peripheral Blood Qualitative Discussion. *The Journal of Japanese Association of Physical Medicine, Balneology and Climatology*, **65**, 207-211.

[15] Wang, X.X., Katoh, S. and Liu, B.X. (1998) Effect of Physical Exercise on Leukocyte and Lymphocyte Subpopulations in Human Peripheral Blood. *Cytometry Research*, **8**, 53-61.

[16] Kitada, Y., Wan, W., Matsui, K., Shimizu, S. and Yamaguchi, N. (2000) Regulation of Peripheral White Blood Cells in Numbers and Functions through Hot-Spring Bathing during a Short Term Studies in Control Experiments. *Journal of the Japanese Society of Balneology, Climatology and Physical Medicine*, **63**, 151-164.

[17] Yamaguchi, N., Takahashi, T., Sugita, T., Ichikawa, K., Sakaihara, S., Kanda, T., Arai, M. and Kawakita, K. (2007) Acupuncture Regulates Leukocyte Subpopulations in Human Peripheral Blood. *Evidence-Based Complementary and Alternative Medicine*, **4**, 447-453.

[18] Yamaguchi, N., Shimizu, S. and Izumi, H. (2004) Hydrotherapy Can Modulate Peripheral Leukocytes: An Approach to Alternative Medicine. In: *Complementary and Alternative Approaches to Biomedicine*, Kluwer Academic/Plenum Publishers, New York, 239-251. http://dx.doi.org/10.1007/978-1-4757-4820-8_18

[19] Gorantla, S., Dou, H., Boska, M., Destache, C.J., Nelson, J., Poluektova, L., Rabinow, B.E., Gendelman, H.E. and Mosley, R.L. (2006) Quantitative Magnetic Resonance and SPECT Imaging for Macrophage Tissue Migration and Nanoformulated Drug Delivery. *Journal of Leukocyte Biology*, **80**, 1165-1174. http://dx.doi.org/10.1189/jlb.0206110

[20] Stoika, R.S., Lutsik, M.D., Barska, M.L., Tsyrulnyk, A.A. and Kashchak, N.I. (2002) *In Vitro* Studies of Activation of Phagocytic Cells by Bioactive Peptides. *Journal of Physiology and Pharmacology*, **53**, 675-688.

[21] Elbim, C., Pillet, S., Prevost, M.H., Preira, A., Girard, P.M., Rogine, N., Hakim, J., Israel, N. and Gougerot-Pocidalo, M.A. (2001) The Role of Phagocytes in HIV-Related Oxidative Stress. *Journal of Clinical Virology*, **20**, 99-109. http://dx.doi.org/10.1016/S1386-6532(00)00133-5

[22] Speer, C.P., Gahr, M. and Pabst, M.J. (1986) Phagocytosis-Associated Oxidative Metabolism in Human Milk Macrophages. *Acta Paediatrica*, **75**, 444-451. http://dx.doi.org/10.1111/j.1651-2227.1986.tb10228.x

[23] Waitzberg, D.L., Bellinati-Pires, R., Salgado, M.M., Hypolito, I.P., Colleto, G.M., Yagi, O., Yamamuro, E.M., Gama-Rodrigues, J. and Pinotti, H.W. (1997) Effect of Total Parenteral Nutrition with Different Lipid Emulsions on Human Monocyte and Neutrophil Functions. *Nutrition*, **13**, 128-132. http://dx.doi.org/10.1016/S0899-9007(96)00386-3

[24] Kaplan, S.S., Basford, R.E., Jeong, M.H. and Simmons, R.L. (1996) Biomaterial-Neutrophil Interactions: Dysregulation of Oxidative Functions of Fresh Neutrophils Induced by Prior Neutrophil-Biomaterial Interaction. *Journal of Biomedical Materials Research*, **30**, 67-75. http://dx.doi.org/10.1002/(SICI)1097-4636(199601)30:1<67::AID-JBM9>3.0.CO;2-P

[25] Cohen, M.S., Britigan, B.E., Chai, Y.S., Pou, S., Roeder, T.L. and Rosen, G.M. (1991) Phagocyte-Derived Free Radicals Stimulated by Ingestion of Iron-Rich *Staphylococcus aureus*: A Spin-Trapping Study. *Journal of Infectious Diseases*, **163**, 819-824. http://dx.doi.org/10.1093/infdis/163.4.819

[26] Mege, J.L., Martin, C., Saux, P., Charrel, J., Mallet, M.N. and Bongrand, P. (1989) Phagocyte-Pathogen in the Infected Host. *Critical Care Medicine*, **17**, 1247-1253.

[27] Root, R.K., Rosenthal, A.S. and Balestra, D.J. (1972) Abnormal Bactericidal, Metabolic, and Lysosomal Functions of Chediak-Higashi Syndrome Leukocytes. *Journal of Clinical Investigation*, **51**, 649-665. http://dx.doi.org/10.1172/JCI106854

[28] Jerne, N.K. and Nordin, A.A. (1963) Plaque Formation in Agar by Single Antibody Producing Cells. *Science*, **140**, 405.

[29] Jerne, N.K., Nordin, A.A. and Henry, C. (1963) The Agar Technique for Recognizing Antibody Producing Cells. In: Amons, B. and Kaprowski, H., Eds., *Cell-Bound Antibodies*, The Wistar Institute Press, Philadelphia, 109-125.

[30] Shih, C.C., Liao, C.C., Su, Y.C., Tsai, C.C. and Lin, J.G. (2012) Gender Differences in Traditional Chinese Medicine

Use among Adults in Taiwan. *PLoS ONE*, **7**, e32540. http://dx.doi.org/10.1371/journal.pone.0032540

[31] Lin, M.H., Chou, M.Y., Liang, C.K., Peng, L.N. and Chen, L.K. (2010) Population Aging and Its Impacts: Strategies of the Health-Care System in Taipei. *Ageing Research Reviews*, **9**, S23-S27. http://dx.doi.org/10.1016/j.arr.2010.07.004

[32] Lin, Y.H. and Chiu, J.H. (2011) Use of Chinese Medicine by Women with Breast Cancer: A Nationwide Cross-Sectional Study in Taiwan. *Complementary Therapies in Medicine*, **19**, 137-143. http://dx.doi.org/10.1016/j.ctim.2011.04.001

[33] Navo, M.A., Phan, J., Vaughan, C., Lynn Palmer, J., Michaud, L., Jones, K.L., *et al.* (2004) An Assessment of the Utilization of Complementary and Alternative Medication in Women with Gynecologic or Breast Malignancies. *Journal of Clinical Oncology*, **22**, 671-677.

[34] Liao, H.L., Ma, T.C., Chiu, Y.L., Chen, J.T. and Chang, Y.S. (2008) Factors Influencing the Purchasing Behavior of TCM Outpatients in Taiwan. *Journal of Alternative and Complementary Medicine*, **14**, 741-748. http://dx.doi.org/10.1089/acm.2007.7111

[35] Liu, J.P., Yang, H., Xia, Y. and Cardini, F. (2009) Herbal Preparations for Uterine Fibroids. *Cochrane Database of Systematic Reviews*, **2009**, Article ID: 005292. http://dx.doi.org/10.1002/14651858.CD005292.pub2

[36] Abo, T., Kawate, T., Itoh, K. and Kumagai, K. (1981) Studies on the Bioperiodicity of the Immune Response. 1. Circadian Rhythms of Human T, B and K Cell Traffic in the Peripheral Blood. *Journal of Immunology*, **126**, 1360-1363.

[37] Abo, T. and Kumagai, T. (1978) Studies of Surface Immunoglobulins on Human B Lymphocytes. III. Physiological Variations of $SIg^+$ Cells in Peripheral Blood. *Clinical & Experimental Immunology*, **33**, 441-452.

[38] Suzuki, S., Toyabe, S., Moroda, T., Tada, T., Tsukahara, A., Iiai, T., *et al.* (1997) Circadian Rhythm of Leukocytes and Lymphocytes Subsets and Its Possible Correlation with the Function of the Autonomic Nervous System. *Clinical & Experimental Immunology*, **110**, 500-508. http://dx.doi.org/10.1046/j.1365-2249.1997.4411460.x

[39] Ignarro, L.J. and Colombo, C. (1973) Enzyme Release from Polymorphonuclear Leukocyte Lysosomes: Regulation by Autonomic Drugs and Cyclic Nucleotides. *Science*, **180**, 1181-1183. http://dx.doi.org/10.1126/science.180.4091.1181

[40] Elenkov, I.J. and Crousos, G.P. (1999) Stress Hormones, Th1/Th2 Patterns, Pro/Anti-Inflammatory Cytokines and Susceptibility to Disease. *Trends in Endocrinology and Metabolism*, **10**, 359-368.

[41] Landmann, R.M.A., Muller, F.B., Perini, C., Wesp, M., Erne, P. and Buhler, F.R. (1984) Changes of Immunoregulatory Cells Induced by Psychological and Physical Stress: Relationship to Plasma Catecholamines. *Clinical & Experimental Immunology*, **58**, 127-135.

## Abbreviations

BYT: Bu-Zong-Ye-Qi-Tang. A famous TCM formula for augment blood cell in number and function.
CAM: Complementary and alternative medicine. Beside the western medicine, there are many traditional medicine and/or health promoting menu all over the world.
CD: Cluster of differentiation. Each lymphocyte has name that expressed CD number, for example CD2, CD4, etc.
PFC: Plague forming cell. Detecting method for antibody producing cell.
SRBC: Sheep red blood cell. Good T-dependent antigen for detecting PFC.
SPC: Spleen cell. Cells from central organ where antibody secreting cells develop.
SDT: Shi-Quan-Da-Bu-Tang. A famous TCM formula for augment blood cell in number and function.
sCRT: Shao-Chin-Rong-Tang. A famous TCM formula for suppressed leukocyte in number and function.

7

# Aspect of QOL Assessment and Proposed New Scale for Evaluation

**Nobuo Yamaguchi[1,2*], Matsuo Arai[2], Tsugiya Murayama[2,3]**

[1]Department of Fundamental Research for CAM, Kanazawa Medical University, Ishikawa, Japan
[2]Ishikawa Natural Medicinal Products Research Center, Ishikawa, Japan
[3]Faculty of Pharmaceutical Sciences, Department of Microbiology and Immunology, Hokuriku University, Ishikawa, Japan
Email: *serumaya@kanazawa-med.ac.jp

## Abstract

**According to the reports from Ministry of Health in each country, the average life span is elongated over the past decade. This trend is expected to be keeping constant further in the future and at the same time continued efforts should be made. Next, it is necessary for us to consent about improving the quality of life. In an effort of improving the quality of life, other than the western medicine, we have attempted to introduce many traditional medical practices, including the oriental medicine, from various parts of the world into the medical field as a complementary & alternative medicine (CAM). Judging both positive and negative aspects by the evaluation standard of the Western medicine, we try to obtain numerical aspects in termed of QOL. Some methods of alternative medicine involved in this review are acupuncture, moxibustion, TCM and other traditional medicine. Above all, WHO suggests selecting the suzerain nation of acupuncture moxibustion, which has been developed in the oriental countries as a specialized cure, by identifying merits & demerits and ascertaining which nation can be a the best model for special field. At the moment for evaluating CAM, for example, what kind of methods is/are suitable for evaluating each CAM. We have been trying to propose the peripheral leukocyte, that is one of the best marker for evaluating CAM. Our trial is a hot spring hydrotherapy, acupuncture and moxibution, light exercise and Ondle/floor heating etc. In these trials, we find the common results from leukocyte effects which exhibit a strong correlation for the regulation in number and function, as a new scale for evaluating QOL. The contents are the result from the data showing the much in number of volunteer tend to down regulate, on the other hand, lower number of volunteer is up-regulated at next day by each menu of CAM as a constitution dependent manner. However, even in western medical methodology, double blind and cross over system are the better way to evaluation even in CAM. The responsibility in human to each CAM therapy is different in individually, so to say according to constitution. In other words, there are so many vectors within the group, including at least three**

*Corresponding author.

**groups, up-regulating, down regulating and stand stilled one. So we have no positive results by the method by sum-up and made mean. According to this system, individual vector is cancelled each other and real effect is not exhibited as a final result. So, we would like to present more smart way to access the efficacy for CAM menu. That is trial to plot each individual effect on the linear function and making slant/co-efficiency that plot each variable vector which is derived from the relative value compared to that of the day before. This procedure is easy to compare between each impact to the volunteer. We would like to propose this evaluation system as Super Constitution System: SCS. This kind of regulation showed within a 24 hours, for the leukocyte subsets, granulocyte and lymphocyte are changed even if they are under control of the circadian rhythm. So, for the purpose of evaluating leukocyte deviation, we set the point for evaluation at the same time-zone from the first set of evaluation to the next time-zone of evaluation. Under these conditions, we get a same result reproductively that the whole number of leukocyte, and its subset, granulocyte and lymphocyte also regulate within a 24 hours. This kind of phenomenon is the case that we confirm a lot of kind of CAM with repetition. This kind of regulation is confirmed in the content of the emotional hormone regulation. Within a hormonal change, adrenalin and dopamine are just under the regulation in the mode of SCS. However, the life span of leukocyte are at lease 3 - 4 days in rapid group of leukocytes, and no such a drastic apoptosis is induced by such a stimulation. For the purpose of scientific explanation, we also propose that the emotional hormone is concerned this change of leukocytes population. For the results of this hypothesis, there are reasonable changes in the peripheral blood about emotional hormone, adrenaline and dopamine. Other hormone concern thyroid grand is not changed significantly. In the final part of this chapter, we also propose that the suitable approach for anti-oxidative assessment and the effective pathway of complement for enabling some historical food supplement activate the whole body cell that expresses a complement receptor. This is not a case of infection but another stage of complement activation by fragmented polysaccharides for historical human use as foods. The protein materials are also fermented and served as digestive food around the world. Almost all the products have some distinctive smell but accompanying some effects through independent digestive rout for intact protein itself. With these aspects, we try to emphasize SCS and discuss by showing evident based manner with various menu of CAM.**

## Keywords

**QOL, Leukocyte Subset, Granulocyte, Lymphocyte, Constitution Dependent Assay System, Double Blind-Cross Over System, Immunological Factors, Emotional Hormone, Adrenalin, Dopamine, Anti-Oxidative Assay by Macrophage, Immunological Factors**

## 1. Introduction

There are two primary systems: innate and adaptive. Despite this defenses system in the overwhelming problems of possessing this dual system, the innate and adoptive do not seem to guard or even prevent the development of one internal threat to survival, However, every individual in the world exposes to the lisk of immunodeficiency in daily life with both internal and externals. The factors that influence the acquired immune activity are systemic metabolic disorder such as diabetes mellitus, malnutrition, extreme exhaustion, stress, aging and medical side effect in cancer [1]-[12]. So we have to select appropriate menu to regulate immune function through leukocyte storage. The menu has been summarized and listed as CAM: complementary and alternative medicine.

In this review, we plan to collect evidence and judge them with the content suggested in the case of eCAM setup. In other words, as a judging standard, setting immunologic factors as main items, we will judge superior and inferior of methods in each country.

Recommending not only quantitatively, but also qualitatively to evaluate "balance of the lymphocyte which is the associate of the white blood corpuscle and the polymorph" as a standard of the alternative medicine.

Every creature in the world including human exposes to the lisk of immunodeficiency in daily life [1]-[10]. The factors that influence the acquired immune activity are systemic metabolic disorder such as diabetes meritus, mal-nutrition, extreme exhaustion and stress, senile and side effect in cancer. So we have to select a daily appropriate menu to regulate immune function through leukocyte storage. The menu has been summarized and listed as CAM: complementary and alternative medicine. One of the major menus is TCM in western medicine world, some trying to integrate Western Medicine and Eastern Medicine (**Figure 1**).

## 2. The Urgent Need for QOL Assessment

1) A choice of health menu in conjunction with each constitution is in a quandary due to lack of information concerning these cross-interactions among general public and lack of information among the health professionals resulting with a potentially significant health scale.
2) A vertebrate animal acquired two ontogenically and phylogenically defense systems and ontogenetically, innate and adaptive. Despite these defense systems overwhelming problems of possessing these dual systems, the innate and adoptive does not seem to guard or even prevent the development of one internal threat to survival. However, every individual expose to the risks of immunodeficiency status in daily life with both internal and externals [1]-[12]. The factors that influence the acquired immune activity are systemic metabolic disorder such as diabetes mellitus, malnutrition, extreme exhaustion, extensive stress, aging and medical side effects [1]-[12]. So we have to select appropriate menu to regulate immune function through leukocyte storage.

In other words, no tentative scale for evaluate the intense of each trial. We have been reported the best tailored scale by different menu through leukocyte regulation in number and function [13]. We have been trying to regulate the immune responsiveness through much mature for fragile in daily stress and so on. The main menu from our trials were, acupuncture, hot-spring hydrotherapy, light exercise Ondel heating etc. In this article, we would like to show the regulatory mechanism of the hot spring hydrotherapy. The circumstance, the balneotherapy using the effectiveness of hot-springs hydrotherapy, except for cases of contraindication, has been medically useful approved to be effective in many stress-related disorders and the improvement of dysfunction of the biological rhythm disturbance as well as chronic disease. The mechanism of effects has been reported in many studies, but many things are still unclear. Balneotherapy needs to be treated in general a period of time, but the

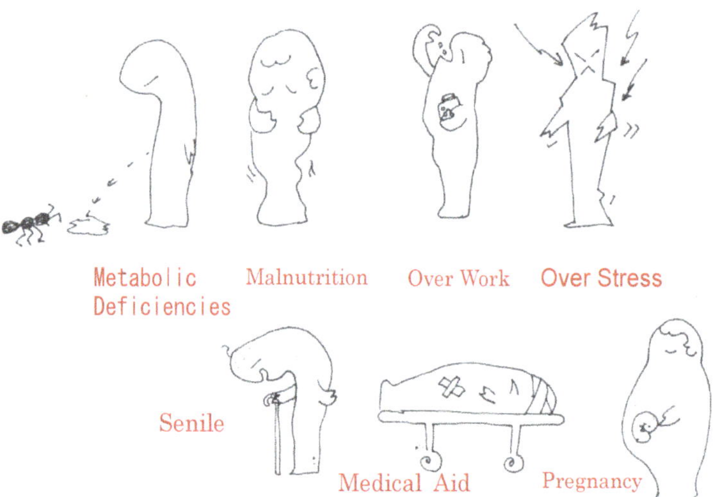


**Figure 1.** Acquired Immunodeficiency in Daily Life. The lists for causative factors induce acquired immune-deficiency.in daily life. We had prepared the native non-specific gourd line outside of the skin and/or mucous membrane. However, the gourd line is easily broken by accidental affair. However, non-specific and specific attack system had been prepare as lympho-reticular line of defuse. This defense lines are accidentally broken by the factor listed in this figure.

effectiveness has been suggested even if the short duration hot-springs hydrotherapy. We examined the effect of hot spring hydrotherapy for a short duration on immune system and reported about the quantitative and qualitative variation of immuno-competent cells [11]-[14]. The mechanism is suggested the association with an autonomic nervous system and the endocrine system. Hot spring hydrotherapy for a short duration was expected to stimulate sympathetic nerve or parasympathetic nerve and to change the levels of catecholamines (adrenalin, noradrenaline, and dopamine), which are neurotransmitters and hormones, as well as the number and function of immune cells (**Figure 2**).

## 3. A Simple Sum-Up & Make Mean Fade out the Important Changes, in a System Double-Blind & Cross over

There are many experimental system for evaluating QOL on the basis of western medicine. Almost all the experimental protocols are recommended to double blind and cross over system as a better evaluating system. However, simple sum up and make mean for comparison of efficacy before and after the administrating some menu. Our evidence from light exercise, walking, hot spring hydrotherapy etc., we had no result by the method, making summing up and make mean in all the menu of CAM (**Figure 3**). For at least three types of individuals that responded to up-regulation, down regulation and no changed one. So simple summing up is cancelled the each vector of individual. The X-axis according to the value before each CAM menu. As shown in the Figures, the data could represent by linear slant. The value correlation/tangent was represented the each result from CAM menu/walking. We tried to compare the best impact for each individual, we set up two sort of impact. The one was walking 4 km/hour (4 mets), and the other was 8 km/hour (8 mets) to the same volunteer at the different day after the cooling of the former menu (one month interval).

In order to establish some effect from each designed experiment, one usually recommended to make experimental system as double blind and crossing over system. Hot Spring Hydrotherapy Regulate Peripheral Leukocyte Together with Emotional Hormone and Receptor Positive Lymphocytes According to Each Constitu-

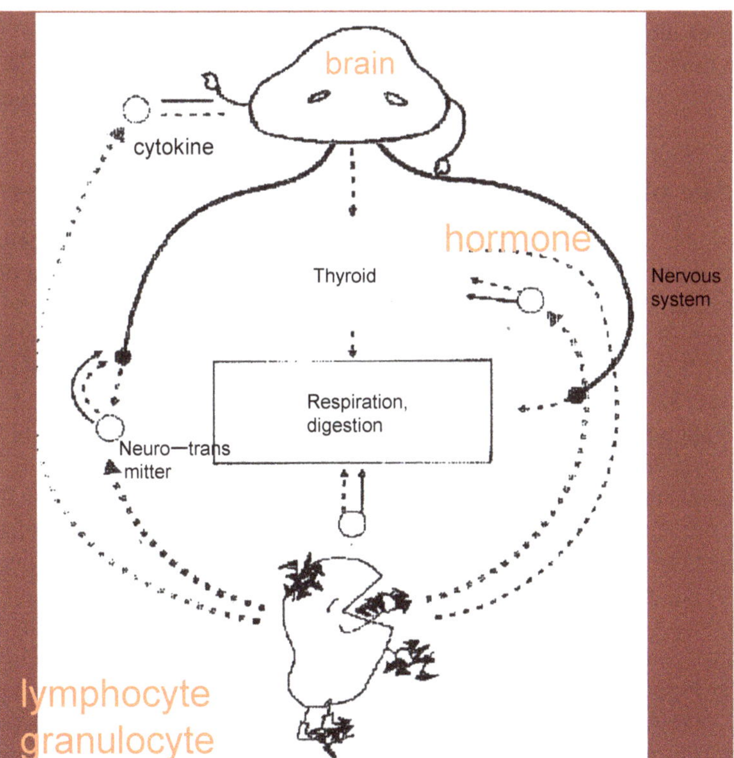


**Figure 2.** The illustration showed a close network between brain, hormone and peripheral leukocyte. In this review, peripheral leukocyte and hormone level were tie-up each other so to in a constitution dependent manner, especially in emotional hormone, adrenalin and dopamine.

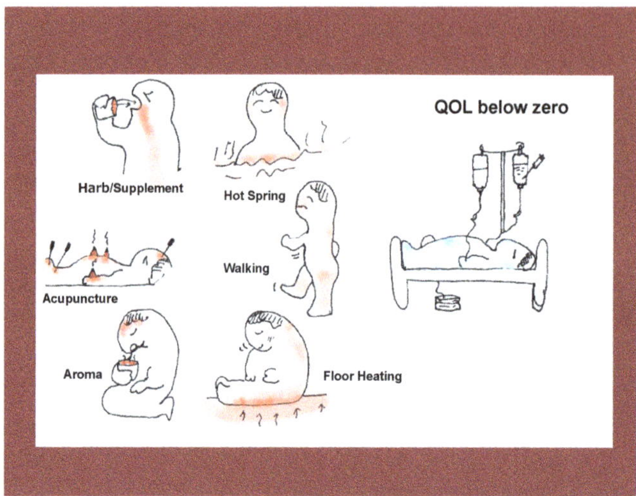


**Figure 3.** The CAM menu that introduced in this article with evidence based manner on the basis of each constitution/condition. We tried to express the effect of peripheral total leukocyte number by individual level of change and plot in the X-axis as in each age. The confirmed menu were, hot-spring hydrotherapy, supplement administration especially with fomented polysaccharide and depredated protein, light exercise, acupuncture, floor heating and aroma therapy Variations in leukocyte subpopulations in the peripheral blood before and after each CAM therapy.

tion/Condition is important to conscious of circadian rhythm. Abo reported that it was possible to sort the constitution, granulocyte-rich individual and lymphocyte-rich one with the peripheral leukocyte [15]-[26].

Each population of subset is depending on a circadian rhythm. Within a same individual, granulocyte increase in the daytime, on the other hand, lymphocyte increased in the nighttime in a cycle 24 hrs. So we have to compare the effect of each menu for the peripheral leukocyte on the same time before and after the menu. **Figures 3-6**.

## 4. The Best Scale of QOL Assessment for Constitutionally Different in Human

Our results showed that within 24 hours after hot spring hydrotherapy, the white blood cells in peripheral blood had changed significantly, not only in cell count but also cell function. We hope that our work will attract more attention to the mechanisms of which hot spring hydrotherapy regulates the human immune system. Abo reported that according to the lymphocyte subset content, lymphocyte rich type showed over 40% on the other hand granulocyte rich type show over 60% of granulocyte [27] [28]. Each type exhibited different character even in the same age, sexuality and each age. In the Figures, within the same age and the sex, even in mankind can sorts out as G-rich type (granulocyte 60%), and L-rich type (lymphocyte 40%). On the other hand, as a stand point of sex difference, the lady belongs to L-rich type.

Hot Spring Hydrotherapy Regulate Peripheral Leukocyte Together with Emotional Hormone and Receptor Positive Lymphocytes according to each constitution/condition but the gentleman belongs G-rich type. According to the age-related change, G-rich type of young man change to L-rich type according getting older.

We have been trying to regulate the immune responsiveness through much mature for fragile daily condition from circumstance stress and so on. The main menu were, acupuncture, hot-spring hydrotherapy, light exercise etc. In this article, we would like to show the regulatory mechanism of the hot spring hydrotherapy.

As shown in the **Figure 7** and **Figure 8**, Leucocyte subsets, granulocyte and Lymphocyte are regulated by each CAM menu. Moreover, we tried to select emotional hormone in order to catch a possibility to show regulational factor dependent on each condition and constitution. We had selected 5 hormones for possible candidate, adrenalin, nor-adrenalin dopamine, ACTH, T4 and T5, adrenalin and dopamine were completely dependent on the condition and constitution.

In the Figures, the regulational bias was also could indicated as slant, correlation efficiency, possible to express one key word of number, easy to compare the efficacy of each menu. For example, we selected the light

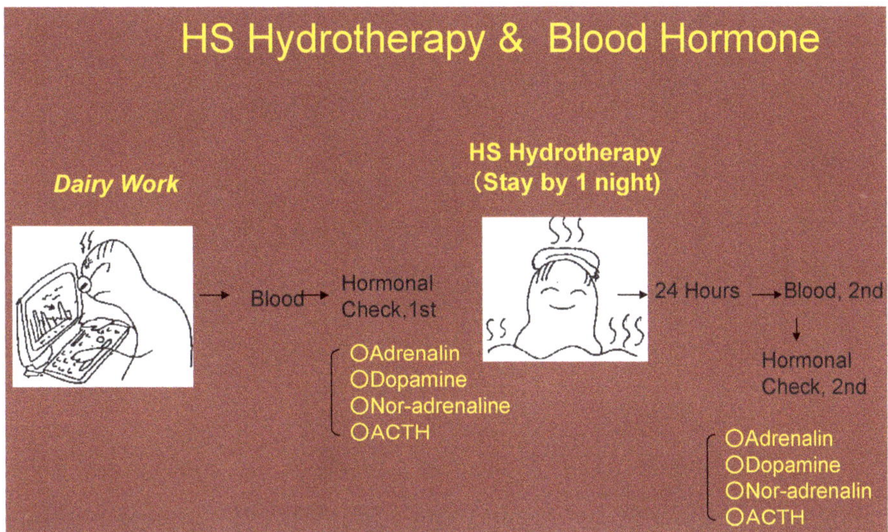


**Figure 4.** General experimental design to evaluate each CAM therapy. General style for the experiment was designed to collect factors before and after the CAM menu. However, the impotent sings to collect the factor have to keep the time lag is 24 hours in order to avoid the circadian rhythm. Twenty-four hours change of leukocyte counts on the bases of group comparison between pre/post therapy. We sampled peripheral blood from each volunteer before and after CAM therapy, at the same time on each day, in accordance with the consideration of circadian rhythm of leukocyte in this figure, we tried to show the date simply pooled and make mean, then compared.

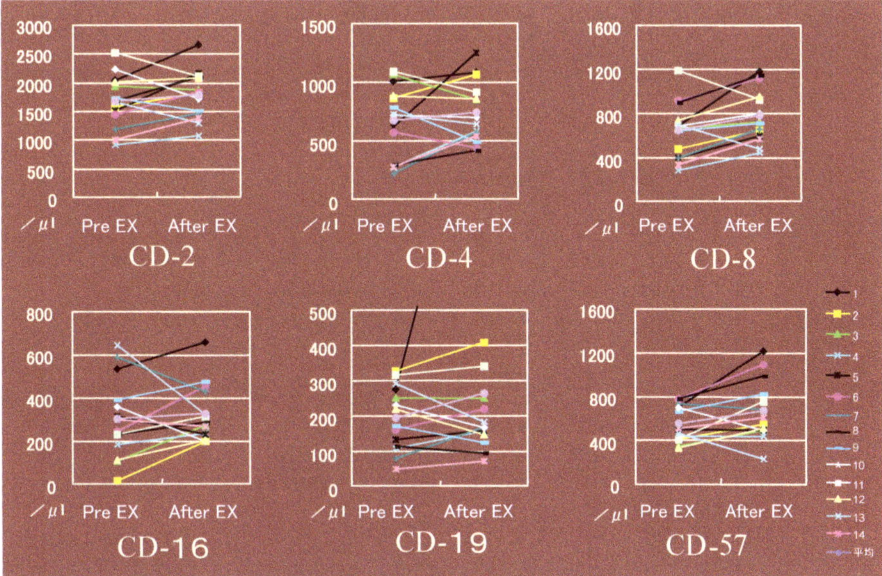


**Figure 5.** Simple & conventional presentation of the effect by walking, 4 mets. We first got the data from leukocyte regulation from 24 hours interval. But there were many constitutional difference. For example, up-regulated group, down-regulated and no-changed group. So, in this presentation style, simple sum-up and make mean got the result as no change from this figure.

walking for regulative menu for leukocyte regulation. We had planned two type of impact. One is for waking around 4 km/hour hour and the other was 8 km /hour. 8 mets of walking brought ideal regulation, co-efficiency (**Figure 9**). However, 8 met excursive was not so effective and clearly compared by the value calculated. Moreover, the presentation is one of the scale for appropriate suggestion for someone ask his/her impact of walking.

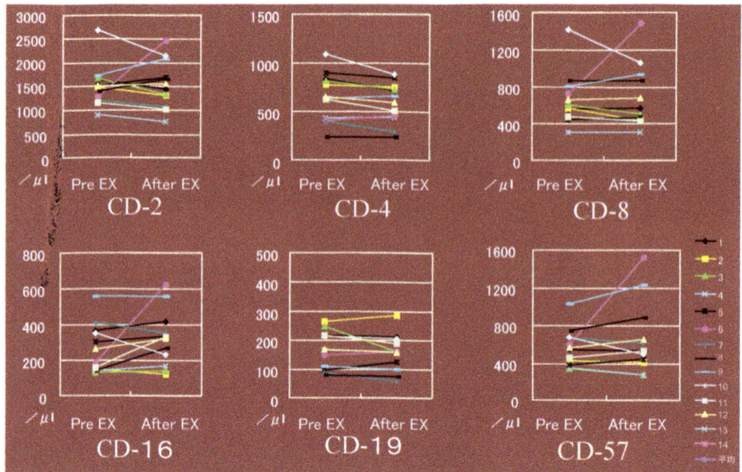


**Figure 6.** Simple & conventional presentation of the effect by walking 8 mets. We first got the data from leukocyte regulation from 24 hours interval. But there were many constitutional difference. For example, up-regulated group, down-regulated and no-changed group. So, in this presentation style, simple sum-up and make mean also got the result as no change from this figure.

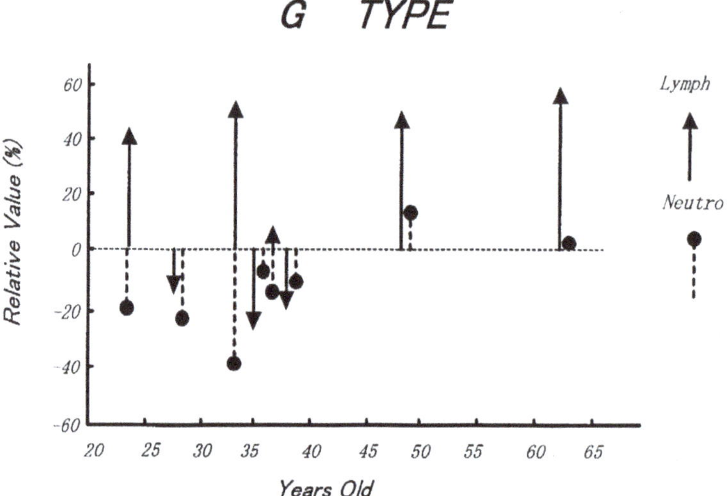


**Figure 7.** We reported that according to the lymphocyte subset content, lymphocyte rich type showed over 40% on the other hand granulocyte rich type show over 60% of granulocyte. Each type exhibited different character even in the same age; sexuality and each age (see **Figure 10**). In the figure, within the same age and the sex, even in mankind can sorts out as G-rich type (granulocyte 60%; ---➔), and L-rich type (lymphocyte 40%; ----⓫).On the other hand, as a stand point of sex difference, According to this figure, G-rich type changed to increase lymphocyte number, on the other hand, L-rich type increase granulocyte/neutrophyle. It was prominent that the young aged G-type decreased the granulocyte.

For example haw many speed and how many km should do for the best impact? The circumstance, the balneotherapy using the effectiveness of hot-springs hydrotherapy, except for cases of contraindication, has been medically useful approved to be effective in many stress-related disorders and the improvement of dysfunction of the biological rhythm disturbance as well as chronic disease. The mechanism of effects has been reported in many studies, but many things are still unclear. Balneotherapy needs to be treated in general a period of time, but the effectiveness has been suggested even if the short duration hot springs hydrotherapy. We examined the

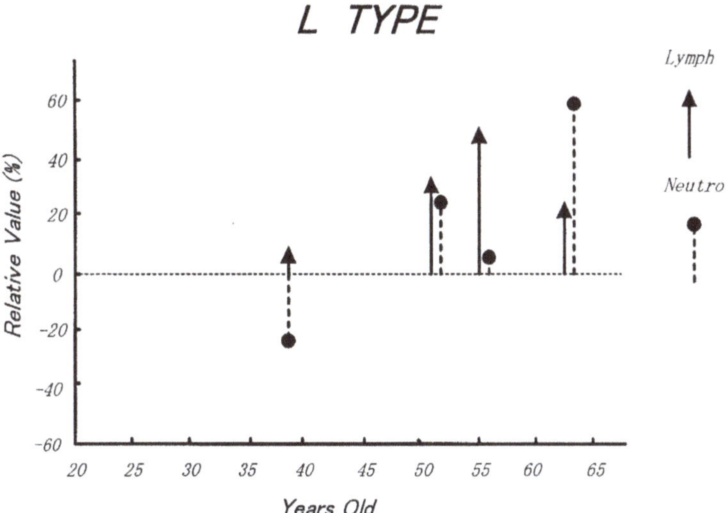


**Figure 8.** We reported that according to the lymphocyte subset content, lymphocyte rich type showed over 40% on the other hand granulocyte rich type show over 60% of granulocyte. Each type exhibited different character even in the same age; sexuality and each age (see **Figure 10**). In the figure, within the same age and the sex, even in mankind can sorts out as L-rich type (granulocyte 60%; ---➔), and L-rich type (lymphocyte 40%; ----⓫).On the other hand, as a stand point of sex difference, According to this figure, G-rich type changed to increase lymphocyte number, on the other hand, L-rich type in crease granulocyte/neutrophyle. It was prominent that the young aged G-type decreased the granulocyte.

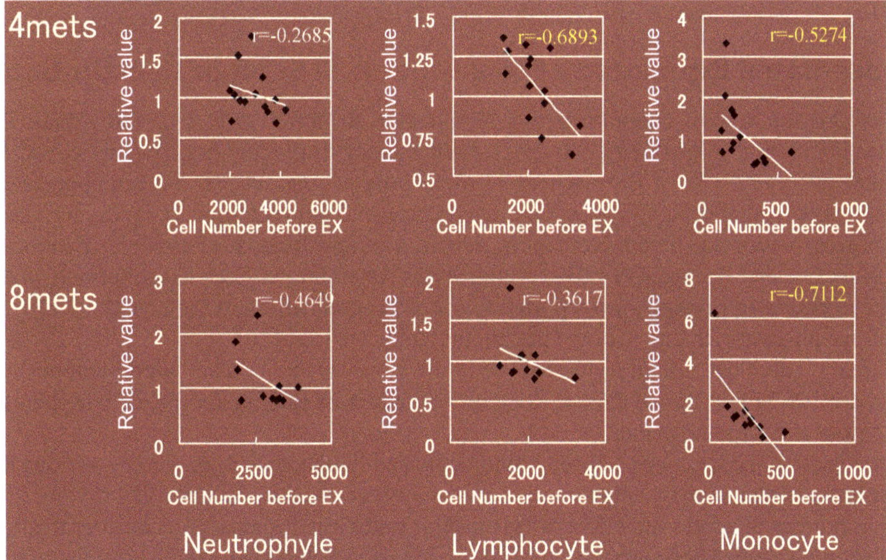


**Figure 9.** The constitution/condition dependent regulation of hot spring hydrotherapy in L-rich type. We reported that according to the lymphocyte subset content, lymphocyte rich type showed over 40% on the other hand granulocyte rich type show over 60% of granulocyte. Each type exhibited different character even in the same age, sexuality and each age. In the figure, within the same age and the sex, even in mankind can sorts out as G-rich type (granulocyte 60%; ---➔), and L-rich type (lymphocyte 40%; ----⓫). On the other hand, as a stand point of sex difference, According to this figure, L-rich type increase granulocyte/neutrophyl but decreased lymphocyte percentage. This type was the major group in senile that regulated to increase both lymphocyteand granulocytes.

effect of hot spring hydrotherapy for a short duration on immune system and reported about the quantitative and qualitative variation of immuno-competent cells [4] [13] [14] [18] [20]. The mechanism is suggested the association with an autonomic nervous system and the endocrine system. Hot spring hydrotherapy for a short duration was expected to stimulate sympathetic nerve or parasympathetic nerve and to change the levels of catecholamines (adrenalin, noradrenaline, and dopamine), which are neurotransmitters and hormones, as well as the number and function of immune cells.

The adrenaline and noradrenaline are secreted by various stress (stimulation); the former from the adrenal medulla and the latter from both the adrenal medulla and the end of sympathetic nerve. They express these functions through the adrenergic receptors (ARs) and regulate the target organ. The adrenergic receptor has two types of $\alpha$ and $\beta$, and there are multiple subtypes ($\alpha_1$, $\alpha_2$, $\beta_1$, $\beta_2$, $\beta_3$) [21]. These subtypes present the vascular ($\alpha_1$), the presynaptic terminal ($\alpha_2$), the heart ($\beta_1$), the bronchial muscle of the lung ($\beta_2$), fat cells ($\beta_3$), respectively. The $\alpha$-receptor stimulation causes Broncho-dilatation and vasodilatation, the $\beta 1$-receptor stimulation causes an increase in heart rate and lipolysis, and the $\beta_2$-receptor stimulation causes bronchoconstriction, vasodilatation, and muscle glycogen resolution. The adrenaline provides heart activation by effect on $\alpha$- and $\beta$-receptors, and the noradrenaline provides blood pressure rises by strongly effect on $\alpha$-receptors. In addition to the above, it has been reported that the ARs are present on leucocyte membranes [21]-[24] and that the level of expression of $\beta$-ARs in lymphocytes was examined by radio ligand (125I-iodopindolol) binding, but the details of subtype of $\beta$-receptors have not been disclosed. The subtypes of the AR are able to be analyzed by flow cytometry (FCM) method. In this study, we described how hot spring hydrotherapy influences leukocyte, lymphocyte subpopulations expressing $\beta_2$-AR and the levels of catecholamine in human peripheral blood.

Abo reported that according to the lymphocyte subset content, lymphocyte rich type showed over 40% on the other hand granulocyte rich type show over 60% of granulocyte. Each type exhibited different character even in the same age, sexuality and each age.

In the Figures, within the same age and the sex, even in mankind can sorts out as G-rich type (granulocyte 60%), and L-rich type (lymphocyte 40%).

On the other hand, as a standpoint of sex difference, the ladies belong to L-rich type but the man belongs G-rich type. According to the age-related change, G-rich type of man change to L-rich type within the same sex (**Figure 10**).

## 5. Evidence-Based Expression of Constitution, SCS; Super Constitution System

Abo reported that the ratio of granulocyte and lymphocyte are different in each individual. This difference reveals the sexual different (**Figure 10**). Moreover, both leucocyte are daily regulated by circadian rhythm and the environmental factors [23] [24]. But each cycle of leukocyte, granulocyte and lymphocyte are different each other. So the experimental design is necessary to synchronized with the time to check, for example, the number of leukocyte from peripheral blood. Hot Spring Hydro Therapy Regulate Peripheral Leukocyte Together with Emotional Hormone and Receptor Positive Lymphocytes According to Each Constitution/Condition is important to conscious of circadian rhythm. Abo reported that it was possible to sort the constitution, granulocyte-rich individual and lymphocyte-rich one with the peripheral leukocyte [25] [26].

Within a same individual, granulocyte increase in the daytime, on the other hand, lymphocyte increased in the nighttime in a cycle 24 hrs. So we have to compare the effect of each menu for the peripheral leukocyte on the same time before and after the menu.

It was reported that the leukocyte subset, granulocyte and lymphocyte regulated by various factors. One major point is that they are regulated by autonomous nervous system, resulting in circadian rhythm [23].

Therefore, in order to access the effect within a short time, it is necessary to consider this factor to adjust the time to collect the sample. For example, efficacy and impact of walking exercise has been widely recognized. However, the majority of walkers did not have a scientific background to know the best exercise menu for the one' QOL; quality of life. The purpose of this study was to demonstrate the best menu of walking that regulates the peripheral white blood cells in number and function as a marker of QOL expression **Figure 9** and **Figure 10**.

## 6. Granulocyte/Lymphocyte Ratio Reveals Constitution

Traditionally, each heat therapy has its own character and efficacy for various complaints. Through the years, each water source was evaluated for its specific properties and with the advent of better transportation in our mountainous land, even remote springs in the mountains were visited for their specific medicinal effect. For

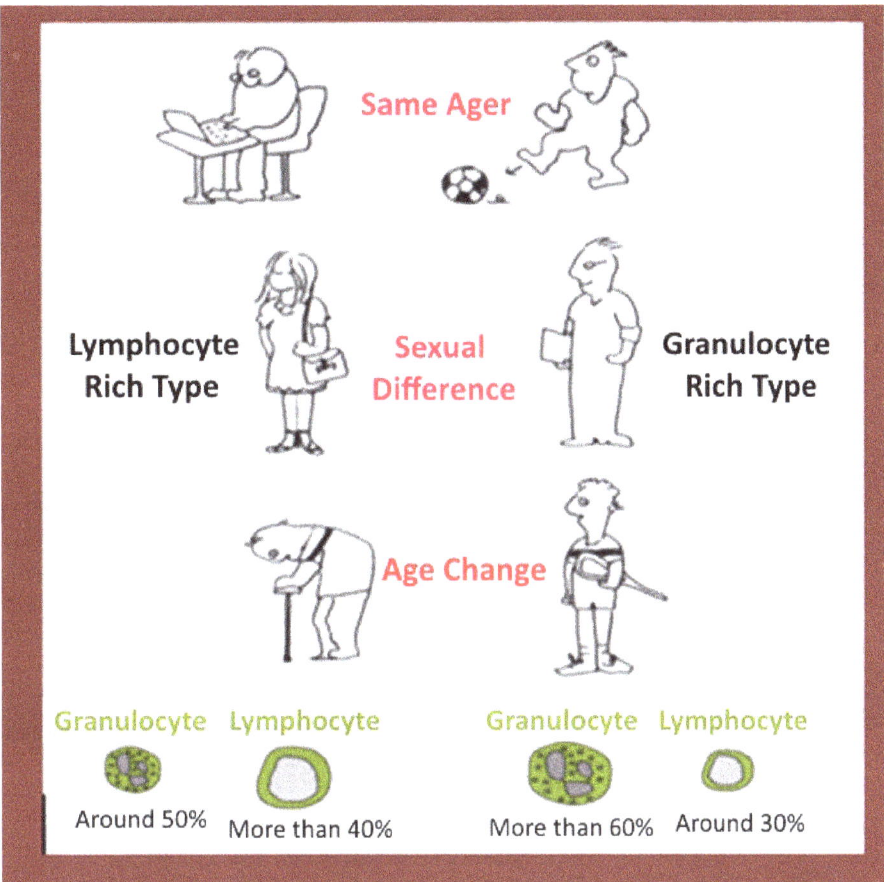


**Figure 10.** An ontogenical and phyogenetical consideration of constitution, for the best condition and the best QOL. In the figure, within the same age and the sex, even in mankind can sorts out as G-rich type (granulocyte 60%), and L-rich type (lymphocyte 40%). On the other hand, as a stand point of sex difference, the ladies belong to L-rich type but the man belongs G-rich type. According to the age-related change, G-rich type of man change to L-rich type within the same sex.

example, the hot spring of Yuwaku-Onsenn, which is located just below our research facility, was known all over the area to cure hemorrhoids. However, almost all the judgments of efficacy are VAS (visual analog scale). The proprietors of the hot spring inns say that many of the guests came to cure that sort of ailment since about 20 years ago. Now in Japan, hot spring hydrotherapy is often used as a supplementary therapy for many diseases [21] [28] [29]. It has shown to reduce surgical complaints such as shoulder pain, amyloidosis and various rheumatic problems. It can also lighten the burden to the heart and improve the condition of patients who suffer from emphysema as well as other respiratory ailments. Hot springs have also traditionally functioned as places to relax and enjoy oneself, even though resort-type hot springs always exist along with those for illnesses. In recent years, trends have been seen that even remote hot springs, such as the one below our facility, transform into fashionable resorts for the healthy to visit for relaxation and stress release. It is interesting to note that this historical duplicity encompassed by hot springs has also entered the world.

## 7. An Importance to Regulate Neutral in Both Leucocyte in Number

Each volunteer was prepared their blood before start to visit hot spring village after informed consented to the experimental purpose by written Ethics of the Committee in Kanazawa Medical University. After lodging the hotel, volunteers enjoyed Japanese type hot spring bath system, with no under wear in the bath room/pool separately prepared for ladies and gentleman. We suggested taking a bath totally 2 - 3 times within two days for the aim of trial. Beside the advance of VAS: visual analog scale in our investigation, we measured the total number of leukocyte and two major subsets, granulocyte and lymphocytes regulated before and after hot spring hydrotherapy.

We tried to express the effect of peripheral total leukocyte number by individual level of change and plot in the x-axis as in each age. As was in **Figure 11**, the groups was separated in to two, up-regulated individuals and down-regulated one. The correlation of change was expressed as a linear function. **Figure 11** was ideal change of effect with hot spring hydrotherapy, showing the best inclination. The results showed that these subsets could reflect the number and function of immuno-competent cells. For example, in an individual with a low granulocyte number, the number increased after treatment, while it decreased in another individual with a higher cell number (**Figure 12**).

We sampled peripheral blood from the 12 volunteers before and after hot sand/hydro therapy, at the same O'clock on the day, with the respect of circadian rhythm [25] [27] of leukocyte. These subjects participated in this study after giving their informed consent. We conducted the experiment at Yuwaku Onsen Spa (Kanazawa, Ishikawa Pref., Japan) in one night of the day. The spring quality is a weak sodium chloride with sodium carbohydrate of the water temperature 41˚C ± 1˚C. During the night and in the morning of the next day, they had a bath in the hot spring two or three times, for 20 - 30 minutes each time. Hot sand spa had performed and bathing for 40 mins. Time interval of blood sampling between before and after hot-spring hydrotherapy was approximately 24 hours. Measurements of the total and differential leukocyte counts and 3 catecholamines levels in the peripheral blood.

We ordered on the laboratory of Ishikawa Prefecture Preventive Medicine Association about the total and differential leukocyte counts and the levels of 3 catecholamines (adrenaline, noradrenaline, and dopamine) in the peripheral blood from the subjects. The total and differential leukocyte counts were measured by the automated hematology analyzer XE-2100 (Sysmex, Inc., Kobe, Japan). The levels of catecholamines were measured by high performance liquid chromatography (HPLC) system (Tosoh Co. and Hitachi High-Technologies Co., ToKyo) The immune system is a totally integrative system. It includes brain, endocrine and immune system. For example, an immune system contains various cells, tissues and organs that protect organisms against potentially

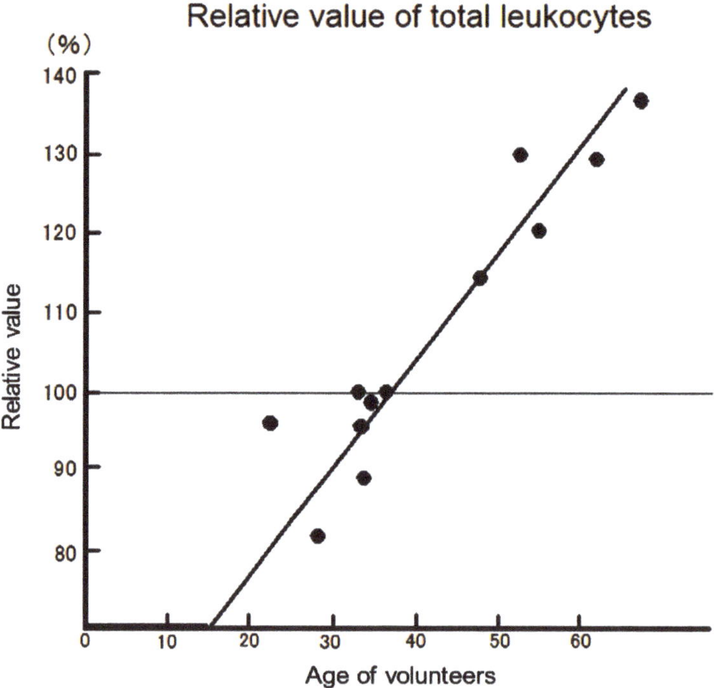


**Figure 11.** The constitution/condition dependent regulation and presentation by linear slant and judging by their tangent value/ co-efficiency. In the figure, the trial was made to show the each slant as a representative of the regulational effect to CD positive lymphocyte. The figure shows after light excursive/walking 4 mets and 8 mets.

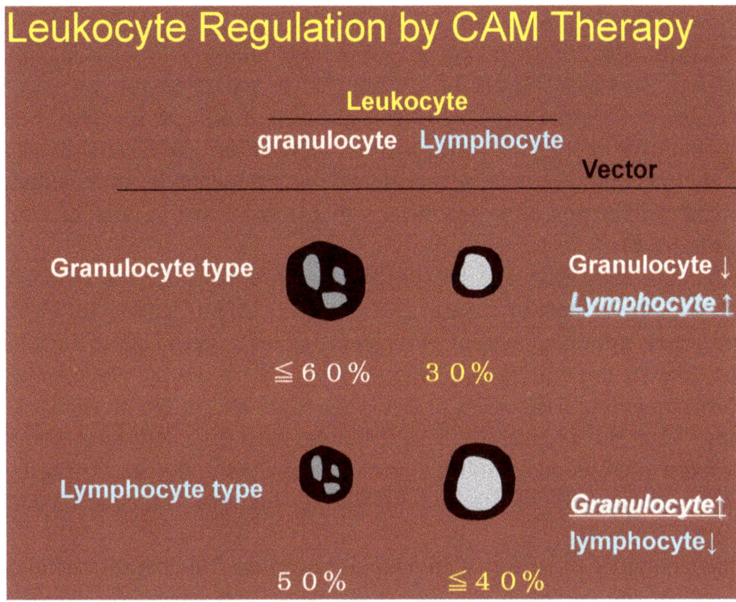


**Figure 12.** A graphical presentation for the summary of the hot spring hydro-therapy. We tried to express the effect of peripheral total leukocyte number by individual level of change and plot in the X-axis as in each age. Variations in leukocyte subpopulations in the peripheral blood before and after each CAM therapy.

harmful pathogens from the external environment. The present concept of the word immunity has proposed considerably from its original definition to the standard scale for CAM (complementary and alternative medicine). Quite literally, its earlier usage referred to exemption from military service or the paying of taxes. Now, immunity not only "frees" one from disease but also the standard scale for CAM (**Figure 3**, **Figure 10**, **Figure 12**).

## 8. Constitution Dependent Regulations Are Important for QOL

The recent excessive commercialization is particularly confusing for patients and doctors who seek remedies for heretofore undefined symptoms. Furthermore, since these treatments have not undergone strict testing, they are not always safe and the same drug may have different effects according to the individual patient and dosage. Complicated considerations are necessary for the application of practices such as those found in Chinese traditional medicine.

Recently, alternative and complementary medicines together with oriental and traditional medicines have attracted much attention. This new interest includes aromatherapy and herbal medications, acupuncture, moxibustion and yoga.

However, these therapies have not been well defined. Some are simply based on legend or belief while others are traditionally applied but without scientific evidence. Then the assessment of each therapy and remedy need for their capacity through a scientific methods especially developed by Western Medicine. Although the word Alternative & Complementary Medicine is not popular enough in Japan than US and European countries, because in oriental countries so called Alternative and Complementary Medicine in Europe and north America is authorized medicine but not alternative one in the long histories in the world. Here I would like to introduce you where the alternative and complementary medicine now in Japan as well as in each country in the world and where should it be going in the future.

Each volunteer was prepared their blood before start to visit hot spring village after informed consented to the experimental purpose by written Ethics of the Committee in Kanazawa Medical University. After lodging the hotel, volunteers enjoyed Japanese type hot spring bath system, with no under wear in the bath room/pool separately prepared for ladies and gentleman. We suggested taking a bath totally 2 - 3 times within two days for the aim of trial. Beside the advance of VAS: visual analog scale in our investigation, we measured the total number of leukocyte and two major subsets, granulocyte and lymphocytes regulated before and after hot spring hydrotherapy.

We tried to express the effect of peripheral total leukocyte number by individual level of change and plot in the x-axis as in each age. As was in **Figure 11**, the groups was separated in to two, up-regulated individuals and down-regulated one. The correlation of change was expressed as a linear function. **Figure 11** was ideal change of effect with hot spring hydrotherapy, showing the best inclination. The results showed that these subsets could reflect the number and function of immuno-competent cells. For example, in an individual with a low granulocyte number, the number increased after treatment, while it decreased in another individual with a higher cell number (**Figure 7**, **Figure 8**).

We sampled peripheral blood from the 12 volunteers before and after hot sand/hydro therapy, at the same O'clock on the day, with the respect of circadian rhythm [25] [27] of leukocyte. These subjects participated in this study after giving their informed consent. We conducted the experiment at Yuwaku Onsen Spa (Kanazawa, Ishikawa Pref., Japan) in one night of the day. The spring quality is a weak sodium chloride with sodium carbohydrate of the water temperature 41˚C ± 1˚C. During the night and in the morning of the next day, they had a bath in the hot spring two or three times, for 20 - 30 minutes each time. Hot sand spa had performed and bathing for 40 mins. Time interval of blood sampling between before and after hot spring hydrotherapy was approximately 24 hours. Measurements of the total and differential leukocyte counts and 3 catecholamines levels in the peripheral blood.

We ordered on the laboratory of Ishikawa Prefecture Preventive Medicine Association about the total and differential leukocyte counts and the levels of 3 catecholamines (adrenaline, noradrenaline, and dopamine) in the peripheral blood from the subjects. The total and differential leukocyte counts were measured by the automated hematology analyzer XE-2100 (Sysmex, Inc., Kobe, Japan). The levels of catecholamines were measured by high performance liquid chromatography (HPLC) system (Tosoh Co. and Hitachi High-Technologies Co.).

As we here took an overview about the today's QOL assessment for the medicine in the east and the west, I think it is high time this medicine should be standardized uniformly and Japan could play an important roll in this task.

In Japan, the Eastern Medicine especially the herbal medicine was once the central medical care for long time until the Meiji Government decided to import the Western medicine as the ordinary medical care. Thus in Japan not only the Western but also the Eastern medicine could have been developed, and Japan now takes great pride in the longevity. This is why I suppose Japan should take the initiative for the standardization of the alternative and complementary medicine.

The problem is how it should be standardized. Here I would like you to propose something. Most of the alternative medicine works through affecting the regularly system inside the body. For example, recent studies revealed the herbal medicine caused the interaction between the immune system, the endocrine system and the nervous system. Therefore observing the immune system by like sampling the peripheral blood might be an indicator for the standardization of the alternative medicine. Due to the above difficulties, this realm of medicine has often been shut out of the serious journals of western medicine. A new Journal concerning around complementary, alternative and traditional medicine" will be launched in a desire to ameliorate this situation, by encouraging the publication of original scientific papers based on sound scientific guidelines, but without prejudice against the possible efficacy of these new and ancient treatments (**Figure 3**).

## 9. Leucocytes Subsets Regulated in the Number and Function

The immune system shares with the nervous system at least two characteristics. The young individual is born with a certain potential to learn and to react to numerous and varied environmental stimuli both systems can lean. Once information is learned by the immune and nervous systems, it becomes in a sense imprinted, and each system retains the information in varying degrees, a process defined as memory. Despite the intense learning that young systems must do subsequent to birth and will continue to do throughout their life time, infants are born into the world with certain innate behavior patterns controlled by the nervous system, and certain innate or characteristic natural immunities. Innate or natural, immunity includes all non-specific resistance or specific immune responses.

Nonspecific reaction of the PE fluorescence was found in the isotype control. Therefore, the real values of the AR expressing cell counts were calculated by subtracting control values. The $CD19^+$ cells were observed non-specific reaction which seems to response of the second antibody. However, the significant variation was not seen from the comparison of $\beta_2$-AR expressing cells before and after hot-spring hydrotherapy. The mean % of $\beta_2$-AR expressing cells in the lymphocyte subsets was 18-19% in $CD3^+$ cells, 5% in $CD4^+$ cells, 57% - 63% in $CD8^+$ cells, and 93% - 95% in $CD56^+$ cells. That in $CD19^+$ cells was approximately 100% (data not shown), but we were not able to be confirmed because it was very likely to be the nonspecific reaction. The adrenaline and noradrenaline are secreted by various stress (stimulation); the former from the adrenal medulla and the latter from both the adrenal medulla and the end of sympathetic nerve. They express these functions through the adrenergic receptors (ARs) and regulate the target organ. The adrenergic receptor has two types of $\alpha$ and $\beta$, and there are multiple subtypes ($\alpha_1$, $\alpha_2$, $\beta_1$, $\beta_2$, $\beta_3$) [4]. These subtypes present the vascular ($\alpha_1$), the pre- synaptic terminal ($\alpha_2$), the heart ($\beta_1$), the bronchial muscle of the lung ($\beta_2$), fat cells ($\beta_3$), respectively. The $\alpha$-receptor stimulation causes bronchodilatation and vasodilatation, the $\beta$1-receptor stimulation causes an increase in heart rate and lipolysis, and the $\beta_2$-receptor stimulation causes bronchoconstriction, vasodilatation, and muscle glycogen resolution. The adrenaline provides heart activation by effect on $\alpha$- and $\beta$-receptors, and the noradrenaline provides blood pressure rises by strongly effect on $\alpha$-receptors. In addition to the above, it has been reported that the ARs are present on leucocyte membranes [20] [21] and that the level of expression of $\beta$-ARs in lymphocytes was examined by radioligand (125I-iodopindolol) binding, but the details of subtype of $\beta$-receptors have not been disclosed. The subtypes of the AR are able to be analyzed by flow cytometry (FCM) method. In this study, we described how hot spring hydrotherapy influences leukocyte, lymphocyte subpopulations expressing $\beta_2$-AR and the levels of catecholamine in human peripheral blood.

The recent excessive commercialization is particularly confusing for patients and doctors who seek remedies for heretofore undefined symptoms. Furthermore, since these treatments have not undergone strict testing, they are not always safe and the same drug may have different effects according to the individual patient and dosage. Complicated considerations are necessary for the application of practices such as those found in Chinese traditional medicine. Recently, alternative and complementary medicines together with oriental and traditional medicines have attracted much attention. This new interest includes aromatherapy and herbal medications, acupuncture, moxibustion and yoga. However, these therapies have not been well defined. Some are simply based on legend or belief while others are traditionally applied but without scientific evidence. Then the assessment of each therapy and remedy need for their capacity through a scientific methods especially developed by Western Medicine. Although the world Alternative & Complementary Medicine is not popular enough in Japan than US and European countries, because in oriental countries so called Alternative and Complementary Medicine in Europe and north America is authorized medicine but not alternative one in the long histories in the world. Here I would like to introduce you where the alternative and complementary medicine now in Japan as well as in each country in the world are and where should it be going in the future (**Figure 3**).

## 10. The Impact of Regulation Can Makes Linear Slant, SCS

The immune system is a totally integrative system. It includes brain, endocrine and immune system. For example, an immune system contains various cells, tissues and organs that protect organisms against potentially harmful pathogens from the external environment. The present concept of the word immunity has proposed considerably from its original definition to the standard scale for CAM (complementary and alternative medicine). Quite literally, its earlier usage referred to exemption from military service or the paying of taxes. Now, immunity not only "frees" one from disease but also the standard scale for CAM.

The immune system shares with the nervous system at least two characteristics. The young individual is born with a certain potential to learn and to react to numerous and varied environmental stimuli both systems can lean. Once information is learned by the immune and nervous systems, it becomes in a sense imprinted, and each system retains the information in varying degrees, a process defined as memory. Despite the intense learning that young systems must do subsequent to birth and will continue to do throughout their life time, infants are born into the world with certain innate behaviour patterns controlled by the nervous system, and certain innate or characteristic natural immunities. Innate or natural, immunity includes all non-specific resistance or immune mechanisms, whereas specific active acquired immunity is immunity deliberately induced by immunization (e.g. immunity to bacteria and virus).

Man, other complex vertebrates, and even many invertebrates have evolved a system of internal transport for communicating components of the immune system. It is the blood, within the circulatory system, that executes these tasks. The blood contains two major types of cells: erythrocytes, or red blood cells, and leukocytes, or white blood cells. Leukocytes play important roles in the immune system. There are two basic types of leukocytes: the non-granular and the granular. The non-granular (agranular) leukocytes are further divided into two types: lymphocytes and monocytes.

Lymphocytes possess antibody receptors for antigens on their surfaces, and are thus vital to specific immune response throughout the entire body, where they freely move about. Monocytes are produced in the bone marrow, but like other blood cells they are eventually found in the blood. They frequently exhibit amoeboid movement, and they are voracious phagocytes when they enter connective tissues as macrophages from the blood. Both are important for quick, on the spot, phagocytosis (**Figure 12**).

## 11. Factors Affect the Lymphocyte Ratio

### 11.1. Total and Differential Leukocyte Counts

The total and differential leukocyte counts in the peripheral blood of 9 subjects tended to decrease after hot spring hydrotherapy and the granulocyte counts significantly decreased ($p < 0.05$) judging from simple sum up and mean (**Figure 5**, **Figure 6**, **Figure 12**).

### 11.2. Catecholamines Levels in the Peripheral Blood

The adrenaline levels significantly decreased after hot spring hydrotherapy ($p < 0.05$); the noradrenaline and dopamine levels ten to decrease (**Figure 13**). The constitution dependent analysis, the detail change and vector

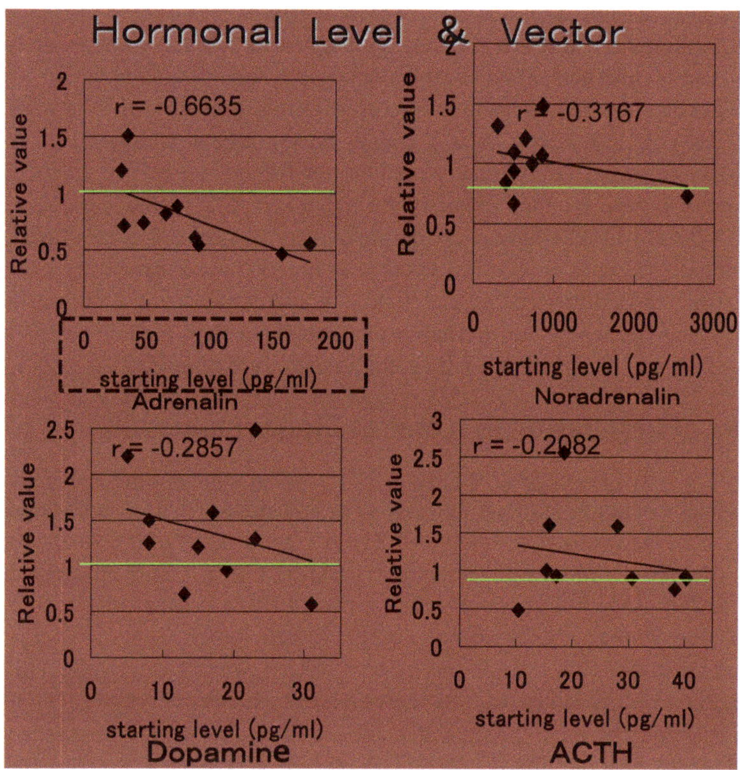


**Figure 13.** A emotional hormone also regulated by CAM therapy. The constitution dependent analysis for (adrenaline and dopamine). Each spot were obtained from the calculation comparing relative value from before and after levels in the serum, catecholamines levels in the peripheral blood within the figure, adrenalin and dopamine were regulated as was the same in leukocyte regulation. The clear slant was made from the data especially, in regulation in adrenalin, overall trend was decrease but was dose dependent manner of the value the day before. Also, dopamine was increased but also dose dependent manner as slant making.

of each change could find from individual data, showing higher value volunteer down regulated much more than lower leveled one. The results indicate that the hot-spring hydrotherapy may influence the secretion of adrenaline from the adrenal medulla.

### 11.3. FCM Analysis of $\beta_2$-AR Expresszion in Lymphocyte Subsets

The analysis of $\beta_2$-AR expressing cells and CD positive cells by FCM was measured by gating in the lymphocytes region on the scattered gram. Nonspecific reaction of the PE fluorescence was found in the isotype control. Therefore, the real values of the AR expressing cell counts were calculated by subtracting the control values. The CD19$^+$ cells were observed nonspecific reaction which seems to response of the second antibody. The comparison of each lymphocyte subpopulations before and after hot spring hydrotherapy showed that the CD8$^+$ cell and CD56$^+$ cell counts tended to increase (**Figure 14**). However, the significant variation was not seen from the comparison of $\beta_2$-AR expressing cells before and after hot-spring hydrotherapy. The mean % of $\beta_2$-AR expressing cells in the lymphocyte subsets was 18% - 19% in CD3$^+$ cells, 5% in CD4$^+$ cells, 57% - 63% in CD8$^+$ cells, and 93% - 95% in CD56$^+$ cells. That in CD19$^+$ cells was approximately 100% (data not shown), but we were not able to be confirmed because it was very likely to be the nonspecific reaction.

We examined the correlation with the rate of change in adrenaline levels and the rate of change in $\beta_2$-AR expressing cell counts of each subset or that in each CD-positive cell counts before and after hot-spring hydrotherapy. In the CD-positive cells, the rate of change in adrenaline levels was a positive correlation with that in the levels of CD56$^+$ cells, CD8$^+$ cells, and CD3$^+$ cells; in particular, a correlation with CD56$^+$ and CD8$^+$ cells was high. In $\beta_2$-AR expressing cells, the rate of change in adrenaline levels was a positive correlation with the rate of change in the levels of $\beta_2$-AR$^+$ CD56$^+$ cells. These results suggested that the variation in adrenaline levels is correlated with CD56$^+$ cells.

Each volunteer was prepared their blood before start for trial and after informed consented to the experimental purpose by written Ethics of the Committee in Kanazawa Medical University. We tried to exhibit the effect of peripheral total leukocyte number by individual level of change and plot in the x-axis as in each value before the exercise. As was in **Figure 9**, the relative value (%) was calculated before and after the exercise and plotted in figure of the X-axis according to the value before exercise. As a result of the trial, there found three groups,

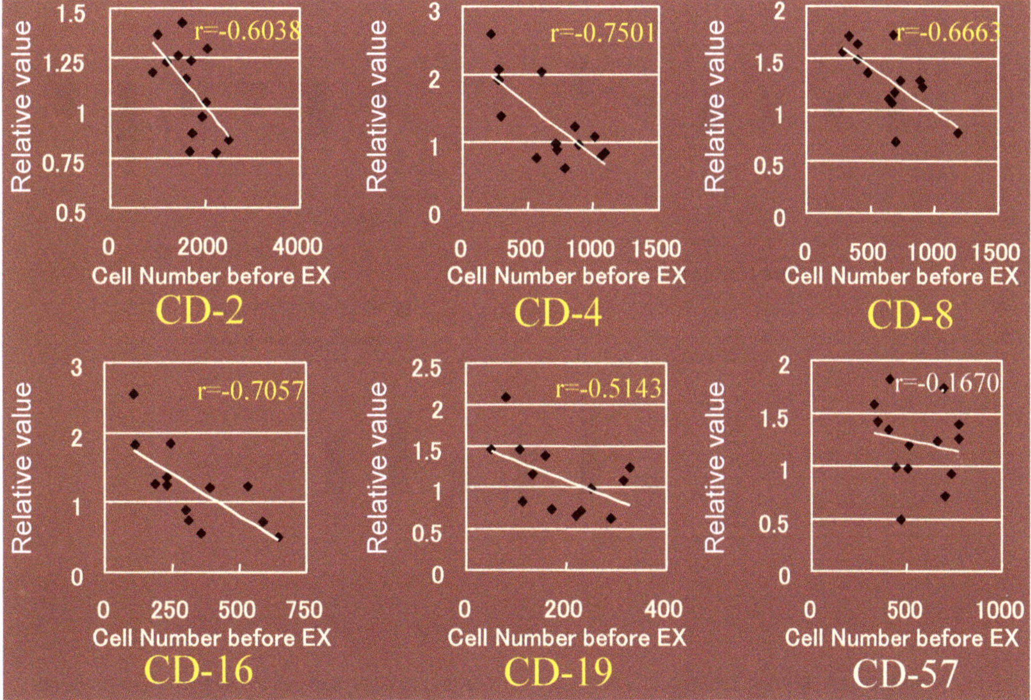


**Figure 14.** In the figure, the trial was made to show the each slant as an representatives of the regulational effect to CD positive lymphocyte. The figure show after hot spring hydro therapy.

separated, up-regulated individuals and down-regulated one and was no change. The correlation of change was expressed as a linear function and significant reverse correlation, -0.6893 indicating ideal value of correlative index −0.5 (**Figure 14**). The data obtained from 4mets exercise was brought ideal regulation. However, 8 mets could not bring such a effect significantly. About the leukocyte subset, the ideal regulation of lymphocyte and monocyte were found by floor heating room.

## 11.4. Twenty-Four Hours Change of Leukocyte Counts after Heating by Hot Air from Overhead

None of volunteer was dropped out with any serious problem. In trial, we set up room temperature also 18C at the 150 cm in high from floor, we tried to express the effect of peripheral total leukocyte number by individual level of change and plot in the X-axis as in each value before the exercise as is in 3.1. As shown in lower panel of **Figure 15**, the correlation was exhibited on a linear function but good correlation was retreated from the results the data obtained from 8 mets exercise was lesser regulatory effect than that compared by 4mets of exercise. About the leukocyte subset, the regulation by lymphocytes were more remarkable. However, only the monocyte exhibited significant change by both.

## 11.5. Leukocyte Subsets Regulation by Floor Heating

After one-weeks of working in the conditioned room as HCFH or HHFC, we set up the different mode of trial at the same course and by the same volunteers. None of volunteer was dropped out with any serious problem. In this time, we set up HCFH system, asking to work about for 5 days. We selected four hormones and accessed the effect of HCFH or HHFC conditioned room. After working about regular desk working in the HCFH conditioned room, each volunteer was down regulated the adrenaline, cortisone and nor-adrenalin. However, dopamine level was up-regulated for all the individuals tested. On the other hand, HHFC system showed reversed effect for all the hormones in this text (**Figure 16**).

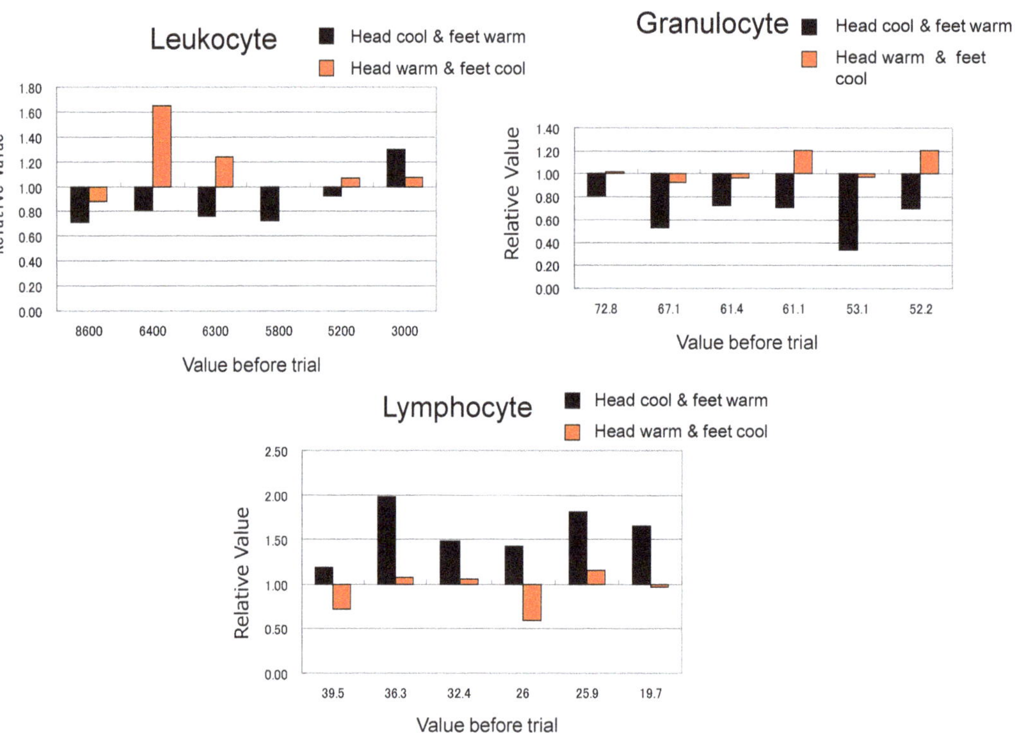


**Figure 15.** We tried to express the effect of peripheral total leukocyte number by individual level. The results were plotted in the x-axis as in each value before the trial. The relative value (%) of post trial was calculated with before and after and plotted in the Y-axis. Total leukocytes, Leukocyte subset, granulocyte and lymphocyte were also traced in the Figures.

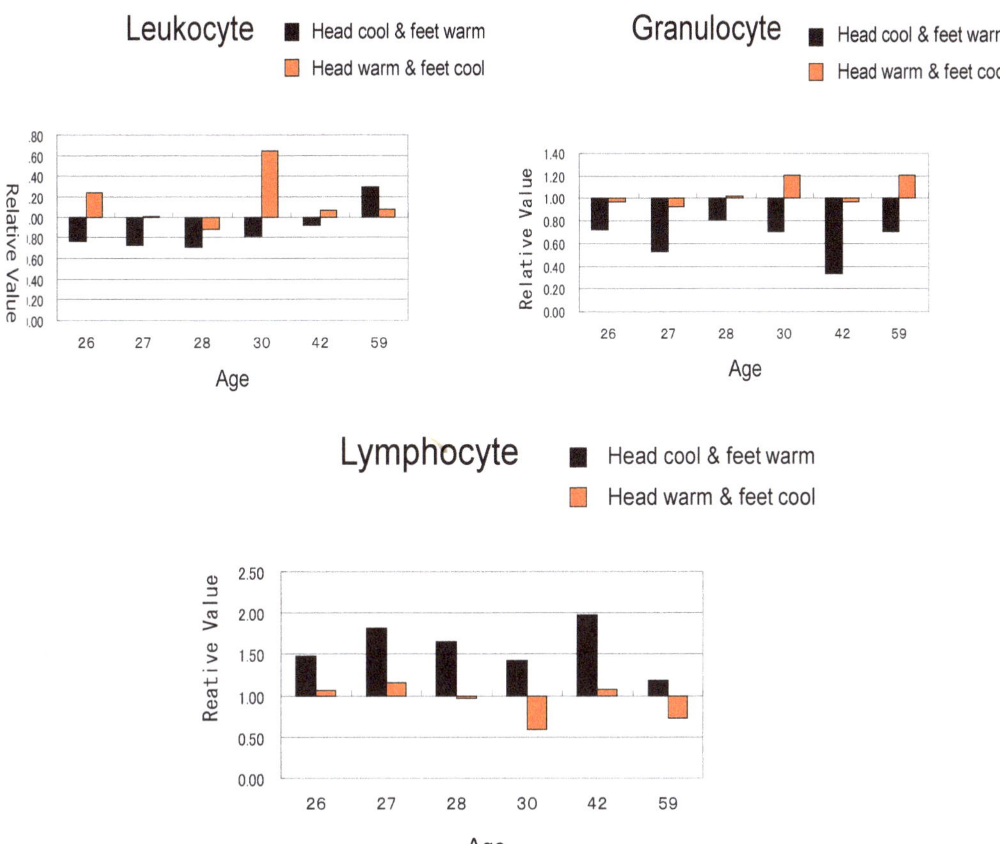


**Figure 16.** We tried to express the effect of peripheral total leukocyte number by individual level of change and plot in the x-axis as in each value according to the age. The relative value (%) of post trial was calculated with before and after and plotted in the y-axis. Leukocyte subset, granulocyte and lymphocyte were also traced in the Figures.

## 12. An Importance to Regulate Neutral in Both Leucocytes Subsets in Number

The results varied among the lymphocyte subsets before and after hot spring hydrotherapy. After hydrotherapy, the $CD16^+$, $CD8^+$ and $CD19^+$ cells increased in the younger group. Meanwhile, the $CD16^+$ cells increased in the older group while the $CD19^+$ cells decreased remarkably (**Figure 14**, **Figure 17**). This quantitative change in lymphocytes is shown in **Figure 14**. Except for $CD8^+$ cells, the $CD2^+$, $CD4^+$, $CD16^+$, $CD19^+$ and $CD56^+$ cells all showed negative variations.

There was a strong correlation between the variable ratio and the value before hydrotherapy: high values tended to decrease and low values tended to increase.

A comparison of the $CD4^+/CD8^+$ cells and $CD16^+/CD56^+$ cells between the two groups was shown. All the ratios of the $CD16^+/CD56^+$ cells increased in both groups. The changes in the $CD4^+/CD8^+$ cells, however, were different: the younger group showed a decrease while the older group showed an increase.

*Hot spring hydrotherapy regulated the leukocyte count differently in G- and L-type individuals.* In order to clarify the effect on individuals according to the type of regulation, we divided the volunteers into two groups: the G-type group had a granulocyte count over 70% and the L-type group had a lymphocyte count over 40 %. **Figure 11** shows that after hydrotherapy, the lymphocytes or lymphocyte subsets increased in the G-type group, accompanied by a decrease in granulocytes. However, in the L type group, the granulocytes increased notably as did the number of lymphocyte populations.

*Hot spring hydrotherapy affected the functional changes in cytokine-containing cells.* To test whether hot spring hydrotherapy affected the functional maturation of immunocytes, we further investigated the number of cytokine containing cells by FACS analysis. The results showed the effect of hot spring hydrotherapy on cyto-

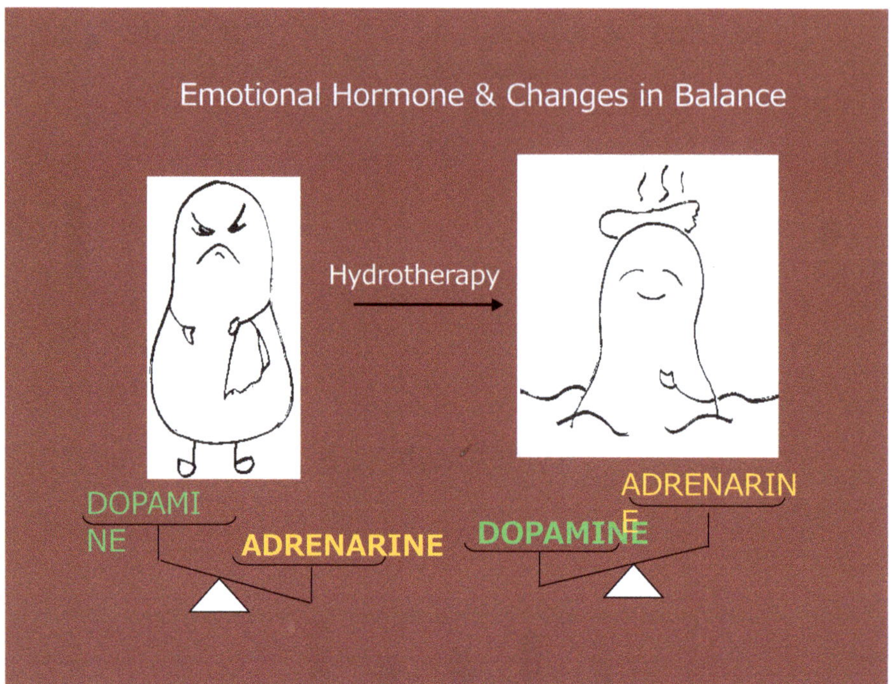


**Figure 17.** An illustrative presentation of hormonal regulation by hot Spring hydrotherapy. The clear slant was made from the data especially, in regulation in adrenalin, overall trend was decrease but was dose dependent manner of the value the day before. Also, dopamine was increased but also dose dependent manner as slant making.

kine production. Even though the increase in IFN-$\gamma$ containing cells had no statistical significance, the increase in IL-4 was remarkable ($r = 0.560$, $p < 0.01$) while the IL-1$\beta$ containing cell counts showed a decrease. In addition, before and after hydrotherapy, the levels of IFN-$\gamma$ and IL4 or IL-1$\beta$ also had meaningful negative changes. After hydrotherapy, there was a decrease of cytokine-producing cells in the subjects who had previously had a higher level.

The changes depended on the basic level of the white blood cells in the blood of the individuals.

*Hot spring hydrotherapy changes hormonal level in blood.* The peripheral blood was sampled twice from the volunteers at before and after 24 hours of the hydrotherapy. As a measurement item, thyroid hormone and 4 kinds of hormone reported to related emotion were measured. As a result of measuring the blood hormonal level around the hot spring hydrotherapy, adrenalin quantity showed the tendency in decrease in most individuals, while dopamine level showed the tendency in increase. On the other hormonal level, the fluctuation could not be observed (**Figure 12**). We also found a negative correlation between the variable ratio and the value before hydrotherapy in adrenalin level (**Figure 12**): high values tended to decrease and low values tended to increase ($r = -0.62016$, $p < 0.001$).

### 12.1. Twenty-Four Hours Change of Total Peripheral Leukocyte Count on the Basis of Each Individual

Each volunteer was prepared their blood before start to visit hot spring village after informed consented to the experimental purpose by written Ethics of the Committee in Kanazawa Medical University. After lodging the hotel, volunteers enjoyed Japanese type hot spring bath system, with no under wear in the bath room/pool separately prepared for ladies and gentleman. We suggested taking a bath totally 2 - 3 times within two days for the aim of trial. Beside the advance of VAS: visual analog scale in our investigation, we measured the total number of leukocyte and two major subsets, granulocyte and lymphocytes regulated before and after hot spring hydrotherapy.

We tried to express the effect of peripheral total leukocyte number by individual level of change and plot in the X-axis as in each age. As was in **Figure 3**, the groups was separated in to two, up-regulated individuals and down-regulated one. The correlation of change was expressed as a linear function. **Figure 10** was ideal change of effect with hot spring hydrotherapy, showing the best inclination. The results showed that these subsets could reflect the number and function of immuno-competent cells. For example, in an individual with a low granulocyte number, the number increased after treatment, while it decreased in another individual with a higher cell number (**Figure 5** and **Figure 6**).

We sampled peripheral blood from the 12 volunteers before and after hot sand/hydro therapy, at the same O'clock on the day, with the respect of circadian rhythm [25] [27] of leukocyte. These subjects participated in this study after giving their informed consent. We conducted the experiment at Yuwaku Onsen Spa (Kanazawa, Ishikawa Pref., Japan) in one night of the day. The spring quality is a weak sodium chloride with sodium carbohydrate of the water temperature 41˚C ± 1˚C. During the night and in the morning of the next day, they had a bath in the hot spring two or three times, for 20 - 30 minutes each time. Hot sand spa had performed and bathing for 40 mins. Time interval of blood sampling between before and after hot spring hydrotherapy was approximately 24 hours. Measurements of the total and differential leukocyte counts and 3 catecholamines levels in the peripheral blood.

We ordered on the laboratory of Ishikawa Prefecture Preventive Medicine Association about the total and differential leukocyte counts and the levels of 3 catecholamines (adrenaline, noradrenaline, and dopamine) in the peripheral blood from the subjects. The total and differential leukocyte counts were measured by the automated hematology analyzer XE-2100 (Sysmex, Inc., Kobe, Japan). The levels of catecholamines were measured by high performance liquid chromatography (HPLC) system (Tosoh Co. and Hitachi High-Technologies Co., Japan).

### 12.2. Twenty-Four Hours Change of Leukocyte Counts on the Bases of Group Comparison between Pre/Post Hydrotherapy

Despite the expression in the Section 3.1, when we tried to explain these values into the grouped value before and after the hydrotherapy, we got only one positive result from the granulocyte change that was the major population of peripheral leukocytes. The other factor did not exhibit as positive result.

The total and differential leukocyte counts in the peripheral blood of 12 subjects tended to decrease after hot-spring hydro-therapy. The statistically significant result only obtained that the granulocyte counts significantly decreased ($p < 0.05$). Another minor group lymphocyte did not changed significantly by judging from simple. Hot Spring Hydro Therapy Regulate Peripheral Leukocyte Together with Emotional Hormone and Receptor Positive Lymphocytes According to Each Constitution/Condition 6.

*The effect of hot spring hydrotherapy on the leukocyte count correlated with the age and original basic count of the individuals.* **Figure 2** shows the total numbers of leukocytes, granulocytes and lymphocytes from peripheral blood collected before and after hot spring hydrotherapy in the older and younger groups. The quantitative variation of the two groups differed. In the younger group, the total number of WBC ($p < 0.05$) and granulocytes ($p < 0.01$) clearly decreased. On the other hand, the total number of WBC and lymphocytes significantly increased ($p < 0.01$) after hydrotherapy in the older group. Furthermore, the results show that changes in the leukocyte count and subset count had a negative relationship before and after hydrotherapy. In other words, subjects who had a higher cell count level before hydrotherapy tended to show a decrease in the number of WBC 24 hrs after hydrotherapy. There was a significant correlation between age and rate of change (**Figure 2**, $r = 0.91$, $p < 0.001$). Since the turning point occurred at 35 years old, we separated the participants into a younger (under 35) and an older (over 36) group.

## 13. Leucocytes Subsets Regulated the Number and Function

### 13.1. Twenty-Four Hours Change of Total Peripheral Leukocyte Count on the Basis of Each Individual

Each volunteer was prepared their blood before start to visit hot spring village after informed consented to the experimental purpose by written Ethics of the Committee in Kanazawa Medical University. After lodging the hotel, volunteers enjoyed Japanese type hot spring bath system, with no under wear in the bath room/pool separately prepared for ladies and gentleman. We suggested taking a bath totally 2 - 3 times within two days for the aim of trial. Beside the advance of VAS: visual analog scale in our investigation, we measured the total number of leukocyte and two major subsets, granulocyte and lymphocytes regulated before and after hot spring hydrotherapy.

We tried to express the effect of peripheral total leukocyte number by individual level of change and plot in the X-axis as in each age. As was in **Figure 3**, the groups was separated in to two, up-regulated individuals and down-regulated one. The correlation of change was expressed as a linear function. **Figure 10** was ideal change of effect with hot spring hydrotherapy, showing the best inclination. The results showed that these subsets could reflect the number and function of immuno-competent cells. For example, in an individual with a low granulocyte number, the number increased after treatment, while it decreased in another individual with a higher cell number.

We sampled peripheral blood from the 12 volunteers before and after hot sand/hydro therapy, at the same O'clock on the day, with the respect of circadian rhythm [25] [27] of leukocyte. These subjects participated in this study after giving their informed consent. We conducted the experiment at Yuwaku Onsen Spa (Kanazawa, Ishikawa Pref., Japan) in one night of the day. The spring quality is a weak sodium chloride with sodium carbohydrate of the water temperature 41˚C ± 1˚C. During the night and in the morning of the next day, they had a bath in the hot spring two or three times, for 20 - 30 minutes each time. Hot sand spa had performed and bathing for 40 mins. Time interval of blood sampling between before and after hot-spring hydrotherapy was approximately 24 hours. Measurements of the total and differential leukocyte counts and 3 catecholamines levels in the peripheral blood.

We ordered on the laboratory of Ishikawa Prefecture Preventive Medicine Association about the total and differential leukocyte counts and the levels of 3 catecholamines (adrenaline, noradrenaline, and dopamine) in the peripheral blood from the subjects. The total and differential leukocyte counts were measured by the automated hematology analyzer XE-2100 (Sysmex, Inc., Kobe, Japan). The levels of catecholamines were measured by high performance liquid chromatography (HPLC) system (Tosoh Co. and Hitachi High-Technologies Co., Japan).

### 13.2. Twenty-Four Hours Change of Leukocyte Counts on the Bases of Group Comparison between Pre/Post Hydrotherapy

Despite the expression in the Section 3.1, when we tried to explain these values into the grouped value before and after the hydrotherapy, we got only one positive result from the granulocyte change that was the major population of peripheral leukocytes. The other factor did not exhibit as positive result.

The total and differential leukocyte counts in the peripheral blood of 12 subjects tended to decrease after hot-spring hydro-therapy. The statistically significant result only obtained that the granulocyte counts significantly decreased ($p < 0.05$). Another minor group lymphocyte did not changed significantly by judging from simple.

Hot Spring Hydro Therapy Regulate Peripheral Leukocyte Together with Emotional Hormone and Receptor Positive Lymphocytes According to Each Constitution/Condition.

**Figure 18** shows the total numbers of leukocytes, granulocytes and lymphocytes from peripheral blood collected before and after hot spring hydrotherapy in the older and younger groups. The quantitative variation of the two groups differed. In the younger group, the total number of WBC ($p < 0.05$) and granulocytes ($p < 0.01$) clearly decreased. On the other hand, the total number of WBC and lymphocytes significantly increased ($p < 0.01$) after hydrotherapy in the older group. Furthermore, the results show that changes in the leukocyte count and subset count had a negative relationship before and after hydrotherapy. In other words, subjects who had a higher cell count level before hydrotherapy tended to show a decrease in the number of WBC 24 hrs after hydrotherapy. There was a significant correlation between age and rate of change (**Figure 2**, $r = 0.91$, $p < 0.001$). Since the turning point occurred at 35 years old, we separated the participants into a younger (under 35) and an older (over 36) group.

## 14. The Slant Suggest the Efficacy of Each CAM Menu

### 14.1. In Case of Hot Spring Hydrotherapy

Each volunteer was prepared their blood before start to visit hot spring village after informed consented to the experimental purpose by written Ethics of the Committee in Kanazawa Medical University. After lodging the hotel, volunteers enjoyed Japanese type hot spring bath system, with no under wear in the bath room/pool separately prepared for ladies and gentleman. We suggested taking a bath totally 2 - 3 times within two days for the aim of tryal. Beside the advance of VAS: visual analog scale in our investigation, we measured the total number of leukocyte and two major subsets, granulocyte and lymphocytes regulated before and after hot spring hydrotherapy.

We tried to express the effect of peripheral total leukocyte number by individual level of change and plot in the X-axis as in each age. As was in **Figure 2**, the groups was separated in to two, up-regulated individuals and down-regulated one. The correlation of change was expressed as a linear function. **Figure 10** was ideal change of effect with hot spring hydrotherapy, showing ideal inclination. The results showed that these subsets could reflect the number and function of immuno-competent cells. For example, in an individual with a low granulocyte number, the number increased after treatment, while it decreased in another individual with a higher cell number.

We sampled peripheral blood from the 12 volunteers before and after hot sand/hydro therapy, at the same O'clock on the day, with the respect of circadian rhythm [21] [30] of leukocyte. These subjects participated in this study after giving their informed consent. We conducted the experiment at Yuwaku Onsen Spa (Kanazawa, Ishikawa Pref., Japan) in one night of the day. The spring quality is a weak sodium chloride with sodium carbohydrate of the water temperature 41˚C ± 1˚C. During the night and in the morning of the next day, they had a bath in the hot spring two or three times, for 20 - 30 minutes each time. Hot sand spa had performed and bathing for 40 mins. Time interval of blood sampling between before and after hot-spring hydrotherapy was approximately 24 hours. Measurements of the total and differential leukocyte counts and 3 catecholamines levels in the peripheral blood.

We ordered on the laboratory of Ishikawa Prefecture Preventive Medicine Association about the total and differential leukocyte counts and the levels of 3 catecholamines (adrenaline, noradrenaline, and dopamine) in the peripheral blood from the subjects. The total and differential leukocyte counts were measured by the automated hematology analyzer XE-2100 (Sysmex, Inc., Kobe, Japan). The levels of catecholamines were measured by high performance liquid chromatography (HPLC) system (Tosoh Co. and Hitachi High-Technologies Co., Japan).

## 14.2. Emotional Hormones Also Regulated with Condition/Constitution Dependent Manner

We had been observed the reputational effect of hydrotherapy could be evidenced within a short period. But the possibility still remain that the leukocyte change was happen to emerge for the dairy life as accidental factor,

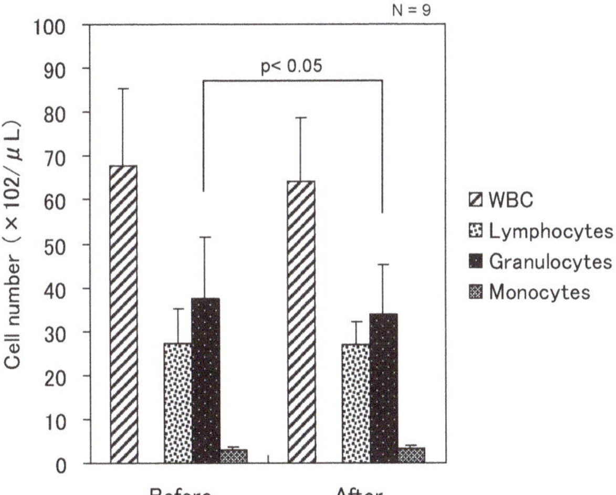


**Figure 18.** Twenty-four hours change of leukocyte counts on the bases of group comparison between pre/post hydrotherapy. We sampled peripheral blood from the 12 volunteers before and after hot spring hydrotherapy, at the same time on each day, in accordance with the consideration of circadian rhythm of leukocyte In this Figure, we tried to show the date simply pooled and make mean, then compared.

such as stress and so on. In order to avoid such possibility, then we tried to show the change of the peripheral leukocyte number was the result of another network system of the inner system such as peripheral leukocyte, endocrine and brain system. We sampled peripheral blood from the 12 volunteers before and after hot sand/hydro therapy, at the same time on the next day, with the respect of circadian rhythm of leukocyte [21]. These subjects participated in this study after giving their informed consent. We conducted the experiment at Yuwaku Onsen Spa (Kanazawa, Ishikawa Pref., Japan) in one night of the day. The spring quality is a weak sodium chloride with sodium carbohydrate of the water temperature 41˚C ± 1˚C. During the night and in the morning of the next day, they had a bath in the hot spring two or three times, for 20-30 minutes each time. Time interval of blood sampling between before and after hot spring hydrotherapy was approximately 24 hours. Measurements of the total and differential leukocyte counts and 3 catecholamines levels in the peripheral blood

The adrenaline and nor-adrenaline are secreted by various stress (stimulation); the former from the adrenal medulla and the latter from both the adrenal medulla and the end of sympathetic nerve. They express these functions through the adrenergic receptors (ARs) and regulate the target organ. The adrenergic receptor has two types of $\alpha$ and $\beta$, and there are multiple subtypes ($\alpha_1$, $\alpha_2$, $\beta_1$, $\beta_2$, $\beta_3$) (4). These subtypes present the vascular ($\alpha_1$), the presynaptic terminal ($\alpha_2$), the heart ($\beta_1$), the bronchial muscle of the lung ($\beta_2$), fat cells ($\beta_3$), respectively. The $\alpha$-receptor stimulation causes bronchodilatation and vasodilatation, the $\beta_1$-receptor stimulation causes an increase in heart rate and lipolysis, and the $\beta_2$-receptor stimulation causes bronchoconstriction, vasodilatation, and muscle glycogen resolution. The adrenaline provides heart activation by effect on $\alpha$- and $\beta$-receptors, and the nor-adrenaline provides blood pressure rises by strongly effect on $\alpha$-receptors. In addition to the above, it has been reported that the ARs are present on leucocyte membranes [21]-[23] and that the level of expression of $\beta$-ARs in lymphocytes was examined by radioligand ($^{125}$iodopindolol) binding, but the details of subtype of $\beta$- receptors have not been disclosed. The subtypes of the AR are able to be analyzed by flow cytometry (FCM) method. In this study, we described how hot spring hydrotherapy influences leukocyte, lymphocyte subpopulations expressing $\beta_2$-AR and the levels of catecholamine in human peripheral blood (**Figure 19**).

## 14.3. CD Positive Lymphocytes Correlate with Serum Adrenaline Level, as a Result of the Regulation by Hot Spring Hydrotherapy

The analysis of CD positive cells by FCM was measured by gating in the lymphocytes region on the scattered gram. **Figure 8** shows an example analysis. Nonspecific reaction of the PE fluorescence was found in the isotype control. Therefore, the real values of the AR expressing cell counts were calculated by subtracting the control values. The CD19$^+$ cells were observed nonspecific reaction which seems to response of the second antibody. The comparison of each lymphocyte subpopulations before and after hot spring hydrotherapy showed that the CD8$^+$ cell and CD56$^+$ cell counts tended to increase (**Figure 5**, **Figure 6**). However, the significant variation was not seen from the comparison of $\beta_2$-AR expressing cells before and after hot-spring hydrotherapy. The mean % of $\beta_2$-AR expressing cells in the lymphocyte subsets was 18% - 19% in CD3$^+$ cells, 5% in CD4$^+$ cells, 57% - 63% in CD8$^+$ cells, and 93% - 95% in CD56$^+$ cells. That in CD19$^+$ cells was approximately 100% (data not shown), but we were not able to be confirmed because it was very likely to be the nonspecific reaction.

We examined the correlation with the rate of change in adrenaline levels and the rate of change in $\beta_2$-AR expressing cell counts of each subset or that in each CD-positive cell counts before and after hot spring hydrotherapy. In the CD-positive cells, the rate of change in adrenaline levels was a positive correlation with that in the levels of CD56$^+$ cells, CD8$^+$ cells, and CD3$^+$ cells; in particular, a correlation with CD56$^+$ and CD8$^+$ cells was high. In $\beta_2$-AR expressing cells, the rate of change in adrenaline levels was a positive correlation with the rate of change in the levels of $\beta_2$-AR$^+$ CD56$^+$ cells (**Figure 20**, **Figure 21** and **Figure 22**). These results suggested that the variation in adrenaline levels is correlated with CD56$^+$ cells.

## 14.4. $\beta_2$-AR$^+$ Receptor Positive Lymphocytes Correlate with Adrenaline Level, as a Result of the Regulation by Hydrotherapy

The adrenaline and noradrenaline are secreted by various stress (stimulation); the former from the adrenal medulla and the latter from both the adrenal medulla and the end of sympathetic nerve. They express these functions through the adrenergic receptors (ARs) and regulate the target organ. The adrenergic receptor has two types of $\alpha$ and $\beta$, and there are multiple subtypes ($\alpha_1$, $\alpha_2$, $\beta_1$, $\beta_2$, $\beta_3$). These subtypes present the vascular ($\alpha_1$), the presynaptic terminal ($\alpha_2$), the heart ($\beta_1$), the bronchial muscle of the lung ($\beta_2$), fat cells ($\beta_3$), respectively. The $\alpha$-

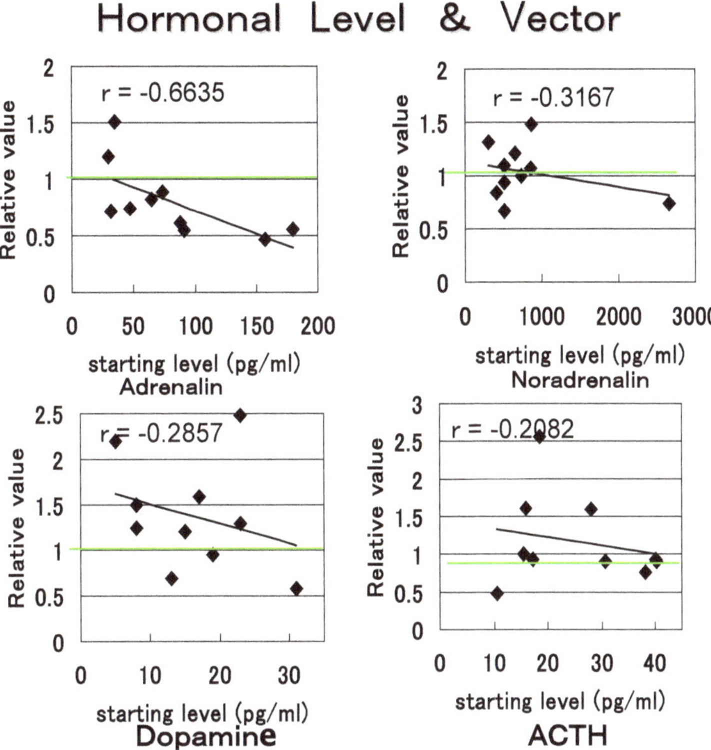


**Figure 19.** The constitution dependent analysis for (adrenaline and dopamine). Each spot were obtained from the calculation comparing relative value from before and after levels in the serum, catecholamines levels in the peripheral blood Relative value 1 shows no change before and after the menu. The constitution dependent analysis, the detail change and vector of each change could find from individual data, showing higher value volunteer down regulated much more than lower leveled one (**Figure 20**).

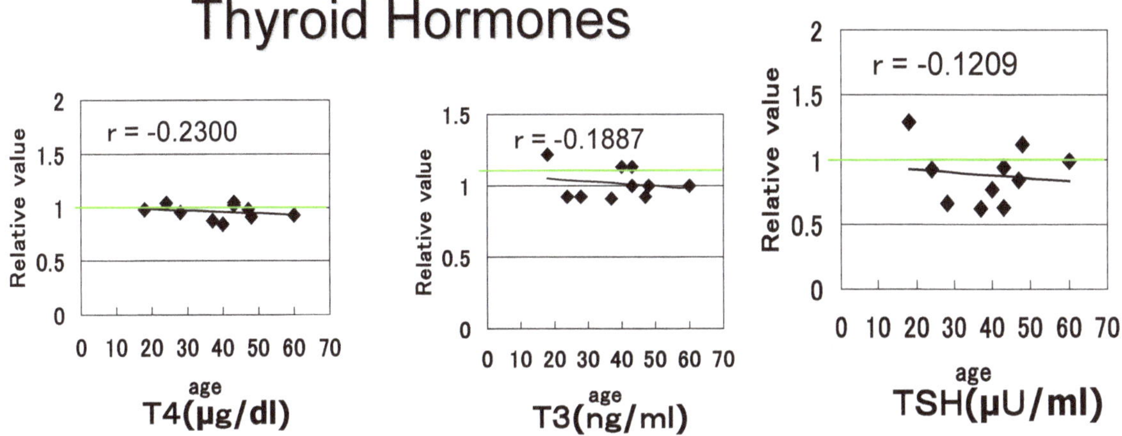


**Figure 20.** The constitution dependent analysis for thyroid hormones (T3, T4 and TSH). Each spot were obtained from the calculation comparing relative value from before and after levels in the serum.

receptor stimulation causes bronchodilatation and vasodilatation, the $\beta_1$-receptor stimulation causes an increase in heart rate and lipolysis, and the $\beta_2$-receptor stimulation causes bronchoconstriction, vasodilatation, and muscle glycogen resolution. The adrenaline provides heart activation by effect on $\alpha$- and $\beta$-receptors, and the noradrenaline provides blood pressure rises by strongly effect on $\alpha$-receptors. In addition to the above, it has been

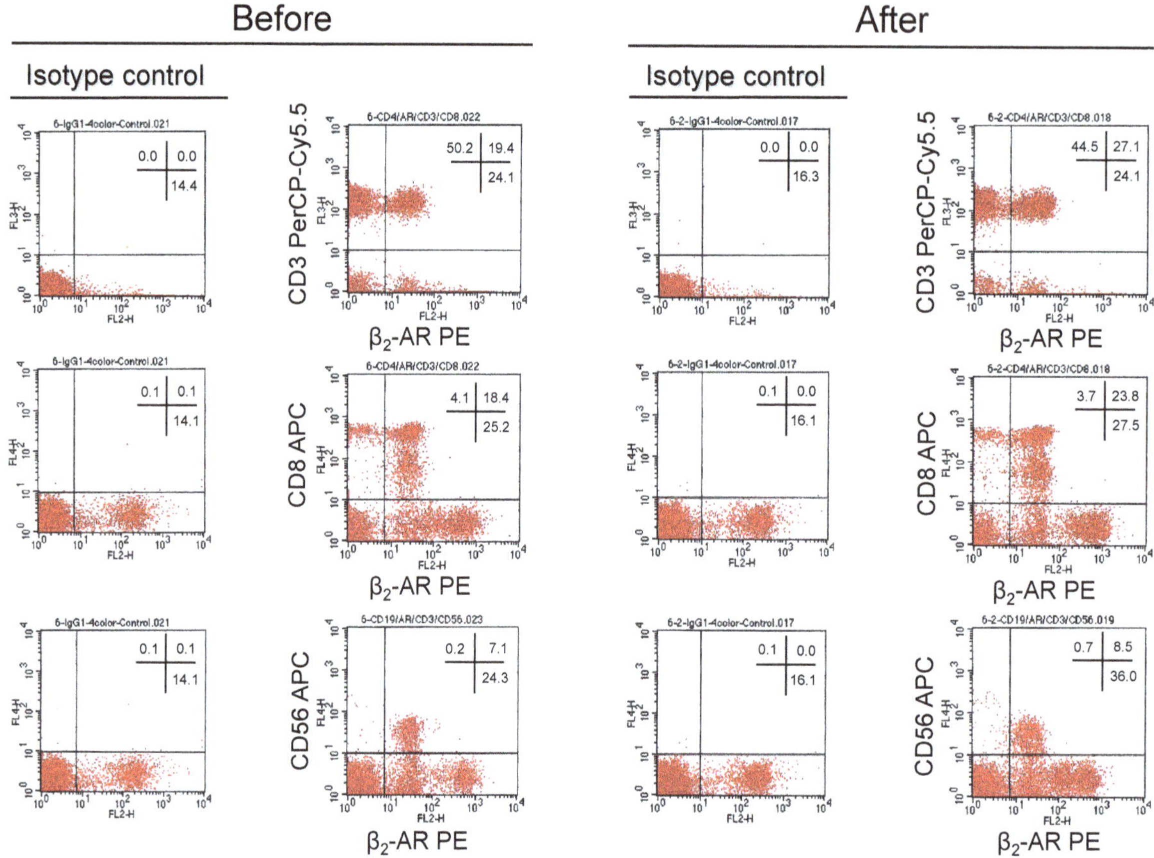


**Figure 21.** FACS analyses of $\beta_2$-AR$^+$ cells in lymphocyte subpopulations before and after hot spring hydrotherapy. The analysis of $\beta_2$-AR expressing cells and CD positive cells by FCM was measured by gating in the lymphocytes region on the scattered gram.

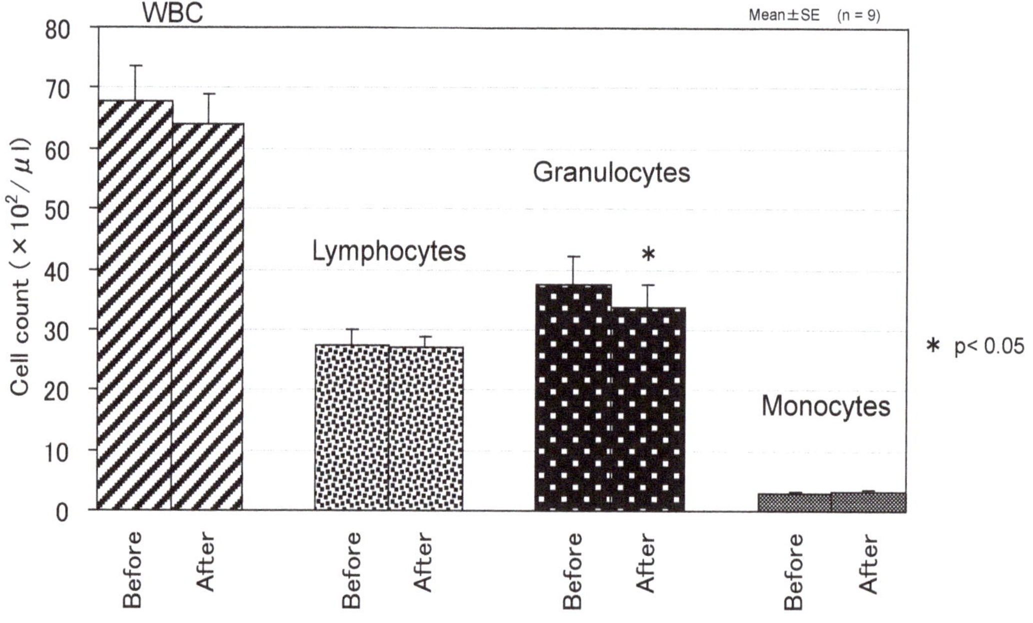


**Figure 22.** Non-constitutional Comparison of WBC and Subsets Number by Hydrotherapy.

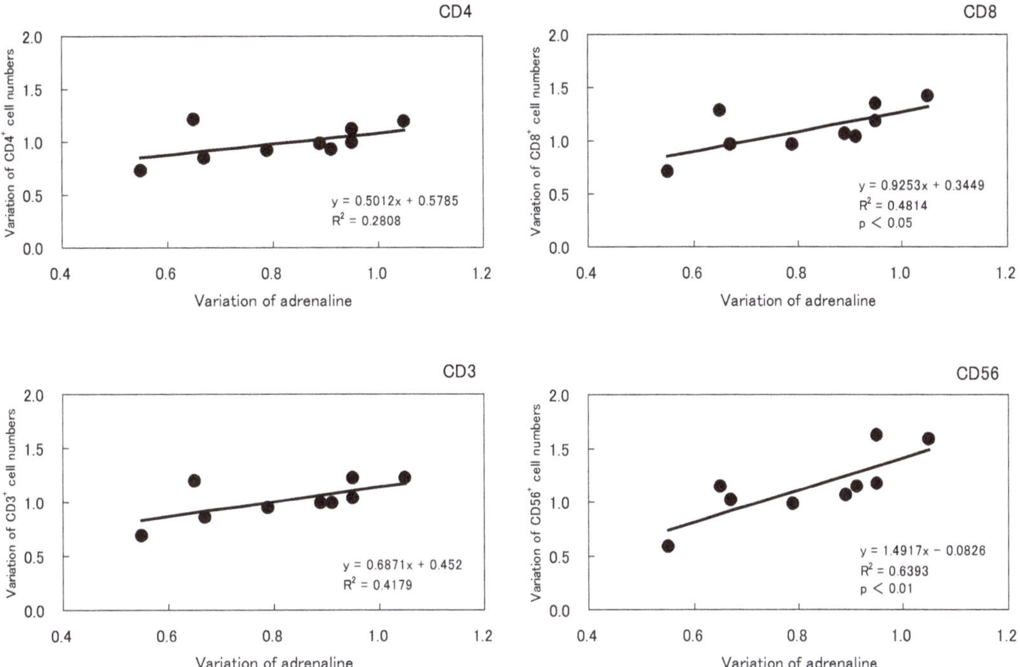


**Figure 23.** Relationship between the rate of change in adrenaline levels and the rate of change in the levels of CD-positive cells before and after hydrotherapy.

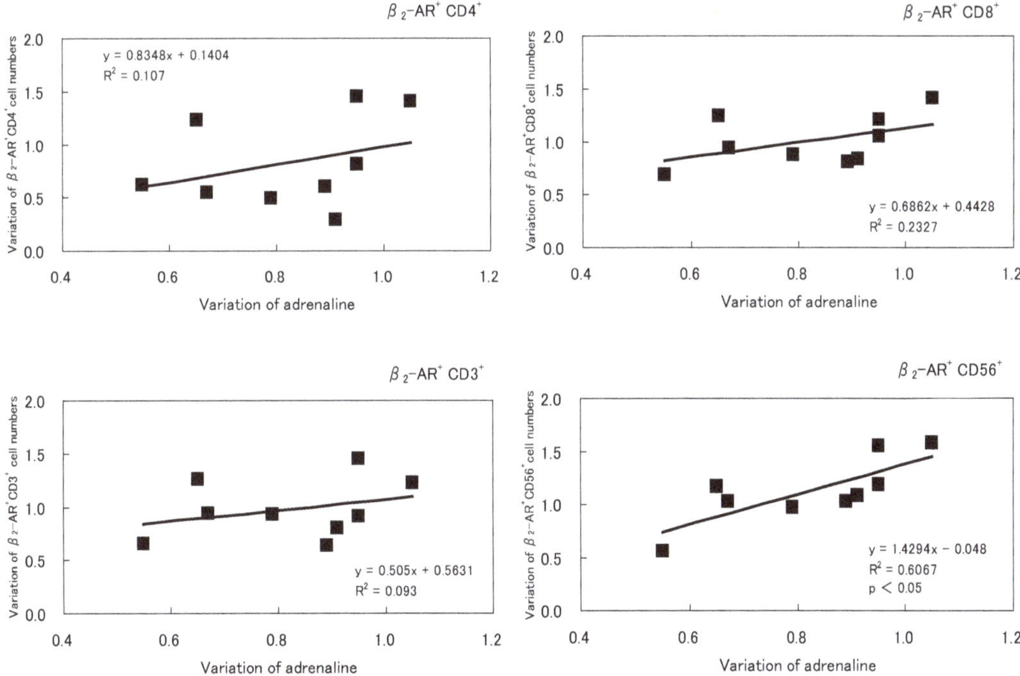


**Figure 24.** Variations in the number of $\beta_2$-AR$^+$ cells in lymphocyte subpopulations. And adrenaline levels in the peripheral The analysis of $\beta_2$-AR receptor expressing cells and CD positive cells by FCM was measured by gating in the lymphocytes region on the scattered gram. s an example analysis (**Figure 23**, **Figure 24**).

reported that the ARs are present on leucocyte membranes and that the level of expression of $\beta$-ARs in lymphocytes was examined by radioligand ($^{125}$I-iodopindolol) binding, but the details of subtype of $\beta$-receptors have not been disclosed. The subtypes of the AR are able to be analyzed by flow cytometry (FCM) method. In this study, we described how hot spring hydrotherapy influences leukocyte, lymphocyte subpopulations expressing $\beta_2$-AR and the levels of catecholamine in human peripheral blood (**Figure 25**).

The analysis of $\beta_2$-AR expressing cells and CD positive cells by FCM was measured by gating in the lymphocytes region on the scattered gram. Figure showed an example analysis. Nonspecific reaction of the PE fluorescence was found in the isotype control. Therefore, the real values of the AR expressing cell counts were calculated by subtracting the control values. The CD19$^+$ cells were observed nonspecific reaction which seems to response of the second antibody. The comparison of each lymphocyte subpopulations before and after hot spring hydrotherapy showed that the CD8$^+$ cell and CD56$^+$ cell counts tended to increase. However, the significant variation was not seen from the comparison of $\beta_2$-AR expressing cells before and after hot-spring hydrotherapy. The mean % of $\beta_2$-AR expressing cells in the lymphocyte subsets was 18% - 19% in CD3$^+$ cells, 5% in CD4$^+$ cells, 57% - 63% in CD8$^+$ cells, and 93-95% in CD56$^+$ cells. That in CD19$^+$ cells was approximately 100% (data not shown), but we were not able to be confirmed because it was very likely to be the nonspecific reaction.

We examined the correlation with the rate of change in adrenaline levels and the rate of change in $\beta_2$-AR expressing cell counts of each subset or that in each CD-positive cell counts before and after hot spring hydrotherapy. In the CD-positive cells, the rate of change in adrenaline levels was a positive correlation with that in the levels of CD56$^+$ cells, CD8$^+$ cells, and CD3$^+$ cells; in particular, a correlation with CD56$^+$ and CD8$^+$ cells was high (**Figure 20**). In $\beta_2$-AR expressing cells, the rate of change in adrenaline levels was a positive correlation with the rate of change in the levels of $\beta_2$-AR$^+$ CD56$^+$ cells. These results suggested that the variation in adrenaline levels is correlated with CD56$^+$ cells.

## 15. The Results in Light Exercise/Walking

### Emotional Hormones Also Regulated with Condition/Constitution Dependent Manner

We had been observed the reputational effect of hydrotherapy could be evidenced within a short period. But the possibility still remain that the leukocyte change was happen to emerge for the dairy life as accidental factor, such as stress and so on. In order to avoid such possibility, then we tried to show the change of the peripheral leukocyte number was the result of another network system of the inner system such as peripheral leukocyte, endocrine and brain system. We sampled peripheral blood from the 12 volunteers before and after hot sand/hydro therapy, at the same time on the next day, with the respect of circadian rhythm of leukocyte [25]-[27]. These subjects participated in this study after giving their in- formed consent. We conducted the experiment at Yuwaku Onsen Spa (Kanazawa, Ishikawa Pref., Japan) in one night of the day. The spring quality is a weak sodium chloride with sodium carbohydrate of the water temperature 41˚C ± 1˚C. During the night and in

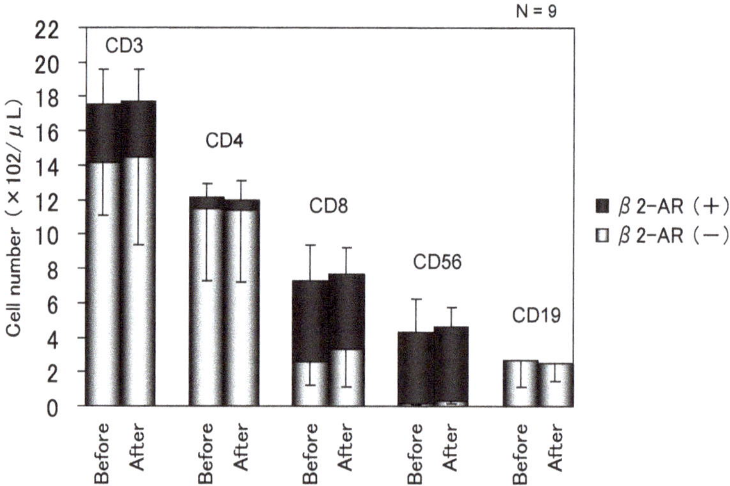


**Figure 25.** Individual comparison of adrenalin levels and CD positive cells in the peripheral blood Time interval of blood sampling between before and after hot spring hydrotherapy was approximately 24 hours. Measurements of the total and differential leukocyte counts and 3 adrenergic receptors (ARs) levels in the peripheral blood.

the morning of the next day, they had a bath in the hot spring two or three times, for 20 - 30 minutes each time. Time interval of blood sampling between before and after hot spring hydrotherapy was approximately 24 hours. Measurements of the total and differential leukocyte counts and 3 catecholamines levels in the peripheral blood.

The adrenaline and noradrenaline are secreted by various stress (stimulation); the former from the adrenal medulla and the latter from both the adrenal medulla and the end of sympathetic nerve. They express these functions through the adrenergic receptors (ARs) and regulate the target organ. The adrenergic receptor has two types of $\alpha$ and $\beta$, and there are multiple subtypes ($\alpha_1$, $\alpha_2$, $\beta_1$, $\beta_2$, $\beta_3$) [21]. These subtypes present the vascular ($\alpha_1$), the pre-synaptic terminal ($\alpha_2$), the heart ($\beta_1$), the bronchial muscle of the lung ($\beta_2$), fat cells ($\beta 3$), respectively. The $\alpha$-receptor stimulation causes bronchodilatation and vasodilatation, the $\beta 1$-receptor stimulation causes an increase in heart rate and lipolysis, and the $\beta_2$-receptor stimulation causes bronchoconstriction, vasodilatation, and muscle glycogen resolution. The adrenaline provides heart activation by effect on $\alpha$- and $\beta$-receptors, and the noradrenaline provides blood pressure rises by strongly effect on $\alpha$-receptors. In addition to the above, it has been reported that the ARs are present on leucocyte membranes [22]-[24] and that the level of expression of $\beta$-ARs in lymphocytes was examined by radioligand (125I-iodopindolol) binding, but the details of subtype of $\beta$-receptors have not been disclosed. The subtypes of the AR are able to be analyzed.

The adrenaline and noradrenaline are secreted by various stress (stimulation); the former from the adrenal medulla and the latter from both the adrenal medulla and the end of sympathetic nerve. They express these functions through the adrenergic receptors (ARs) and regulate the target organ. The adrenergic receptor has two types of $\alpha$ and $\beta$, and there are multiple subtypes ($\alpha_1$, $\alpha_2$, $\beta_1$, $\beta_2$, $\beta_3$) [21]. These subtypes present the vascular ($\alpha_1$), the pre- synaptic terminal ($\alpha_2$), the heart ($\beta_1$), the bronchial muscle of the lung ($\beta_2$), fat cells ($\beta_3$), respectively. The $\alpha$-receptor stimulation causes bronchodilatation and vasodilatation, the $\beta 1$-receptor stimulation causes an increase in heart rate and lipolysis, and the $\beta_2$-receptor stimulation causes bronchoconstriction, vasodilatation, and muscle glycogen resolution. The adrenaline provides heart activation by effect on $\alpha$- and $\beta$-receptors, and the noradrenaline provides blood pressure rises by strongly effect on $\alpha$-receptors. In addition to the above, it has been reported that the ARs are present on leucocyte membranes [22]-[24] and that the level of expression of $\beta$-ARs in lymphocytes was examined by radioligand (125I-iodopindolol) binding, but the details of subtype of $\beta$-receptors have not been disclosed. The subtypes of the AR are able to be analyzed by flow cytometry (FCM) method. In this study, we described how hot spring hydrotherapy influences leukocyte, lymphocyte subpopulations expressing $\beta_2$-AR.

## 16. In Case of Light Exercise/Walking, for the Best Menu to Each Freak

We selected 14 healthy volunteers (mean age, 41 ± 15.2 years, ranging 19 - 60 years old in both sexualities) and informed consented according to the Ethics Committee of Kanazawa Medical University. The contents of sexuality were 56.25% of the lady and 43.75% for gentleman. They were the students of Medical University and the stuff for the school of medicine. None of them was a specialist for athletic field. The group was set up into two groups according to the intense of walking, 4 mets and 8 mets.

### 16.1. Walking Exercise by 4 Mets

These subjects participated in this study after giving their informed consent. We conducted the walking exercise at the country side of Japan. The course of exercise located at 40 meter in high and 1015 mb of atmospheric pressure. We sampled peripheral blood from the 14 volunteers before and after exercise, at the same time on each day, in consideration of circadian rhythm [21] [22] of leukocyte. The exercise start at ten o'clock for about one hour, corresponding 4 metabolic rates; mets [23] [24]. Time interval of blood sampling between before and after exercise was approximately 24 hours. Measurements of the total leukocyte were assessed for differential leukocyte counts and granlocyte and lymphocyte ratio in the peripheral blood.

We ordered to the laboratory of Ishikawa Prefecture Preventive Medicine Association for precise counts for the total and differential leukocyte counts in the peripheral blood from the subjects. The total and differential leukocyte counts were measured by the automated hematology analyzer XE-2100 (Sysmex, Inc., Kobe, Japan).

### 16.2. Walking Exercise by 8 Mets

After two weeks of cooling down for all volunteers, we set up again for the same exercise except for the intense of walking was 8 km/hour for the same kilo-meter of the same course (8 mets). We prepared peripheral blood from the same 14 volunteers before and after the exercise, at the same time on each day, in consideration of circadian rhythm [21] [30] of leukocyte. We conducted the walking exercise at the same course in country side of Japan (**Figure 26**).

## 16.3. Assessment of Lymphocyte Subsets by FCM

For the purpose of estimating CD positive cell, the whole blood obtained from the subjects by blood collection tube containing an anticoagulant EDTA-2K. 100 μl of whole blood were added the antibody. After washing with PBS, the suspensions were mixed phycoerythrin (PE)-conjugated streptavidin (Beckman Coulter Inc. France) and fluorescence monoclonal antibody: peridinin chlorophyll protein-cyanin 5.5 (PerCP-Cy5.5)-conjugated CD2, flu conjugated CD19, FITC-conjugated CD57 (each Becton Dickinson Co. USA), allophycocyanin (APC)-conjugated CD8, and APC-conjugated CD57 (each Beckman Coulter). The negative controls were added PE-conjugated streptavidin and the isotype control antibodies to the CD antibodies. After incubation for 30 minutes at 4°C, these samples were hemolyzed using a 10-times dilution FACS Lysing Solution (Becton Dickinson). After washing with PBS, the cell suspensions were fixed using a 10-times dilution CellFIX (Becton Dickinson) and analyzed by flow cytometer FACS Caliber (Becton Dickinson) [25] [27].

## 16.4. Statistical Analysis

The statistical comparisons between two groups (before and after walking) for the test of significant difference were performed using paired t-test and wilcoxon signed-ranks test. Further, the test of the correlation were performed a spearman's correlation coefficient by rank test. Data are expressed as means ± standard error of mean (SE). A $p$ value < 0.05 was considered to be statistically significant. The Kendall tau rank correlation and the two-sided $p$-value ($H_0$: tau = 0). The ordinary scatterplot and the scatterplot between ranks of X & Y are also shown [28].

## 16.5. Twenty-Four Hours Change of Leukocyte Counts after 4 Mets of Walking

Each volunteer was prepared their blood before start for exercise and after informed consented to the experimental purpose by written Ethics of the Committee in Kanazawa Medical University. After warming up for 5 minutes by Radio exercise by NHK. We suggested taking a walk for one hour for 4km of the curse (4 mets). We tried to exhibit the effect of peripheral total leukocyte number by individual level of change and plot in the X-axis as in each value before the exercise. As was in **Figure**, the relative value (%) was calculated before and after the exercise and plotted in the Figures of the X-axis according to the value before exercise. As a result of the exhibition, there found three groups, separated, up-regulated individuals and down-regulated one and was no change. The correlation of change was expressed as a linear function and significant reverse correlation, −0.6893 indicating ideal value of correlative index −0.5 (**Figure 27**). The data obtained from 4mets exercise was brought ideal regulation. However, 8 mets could not bring such an effect significantly. About the leukocyte sub-orescein isothiocyanate (FITC)-conjugated CD4, FITC-conjugated CD8, FITC-conjugated CD16, FITC-

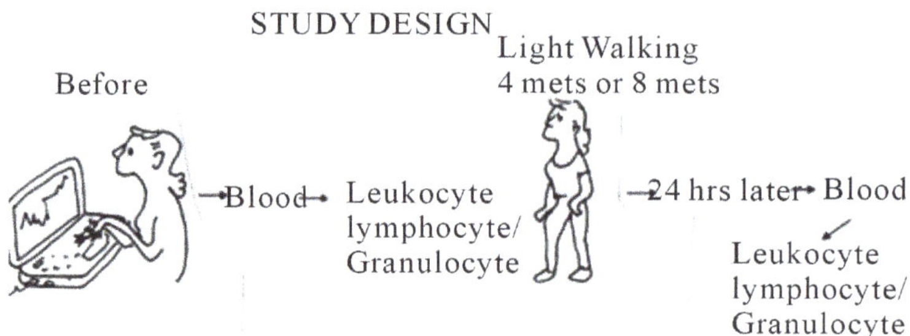


**Figure 26.** Experimental design of this report. We sampled peripheral blood from the 16 volunteers before and after walking exercise, at the same time on each day, in accordance with the consideration of circadian rhythm of leukocyte. We sampled peripheral blood from the 14 volunteers before and after exercise, at the same time on each day, in consideration of circadian rhythm of leukocyte. These subjects participated in this study after giving them informed consent.

set, the ideal regulation of lymphocyte and monocyte were found by 4 mets, but not in granulocyte (**Figure 27**).

## 16.6. Twenty-Four Hours Change of Leukocyte Counts after 8 Mets of Walking

After 2-weeks of cooling down, we set up the same mode of trial at the same course and by the same volunteers. None of volunteer was dropped out with any serious problem. In this time, we set up 8 mets impacts of exercise, asking to walk out by half an hour for the same course of 4 kilometers (8 mets). Preparing 5-min. warming up, we tried to express the effect of peripheral total leukocyte number by individual level of change and plot in the x-axis as in each value before the exercise as is in 3.1. (**Figure 27**). As shown in lower panel in **Figure 28**, the correlation was exhibited on a linear function but good correlation was retreated from the results by the case by 8 mets. The slant value was −0.3617. The data obtained from 8mets exercise was lesser regulatory effect than that compared by 4 mets of exercise. About the leukocyte subset, the regulation by lymphocytes were more remarkable. However, only of the monocyte exhibited significant change by both impact 4 and 8 mets.

## 16.7. Lymphocyte Subsets Regulation by 4 Mets

We had been observed the reputational effect of exercise could be evidenced within a short period. But the possibility still remain that the leukocyte change was happen to emerge for the dairy life as accidental factor, such as stress and so on. In order to avoid such possibility, then we tried to show the change of the peripheral leukocyte number was the result of another network system of the inner system such as peripheral leukocyte, endocrine and brain system. We tried to access the effect CD positive lymphocyte. They were CD2, CD CD4, CD8, CD16, CD19, CD57 within those CD positive cells, CD2, CD4, CD8, CD19 cells were regulated significantly as in number of each CD marker positive cells by 4 mets of excercise.

## 16.8. Twenty-Four Hours Change of Lymphocyte Subsets by 8 Mets

After 2-weeks of cooling down, we set up the same mode of trial at the same course and by the same volunteers. None of volunteer was dropped out with any serious problem. In this time, we set up 8 mets impacts of exercise, asking to walk out by half an hour for the same course of 4 kilometers (8 mets). Preparing 5-min. warming up, we tried to express the effect on lymphocyte subsets as CD positive number. They were CD2, CD 4, CD 8, CD 16, CD 19, CD57. As shown in the **Figure 29**, the regulatory effect was overwealed 27 in the all the subset in 8 mets of exercise.

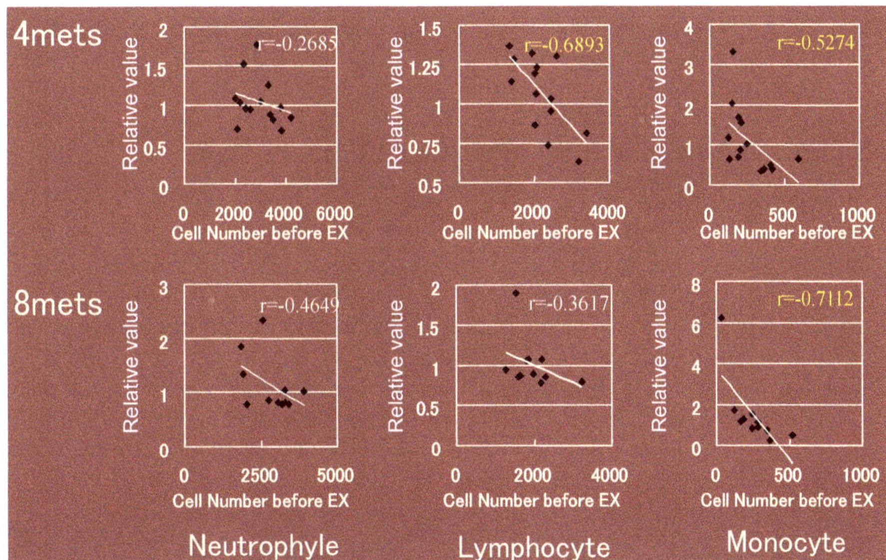


**Figure 27.** We tried to express the effect of peripheral total leukocyte number by individual level of change and plot in the x-axis as in each value before the exercise. The relative value (%) of post walking was calculated with before and after and plotted in the X-avis. The statistically significant value of slope were Indicated in yellow.

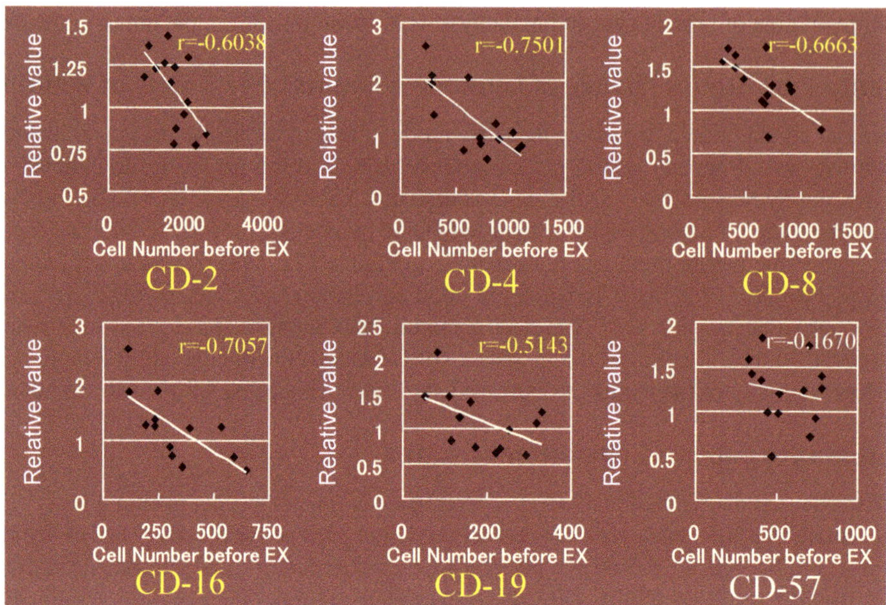


**Figure 28.** For the purpose of estimating CD positive cell, the whole blood obtained from the subjects by blood collection tube containing anticoagulant EDTA-2K. 100 μl of whole blood were added the antibody. After washing with PBS, the suspensions were mixed phycoerythrin (PE)-conjugated streptavidin: peridinin chlorophyll protein-cyanin 5.5 (PerCP-Cy5.5)-conjugated CD2, CD4, CD8, CD16, CD19, CD57. We tried to express the effect of peripheral total leukocyte number by individual level of change and plot in the x-axis as in each value before the exercise. The relative value was calculated before and after the exercise and plotted in the figure of the X-axis for the value before exercise. The statistically significant value of slope were indicated in yellow.

### 16.9. Simple Sum up & Make Mean, Get No Meaning after 24 Hours Change of Lymphocyte Subsets by Both 4 & 8 Mets

As shown in **Figure 27** and **Figure 28**, we can compared and got the result that of 4mets of exercise was more effective to regulate lymphocyte and lymphocyte subset by individual change by plotting the linear function. We tried to exhibit the same data with grouped and tried to make mean. From the results, there was no significant change.

### 16.10. The Tailored Assessment Was Provided by Linear Slant

Our results showed that within 24 hours after light exercise, the white blood cells in peripheral blood had regulated significantly, not only in leukocyte subset but also lymphocyte subset. The results showed that these subsets could reflect the number and function of immuno-competent cells [13]-[19]. For example, in an individual with a low granulocyte number, the number increased after treatment, while it decreased in another individual with a higher cell number. Our results led us to believe that leukocyte subsets could be an interesting indicator for the evaluation of alternative therapies. Many systems are in place to evaluate Western therapies that aim at healing the symptoms of an illness. We hope that our work will attract more attention to the mechanisms of which each CAM menu regulates the human immune system. Abo reported that according to the lymphocyte subset content, lymphocyte rich type showed over 40% on the other hand granulocyte rich type show over 6o% of granulocyte. Each type exhibited different character even in the same age, sexuality and different age. Within the same age and the sexuality, even in gentleman can sorts out as G-rich type (granulocyte 60%), and L-rich type (lymphocyte 40%). On the other hand, as a stand point of sexuality difference, the lady belongs to L-rich type but the gentleman belongs G-rich type. According to the age-related change, G-rich type of young man change to L-rich type according to getting older [21] [29].

We have been trying to regulate the immune responsiveness through much mature by fragile daily condition from circumstance stress and so on. The main menu were, acupuncture, hot-spring hydrotherapy, light exercise etc. In this article, we would like to show the regulatory mechanism of the light exercise walking as a tailored scale. The circumstance, except for cases of contraindication, has been medically useful approved to be effective in many stress-related disorders and the improvement of dysfunction of the biological rhythm disturbance as well as chronic disease. The mechanism of effects has been reported in many studies, but many things are still unclear.

## 16.11. The Grouped Comparison by Conventional Assessment

In order to assess correctly to the changes after the menu, it is important to conscious of circadian rhythm. Abo also reported that it was possible to sort the constitution, granulocyte-rich individual and lymphocyte-rich one with the peripheral leukocyte [22] [31]-[33].

Each population of subset is depends on a circadian rhythm. Within a same individual, granulocyte increase in the daytime, on the other hand, lymphocyte increased in the night time in a cycle 24 hrs. So we have to compare the effect of each menu for the peripheral leukocyte on the same time before and after the menu.

With our report, simple comparison of grouped value did not exhibit the valuable change in each individual. So this style of presentation was suggestive to the patient for immunodeficy such as in DM [34]-[56].

It was reported that the leukocyte subset, granulocyte and lymphocyte regulated by various factors. One major point is that they are regulated by autonomous nervous system, resulting in circadian rhythm [23] [24]. Therefore, in order to access the effect within a short time, it is necessary to consider this factor to adjust the time to collect the sample. For example, efficacy and impact of walking exercise has been widely recognized. However, the majority of walkers did not have a scientific background to know the best exercise menu for the one' QOL; quality of life. The purpose of this study was to demonstrate the best menu of walking that regulates the peripheral white blood cells in number and function as a marker of QOL expression [21] [57].

However, almost all the judgments of efficacy are VAS (visual analog scale). Moreover, simple processing by grouped value and make mean fadeout the precise regulation according to each constitution. Therefore, we hope our tailored scale can suggest to assess every CAM therapies in the world for competition.

## 16.12. Twenty-Four Hours Change of Leukocyte Counts after Heating by Hot Air from Overhead

None of volunteer was dropped out with any serious problem. In trial, we set up room temperature also 18C at

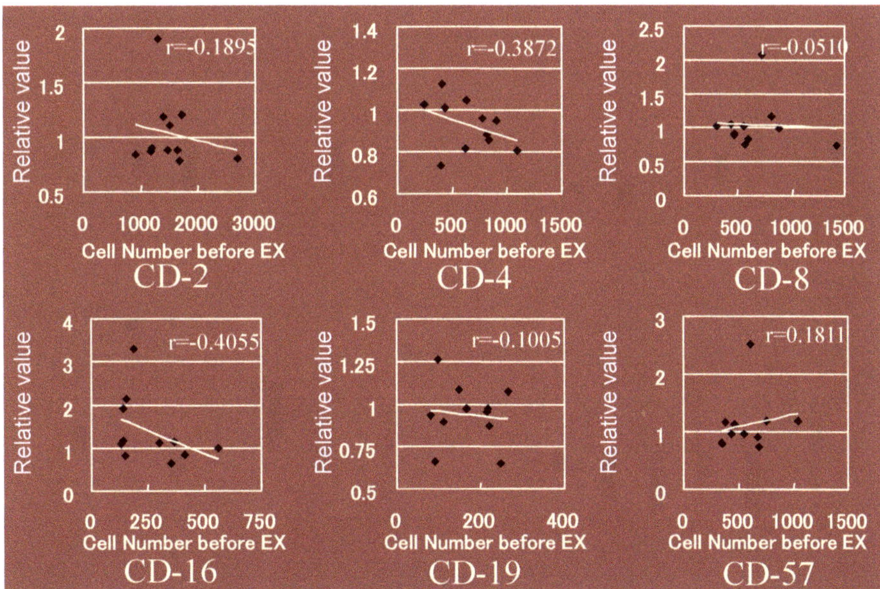


**Figure 29.** For the purpose of estimating CD positive cell, the whole blood obtained from the subjects by blood collection tube containing an anticoagulant EDTA-2K. The contents were the same in **Figure 4** except that the data were from the volunteers from 8 mets of walking. The statistically significant value of slope were indicated in yellow.

the 150 cm in high from floor, we tried to express the effect of peripheral total leukocyte number by individual level of change and plot in the X-axis as in each value before the exercise as is in 3.1. As shown in lower panel in **Figure 30**, the correlation was exhibited on a linear function but good correlation was retreated from the results. About the leukocyte subset, the regulation by lymphocytes were more remarkable. However, only the

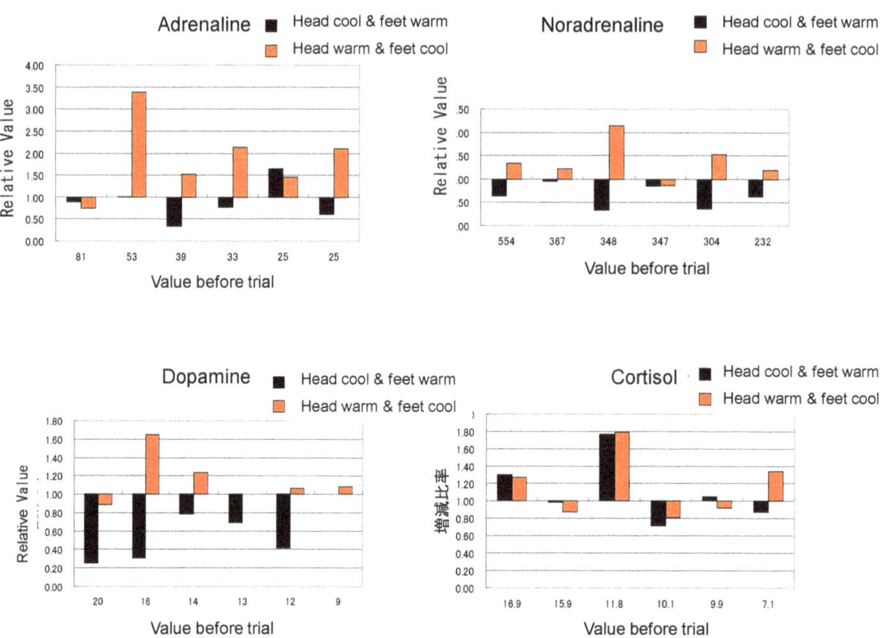


**Figure 30.** We tried to express the effect of peripheral total leukocyte number by individual level. The results were plotted in the X-axis as in each value before the trial. The relative value (%) of post trial was calculated with before and after and plotted in the Y-axis. Total leukocytes, Leukocyte subset, granulocyte and lymphocyte were also traced in the Figures.

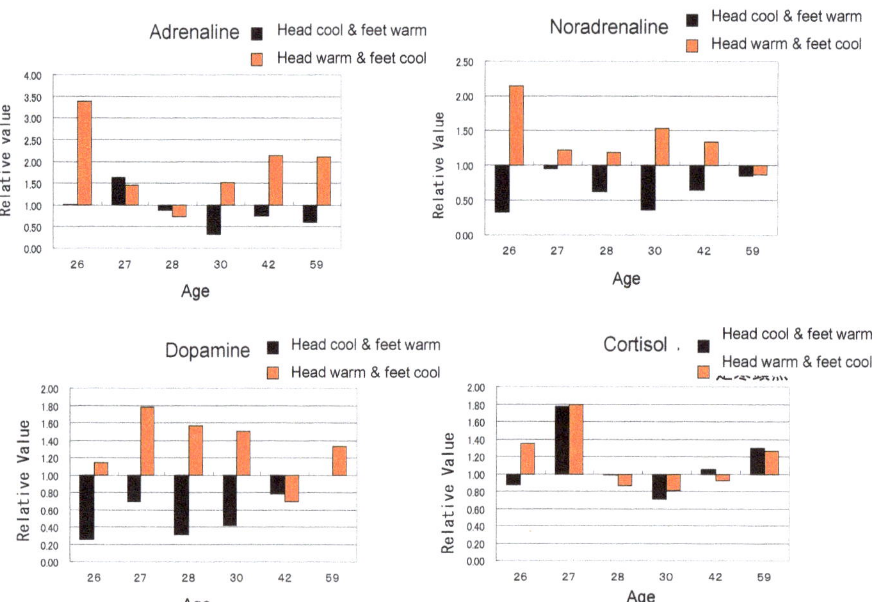


**Figure 31.** We tried to express the effect of peripheral total leukocyte number by individual level of change and plot in the x-axis as in each value according to the age. The relative value (%) of post trial was calculated with before and after and plotted in the Y-axis. Leukocyte subset, granulocyte and lymphocyte were also traced in the Figures.

monocyte exhibited significant change by both.

## 16.13. Leukocyte Subsets Regulation by Floor Heating

After one-weeks of working in the conditioned room as HCFH or HHFC, we set up the different mode of trial at the same course and by the same volunteers. None of volunteer is dropped out with any serious problems. In this time, we set up HCFH system, asking to work about for 5 days. We select four hormones and access the effect of HCFH or HHFC conditioned room. After working about regular desk working in the HCFH conditioned room, each volunteer is down-regulated the adrenaline, cortisone and nor-adrenalin. However, dopamine level is up-regulated for all the individuals being tested. On the other hand, HHFC system shows a reversed effect for all the hormones in this text [21] [57] (**Figure 31**).

## References

[1] Kurashige, S., Yoshida, T. and Mitsuhashi, S. (1980) Immune Response in Sarcoma 10-Bearing Mice. *Annual Report of Gunnma University*, **1**, 36-44.

[2] Miyazaki, S. (1977) Immunodificiency in Clinical Origin. *Clinical Pediatrics*, **1**, 1001-1006.

[3] Kishida, K., Miyazaku, S., Take, H., Fujimoto, T., Shi, H., Sasaki, K. and Goya, N. (1978) Granial Irradiation and Lymphocyte Subpopulation in Acute Lymphatic Leukemia. *Journal of Pediatrics*, **92**, 785-786. http://dx.doi.org/10.1016/S0022-3476(78)80155-3

[4] Yamaguchi, N., Takei, T., Chen, R., Wushuer, P. and Wu, H.W. (2013) Maternal Bias of Immunity to Her Offspring: Possibility of an Autoimmunity Twist out from Maternal Immunity to Her Young. *Open Journal of Rheumatology and Autoimmune Diseases*, **3**, Article ID: 28147.

[5] Murgita, R.A. and Tomasi Jr., T.B. (1975) Suppression of the Immune Response by Alpha-Fetoprotein. *The Journal of Experimental Medicine*, **141**, 269-286. http://dx.doi.org/10.1084/jem.141.2.269

[6] Paul, G., Margaret, S., Liew, Y.F. and Allan, M.M. (1995) $CD4^+$ but Not $CD8^+$ T Cells Are Required for the Induction of Oral Tolerance. *International Immunology*, **7**, 501-504. http://dx.doi.org/10.1093/intimm/7.3.501

[7] Koshimo, H., Miyazawa, H.Y., Shimizu, Y. and Yamaguchi, N. (1989) Maternal Antigenic Stimulation Actively Produces Suppressor Activity in Offspring. *Developmental & Comparative Immunology*, **13**, 79-85. http://dx.doi.org/10.1016/0145-305X(89)90020-7

[8] Zoeller, M. (1988) Tolerization during Pregnancy: Impact on the Development of Antigen-Specific Help and Suppression. *European Journal of Immunology*, **18**, 1937-1943. http://dx.doi.org/10.1002/eji.1830181211

[9] Auerback, R. and Clark, S. (1975) Immunological Tolerance: Transmission from Mother to Offspring. *Science*, **189**, 811-813. http://dx.doi.org/10.1126/science.1162355

[10] Shinka, S., Dohi, Y., Komatsu, T., Natarajan, R. and Amano, T. (1974) Immunological Unresponsiveness in Mice. I. Immunological Unresponsiveness Induced in Embryonic Mice by Maternofetal Transfer of Human-Globulin. *Biken Journal*, **17**, 59-72.

[11] Aase, J.M., Noren, G.R., Reddy, D.V. and Geme Jr., J.W. (1972) Mumps-Virus Infection in Pregnant Women and the Immunologic Response of Their Offspring. *The New England Journal of Medicine*, **286**, 1379-1382. http://dx.doi.org/10.1056/NEJM197206292862603

[12] Cramer, D.V., Kunz, H.W. and Gill III, T.J. (1974) Immunologic Sensitization Prior to Birth. *American Journal of Obstetrics & Gynecology*, **120**, 431-439.

[13] Wang, X.X., Kitada, K., Matsui, S., Ohkawa, T., Sugiyama, H., Kohno, S., Shimizu, S., Lai, J.-., Matsuno, H. and Yamaguchi, N. (1999) Variation of Cell Populations Taking Charge of Immunity in Human Peripheral Blood Following Hot Spring Hydrotherapy Quantitative Discussion. *The Journal of Japanese Association of Physical Medicine, Balneology and Climatology*, **62**, 129-134.

[14] Matsuno, H., Wang, X.X., Wan, W., Matsui, K., Ohkawa, S., Sugiyama, T., Kohno, H., Shimizu, S., Lai, J.-E. and Yamaguchi, N. (1999) Variation of Cell Populations Taking Charge of Immunity in Human Peripheral Blood Following Hot Spring Hydrotherapy Qualitative Discussion. *The Journal of Japanese Association of Physical Medicine, Balneology and Climatology*, **62**, 135-140.

[15] Yamaguchi, N., Hashimoto, H., Arai, M., Takada, S., Kawada, N., Taru, A., Li, A.L., Izumi, H. and Sugiyama, K. (2002) Effect of Acupuncture on Leukocyte and Lymphocyte Subpopulation in Human Peripheral Blood-Quantitative Discussion. *The Journal of Japanese Association of Physical Medicine, Balneology and Climatology*, **65**, 199-206.

[16] Wan, W., Li, A.L., Izumi, H., Kawada, N., Arai, M., Takada, A., Taru, A., Hashimoto, H. and Yamaguchi, N. (2002) Effect of Acupuncture on Leukocyte and Lymphocyte Sub-Population in Human Peripheral Blood Qualitative Discus-

sion. *The Journal of Japanese Association of Physical Medicine, Balneology and Climatology*, **65**, 207-211.

[17] Wang, X.X., Katoh, S. and Liu, B.X. (1998) Effect of Physical Exercise on Leukocyte and Lymphocyte Subpopulations in Human Peripheral Blood. *Cytometry Research*, **8**, 53-61.

[18] Kitada, Y., Wan, W., Matsui, K., Shimizu, S. and Yamaguchi, N. (2000) Regulation of Peripheral White Blood Cells in Numbers and Functions through Hot-Spring Bathing during a Short Term Studies in Control Experiments. *Journal of Japanese Society Balneology Climatology Physiological Medicine*, **63**, 151-164.

[19] Yamaguchi, N., Takahashi, T., Sugita, T., Ichikawa, K., Sakaihara, S., Kanda, T., Arai, M. and Kawakita, K. (2007) Acupuncture Regulates Leukocyte Subpopulations in Human Peripheral Blood. *Evidence-Based Complementary and Alternative Medicine*, **4**, 447-453. http://dx.doi.org/10.1093/ecam/nel107

[20] Yamaguchi, N., Shimizu, S. and Izumi, H. (2004) Hydrotherapy Can Modulate Peripheral Leukocytes: An Approach to Alternative Medicine, Complementary and Alternative Approaches to Biomedicine. Ishikawa, 239-251.

[21] Yamaguchi, N., Chen, R., Okamoto, K., Takei, T., Tsubokawa, M., Sakamoto, D., Jia, X.F., Wan, W. and Murayama, T. (2013) Quantitative Regulation of Peripheral Leukocyte by Light Exercise and Tailored Scale for Assessment. *Open Journal of Immunology*, **3**, 175-183.

[22] Yamaguchi, N., Wan, W., Sakamoto, D., Nurmuhammad, A., Matsumoto, K., Takei, T., Okuzumi, K., Murayama, T. and Takahashi T. (2013) Regulative Effect for Natural Killer Cell by Hot Spring Hydrotherapy—Quantitative and Qualitative Discussion. *Open Journal of Immunology*, **3**, 201-209.

[23] Abo, T., Kawate, T., Itoh, K. and Kumagai, K. (1981) Studies on the Bioperiodicity of the Immune Response. 1. Circadian Rhythms of Human T, B and K Cell Traffic in the Peripheral Blood. *Journal of Immunology*, **126**, 1360-1363.

[24] Abo, T. and Kumagai, T. (1978) Studies of Surface Immunoglobulins on Human B Lymphocytes. III Physiological Variations of Sig+ Cells in Peripheral Blood. *Clinical Experimental Immunology*, **33**, 441-452.

[25] Suzuki, S., Toyabe, S., Moroda, T., Tada, T., Tsukahara, A. and Iiai, T. (1997) Circadian Rhythm of Leukocytes and Lymphocytes Subsets and Its Possible Correlation with the Function of the Autonomic Nervous System. *Clinical Experimental Immunology*, **110**, 500-508. http://dx.doi.org/10.1046/j.1365-2249.1997.4411460.x

[26] Bylund, D.B., Eikenberg, D.C., Hieble, J.P., Langer, S.Z., Lefkowitz, R.J. and Minneman, K.P. (1994) Intenational Union of Pharmacology Nomenclature of Adrenoceptors. *Pharmacological Review*, **46**, 121-136.

[27] Dulis, B.H. and Wilson, I.B. (1980) The $\beta$-Adrenergic Receptor of Live Human Polymorphonuclear Leukocytes. *Journal of Biological Chemistry*, **255**, 1043-1048.

[28] Maisel, A.S., Harris, T., Rearden, C.A. and Michel, M.C. (1990) Beta-Adrenergic Receptors in Lymphocyte Subsets after Exercise. Alterations in Normal Individuals and Patients with Congestive Heart Failure. *Circulation*, **82**, 2003-2010. http://dx.doi.org/10.1161/01.CIR.82.6.2003

[29] Sanders, V.M., Baker, R.A., Ramer-Quinn, D.S., Kasprowicz, D.J., Fuchs, B.A. and Street, N.E. (1997) Differential Expression of the $\beta_2$-Adrenaergic Receptor by Th1 and Th2 Clones. *Journal of. Immunology*, **158**, 4200-4210.

[30] Yamaguchi, N., Ueyama, T., Amat, N., Yimit, D., Hoxur, P., Sakamoto, D., Katoh, Y., Watanabe, I. and Su, S.Y. (2015) Bi-Directional Regulation by Chinese Herbal Formulae to Host and Parasite for Multi-Drug Resistant *Staphylococcus aureus* in Humans and Rodents. *Open Journal of Immunology*, **4**, 18-32. http://dx.doi.org/10.4236/oji.2015.51003

[31] Gorantla, S., Dou, H., Boska, M., Destache, C.J., Nelson, J., Poluektova, L., Rabinow, B.E., Gendelman, H.E. and Mosley, R.L. (2006) Quantitative Magnetic Resonance and SPECT Imaging for Macrophage Tissue Migration and Nanofor-Mulated Drug Delivery. *Journal of Leukocyte Biology*, **80**, 1165-1174. http://dx.doi.org/10.1189/jlb.0206110

[32] Stoika, R.S., Lutsik, M.D., Barska, M.L., Tsyrulnyk, A.A. and Kashchak, N.I. (2002) *In Vitro* Studies of Activation of Phagocytic Cells by Bioactive Peptides. *Journal of Physiology and Pharmacology*, **53**, 675-688.

[33] Elbim, C., Pillet, S., Prevost, M.H., Preira, A., Girard, P.M., Rogine, N., Hakim, J., Israel, N. and M. Gougerot-Pocidalo, A. (2001) The Role of Phagocytes in HIV-Related Oxidative Stress. *Journal of Clinical Virology*, **20**, 99-109.

[34] Speer, C.P., Gahr, M. and Pabst, M.J. (1986) Phagocytosis Associated Oxidative Metabolism in Human Milk Macrophages. *Acta Paediatrica Scandinavica*, **75**, 444-451. http://dx.doi.org/10.1111/j.1651-2227.1986.tb10228.x

[35] Iqbal, M., Sharma, S.D., Okazaki, Y., Fujisawa, M. and Okada, S. (2003) Dietary Supplementation of Curcumin Enhances Antioxidant and Phase II Metabolizing Enzymes in ddY Male Mice; Possible Role in Protection against Chemical Rall Estimation of Anti-Oxidant Activity by Mammal Macrophage Carcinogenesis and Toxicity. *Pharmacology & Toxicology*, **92**, 33-38. http://dx.doi.org/10.1034/j.1600-0773.2003.920106.x

[36] Kohno, H., Tanaka, T., Kawabata, K., Hirose, Y., Sugi, S., Tsuba, H. and Mori, H. (2002) Silymarin, a Naturally Occurring Polyphenolic Anotioxidant Flavionoid, Inhibits Azoxymethane-Inbuced Colon Carcinogenesis in Male F344 Rats. *Oxidative Stress in Dermatology*, In: Fuchs, J. and Packer, L., Eds., Marcel Dekker, New York, 461-468. http://dx.doi.org/10.1002/ijc.10625

[37] Karbownik, M., Tan, D., Manchester, L.C. and Reiter, R.J. (2000) Renal Toxicity of the Carcinogen Delta-Aminolevulinic Acid: Antioxidant Effects of Melatonin. *Cancer Letters*, **161**, 1-7. http://dx.doi.org/10.1016/S0304-3835(00)00568-1

[38] Harman, D. (1956) Aging: A Theory Based on Free Radical and Radiation Chemistry. *Journal of Gerontology*, **11**, 293-300. http://dx.doi.org/10.1093/geronj/11.3.298

[39] Inoue, M. (2002) Free Radical Theory of Aging. *Nippon Ronen Igakkai Zasshi*, **39**, 36-38.

[40] Biesalski, H.K. (2002) Free Radical Theory of Aging. *Current Opinion in Clinical Nutrition and Metabolic Care*, **5**, 5-10. http://dx.doi.org/10.1097/00075197-200201000-00002

[41] Wei, Y.H. and Lee, H.C. (2002) Oxidative Stress, Mitochondrial DNA Mutation, and Impairment of Antioxidant Enzymes in Aging. *Experimental Biology and Medicine* (*Maywood*), **227**, 671-682.

[42] Sanz, N., Diez-Fernandez, C., Andres, D. and Cascales, M. (2002) Hepatotoxicity and Aging: Endogenous Antioxidant Systems in Hepatocytes from 2-, 6-, 12-, 18- and 30- Month-Old Rats Following a Necrogenic Dose of Thioacetamide. *Biochimica et Biophysica Acta*, **1587**, 12-20. http://dx.doi.org/10.1016/S0925-4439(02)00048-0

[43] Diamond, J., Skaggs, J. and Manaligod, J.M. (2002) Free-Radical Damage: A Possible Mechanism of Laryngeal Aging. *Ear, Nose & Throat*, **81**, 531-533.

[44] Melov, S. (2002) Animal Models of Oxidative Stress, Aging, and Therapeutic Antioxidant Interventions. *International Journal of Biochemistry & Cell Biology*, **34**, 1395-1400. http://dx.doi.org/10.1016/S1357-2725(02)00086-9

[45] Arockia-Rani, P.J. and Panneerselvam, C. (2001) Carnitine as a Free Radical Scavenger in Aging. *Experimental Gerontology*, **36**, 1713-1726.

[46] Kasapoglu, M. and Ozben, T. (2001) Alterations of Antioxidant Enzymes and Oxidative Stress Markers in Aging. *Experimental Gerontology*, **36**, 209-220. http://dx.doi.org/10.1016/S0531-5565(00)00198-4

[47] Perchellet, J.P. and Perchellet, M. (1989) Antioxidants and Multistage Carcingenesis in Mouse Skin. *Free Radical Biology and Medicine* (*Medsci*), **7**, 377-408. http://dx.doi.org/10.1016/0891-5849(89)90124-X

[48] Edsmyr, F. (1982) Super Oxide Anion Dismutase Efficacy in Ameliorating Side Effects of Radiation Therapy. *Pathology of Oxygen*, Academic Press, New York, 315-326.

[49] Johansson, M.H., Deinum, J., Marklund, S.L. and Sjoquist, P.O. (1990) Recombinant Human Extra-Celluar Super Oxide Anion Dismutase Reduces Concentration of Oxygen Free Redicals in the Reperfusedret Heart. *Cardiouas*, **24**, 500-503.

[50] Venugopal, S.K., Devaraj, S., Yang, T. and Jialal, L. (2002) Alpha-Tocopherol Decreases Superoxide Anion Release in Human Monocytes under Hyperglycemic Conditions via Inhibition of Protein Kinase C-Alpha. *Diabetes*, **51**, 3049-3054. http://dx.doi.org/10.2337/diabetes.51.10.3049

[51] Nayak, D.U., Karmen, C., Frishman, W.H. and Va-kili, B.A. (2001) Antioxidant Vitamins and Enzymatic and Synthetic Oxygen-Derived Free Radical Scavengers in the Prevention and Treatment of Cardiovascular Disease. *Heart Disease*, **3**, 28-45. http://dx.doi.org/10.1097/00132580-200101000-00006

[52] Miyachi, Y. (1993) Skin Diseases Associated with Oxidative Injury. *Oxidative Stress in Dermatology*, 323-331.

[53] De Beer, D., Joubert, E., Gelderblom, W.C. and Manley, M. (2003) Antioxidant Activity of South African Red and White Cultivar Wines: Free Radical Scavenging. *Journal of Agricultural and Food Chemistry*, **51**, 902-909. http://dx.doi.org/10.1021/jf026011o

[54] Lee, S.E., Ju, E.M. and Kim, J.H. (2001) Free Radical Scavenging and Antioxidant Enzyme Fortifying Activities of Extracts from Smilax China Root. *Experimental and Molecular Medicine*, **33**, 263-268. http://dx.doi.org/10.1038/emm.2001.43

[55] Joshi, R., Adhikari, S., Patro, B.S., Chattopadhyay, S. and Mukherjee, T. (2001) Free Radical Scavenging Behavior of Folic Acid: Evidence for Possible Antioxidant Activity. *Free Radical Biology & Medicine*, **30**, 1390-1399. http://dx.doi.org/10.1016/S0891-5849(01)00543-3

[56] Lin, C.C., Hsu, Y.F. and Lin, T.C. (2001) Antioxidant and Free Radical Scavenging Effects of the Tannins of *Terminalia catappa* L. *Anticancer Research*, **21**, 237-243.

[57] Shimizu, S., Kitada, H., Yokota, H., Yamakawa, J., Murayama, T., Sugiyama, K., Izumi, H. and Yamaguchi, N. (2002) Activation of the Alternative Complement Pathway by Agaricus Blazei Murill. *Phytomedicine*, **9**, 536-545.

# 8

# General Guide for Korean Acupuncture & Moxibustion

**Hyo-Jung Kwon, Yong-Suk Kim***

Department of Acupuncture & Moxibustion, (Brain & Neurological Disorders and Pain), Kangnam Korean Hospital, Kyung Hee University, Seoul, Korea
Email: *ackys@hanmail.net

## Abstract

**As ancient Korean and Chinese dynasties held close relationships in politics and culture throughout history, the medicine of the two nations were developed in mutual influence. For instance, the current version of *Lingshu*, the second half of the *Huangdineijing*, was transcribed from The Bible of Acupuncture, which was brought to the Chinese Song dynasty from the Korean Koryo dynasty in 1092. While maintained a close relationship with traditional Chinese medicine, Korean medicine had continued to develop unique systems on its own over the history and established typical types of acupuncture methods, which are different from those of traditional Chinese medicine [1]. In the 17th century, a royal physician by the name of Dr. Heo Jun wrote *Donguibogam*, the first encyclopedia of Korean medicine in Korea. It remained to be a book of instruction for Korean Medicine Doctors. Another book called *Donguisusebowon* was published in 1901 on the basis of the theory of four constitutions by Dr. Lee Je-Ma at the end of the Chosun dynasty [2]. There were two other representative Korean acupuncture methods: Saam acupuncture and Constitutional acupuncture (Taeguek acupuncture). Theories of Korean acupuncture applied a summarized framework for each individual to diagnose a physical condition, explaining the biologic phenomena within the concept of constitutional medicine [1]. The diagnosis systems of several Korean acupuncture styles were focused on simplifying the understanding of the body's core imbalances, and the resulting diagnosis enabled practitioners to devise therapeutic strategies that were based on constitutional energy traits. Saam acupuncture used 12 energy (or *Qi*) traits, mainly controlled by the 12 corresponding Meridians, that underlie diverse superficial biologic phenomena [2] [3]. It was suggested that these 12 energies determined the inclinations of the whole body, and they were targeted to recover the balance of the body's constancy. Taegeuk acupuncture was identified by Sasang constitutional medicine according to the patient's innate constitution. Sasang constitutional medicine identified four constitutions according to the individual's inherent disparities among major Organ energies, expressed as the size of the Organs, all of which determined the physiologic characteristics of the individual patient and served as a major imbalance succeeding diverse pa-**

*Corresponding author.

**thologic processes. These constitutional traits were suggested to be the source of individual differences in apparently similar physiologic or pathologic reactions [2]. As Meridian theory is based on the *Qi* thesis of *Yin-Yang* and Five Elements among Organs, acupuncture treatment couldn't be separated from these viewpoints. Saam acupuncture was based on the control of *Qi* and Blood among Organs and channels, and thus the clinical use of Saam acupuncture treatments seemed to be core to oriental medicine [4]. As the creation of Blood originates from *Qi*, one could argue that *Qi* included Blood, thereby stating that the effect of Saam acupuncture was achieved by harmonizing the function and flow of *Qi*. The treatment protocol of Saam acupuncture mainly focused on tonification and sedation of the Five *Shu* points ("five transport points"), firmly based on regular pattern. It had a strong effect on imbalances of the Five Organs, but on the other hand could be said to have little effect on disease of interruption such as stagnation and irregularities in Meridian networks. Thus, acupoints other than the Five *Shu* points were used as well.**

## Keywords

**Saam Acupuncture, Constitutional Acupuncture, Five Elements, Taegeuk Acupuncture**

## 1. Introduction

Saam acupuncture is one of unique Korean acupuncture styles and its technique is widely adopted by clinicians and educational institutions in Korea today. It originated in the 17th century, probably by a Buddhist monk called "Saam". Saam acupuncture provides basic acupuncture prescriptions for the imbalances of each of the twelve Meridians. The main energy traits of the 12 Meridians are employed by applying the promotion cycle (*Sheng*, creation, "nourishing") and control cycle (*Ke*, governor, "suppressing") relationships of the Five Elements (or "Five Phases") theory onto the Five *Shu* points and 12 Meridians [3] [4]. Saam acupuncture summarizes diverse physiological or pathologic processes into 12 images of *Qi* imbalance corresponding to the 12 Meridians and expands the use of the Five *Shu* points. The manuscripts of Saam acupuncture carry clinical applications and modifications of the basic acupuncture prescriptions [5].

Five Elements acupuncture consists of tonification and sedation using Five *Shu* points. Five Elements acupuncture, also known as "tonification and sedation in self-Meridian" on the basis of the creation cycle, was first proposed by Gao-wu during the Ming dynasty in China. Saam developed this technique further by extending it into another Meridian and using the governor cycle in self- and other-Meridians.

Gao-Wu, during the Ming Dynasty (1519 AD), was the first and foremost medical acupuncturist to tonify deficiency and sedate the excess on the basis of either depletion or repletion of the promotion cycle, which is explained in "The Four Needle method" by Ross [6] [7]. Saam acupuncture [8] proposes the Five Elements acupuncture style that simultaneously uses the Five *Shu* points of the promotion and the control cycles, called the "Four Needle technique" by Hicks *et al.* [9] and the "eight Needle methods" by Ross [6].

Gao-Wu described the use of "tonification and sedation points" along the self Meridian using the Five *Shu* points. The basis of Gao-Wu's treatment was the creation (mother-child) cycle and is included in the "Four Needle method" with the following rules: to determine the tonification point for a Meridian, select the Mother Element on the Meridian in question, and to determine the sedation points, select the Child Element. But Saam acupuncture, on the basis of Gao-Wu's treatment, created a Five Element acupuncture therapy by adding the control (grandmother-grandchild) cycle, as well as selecting acupuncture points among other related Meridians. From the above approach, this theory consisted of two tonifications and two sedation points, which were selected from among the Five *Shu* points. The Five *Shu* points had characteristics of their particular Five Elements theory according to the difficult issues in *Nan-Ching*.

The principles of Saam acupuncture originated from the creation and controlled cycles among the Five Elements and had the following rules: to determine the tonification and sedation points for a Meridian in deficiencies, first tonified the mother Element Five *Shu* points on the Meridian in question as well as the master point (Five *Shu* points of same Element as the Meridian) on the mother Element Meridian, and then sedated the Controller Element Five *Shu* points on the affected Meridian as well as the master point on the Controller Element

Meridian; to determine the tonification and sedation points for a Meridian in excesses, first sedated the child Element Five *Shu* points on the affected Meridian, and then tonified the Controller Element Five *Shu* points on the affected Meridian as well as the master point on the Controller Meridian.

There also exists another setting of tonification and sedation system called the "coldness-heat acupuncture treatment", derived from the "deficiency-excesses acupuncture treatment", that is simple and rarely used because it selects only the Water and Fire Element Five *Shu* points among a Meridian and has the following rules: for cold symptoms, to determine the tonification and sedation points for a Meridian, first tonify the Fire Element Five *Shu* points on the affected Meridian as well as the Fire point on the Fire Meridian—namely HT8 for *Yin* Meridians and SI5 for *Yang* Meridians, and then sedate the Water Element Five *Shu* points on the affected Meridian as well as the Water point on the Water Meridian—namely KI10 for *Yin* Meridians and BL66 for *Yang* Meridians.

For heat symptoms, to determine the tonification and sedation points for a Meridian, first sedate the Fire Element Five *Shu* points on the affected Meridian as well as the Fire point on the Fire Meridian, and secondly tonify the Water Element Five *Shu* points on the affected Meridian as well as the Water point on the Water Meridian.

## 1.1. Acupoints Used in Saam Acupuncture

The Five *Shu* points, located below the elbow and knee joints, could be used corresponding to the Five Elements for imbalances in correlation to tonification and sedation [10] (**Table 1**). Every acupuncture point has an effect on disturbances of the corresponding channel and the coupled channel as well as on the illness of the corresponding Organ, the allocated tissues and sensory Organs [11]. Acupuncture points have an effect on the related channel axis, for example, ST38 along the *Yangming* Meridian on the shoulder, more namely the Stomach Meridian and the Large Intestine Meridian.

Giovanni [12]: "The sections of channel between fingers/toes and elbows/knees are more superficial than the rest, which is one of the reasons for the importance of the points lying along its path. The energetic action of the points along a section of such a channel is much more dynamic than other points, which explains their frequent use in clinical practice. Another reason for the dynamism of these points is that, at the tips of fingers and toes, the energy changes polarity from *Yin* to *Yang* or vice versa and, due to this polarity change, the *Qi* of the channel is more unstable and thus more easily influenced. The progression of the Five Element points along the channel is probably in relation to this change of polarity, as the second point belongs to the Fire in the *Yin* channels and the Water in the *Yang* channels. Five points situated along this channel section are particularly important and are

**Table 1.** Five *Shu* Points.

| ***Yin* Meridian** | **Wood (well)** | **Fire (spring)** | **Earth (stream)** | **Metal (river)** | **Water (sea)** |
|---|---|---|---|---|---|
| **Lung (Metal)** | LU11 | LU10 | LU9 | LU8 | LU5 |
| **Heart (Fire)** | HT9 | HT8 | HT7 | HT4 | HT3 |
| **Pericardium (Fire)** | PC9 | PC8 | PC7 | PC5 | PC3 |
| **Spleen (Earth)** | SP1 | SP2 | SP3 | SP5 | SP9 |
| **Kidney (Water)** | KI1 | KI2 | KI3 | KI7 | KI10 |
| **Liver (Wood)** | LR1 | LR2 | LR3 | LR4 | LR8 |
| ***Yang* Meridian** | **Metal (well)** | **Water (spring)** | **Wood (stream)** | **Fire (river)** | **Earth (sea)** |
| **Large Intestine (Metal)** | LI1 | LI2 | LI3 | LI5 | LI11 |
| **Small Intestine (Fire)** | SI1 | SI2 | SI3 | SI5 | SI8 |
| **Triple Energizer (Fire)** | TE1 | TE2 | TE3 | TE6 | TE10 |
| **Stomach (Earth)** | ST45 | ST44 | ST43 | ST41 | ST36 |
| **Bladder (Water)** | BL67 | BL66 | BL65 | BL60 | BL54 |
| **Gall Bladder (Wood)** | GB44 | GB43 | GB41 | GB38 | GB34 |

called the Five Transporting points; they also coincide with what are called the Elements points. However, the dynamic of these points is irrespective of their Five Elements character".

Yun-Tao-Ma [13]: "An interesting neurological fact is that the limbs below the elbows and knees occupy large regions in the brain sensory gyrus. Thus, the acupoints below the elbows and knees also occupy a large region in the cortical representation of the brain's post-central sensory gyrus. This correlation may explain the reason why the acupoints below the elbows and knees contain more sensory receptors and needling stimulation of these points can induce a greater reaction and activity in the brain. This principle clearly supports the concept of using certain acupoints below the elbows and knees as diagnosis and treatment points during acupuncture treatment".

Most illnesses are caused by interruptions of *Qi* and blood manifested by stagnation and irregularities. Illnesses are also caused by imbalances of Organs brought on by deficiency and excess through the Meridian network. Acupuncture treatments, therefore, must cover these two aspects of illness to achieve acupoint efficacy and functions of tonification and sedation. In order to gain greater efficacy, acupuncture based on acupoint efficacy and Saam acupuncture can be combined to simultaneously correct interruptions and imbalances as well as have tonification-sedation effects. In relations to the principles of acupuncture treatments, the acupuncture procedures based on acupoint efficacy to correct interruptions can be assumed as "branch treatment", and acupuncture based on tonification-sedation effects to correct imbalances can be assumed as "root treatment". Effective acupuncture treatment, therefore, is a combination of acupoint efficacy with Five Element acupuncture [2].

It can be said that a local acupoint directs the treatment strategy to the affected energetic functional sphere or zone (in internal energetic disturbances), while the distal acupoints serve to determine the nature of the energetic manipulation (such as tonification, dispersal, warming, cooling, harmonizing) [14]. The combination of local and distal acupoints forms a pattern of treatment that resembles the pattern of the disharmony being treated. In its most sophisticated application, a treatment pattern and its effects will confirm the diagnosis of the pattern of disharmony. In order to have more effective acupuncture treatment results for other diseases, combination methods that cover local, special and distal acupoints should be used to increase efficacy and serve as tonification or sedation for imbalances. More effective treatment when using Saam acupuncture could be achieved by using it as a root treatment to correct imbalances, while local acupoints, special acupoints and symptomatic treatments are applied as branch treatment to correct interruptions in proper stimulation techniques [4].

## 1.2. Promotion and Control Cycles Leading to the Disease Type of Five Evils

The 50th issue of *Nan-Ching* explains the pathology of the Five Evils [15] [16] and the 69th issue of *Nan-Ching* describes the treatment for these evils. This method consists of, in a broad sense, the method of "tonification-sedation between deficiency and excess" as well as the method of "tonification-sedation between coldness and heat".

Among the illnesses are the Depletion, Repletion, Destroyer, Weakness, and Regular Evils, and distinguished as thus:

1) Those (illnesses) coming from behind represent a Depletion Evil;
2) Those coming from ahead represent a Repletion Evil;
3) Those coming from what cannot be overcome represent a Destroyer Evil;
4) Those coming from what can be overcome represent a Weakness Evil;
5) If the respective depot is afflicted from within itself, it represents a Regular Evil.

In case of depletion, it should be filled, while in case of repletion, it should be drained. When neither repletion nor depletion is present, the illness should be removed from the conduits, meaning that in the case of depletion, one should fill the respective (conduit's) mother, and in case of repletion, one should drain the respective (conduit's) child. One must fill first and then drain afterward (**Table 2**).

One characteristic of Saam acupuncture is the addition of the control (governor) cycle—consisting of grandmother and grandchild elements—to the promotion cycle—consisting of mother and son elements. This method includes a new concept of the "governor Meridian" in the application of the law of the Five Elements based on the inter-destructive cycle.

*Wang Sheng Xiu Qiu Si* is another concept of the Five Elements [17]. *Wang Sheng Xiu* is a family and in a promotion cycle of the Five Elements, while *Qiu Si* is an enemy and in a control cycle of the Five Elements. In promoting the cycle of the Five Elements, a reinforcing method can be done while the control cycle of the Five

**Table 2.** Relationship of Five Elements and Five Evils.

| **Relationship** | Mother | Self | Child | Enemy whom I control | Enemy who controls me |
|---|---|---|---|---|---|
| **Five Evil** | Depletion | Regular | Repletion | Weakness | Destroyer |
| **Wang Sheng** | *Xiu* | *Wang* | *Sheng* | *Qiu* | *Si* |
| **Principle for treatment** | Tonify the mother for deficiency | Self-tonify or self-sedate | Sedate the child for excess | Sedate the enemy for deficiency | Tonify the enemy for excess, sedate for deficiency |

Elements require a reducing method. It is meaningful that each Element promotes like a family in the promoting cycle while each Element reduces like an enemy.

Ross [6] calls acupoint selection of tonification and sedation among its own Meridians "Within Element treatments" and acupoint selection of tonification and sedation among other Meridians "Between Element treatments". This selection, in what is called the Four Needle method, is based on the theory of promotion cycle of the Five Elements. He also explains the Eight Needle method which selects another acupoint based on the theory of the inhibition cycle of the Five Elements, in addition to the Four Needle method. He did not explain the originality of its treatments, but the selection is the same as Saam acupuncture.

## 1.3. The Six Energy Characteristics of Three *Yin* and Three *Yang*

To achieve a comprehensive understanding of the energy controlled by Meridians, both the Five Elements and Six Energy characteristics must be considered. The characteristic energy controlled by the Meridian is determined not only by the Five Elements, but also by the Six Energy attributes. Six Energies are the subdivision of *Yin* and *Yang* energies into three *Yin* and three *Yang*, namely *Jueyin* ("absolute *Yin*"), *Shaoyin* ("lesser *Yin*"), *Taiyin* ("greater *Yin*"), *Shaoyang* ("lesser *Yang*"), *Yangming* ("brilliant *Yang*") and *Taiyang* ("greater *Yang*"). They correspond to Wind, King Fire, Earth, Premier Fire, Metal and Water traits respectively. These Six Energies are subdivided into 12 energies mainly controlled by 12 Meridians that function as energy combined with the Five Elements energy in Meridians located in either the upper or lower extremities. For example, although both the Gall Bladder (GB) and Liver (LR) Meridian energies are Wood, GB energy is *Shaoyang* while LR energy is *Jueyin* from the Six Energy perspective. The LR Meridian energy is *Jueyin* combined with Wood, while the Pericardium (PC) Meridian energy is *Jueyin* combined with Fire (Premier Fire).

## 1.4. Five Elements

Most illness and disturbances are rooted in interruptions or imbalances in a network of Meridians. Interruptions comprise stagnation and irregularities, and imbalances are deficiency and excess [6].

A typical diagnosis in Saam acupuncture is one of four imbalances of a Meridian energy, which are deficiency, excess, cold or heat. A physician should first find out the Meridian in which the core imbalance of energy is located, and then determine which type the imbalance belongs to. For example, when the energy of *Shaoyang*, which is expressed as GB or Triple Energizer (TE) Meridian energy, is excessive it may be expressed as a dogmatic personality, sensitive mind or an inclination to give advice to others. When deficient, this energy may be expressed as an atrocious personality, cold mind or a sense of inferiority. More specifically, the energy of GB is associated with centering energy, bright light, aggressiveness, activeness, braveness, dignity or an arrogant attitude, and with energy often compared to a wind power plant or a thunderbolt [18].

The scope of Saam acupuncture can be extensive because of its diverse laws, such as the promotion and inhibition (control) cycle among the Five Elements and its connected Meridians. A Meridian consists of three parts, that is, arm or foot, the more or less of *Yin* and *Yang*, and one of Six Organs (*Zang*) and Six Bowels (*Fu*). When applying the theory of *Yin-Yang* and the Five Elements, the essence of what we are after is the energetic movements of disharmonies which are fleeting. The Eight Guiding Criteria make it possible to systematically analyze all data that are gathered in a consistent manner, and thus measure a patient's pattern of disharmony against the major patterns of Chinese medical pathology [14].

# 2. Method of Acupuncture Treatment

The Five *Shu* points distal to the elbow and knee correspond to the Five Elements and have been used in clinical treatments depending on each acupoint's different effects and indication. The combination of Five *Shu* Points used in Saam acupuncture includes two tonification points and two sedation points. The former, which correspond to the "mother element" according to the law of the Five Elements, tonify the energy of the corresponding channel and Organ. Therefore, the tonification points are needled with stimulation by the tonifying method in Meridian or Organ deficiency conditions.

Each of the 12 Meridians can be subdivided into four types—deficiency, excess, cold, heat—resulting in 48 basic pre-established acupuncture prescriptions, each of which are selections of the Five *Shu* points. Each Five *Shu* point corresponds to one of the Five Elements. Traditional use of the Five *Shu* points incorporates the promotion cycle relationship of the Five Elements where, for example, Wood nourishes Fire and Fire nourishes Earth. As an example, an energy deficiency of the Heart (HT) Meridian (*i.e.* Fire Meridian) may be corrected by needling on the Wood acupoint (HT9) of the Meridian with a tonification method, based on the above theoretical premise. In Saam acupuncture, acupoints are also selected using the control cycle relationship of the Five Elements as well. For example, Water suppresses Fire and Fire suppresses Metal. To correct the example of Fire deficiency, the Water acupoint (HT3) of the Fire Meridian should be sedated. Saam acupuncture practice would also simultaneously modulate other relative Meridians selected by the theory of the promotion or control cycle relationships, which is necessary for whole-body balance. In the above example, the Wood acupoint of the relevant Wood Meridian (LR1) should be needled using the tonification method, and the Water acupoint of the relevant Water Meridian (KI10) should be needled using the sedation method.

In deficiency condition, tonify the Mother Element. One should select the Mother Element Five *Shu* point on the Meridian in question for tonification. For instance, in the case of Lung Meridian deficiency, the Mother Element of the Lung is Earth (Earth is the Mother of Metal), and thus the tonification point of the Lung Meridian would therefore be the Earth point of the Lung Meridian, namely LU9 [7]. In excesses situation, the Child Element on the Meridian in question should be sedated. In the case of the Lung Meridian, the Child Element of the Lung is Water (Water is the Child of Metal), and thus the sedation point of the Lung Meridian would be the Water point on the Lung Meridian, namely LU5. The same principle holds true for the other eleven regular Meridians. The four needle method [6] consists of the Within-Reinforce-Tonification point and the Within-Reduce-Sedation point, which are tonification and sedation of Gao-Wu [7], as well as the Between-Reinforce-Element point and the Between-Reduce-Element point, which are tonification and sedation among other Meridians. They are used in Saam acupuncture in the same way.

Saam acupuncture makes use of the tonification and sedation points along the promotion cycle as well as points along the control cycle in cases of deficiency and excess; and along the fire and water Meridians in cases of heat and coldness. The basic rules, based on the writings of *Nan-Ching* [15] [16], are those of the promotion and control cycle relationships. In the case of any Meridian's insufficiency (weakness), the points of its mother and its own Meridians should be tonified and the points of its governor and its own Meridians should be sedated. In the case of any Meridian's excessiveness (fullness), the points of its governor and its own Meridians should be tonified and the points of its son and its own Meridians should be sedated [14].

## 2.1. Example in Deficiencies

1) Needle 1: Tonify the deficient Meridian at its mother (tonification) point. With a Lung Meridian deficiency, tonify the Earth point of the Lung Meridian, LU6.
2) Needle 2: Tonify the master point on the Mother Element Meridian. With a Lung Meridian deficiency, the Mother of Metal is Earth, hence the Mother of Lung is Spleen, and the master (Earth) point of the Spleen (Earth) Meridian, SP3, should be tonified.
3) Needle 3: Sedate the Controller Element on the affected Meridian. With a Lung Meridian deficiency, the Controller of Metal is Fire, so the Fire point on the affected Meridian, LU10, should be sedated.
4) Needle 4: Sedate the master point on the Controller Element Meridian. With a Lung Meridian deficiency, the Controller Element is Fire, hence the Controller of Lung is Heart, and the master (Fire) point of the Heart (Fire) Meridian, HT8, should be sedated.

## 2.2. Examples in Excesses

1) Needle 1: Sedate the affected Meridian at its Child Element point. For Liver excess, sedate the Fire (Child) point of the Liver Meridian, LR2.

2) Needle 2: Sedate the master on the Child Element Meridian. For Liver excess, the Child of Wood is Fire; hence the Child of Liver is Heart. The master (Fire) point of the Heart, HT8, should be sedated.
3) Needle 3: Tonify the Controller Element on the affected Meridian. For Liver excess, the Controller of Wood is Metal, so the Metal point on the affected Meridian, LR4, should be tonified.
4) Needle 4: Tonify the master point on the Controller Element Meridian. With Liver excess, the Controller Element is Metal, hence the Controller of Liver is Lung, and the master (Metal) point of the Lung (Metal), LU8, should be tonified.

To summarize the principle for deficiency conditions [19]: Tonify the first two needles—tonify the Mother Element Five *Shu* point on the affected Meridian, and then tonify the master point on the Mother Element Meridian; Sedate the second two needles—sedate the Controller Element Five *Shu* points on the affected Meridian, and then sedate the master point on the Controller Element Meridian.

For example, if the Stomach is believed to be hypounderactive: (1) for Fire tonification, Stomach Meridian-Fire point ST41, Small Intestine Meridian-Fire point SI5; (2) for Wood sedation, Stomach Meridian-Wood point ST43, Gall Bladder Meridian-Wood point GB41 should be used. The other Meridians follow the same rule, as described above.

To summarize the principle for excess conditions: Sedate the first two needles—sedate the Child Element Five *Shu* points on the affected Meridian, and then sedate the master point on the Child Element Meridian; Tonify the second two needles—tonify the Controller Element Five *Shu* points on the affected Meridian, and then tonify the master point on the Controller Element Meridian.

## 2.3. Controller Element Meridian

For example, if the stomach is believed to be overactive: (1) for Metal (son) sedation, Stomach Meridian-Metal point ST45, Large Intestine Meridian-Metal point LI1; (2) for Wood tonification, ST43 and GB41 should be used. The Gall Bladder Meridian is opposed to the Stomach Meridian by the control (destructive) cycle of the law of the Five Elements (the governor Meridian), so the Wood point of Gall Bladder Meridian, GB41, destroys the element of Earth within the self-Meridian. The other Meridians follow the same rule described above (**Table 3**).

Some kinds of diseases are caused by the imbalance between heat and coldness in the body and the corresponding treatments consist of using the Water and Fire Element Five *Shu* points along the Meridian in question, the Water Element Meridian, and the Fire Element Meridian. For a heat symptom, the Water point of the self-

**Table 3.** Saam acupuncture method for symptoms of deficiency and excess.

| Meridian | Deficiency (tonification) | | | | Excess (sedation) | | | |
|---|---|---|---|---|---|---|---|---|
| | Tonify | | Sedate | | Tonify | | Sedate | |
| **Lung** | SP3 | LU9 | HT8 | LU10 | HT8 | LU10 | KI10 | LU5 |
| **Large Intestine** | ST36 | LI11 | SI5 | LI5 | SI5 | LI5 | BL66 | LI2 |
| **Stomach** | SI5 | ST41 | GB41 | ST43 | GB41 | ST43 | LI1 | ST45 |
| **Spleen** | HT8 | SP2 | LR1 | SP1 | LR1 | SP1 | LU8 | SP5 |
| **Heart** | LR1 | HT9 | KI19 | HT3 | KI19 | HT3 | SP3 | HT7 |
| **Small Intestine** | GB41 | SI3 | BL66 | SI2 | BL66 | SI2 | ST36 | SI8 |
| **Bladder** | LI1 | BL67 | ST36 | BL54 | ST36 | BL54 | GB41 | BL65 |
| **Kidney** | LU8 | KI7 | SP3 | KI3 | SP3 | KI3 | LR1 | KI1 |
| **Pericardium** | LR1 | PC9 | KI10 | PC3 | KI10 | PC3 | SP3 | PC7 |
| **Triple Energizer** | GB41 | TE3 | BL66 | TE2 | BL66 | TE2 | ST36 | TE10 |
| **Gall Bladder** | BL66 | GB43 | LI1 | GB44 | LI1 | GB44 | SI5 | GB38 |
| **Liver** | KI10 | LR8 | LU8 | LR4 | LU8 | LR4 | HT8 | LR2 |

Meridian and that of the Water Element Meridian are selected to tonify Water, as well as the Fire points of the self and Fire Element Meridians selected to sedate Fire. For a cold symptom, the Fire points of the self and Fire Element Meridians are selected to tonify Fire, as well as the Water point of the self-Meridian and that of the Water Meridians selected to sedate coldness.

In the case of cold symptoms in the Lung, the coldness symptom can be balanced by both the tonification of heat and sedation of coldness. Accordingly, the Fire points, LU10 of the self-Meridian and HT8 of the Fire Element Meridian, should be tonified to warm "coldness." Conversely, the Water points, LU5 of the self-Meridian and KI10 of the Water Element Meridian, should be repressed. The other Meridians follow the same rules described above.

In the case of heat symptoms in the Lung, the Fire symptom can be controlled by Water, and the Water points, LU5 of the self-Meridian and KI10 of the Water Element Meridian should be tonified. Conversely, the Fire points, LI10 of the self-Meridian and HT8 of the Fire Element Meridian, should be repressed. The other Meridians follow the same rule described above (**Table 4**).

## 3. Method of Tonification and Sedation

Saam acupuncture is applied with stimulation techniques such as respiratory, rotational and directional methods. Each stimulation results in tonification or sedation. Tonification and sedation occur depending upon clockwise or counter-clockwise rotations in accordance with direction of Meridians. Tonification occurs following the insertion of a needle as the patient exhales and removal at inhalation. Sedation occurs on insertion of the needle as the patient inhales and removal on exhalation. Tonification occurs when the needle is inserted in the inclined position following the direction of the flow of *Qi* in the Meridian. By contrast, sedation occurs following insertion of the needle in the inclined position in the opposite direction to the flow of *Qi* in the Meridian [2]. In theory, the use of acupuncture stimulation may be possible in treatment but strong technical movements on acupoints located on shallow body surfaces, such as between finger tips and elbow or tips of toes and knee, may be hard for the practitioner to access. Clinically it is recommended that practitioner do not use strong stimulations. A simple and weak stimulation seems to be enough to gain the acupuncture effect.

## 4. Diagnosis Method

The scope of Saam acupuncture can be extensive because of its diverse laws, such as the promotion and inhibi-

**Table 4.** Saam Acupuncture Method for Symptoms of Cold and Heat.

| Meridian | Symptoms | | | | | | | |
|---|---|---|---|---|---|---|---|---|
| | Cold | | | | Heat | | | |
| | Tonify | | Sedate | | Tonify | | Sedate | |
| Lung | HT8 | LU10 | LU5 | KI10 | LU5 | KI10 | SP3 | LU9 |
| Large Intestine | SI5 | ST41 | LI2 | BL66 | LI2 | BL66 | SI5 | ST41 |
| Stomach | ST41 | SI5 | ST44 | BL66 | ST44 | BL66 | ST36 | BL54 |
| Spleen | SP2 | HT8 | SP9 | KI10 | SP9 | KI10 | SP3 | KI3 |
| Heart | HT8 | KI2 | HT3 | KI10 | HT3 | KI10 | HT8 | KI2 |
| Small Intestine | SI5 | BL60 | SI2 | BL66 | SI2 | BL66 | SI8 | ST36 |
| Bladder | SI5 | BL60 | SI2 | BL66 | SI2 | BL66 | ST36 | BL54 |
| Kidney | HT8 | KI2 | KI10 | HT3 | KI10 | HT3 | SP3 | KI3 |
| Pericardium | HT8 | PC8 | PC3 | HT3 | PC3 | HT3 | SP3 | PC7 |
| Triple Energizer | TE6 | BL60 | TE2 | BL66 | TE2 | BL66 | TE6 | BL60 |
| Gall Bladder | GB38 | SI5 | GB43 | BL66 | GB43 | BL66 | BL54 | GB34 |
| Liver | LR2 | HT8 | KI10 | LR8 | KI10 | LR8 | LR3 | SP3 |

tion (control) cycles among the Five Elements and their corresponding Meridians. A Meridian consists of three parts; that are, upper extremity or lower extremity, more or less of *Yin* and *Yang*, and one of Six Organs (*Zangs* including Pericardium) and Six Bowels (*Fus*). A total of 24 deficiency and excess symptoms exist across the Six Organs and Six Bowels, but theories related to these symptoms are too arbitrary to assist in making a diagnosis. Although there are currently many clinical books on Saam acupuncture in Korea, a definitive general standard for the selection of symptom patterns has not yet been established. The general use of Saam acupuncture has previously been discussed in 1985 [20]. The method can be used mainly from a theoretical viewpoint of the Organs, etiology of disease, as well as the more or less of the three *Yang* and three *Yin*. For example, in the case of knee pain, one can use Liver-tonification (mostly deficiency condition) because, according to the theory of the Organs, the Liver controls the muscles and joints. Secondly, in the case of headache due to increasing Liver-*Yang*, one may use Liver-sedation (mostly excess condition) given the etiology of the disease. Furthermore, in the case of backache due to dampness, we can use either Spleen-sedation (excess condition) to sedate dampness or *Yangming*-tonification (deficiency of Large Intestine or Stomach) to tonify dryness from the principle of the more or less of the three *Yang* and three *Yin*.

The above three viewpoints cannot fully explain Saam acupuncture, so a common differential diagnosis shared by many acupuncturists needs to be determined. Lee [21] was the first to propose a differential diagnosis of deficiency and excess by simultaneously comparing the six pulses of both wrists in the 1960s. However, his diagnosis was only focused on deficiency and excess, neglecting coldness and heat. Although he said that irregular forms of treatments were the manifestation of subtle changes in diseases, signs and symptoms are needed to support his assertions. Lee's comparative pulse diagnosis is very original in that it attempted to determine different symptoms, but a diagnosis made only using the pulse method is difficult. Comparative pulse diagnosis can therefore be an important guide in using Saam acupuncture, despite its weakness.

Kim [22] stated that he proposed the diagnosis method called "Saam Five Elements acupuncture of disease symptoms," which differentiates symptoms by simultaneously comparing the pulse, as he found that the original Saam acupuncture could not cope with changes in diseases. He asserted that a floating pulse showed *Yang* excess and *Yin* deficiency, while a deep pulse demonstrated *Yin* excess and *Yang* deficiency on the basis that the medial pulse is neither floating nor deep, and is the manifestation of health. Kim also proposed, from his clinical experience, that more focus needs to be placed on the symptoms of coldness and heat rather than the symptoms of deficiency and excess when differentiating these two symptom types. This can be achieved by comparing both the right and the left *Guan* pulses. If the right *Guan* pulse is weaker than the left the symptom is related to coldness and heat, while if the left *Guan* pulse is weaker than the right *Guan* pulse the symptom is related to either deficiency or excess. For example, looking at the symptom of either coldness or heat, if the pulse is floating, the main symptom is *Yang* excess and *Yin* deficiency. The treatment is then to first tonify the fire within the *Yin* Meridian and then to sedate the coldness within the *Yang* Meridian. In the heat symptom, if the pulse is deep, the main symptom is *Yin* excess and *Yang* deficiency. The treatment is to first tonify the coldness within the *Yang* Meridian and then to sedate the heat within the *Yin* Meridian.

The method used by Kim is more detailed than that of Lee, in that Kim used differentiation of coldness & heat symptom type and deficiency & excess symptom type, and set the criterion for *Yin-Yang* balance by standardizing medial pulse. Kim's theory is still contentious and not fully accepted as a standard of general treatment as it is difficult to decide differential symptoms by pulse diagnosis only. The merit of Kim's treatment is that it contributed greatly to the objective use of Saam acupuncture [7].

Seem [11] also believes that treatments using the four-needle technique are very powerful, and should only be pursued when a strong energetic manipulation is required, and only when one is certain of the primary diagnosis of the affected Five Elements or Phases. This recommendation is because the four-needle technique tonifies twice, then sedates twice, leading to a very concentrated tonifying or sedating action on the affected Five Elements and Meridian. If one is not certain of the primary affected Element, it is far more conservative to use more gentle tonification and sedation acupoints.

Generally speaking, Saam acupuncture primarily focuses on deficiency and excess symptoms rather than coldness and heat symptoms, although the relationship between the deficiency and excess symptom type and coldness and heat symptom type needs to be studied in detail in order to create reasonable guidelines for effective treatments. As there are many different ways to select Five *Shu* points from the various opinions concerning Five Element acupuncture, we need to determine detailed guidelines for patterns of symptoms in the future.

## 5. Practice of Saam Acupuncture

Saam acupuncture is primarily focused on Five *Shu* points, which contradicts other acupuncture methods. For example, backache can be caused by disturbances of the Bladder Meridian, so one can use tonification or sedation of the Bladder Meridian depending upon deficiency or excess. Backache can also be caused by weakness of the Kidney Meridian, which one can then treat by using tonification of the Kidney Meridian. Finally, backache is caused due to excessive dampness of the Spleen, which can be diagnosed in obese people. One can then use tonification of the dry Large Intestine Meridian or Stomach Meridian in order to dry out dampness. Sedation of the damp Spleen Meridian can also be used on rare occasion. The selection of tonification or sedation depends wholly upon the diagnosing practitioner.

Backache is generally associated with Kidney or Bladder functions. The Governor vessel and Gallbladder Meridian, with little connection to other Meridians, can also be involved in backache. Saam acupuncture treats backache using a novel approach. It relates backache to the malfunction of connected Organs (*i.e.* the Bladder, Kidney and Gall Bladder) to the imbalance of *Yin* and *Yang* (Six *Qi*) while primarily using Five *Shu* acupuncture points. It is a wonder how the combination of the acupoints distal to the painful region and located beneath the elbow and knee joints can treat diseases such as backache, shoulder pain, and whatnot. This wonder may be understood using Yun-Tao-Mao's neurobiological fact: as the limbs below the elbows and knees occupy larger areas in the sensory gyrus in the brain and the acupoints below the elbows and knees contain more sensory receptors, needling stimulation to these points may induce a greater reaction and activity in the brain. This principle clearly supports the concept of using certain acupoints below the elbows and knees, such as the Five *Shu* points, as diagnosis and treatment points during acupuncture treatment.

In cases of interruption, acupoints are selected based on local and special effects in correlation with efficacy. Five *Shu* points are selected for either deficiency or excess conditions to tonify or sedate in cases of imbalance. Overall acupuncture treatment method that covers the treatment of interruptions and imbalances of illnesses should be selected. For instance, more effective treatment result may be achieved if we use Saam acupuncture as a "root treatment" to correct imbalances but then combine it with Meridian style acupuncture, channel therapy acupuncture (which uses local and distal acupoints), special acupuncture points, or symptomatic treatment Meridian therapy, as "branch treatments", to correct interruptions in proper stimulation technique.

The original form of Saam acupuncture can be used from the perspective of the Five Organs, disease etiology, imbalanced *Yin* and *Yang*, the mind-only theory and the comparing-pulse diagnoses such as Lee [21] and Kim [22].

## 6. Saam Acupuncture in Research

It was reported that treatment following Saam acupuncture theory produced a positive effect on the dysarthria symptom of stroke patients, which was more prominent than the effects noted from using body acupuncture common in Korean acupuncture and traditional Chinese medicine [23]. It was also reported that acupuncture following Saam acupuncture treatment combined with conventional body acupuncture produced more pronounced results than those of body acupuncture alone [24].

One recent study [25] reported that Saam acupuncture may attenuate the imbalance between sympathetic and parasympathetic activities induced by night-shift work in nurses. Hwang et al assessed the effects of Saam acupuncture on the autonomic nervous system in night-shift nurses using power-spectral heart-rate variability (HRV) analysis. This study had a $2 \times 4$ cross-over design with a series of six ($n = 1$) controlled trials. Six night-shift nurses were randomly divided into two groups, and each nurse received four acupuncture treatments on the third day of night-shift work. One group started with Saam acupuncture (Gall Bladder-tonification), while the other started with sham acupuncture. Saam acupuncture and sham acupuncture were applied in turn. HRV was measured before and after treatment. For statistical analysis, the results of the two groups were combined, and a Bayesian model was used to compare the changes in HRV values before and after treatment, between Saam and sham acupuncture. As the ratio of low-to high-frequency power (LF/HF) for HRV increased on the third day of night-shift work in the pilot study, HRV measurements were made on the third day. Compared with sham acupuncture, Saam acupuncture reduced sympathetic activity; the overall median treatment effect estimate in LF normalized units decreased by −17.4 (confidence interval (CI): −26.67, −8.725) and that for LF/HF decreased by −1.691 (CI: −3.222, −0.3789). The overall median treatment effect estimate in HF normalized units increased by 17.41 (CI: 6.393, 27.13) with Saam acupuncture, suggesting an increase in parasympathetic activity.

## 7. Taegeuk Acupuncture

Taegeuk acupuncture is based on Sasang constitutional medicine, which makes the Heart the Central Ultimate, or *taichi* ("taegeuk"), of the Organs and classifies the body into four types by the relative size of the Organs. It decides the constitution first and tonifies or sedates the source point of the relevant Organ according to the size of the Organs. For example, Tae-yang (Greater *Yang*) constitution belongs to Metal, Tae-eum (Greater *Yin*) to Wood, So-yang (Lesser *Yang*) to Fire, and So-eum (Lesser *Yin*) to Water, and thus the Fire, Metal, Water, and Earth acupoints (HT8, HT4, HT3, HT7) of the Heart Meridian are tonified, for they are of the Five Elements that control the original dominant Organs. By doing so it compensates for the loss of balance, and can further balance the power of Organs by depleting the source point of the relevant Meridian according to the size of the other Organs, thus helping the patient get over his or her own disease by him or herself.

Sasang constitutional medicine describes four constitutions—Tae-yang, Tae-eum, So-yang and So-eum—which indicate constitutional energy discrepancies among major Organs. According to the Sasang constitutional theory, an aggravated energy discrepancy among major Organ energies is the underlying causative imbalance of superficial pathologic conditions [4] [26]. Lee Je-Ma, founder of the Sasang constitutional medicine, prescribed different combinations of herbs for his patients based on their respective constitutions, even if the patients came to seek him with apparently similar diseases. Rather than dealing with thousands of different diseases, practitioners could deliver four simple types of treatment for diverse illnesses aimed at recovering the energy balance of the constitution. Lee Je-Ma's original system of Sasang constitutional medicine lacked an acupuncture treatment system for the four constitutions.

Taegeuk acupuncture is originated by Lee Byeong-Haeng, as a response to Lee Je-Ma's testament that stated, "A doctor needled LI4 of a patient of So-eum constitution suffering dysarthria from stroke and the effect was astonishing that there may be other diseases that are better cured by acupuncture than medicine. Acupoints may be applied to the four constitutions as well; therefore further research is called for in the future". LI4 is the source point of the Large Intestine Meridian, and theoretically in Sasang constitution the Large Intestine is substituted for Kidney because of the principle that the Kidney should not be sedated. The source point is sedated for Kidney is the large Organ in So-eum constitution.

Taegeuk acupuncture provides acupuncture prescriptions for the correction of the underlying energy discrepancies that are assumed in Sasang constitutional medicine. Lee Byeong-Haeng suggested that observation of reactions to acupuncture stimulation of the Heart Meridian acupoints might be helpful in determining the type of constitution that the patient belongs to, because Heart energy plays a central role in controlling other Organs in the system of Sasang constitutional medicine [4].

For example, the constitutional characteristics of the Tae-yang constitution come from the discrepancy between a large Lung and a small Liver energy. According to the Taegeuk acupuncture theory, Tae-yang constitution is considered to be in a state of Metal excess, which may be regulated by stimulating HT8, the Fire point of the Heart Meridian. Fire suppresses Metal from the perspective of the control cycle relationships of the Five Elements. Similarly, people with the Tae-eum constitution have a large Liver and small Lung energy, and are considered to be in a state of Wood excess, which can be regulated by stimulating HT4, the Metal point of the Heart Meridian.

Kim [27] testifies that in his experience the duration of treatment lasted in average three to four months, and some diseases took six to seven months to cure.

Lee Byeong-Haeng used the rotation method and numbers method to tonify and sedate. Kim added respiratory method to prevent fainting during acupuncture intervention. To tonify, place needle while the patient inhales and rotate clockwise for nine times or the multiple of nine times. To sedate place needle while the patient exhales and rotate counter-clockwise for six times or the multiple of six times. Rotate until *deqi* is attained.

The judgment of the constitution may be the most important step in practicing Taegeuk acupuncture. It is done by tonifying the controlling Five Elements acupoint of the Heart Meridian and tonifying or sedating the source point of the small and large Organs' Meridians of an assumed constitution. After placing those three needles, press the solar plexus to confirm the constitution by the tenderness response. When the needles placed are in accord with the patient's constitution the tenderness is gone about 60% - 70%, and when the acupoints are not relevant with the patient's constitution they reply about 20% - 30% of the tenderness is gone. It is best to do the test 1 - 2 minutes after practicing Taegeuk acupuncture.

The symptoms for which Taegeuk acupuncture is effective are listed below by Lee. The exemplified treatments are for patients with So-yang constitution.

1. A stroke patient with hemiplegia can move his or her limbs when HT3 is tonified.
2. Tinnitus disappears at the site.
3. Headache, stomachache and numbness of hands and feet are cured at the site.
4. Hiccupping stops short.
5. It is hard to confirm the cure of stomach cancer but the pain disappears at the site.
6. Eyesight becomes bright.
7. Fatigue is recovered at the site.
8. Myalgia is reduced.
9. Low back pain is cured at the site.

Kim also summarizes his clinical experience and introduces the response of patients after Taegeuk acupuncture.

1. Taegeuk acupuncture is effective for psychogenic disease with symptoms such as palpitation, forgetfulness, insomnia, anxiety, impatience, chest discomfort, shortness of breath, headache, dizziness, and nausea. They relate to disease such as depression, chronic insomnia, aphasia, tic disorder and deficiency of Heart, Gall Bladder and Spleen.

2. Taegeuk acupuncture is effective for illnesses caused by blood circulation disorder such as blurry eyesight, pallor, headache, dizziness, stiff neck, menstrual pain, morning edema, small joint pain, etc.

3. Taegeuk acupuncture is effective for incurable diseases such as hand tremor, shaky head, facial spasm, convulsion of unknown reason, and for diseases for which standard acupuncture worsens the symptoms.

4. Taegeuk acupuncture can be used alongside standard acupuncture for:

1) Tinnitus or sudden deafness by needling TE21, SI19, TE17 of the affected side;
2) Trigeminal neuralgia by needling ST4-ST6, ST7-TE17, GB14-TE23 (electro-acupuncture) of the affected side;
3) Bell's palsy by needling ST4-ST6, ST7-TE17, GB14-TE23 (electro-acupuncture) of the affected side;
4) Unhealed ankle sprain after 3-6 months by using standard acupuncture following the Meridian of the affected side.

In cases of patients with marked solar plexus tenderness, Taegeuk acupuncture is practiced after the diagnosis of the constitution, regardless of the chief complaint whether it is stiff neck, lower back pain or knee joint pain. The following reaction usually results.

1) The mind is calmed and head becomes clear;
2) Chest discomfort disappears;
3) Vision becomes bright;
4) Digestion is boosted, and one feels hunger;
5) One becomes drowsy;
6) The acupuncture treatment site is painful;
7) One does not notice any difference.

The above 1 - 7 reactions are those of the patients right after one treatment session of Taegeuk acupuncture. After 1 - 2 days of the first treatment, the reactions are as follows:

1) Sleeps well at night after acupuncture treatment;
2) Body feels lighter;
3) Fatigue seems to be less;
4) Chronic and recurrent joint pain such as neck stiffness, knee pain and backache seems to be relieved;
5) Myalgia and spasm seem to be improved;
6) Still not sure of any difference.

In one recent study [28] Taegeuk acupuncture had potential as an effective means of stabilizing mental stress-induced imbalance of autonomic nervous system for So-yang constitution. In this study eight women diagnosed as So-yang constitution participated in a study on reducing mental stress assessed by heart rate variability. They were randomly divided into group A and group B. Each participant went through 3 sessions every week with 1 week of washout period in between each session. HRV was measured three times at every session; at baseline, after administering mentally stressful circumstances and after applying either one of simple rest, So-yang Taegeuk acupuncture or So-eum Taegeuk acupuncture. This study was designed as a crossover clinical trial. After same initial simple resting session for both groups at week 1, acupuncture for group A were executed in the order of So-yang Taegeuk acupuncture and So-eum Taegeuk acupuncture at week 2 and 3 respectively, with acupuncture for group B conducted in reverse order. The simple rest and So-eum Taegeuk acupuncture did not show the significant changes in response to LF(norm) and HF(norm) after stress stimuli. So-yang Taegeuk acupuncture did, however, significantly decrease LF(norm) and increase HF(norm). So-yang Taegeuk acupuncture, compared to So-eum Taegeuk acupuncture, significantly stabilized autonomic nervous system.

## References


[1] Yin, C., Park, H.J., Chae, Y., Ha, E., Park, H.K., Lee, H.S., *et al.* (2007) Korean Acupuncture: The Individualized and Practical Acupuncture. *Neurological Research*, **29**, 10-15. http://dx.doi.org/10.1179/016164107X172301

[2] Kim, D.-H. and Kim, J.-H. (1993) The Literary Study on the Written Date of and the Background of Sa-Ahm's 5 Element Acupuncture Method. Kyungwon University, Kyungki.

[3] Yin, C.-S. Chae, Y.-B., Koh, H.-G., Lee, H.-J., Chun, S.-I., *et al.* (2006) Constitutionally Individualized and Practically Integrated Characteristics of Korean Acupuncture. *Korean Journal of Acupuncture*, **23**, 19-28.

[4] Ahn, C.B., Jang, K.J., Yoon, H.M., Kim, C.H., Min, Y.K., Song, C.H., *et al.* (2010) Sa-Ahm Five Element Acupuncture. *Journal of Acupuncture and Meridian Studies*, **3**, 203-213. http://dx.doi.org/10.1016/S2005-2901(10)60037-4

[5] Lee, T.H. (1996) Essentials of Saam's Acupuncture Theory. Haenglim Publishing, Seoul.

[6] Jeremy, R. (2004) Acupuncture Point Combination. Churchill Livingstone, Edinburgh.

[7] Wu, G. (1980) Gatherings from Eminent Acupuncturists-Zhen Jiu Ju Ying. Shinmunfung Publisher, Taipei.

[8] Heng-pa (1975) The Essence of Sa-Ahm's Acupuncture. Heng-Lim Publisher, Seoul.

[9] Hicks, A.H.J. and Mole, P. (2005) Five Element Constitutional Acupuncture. Churchill Livingstone, Edinburgh, 383-384.

[10] Zhang, Y. (1977) Huang-Ti Nei-Ching Su-Men Ling-Shu Ji-Zhu He-Pian. Tai-Lian Guo-Feng Chu-Ban She, Taipei.

[11] Ahn, C.B., Jang, K.J., Yoon, H.M., Kim, C.H., Min, Y.K., Song, C.H., *et al.* (2009) A Study of the Sa-Ahm Five Element Acupuncture Theory. *Journal of Acupuncture and Meridian Studies*, **2**, 309-320. http://dx.doi.org/10.1016/S2005-2901(09)60074-1

[12] Maciocia, G. (2005) The Foundation of Chinese Medicine. Churchill Livingstone, Edinburgh.

[13] Ma, Y. and Cho, Z. (2005) Biomedical Acupuncture for Pain Management. Churchill Livingstone, Edinburgh.

[14] Seem, M.D. (1991) Acupuncture Energetics. Healing Arts Press, Rochester.

[15] Chang, S. (1912) Chiao-cheng t'u-chu pa-shih-i Nan-Ching. Hung-pao chai shu-chu, Taipei, 6-11.

[16] Unschuld, P.U. (1986) Nan-Ching—The Classic of Difficult Issues. University of California Press, Oakland, 474-617.

[17] Lee, I. (2007) A Study on the Basic Forms and Principles of Saam's 5 Phase of Acupuncture Method. *Journal of the Korean Acupuncture and Moxibustion Society*, **1**, 19-51.

[18] Kim, H.G. (1992) Handbook of Saam Acupuncture. Shinnongbaekcho Press, Seoul.

[19] Kim, D. (2002) Reviewed Sa-Ahm's Acupuncture Treatment with Graphs. So-Gang Pub, Busan.

[20] Ahn, C.B. and Choi, D.Y. (1986) Theoretical Study on Five Element Acupuncture. *Dongguk Journal*, **5**, 287-309.

[21] Lee, J.W. (1958) The Secret of Saam's Acupuncture Based on Yin-Yang and Five Elements. Institute for Studying Five Element Acupuncture, Busan.

[22] Kim, D.P. (1972) Saam's Five Element Acupuncture and Its Usages. *The Journal of the Korean Oriental Medical Society*, Winter Issue, 122-123.

[23] Song, M.S., Kim, Y.H., Jang, S.G., Kim, J.H., Yim, Y.K., Kang, J.H., *et al.* (2003) Clinical Comparison Studies on 20 Cases of Stroke Patients with Dysarthria by Sa-Am and General Acupuncture. *Journal of the Korean Acupuncture and Moxibustion Society*, **20**, 161-167.

[24] Kim, J.H., Park, E.J., Park, C.H., Cho, M.R., Ryu, C.R. and Chae, W.S. (2002) Comparison of the Improvement of Back Pain and Sciatica between Common Acupuncture Treatment Group and Common Acupuncture with Shin Jong Gyuk of Ohaeng Acupuncture Treatment Group. *Journal of the Korean Acupuncture and Moxibustion Society*, **19**, 84-91.

[25] Hwang, D.S., Kim, H.K., Seo, J.C., Shin, I.H., Kim, D.H. and Kim, Y.S. (2011) Sympathomodulatory Effects of Saam Acupuncture on Heart Rate Variability in Night-Shift-Working Nurses. *Complementary Therapies in Medicine*, **19**, S33-S40. http://dx.doi.org/10.1016/j.ctim.2010.11.001

[26] Kuon, D.W. (1965) A Study of Constitution-Acupuncture. *Journal of the International Congress of Acupuncture and Moxibustion*, **10**, 149-167.

[27] Kim, J.K. (2011) Clinical Opinion of Taegeuk Acupuncture Treatment by Sasang (4-Type) Constitutional Medicine. *Journal of the Korean Acupuncture and Moxibustion Society*, **28**, 69-73.

[28] Kim, N.S., Kim, S.J., Ryu, H.J., Nam, S.S. and Kim, Y.S. (2012) Effects of Taegeuk Acupuncture on the Autonomic Nervous System by Analyzing Heart Rate Variability in Soyangin. *Journal of the Korean Acupuncture and Moxibustion Society*, **29**, 81-88.

# 9

# Fermented Black Turmeric Designed by Lactobacillus Rearranged Leukocyte Subsets and Anti-Oxidative Activity

**Yousuke Watanabe[1], Nobuo Yamaguchi[1,2*], Isao Horiuch[3,4], Tsugia Murayama[5]**

[1]Ishikawa Natural Medicinal Products Research Center, Ishikawa, Japan
[2]Department of Fundament Research for CAM, Kanazawa Medical University, Ishikawa, Japan
[3]Traditional Uighur Medicine Department, Xinjiang Medical University, Urumchi, China
[4]Traditional Chinese Medicine Hospital, Xinjiang Medical University, Urumchi, China
[5]Faculty of Pharmaceutical Sciences, Department of Microbiology and Immunology, Hokuriku University, Ishikawa, Japan
Email: [*]serumaya@kanazawa-med.ac.jp

## Abstract

**A plant fermentation was carried out by Yeast and *Lactobaccilli* against fermented black turmeric, *Kaempferia parviflora* (FBT). These materials were proved by as safe in animal safety experiment. We tried to investigate changes of immune-competent cells that commonly utilized FBT, including after administration of immno-suppressed animals, the effects by FBT on the regulated effect on the cells were evaluated. Our results showed that FBT augmented the level of lymphocytes in number, while FBT regulated the level of granulocytes in both number and function. In our clinical study with 20 healthy volunteers, granulocyte and lymphocyte ratio suggesting their constitution as neutral in peripheral blood were increased significantly 30 days after the administration of FBT in rodents, and compromised host was prepared with cancer chemotherapeutic agent (Mytomycin-C). Our observations showed against intracellular parasite, and that FBT augmented intercellular pathogen through humoral immunity. We discussed the significance and mechanism of FBT on the level of leukocyte subsets in number and function that were considered to be potential indicators for the activation of the compromised host. We also proposed an idea that FBT exhibited tonic effects via activating complement components. The evidences were shown by immune-electrophoretic method. Moreover, we tried to access further to the anti-oxidative activities of this FBT. This modification brought to the significant lift up for antibody producing cells and anti-oxidative activity for phagocytic cells.**

[*]Corresponding author.

## Keywords

**Family Turmeric Lactobacillus, Fermentation, *Lactobacilli*, Cancer, Chemotherapeutic Agent, Compromised Host, Complement, Alternative Complement Activation**

## 1. Introduction

In recent years, complementary and alternative medicines (CAM) have achieved more and more attentions since they are able to treat many chronic illnesses, such as fatigue syndrome that plagues the industrialized world. The present team has reported that typical styles of CAM, preparing special molecule for both digestive and easy for activate human complement component.

The activated complement components bound to regulate function of all the leukocytein humanimmune system [1]-[7]. Dietary and fermented formula holds a promise as strong inducers of acquired immunity. While the immune system is working against the local infection of pathogens, cytokine and immuno-competent cells react throughout the body in close connection to the brain, the endocrine and immune system [8]. In this study, we hypothesize that FBT may influence immuno-competent cells qualitatively and quantitatively FBT targeting lymphocytes based on the constitution dependent manner. FBT has been employed as tonic agent and the implication has little been made on the characteristics of the levels of leukocyte subset, such as granulocytes and lymphocytes. In this report, we seek to focus on the identity of FBT formula, comparing to another herbal medicine. The influence of FBT on leukocyte and/or lymphocyte subpopulations in human peripheral blood was also discussed. Moreover, Fragmentation of black turmeric has been made by Lactobacillus and by Yeast Fungus in order to induce active component from original material other than dairy use [9] **Figure 1**, **Figure 2**.

## 2. Materials and Methods

### 2.1. Single Shot and Multiple Shot Toxicity

Ten female seven-week-old ddY mice, were used for the acute oral toxicity study. The tests were carried out according to Ethics of the Organization for Economic Co-operation and Development (OECD) Test Guideline 401. The mice were housed at 24˚C ± 1˚C, 50% relative humidity. Both conventional and charged water were suspended in sterile and administered to mice in free supplemental system, calculating daily consumption. Mice

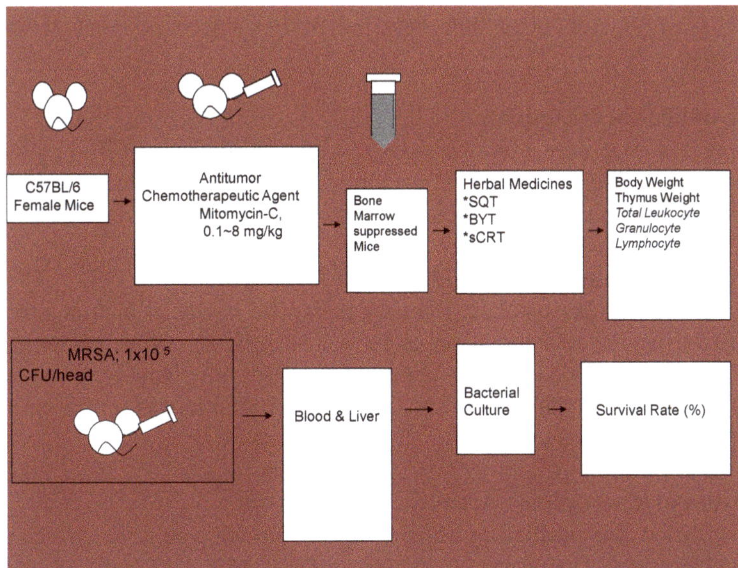


**Figure 1.** Experimental model for the study FBT in immuno-compromised mice.

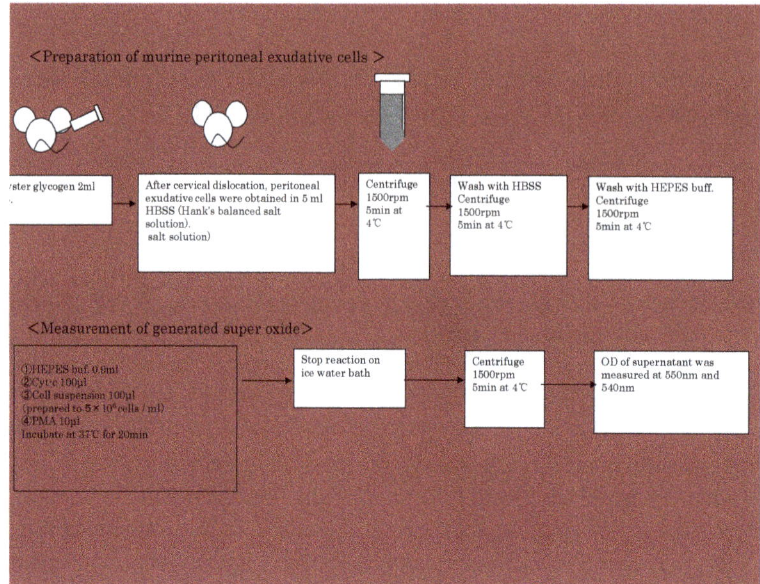


**Figure 2.** The experimental procedure for accessing anti-oxidative of the mice macrophage.

were weighted at 0 - 7 days after administration, and clinical observations were made once a day. Necropsy was performed on all mice seven days after administration.

## 2.2. Experimental Model for Bone Marrow Suppressed Immune-Compromised Mice

In the animal model of immuno-competency reduction, male C57BL/6J mice, aged 8 - 9 weeks, were injected with Mitomycin-C (MMC) (5mg/kg) to inhibit the bone marrow. Then, FBT extracts was administered orally at a dosage of 1 g/kg/day for five consecutive days. *Conventional black turmeric* and *fermented black turmeric* were chosen as controls (**Figure 1**).

### 2.2.1. Recovery of Total Leukocytes and Its Subsets

The bone marrow-suppressed mice were administered herbal decoction FBT 1 g/kg dairy for 5 days and after 1 week later, their blood were withdrawn from their tail vain. Then, the number of leukocytes was counted in Bürker-Türk solution.

### 2.2.2. Regulation of Leukocyte Subsets

Bone marrow-suppressed mice were administered with herbal decoction of FBT (1 g/kg/day) for five days. One week later, the blood from their tail vain was withdrawn. Then the granulocyte and lymphocyte subsets were counted in Bürker-Türk solution.

### 2.2.3. Recovery of Macrophage Activity, Migration

Cells from peritoneal exudates were collect from the peritoneal cavity of bone marrow-suppressed mice. Phagocytes were purified using adherent technique to get cell suspensions which contained more than 95% of phagocytes. The purified cells were loaded to the upper room of Boyden chamber to test migration ability at a concentration of $1 \times 10^4$ cell/ml. Human serum treated at 56˚C for 30 min was for the chemo tactic agent of mouse phagocyte [10]-[18].

### 2.2.4. Augmentation of Macrophage Activity, Phagocytosis

The same cells suspension was purified by adherent technique for phagocyte, which produces cells contained more than 95% of phagocytes. The purified cells were adjusted to $1 \times 10^4$ cell/cm$^2$ and mixed with latex beads that are 5 μm in granule with fluorescence isochianate. After 90 min of incubation, remained granule were washed out from the glass slide. Number of phagocytic cell and their ability to catch up the latex beads were automatically measured by ACAS system, which outputs the result in a digital form (Adeherent cell activity evaluating system; Shimazu, Kyoto, Japan).

#### 2.2.5. A Recovery of Lymphocyte Activity, Antibody Secreting Cell

The bone marrow suppressed mice were administered herbal decoction of FBT (1 g/kg/day) for 5 days. One week later, mice were immunized with sheep red blood cells, ($2 \times 10^8$/mouse) intraperitoneally. Five days later, their spleen cells were collected. Plague-forming cells (PFC) were developed, and the ability of IgM and IgG antibody production was tested by the method reported by Jerne and Nordin [19] [20].

#### 2.2.6. CD Positive Lymphocyte Distribution by FBT against Different Constitution

Whole blood obtained from the subjects was washed twice with PBS. One hundred micro-liters of the suspensions were stained with 20 μl of fluorescent monoclonal antibodies (anti-human $CD2^+$, $CD4^+$, $CD8^+$, $CD11b^+$, $CD14^+$, $CD16^+$, $CD19^+$ and $CD56^+$ antibodies). Ten thousands stained cells were re-suspended in PBS to detect surface markers by flow cytometry (FACS Calibur; Becton Dickinson Immnocytometry Systems, CA, USA).

#### 2.2.7. Distribution of Cytokine Producing Lymphocytes in Different Constitution

The blood cell suspensions were cultured with PMA (phorbol 12-myristate 13-acetate), ionomycin and BSA (bovine serum albumin) for 4 - 5 hours at 37˚C. After that, the cell suspensions were stained using the monoclonal antibodies of PE-IL-4, FITC-IFN-$\gamma$ and FITC-IL-1$\beta$. Then they were analyzed by the FACScan (Becton Dickinson Co. Ltd. USA). The antibodies and reagents used in the test were purchased from Becton Dickinson Immunocytometry System (USA).

#### 2.2.8. Estimation of Macrophage Activity FBT the Examination of Phagocytosis

The peritoneal exudates cells were collect from the peritoneal cavity of bone marrow-suppressed mice. Cell suspensions were purified by adherent technique for phagocyte, getting a suspension which contained over 95% of phagocytes. The purified cells were adjusted to $1 \times 10^4$ cell/ml and loaded at the upper chamber of Boyden chamber for test migration. Human serum with treated at 56˚C for 30 min was for the chemotactic agent for mouse phagocyte.

Phagocytic activity and antibody production of macrophages were analyzed using a classical test that could test the total activity of the immune system by examine chemotaxis, phagocytosis and intracellular degradation of macrophage. For identifying antibody-forming cells, plaque-forming cells were detected using heterogeneous erythrocyte; sheep erythrocyte was a target antigen. Peritoneal macrophages were collected and purified in fetal calf serum (FCS)-coated petri-dishes. The cell population was approximately 97% uniform in function and morphology. These cells were applied to the nuclepore-membrane (pore size: 5 μm; Neuro Probe Co. Ltd., Cabin John MD, USA) with a chemotaxis chamber (Neuro Probe Co. Ltd.). After 90 minutes' incubation, the membrane was vigorously washed with saline (37˚C), fixed, and then stained with methylene blue dye. After counting under a microscope for the total field of the membrane, the average number of migrating cells was expressed as cell counts/mm$^2$.

The same cells suspension was purified by adherent technique for phagocyte, which contained over 95% of phagocytes. The purified cells were adjusted to $1 \times 10^4$ cell/cm$^2$ and mixed with latex beads that were 5 um in granule with FBT fluorescence isochianate. After 90 min of incubation, the remained granule were washed out from the glass slide and counting automatically by ACAS system, which outputs digital presentation, for evaluating phagocytes in number and in their ability to catch up the latex beads (Adherent cell analyzing system, Shimazu, Kyoto, Japan). Latex beads in 5 μm with fluorescence were used to test phagocytic activity and *Candida albicans* was cell killing activity. A macrophage-target cell ratio of 1:10 was considered to be optimum. Ten minutes after incubating phagocytes and target cells, intracellular Candida cells were cultured on an agar dish with conventional medium 1640 until the next day to perform the colony forming assay. In this way, the phagocytic ability of the macrophages was monitored. To document intracellular killing activity, the same procedures were performed excepting that the incubation time was changed to 90 minutes.

#### 2.2.9. Antibody Forming Cell Study

Sheep erythrocyte (SRBC), a T-dependent antigen, was used for antibody formation cell study. Ten days after tumor transplantation, each antigen was intra-peritoneally injected. After four and six days, the antibody-forming cells were detected using localized hemolysis in an agar gel. Plaque-forming cells were developed FBT the method of Jerne and Nordin [19] [20].

## 2.3. Anti-Oxidative Evaluation

### 2.3.1. Experimental Animals

Eight week-old female C57BL/6 were purchased from Sankyo Laboratory Service Corporation (Shizuoka, Japan). All mice were kept under specific pathogen-free conditions. Mice food and distilled water were freely accessible for each mouse. Housing temperature and humidity were controlled 25˚C ± 1˚C and 60%.

### 2.3.2. Reagents and Preparation

As for the basic medium, HEPES buffer (HEPES 17 mM, NaCl 120 mM, Glucose 5 mM, KCl 5 mM, $CaCl_2$ 1 mM, $MgCl_2$ 1 mM) was prepared and sterilized by filtration. Phorbol 12-myristate 13-acetate (PMA, Sigma, USA) was diluted to $10^{-6}$ M by dimethyl sulfoxide DMSO, Sigma, USA) and used as a stimulant for super oxide anion generation for murine peritoneal exudates cells. Cytochrome-c (Sigma, USA) was diluted to 1 mM by HEPES buffer. Since cytochrome-c reduced by super oxide showed maximum absorbance at 550 nm, we used cytochrome-c to measure the amount of super oxide anion generation through spectro-photometrical technique. Oyster glycogen (type II, Sigma, USA) was diluted in the purified water (10% w/v, Wako, Japan) and autoclaved at 120˚C for 20 min. This solution was used for intraperitoneal injection to mice in order to induce peripheral neutrophils into the abdominal cavity (**Figure 2**).

### 2.3.3. The Assessing the Amount of Super Oxide Anion Generated by Murine Peritoneal Exudates Cells

Each drug was orally administered to mice (500 mg/kg) for one week. Two milliliters of 10% Oyster glycogen was injected intraperitoneally 10 hours before the assay. Sufficient murine peritoneal exudative cells were induced ten hours after the stimulation. Mice were euthanized by cervical dislocation, murine peritoneal exudates cells (PEC) suspension was centrifuged twice for 5 minutes at 1500 rpm at 4˚C. Then PEC was prepared to $1 \times 10^6$ cells/ml of HEPES buffer. One hundred microliters of cytochrome-c and 10 μl of PMA were added to the cell suspension and this was incubated for 20 minutes at 37˚C. The reaction mixture was then centrifuged for 10 minutes at 1500 rpm, 4˚C. An OD of supernatant was measured at both 550 nm and 540 nm, the amount of generated super oxide anion was shown in the formula; increased absorbance at 550 nm $(\Delta A_{550\text{-}540})/19.1 \times 10^3$ (mmol/ml). In order to ensure if we really measured the amount of generated super oxide anion or not, we tried to add super oxide anion dismutase (SOD), an enzyme for its anti-oxidative effect, into our experimental system. The result was as expected that the reduction of cytochrome-c was inhibited after the addition of SOD. This showed us that our experimental system could be used properly for measuring the amount of generated super oxide anion.

## 2.4. Statistical Analysis

Data are expressed as means ± standard deviations. The differences between FBT-treated and non-treated conditions were compared using a one-tailed analysis of variance. A $P$ value < 0.05 was considered to be statistically significant.

# 3. Results

## 3.1. Animal Test for FBT

### 3.1.1. Single and Multiple Dose Toxicity study for *Conv.* BT and *Fermented* BT

Ten female seven-week-old ddY mice, were used for the acute oral toxicity study. The tests were carried out according to Ethics of the Organization for Economic Co-operation and Development (OECD) Test Guideline 401. The mice were housed at 24˚C ± 1˚C, 50% relative humidity. Both conventional and charged water were suspended in sterile and administered to mice in free supplemental system, calculating daily consumption. Mice were weighted at 0 - 7 days after administration, and clinical observations were made once a day. Necropsy was performed on all mice seven days after administration.

No deaths or abnormalities of body weight, water and food consumption, or coat condition were observed in the treated mice. Necropsy evaluation of the mice did not reveal any significant differences in thymus, liver, spleen, kidney, adrenal gland and testicle weights between the control group and both conventional water and charged and activated water.

### 3.1.2. Recovery of Whole Body Weight by FBT

The body weight and thymus weight reduced in bone marrow-suppressed mice, resulting in the reduction of peripheral blood leukocyte to around 40%. After administered each herbal decoction 1 g/kg dairy for 5 days and after 1 week later, their blood were recovered to around 90% of normal value

### 3.1.3. Recovery of Thymus Weight by FBT

The bone marrow-suppressed mice were administered FBT 1 g/kg dairy for 5 days, and one week later, their blood was withdrawn from their tail vein. The cell count of the peripheral blood is showed in **Figure 4**. **Table 1** shows that the thymus weight decreased to half of normal control after 5 mg/kg of MMC was injected. However,

**Table 1.** Proteins of the complement system.

| Protein | Molecular Weight | Plasma Concentration | |
|---|---|---|---|
| **Classical Pathway** | | | |
| C1q | 400,000 | 65 | μg/ml |
| C1r | 190,000 | 50 | μg/ml |
| C1s | 88,000 | 40 | μg/ml |
| C4 | 200,000 | 640 | μg/ml |
| C2 | 117,000 | 25 | μg/ml |
| C3 | 185,000 | 1400 | μg/ml |
| **Alternative Pathway** | | | |
| Factor B | 93,000 | 200 | μg/ml |
| Factor D | 23,000 | 2 | μg/ml |
| C3 | 185,000 | 1400 | μg/ml |
| **Membrane Attack Pathway** | | | |
| C5 | 200,000 | 80 | μg/ml |
| C6 | 128,000 | 75 | μg/ml |
| C7 | 121,000 | 55 | μg/ml |
| C8 | 154,000 | 55 | μg/ml |
| C9 | 79,000 | 60 | μg/ml |
| **Regulatory Proteins** | | | |
| C1 Inhibitor | 85,000 | 20 | μg/ml |
| C4b Binding protein | 570,000 | 250 | μg/ml |
| Carboxypeptidase N | 310,000 | 50 | μg/ml |
| Factor H | 150,000 | 500 | μg/ml |
| Factor I | 80,000 | 35 | μg/ml |
| Properdin | 180,000 | 25 | μg/ml |
| S-Protein | 71,000 | 600 | μg/ml |

all the three FBTs recovered thymus weight to about 70% of the control.

#### 3.1.4. Recovery of CD+ Cells and Cytokine Producing Cells by FBT

CD3, CD4 and CD19 cells of MMC treated mice were recovered to almost normal values after the administration of FBTs. As for the functional recovery, IFN-$\gamma$ and IL-4 producing cells were also recovered by FBT. The all three decoction, including FBTs and a functionally depressive agent of TCM. In cytokine producing cells, IFN-$\gamma$ and IL-4 producing cell were recovered with FBT. In all the three FBTs tested, cytokine producing cells were recovered with BT and even fermented BT.

#### 3.1.5. Recovery of Macrophage Activity, Phagocytosis by FBT

The figure shows that MMC clearly suppressed the phagocytic activity of mice both in number and function. After the treatment of FBT, the mice recovered their phagocytic activity to normal range. With a precise observation, the recovery activity was different between BT and FBT, and were the strongest FBT among the four formulae as to augmentation in number and function of phagocytes. On the other hand, the augmentation by BT was less than that by FRT

#### 3.1.6. Recovery of Lymphocyte Activity, Antibody Secreting Cell by FBT

The bone marrow-suppressed mice were administered herbal decoction FBT for five days. One week later, mice were immunized with sheep red blood cells, ($2 \times 10^8$/mouse) intraperitoneally. Four and six days later, their plague-forming cells (PFC) were developed. The ability of IgM and IgG antibody production was tested FBT, the method reported by Jerne and Nordin [19] [20]. In this mouse model, MMC did not reduce the antibody forming cells significantly but the tendency was the same as shown in the former section. In this test, B was the most effective than that of A. FBT was the strongest material to augment antibody secreting cell among the two formulae.

#### 3.1.7. Phagocytic Activity of Macrophage by FBT

So as to detect the supportive effect and important immunological stimulation by the Tonic agent, we traced the augmentation pattern of each remedy. As results of this trial, the phagocytic patterns by the tonic agents, were clearly different from MMC-treated mice. Moreover, augmentation of phagocytes were different between each FBT was prominent in activating phagocytes quantitatively and qualitatively compared to FBT.

We showed the diversity in the recovery pattern of FBTs. Famous tonic remedies in China and Japan, FBT, strongly recovered phagocytic activity in compromised hosts, but the recovery by FBT was much less than that by FBT. The recovery level of phagocytic activity by FBT was between conventional black turmeric and Fermented one.

### 3.2. The Amount of Generated Super Oxide Anion Regulated by FBT

The amount of generated super oxide anion was calculated in the formula shown above. The generated super oxide anion after one week administration of *Agaricus* and *Chlorella* were 2.64 and $1.95 \times 10^{-5}$ mmol/ml, respectively, whereas that was $2.85 \times 10^{-5}$ mmol/ml in control group. The generated super oxide anion after one week administration of BT and FBT were 1.24, 1.25 and $2.88 \times 10^{-5}$ mmol/ml, respectively. The generated super oxide anion after one week administration of Propolis was $2.55 \times 10^{-5}$ mmol/ml. All these drugs, except for FBT, decreased super oxide anion generation after administration for one week in mice.

### 3.3. The Comparison of Generated Super Oxide Anion between the Fermented and Non Fermented Black Turmeric

Since the antioxidative effects of herbal medicine were demonstrated, we investigated the way to reinforce this effect. The fermentation is one of the possibilities. Since the fermentation is preceded by bacterial digestion and degradation, less efficient constituents would be lost than commonly used extraction by hot water. Therefore, we decided to ferment the herbal medicine by yeast (*Saccharomyces cerevisiae*), expecting the enhancement of its antioxidative effects. The generated super oxide anion after one week administration of fermented herbal medicine TCM, FBT, FBT and sCRT were 0.62, 0.84 and $1.50 \times 10^{-5}$ mmol/ml, respectively. All the fermented herbal medicine decreased super oxide anion generation in compare with their corresponding unfermented ones

(**Figure 3**).

### 3.4. The Comparison of Generated Super Oxide Anion between the Fermented and Original Black Turmeric

The antioxidative activity of Propoils has been demonstrated, however, the particle of native Propolis was seen to be gross. In order to reinforce its antioxidative activity from physical constructive view point, we tried to micrified Propolis into 0.5 µm, expecting enlarged attachment area with reaction mixture. The generated super oxide anion after one week administration of micrified Propolis was $2.52 \times 10^{-5}$ mmol/ml, whereas that of non-micrified Propolis was $2.55 \times 10^{-5}$ mmol/ml. The antioxidative activity was slightly enhanced by micrifying the drug.

### 3.5. Antibody Forming Cell Study by Black Turmeric Derivatives

Sheep erythrocyte (SRBC), a T-dependent antigen, was used for antibody formation cell study. Ten days after tumor transplantation, each antigen was intra-peritoneally injected. After four and six days, the antibody-forming cells were detected using localized hemolysis in an agar gel. Plaque-forming cells were developed FBT. The method of Jerne and Nordin [19] [20].

The fermentation is preceded by bacterial digestion and degradation, less of the efficient constituents would be lost than commonly used extraction by hot water. Therefore we decided to ferment the herbal medicine by yeast (*Saccharomyces cerevisiae*), expecting the enhancement of lymphocyte activating effects through antibody forming cells. The antibody forming cells after one week's administration of fermented SQT and FBT were 135% and 140%, respectively. All the fermented herbal medicines from FBT increased PFC.

## 4. Clinical Findings

### 4.1. Changes in Cell Number of Total Leukocyte and Subsets by FBT

Leukocyte numbers have been counted one hour before and 15 days after the treatment of hemopoitic formula. The cell number measured one hour before the administration was set as 100%. Relative percentage of cell number on the 15th day was calculated. No significant changes were observed in G-group after the administration of FBT. However, significant change was found in L-type group (**Table 2**).

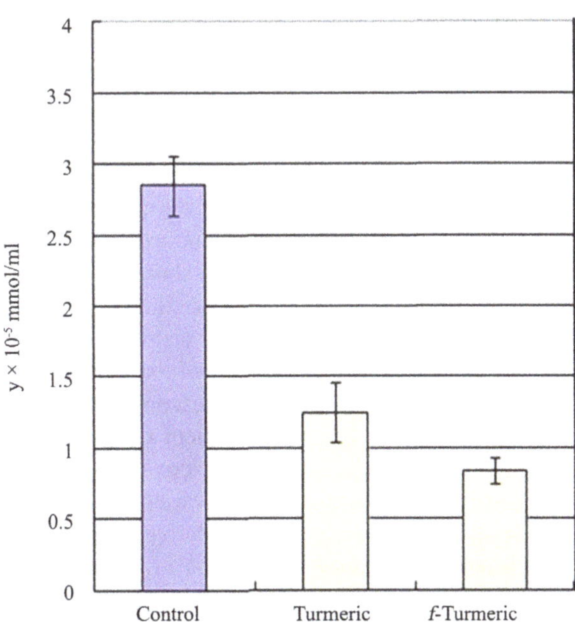


**Figure 3.** Anti-oxidative activity by fermented black turmeric and conventional one.

**Table 2.** Constitution dependent regulation of leukocyte by *Black Turmeric.*

| | G-type individual | | L-type individual | |
|---|---|---|---|---|
| | *Conv. B. Turmeric* | | *f-B. Turmeric* | |
| | Before | After | Before | After |
| Total WBC (×$10^3$ μl) | 6.44 | 5.78 | 3.47 | 5.65 |
| Lymphocyte (%) | 25.6 | 26.8 | 43.6 | 38.7 |
| Granulocyte (%) | 67.5 | 68.5 | 54.8 | 57.5 |
| Neutrophil (%) | 65.5 | 64.3 | 44.6 | 53.1 |
| Eosinophil (%) | 1.5 | 2.9 | 2.5 | 4.2 |
| Basophil (%) | 0.5 | 0.6 | 0.8 | 0.8 |

## 4.2. Dividing Subjects into Two Groups, G-Type and L-Type by Granulocyte and Lymphocyte Proportion

The volunteers were healthy subject, with no drastic change for the total number of leukocytes. However, we tried to check the regulative effect of herbal formulae for two different constitution, G-rich type and L-rich type. Analysis that mixed both groups together showed no significant differences in total leukocyte number except that for FBT; in G-type group, total number of leukocytes was down regulated by *conventional black turmeric.* This was a results of the down regulation of major group of leukocyte, granulocyte.

As for the L-type, no significant changes were found after the treatment of both FBTs. In the L-type group, FBT, on the other hand, increased the tonal leukocyte and granulocyte in number, on the contrary to the down regulation for lymphocytes. To further clarify the influence of hemopoietic formula, we divided the subjects into two groups: the G-type group, who had a granulocyte count over 60%, and the L-type group, who had a lymphocyte count over 40%. In the L-type group, lymphocyte counts tended to decrease on day 15, accompanied by an increase in granulocyte numbers by *conventional black turmeric* but not by FBT. On the contrary, the granulocyte counts of G type group tended to decrease on day 15. The decrease of granulocyte count was raised by *fermented black turmeric*, but not by *conventional black turmeric* on day 15 (**Table 3**).

## 4.3. The Complement System-Another Stage for Focusing by Fragmented Polysaccharide by FBT

We would like to focus on another important factor of immunological component, complement. These proteins are composed of at least 9 components. These proteins are famous for its defensive activity against infections organisms as in the defense immunity. However, we had found that the complement had worked when we introduced fragmented/fermented polysaccharide as complement activator, so called alternative pathway conjunct to Alternative Medicine. So in this chapter, we would like to show the nature of complement and activated mechanism that lead to the activation of all the physical activities through the augmentation of complement receptor positive structure cells. Activation of the complement system results in a cascade of interactions of these proteins, leading to the generation of products that have important biologic activities and that constitute an important humoral mediator system involved in inflammatory reactions. First, coating of particles, such as bacteria or immune complexes, with certain components of complement facilitates the ingestion of the particle by phagocytic cells (opsonic function of complement). Second, the activation event generates many fission products of complement proteins for which specific receptors exist on a variety of inflammatory cells, such as granulocytes, lymphocytes, and other cells. Binding of these complement-derived products to such receptors results in biologic activities such as chemotaxis and hormone-like activation of cellular functions (inflammatory function of complement) [21] [22] (**Figure 4**).

### 4.3.1. Pathways of Complement Activation and Complement Proteins by FBT

The complement component can activate by two separate pathways: the classical and the alternative pathways.

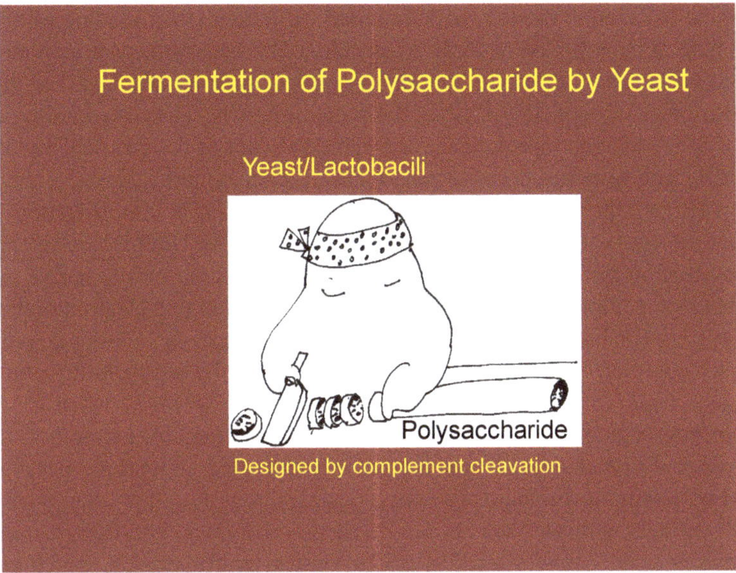


**Figure 4.** An illustrative imaging for degradation of polysaccharide by microorganism.

**Table 2.** Constitution dependent regulation of lymphocyte by *Black Turmeric.*

| CD | G-type individual | | L-type individual | |
|---|---|---|---|---|
| | *Conv. B. Turmeric* | | *f-B. Turmeric* | |
| | **Before (%)** | **After (%)** | **Before (%)** | **After (%)** |
| CD2 | 6.66 | 76.76 | 60.43 | 77.65 |
| CD4 | 19.54 | 28.44 | 31.43 | 45.67 |
| CD8 | 37.65 | 42.57 | 26.38 | 28.63 |
| CD11 | 73.77 | 72.68 | 63.45 | 69.54 |
| CD14 | 0.03 | 0.06 | 0.06 | 0.07 |
| CD16 | 67.65 | 58.55 | 54.24 | 46.67 |
| CD19 | 8.45 | 8.21 | 8.41 | 7.95 |
| CD56 | 1.57 | 1.88 | 1.78 | 2.87 |

Both pathways lead to a common terminal pathway referred to as the pathway of membrane attack complex. Twenty plasma proteins are now known to be constituents of these pathways. These proteins can be divided into functional proteins, which represent the elements of the various pathways, and regulatory proteins, which exhibit each function. The blood level of the proteins in normal human varies a broad range. They are synthesized in the liver but also by cells of the lympho-reticular system, such as lymphocytes and monocytes. Both the classical and the alternative complement pathways can be organized into various operational units: initiation, amplification, and membrane attack. Following an initial recognition event, which leads to initiation of the pathway, an amplification phase takes place that involves the action of proteases and the recruitment of additional molecules; this is followed by a terminal phase of membrane attack during which the cell dies. The recognition unit for the classical pathway, C1, is composed of three separate proteins, Clq, Clr, and Cls. The initiation of this pathway of complement typically involves the reaction of antibody with antigen, which may be soluble or on the surface of a target cell. This antigen-antibody reaction allows the binding of Clq to two or more Fc regions of certain IgG subclasses (IgG1, IgG2, IgG,) or IgM. Activators of the classical pathway. The ultra structure of Clq has been demonstrated by electron microscopy to consist of six subunits similar to a bouquet of six flowers. The central stalks of Clq resemble collagen in primary and secondary structure. Upon binding of one Clq molecule to the Fc regions of two or more antigen-bound antibody molecules, Clr proenzymes are activated. The chemical basis of this activation is the cleavage of a peptide bond by an autocatalytic mechanism, leading to the formation of activated Clr, a protease that subsequently cleaves the proenzyme Cls. Thus, the binding of Clq to an immunoglobulin in complex with the antigen represents the recognition event of the classical pathway, resulting in the activation of Clr and Cls. The final result is the generation of an enzymatically active component, Cls, which will cleave and thereby activate the next proteins in the cascade, leading to amplification of the recognition event. The other activation process, polysaccharide molecule also hits the complement component. Therefore, some polysaccharide molecule hit the complement component in the manner of alternative pathway. Thus, U-164 derivatives activated human complement component and shown by immune elecrophoretic methods.

The enzymatic protein Cls has two physiologic substrates, C4 and C2. C4 is cleaved by Cls into C4a, one of the three anaphylatoxins (molecules that promote increased vascular permeability and smooth muscle contraction), and C4b, which binds to the target cell surface. Cls also cleaves C2 when C2 is in complex with C4b. Cleavage of C2 generates C2b, which is released, and C2a, which remains bound to C4b. The bimolecular complex C4b, 2a is a protease that cleaves C3 and therefore is called C3 convertase. Cleavage of C3 by the C3 convertase generates two important biologically active peptides, C3a (another anaphylatoxin) and cab, which attaches to target cell surfaces and can bind to C5. C5, when in complex with C3b, can be cleaved by the C3 convertase (then referred to as C5 convertase). The C5 convertase hydrolyzes C5, which generates the C5a anaphylatoxin and C5b. C5b is the nucleus for the formation of the membrane attack complex. Immediately following their generation, C3b and C4b exhibit a unique transient ability to covalently bind to target cells ("metastable binding site"). This property has reentry been shown to be due to an intramolecular thioester bond that is present between the sulfhydryl group of a cysteine residue and the gamma carbonyl group of a glutamine residue on C3 and C4. Upon activation of C3 or C4, this thioester becomes highly reactive and can react with a cell surface hydroxyl or amino group. This results in the covalent attachment of C3b or C4b to the target cell. An additional function of the thioester bond is its hydrolysis by water, occurring during activation of the alternative pathway as described below.

The alternative pathway can be activated when a molecule of C3b is bound to a target cell. This C3b molecule combines with the plasma protein Factor B, which is a zymogen, and which, when bound to C3b, can be activated by the plasma protein Factor D by cleavage into two fragments, Ba and Bb. The Bb fragment, which contains the active enzymatic site, remains bound to C3b, as C3b, Bb. This complex, like C4b, 2a in the classical pathway, is a C3 convertase (C3b; Bb); it is stabilized by the binding of another plasma protein, properdin. Thus, the alternative pathway used to be called the properdin pathway. The presence of a single molecule of C3b generates many molecules of C3b, Bb, resulting in a tremendous amplification. The C3 convertase (C3b, Bb) cleaves C3, thereby generating more molecules of C3b, which can combine with other molecules of factor B to give more molecules of cab, Bb, which can, in turn, cleave more molecules of C3. Therefore, the central feature of the alternative pathway is a positive feedback loop that amplifies the original recognition event. As in the classical pathway, attachment of many C3b molecules to the target cell will allow binding of C5 and its cleavage into C5a and C5b by the enzyme C3b, Bb, now referred to as C5 convertase.

Owing to the potential of this positive feedback loop to rapidly use up Factor B and C3, the positive feedback must be carefully regulated. There are two important regulatory proteins in plasma. The first protein, Factor H (formerly referred to as PIH), competes with Factor B for binding to C3b and also dissociates C3b, Bb into C3b and Bb. The second control protein, Factor I (formerly referred to as C3b in activator), cleaves C3b that is bound to Factor H or to a similar protein found on the surface of the host cell. The resulting cleaved C3b, termed C3b, can no longer form a C3 convertase. The action of these two control proteins prevents the consumption of Factor B and C3 in plasma; in addition, these two proteins in activate C3b, Bb on host cell surfaces. In contrast, surfaces of many target cells, such as bacteria and other microorganisms, protect C3b, Bb from in activation by Factors H and I. This protection allows the positive feedback loop to proceed on the surface of the target cell, leading to the activation of the pathway and subsequent cell death. In other words, the alternative pathway is activated by those substances that prevent the inactivation of the positive feedback loop enzyme C3b, Bb. A substance is therefore treated as "foreign" if it restricts the action of Factors H and I and allows the positive feedback loop to continue.

The chemical structures on surfaces of particles and cells responsible for activation or non-activation of the alternative pathway have not been identified. There is some evidence that carbohydrate moieties are involved, particularly sialic acid. The alternative pathway protein(s) responsible for the recognition of these structures also remains to be determined. As pointed out earlier, the activation of the alternative pathway requires a C3b molecule bound to the surface of a target cell. An intriguing question is, "Where does the critical first cab molecule come from?". Although it can be provided by the C3 convertase of the classical pathway or by cleavage of C3 by plasmin and certain bacterial and other cellular proteases, the alternative pathway can generate this first C3b molecule without these proteases. The intramolecular thioester, which is highly reactive in nascent C3b and is responsible for the covalent attachment to targets, is also accessible in native C3 to water molecules. Thus, spontaneous hydrolysis of the thioester bond occurs constantly in plasma at a low rate. The C3 molecules in which the thioester bond has been hydrolyzed behave like C3b, although the C3a domain has not been removed. C3 with a hydrolyzed thioester is called C3 or C3b-like C3. It can bind Factor B and allow Factor D to activated Factor B, which results in formation of a fluid-phase C3 convertase, C3, Bb. This enzyme is continuously formed and produces C3b molecules that can randomly attach to cells. Although these C3b molecules will be rapidly inactivated on host cells by Factors H and I, they will start the positive feedback loop on foreign surfaces, as outlined previously. In other words, the alternative pathway is constantly activated at a low rate, but amplification with subsequent cell death occurs only on foreign particles [21].

With this consept, we tried to demonstrate visually by the immune-electrophoresis. The human serum was prepared after administrating *f-Black Turmeric* together with the sample with befor fermentation. Immuno-electrophoresis was setting up for 90 min, followed by incubating with anti-human whole serum and specific for C3 and Bf component. These specific anti-complement component serum were kindly supplied by Dr. Syunnosuke SAKAI, Cancer Research Institute of Kanazawa University, Japan.

### 4.3.2. Products of Complement Activation by FBT Possessing Biological Activity

Activation of either the alternative or the classical pathway results in the generation of many important peptides involved in inflammatory responses. The anaphylaxis increase of vascular permeability degranulation of mast cells and basophils with release of histamine Degranulation of eosinophils Aggregation of platelets opsonization of particles and solubilization of immune complexes with subsequent facilitation of phagocytosis Release of neutrophils from bone marrow resulting in leukocytosis Smooth muscle contraction Increase of vascular permeability Smooth muscle contraction Increase of vascular permeability Degranulation of mast cells and basophils with release of histamine Degranulation of eosinophils Aggregation of platelets Chemotaxis of basophils, eosinophils, neutrophils, and monocytes Release of hydrolytic enzymes from neutrophils Chemotaxis of neutrophils Release of hydrolytic enzymes from neutrophils Inhibition of migration and indulation of spreading of monocytes and anaphylatoxins C3a, C4a, and C5a are derived from the enzymatic cleavage of C3, C4, and C5 respectively. Historically, C3a and C5a were defined as factors derived from activated serum possessing spasmogenic activity. The anaphylatoxins are now recognized as having many additional biologic functions. Both C3a and C5a are known to induce the release of histamine from mast cells and basophils. As shown in the Figure anaphylatoxins cause smooth muscle contraction and induce the release of vasoactive amines, which cause an increase in vascular permeability.

The effect of C5a anaphylatoxin on neutrophils is of considerable importance in the inaammatory response. Not only can C5a induce neutrophil aggregation, but this anaphylatoxin appears to be the main chemotactic peptide generated by activation of either complement pathway. *In vitro*, nanomolar concentrations of C5a will induce the unidirectional movement of neutrophils. Other inflammatory cells, such as monocytes, eosinophils, basophils, and macrophages, have also been shown to exhibit a chemotactic response to C5a. The removal of the carboxy-terminal arginine from C5a by serum carboxy peptidase N, generating C5a-des-arg, inactivates the spasmogen, yet restoration of full chemotactic activity of C5a-des-are may occur in the presence of serum. Therefore, C5a-des-arg may also be responsible for *in vivo* neutrophil chemotactic activity.

As described earlier, the cleavage of C3 by either the alternative or the classical C3 convertases results in the production of two major split products, the C3a anaphylatoxin and cab. The larger C3b fragment can serve as an opsonin (promoter of phagocytosis) by binding to a target through the thioester mechanism. This renders the particle or cell immediately susceptible to ingestion by a variety of phagocytic cells that carry specific receptors for C3b.

Many recent observations point to additional roles for complement fragments in regulating the activity 9f cells of the immune system. These observations include the presence of receptors on lymphocytes for various complement proteins, including C3 split products and Factor H, affecting B- and T cell function. This is an important area for future research [21] (**Figure 5**).

## 5. Discussion

Our investigation clarified how hemopoitic formula, also known as tonic agent, influenced the immune system (e.g. leukocyte, granulocyte and lymphocyte subsets in particular).

We quantified CD positive cell counts as indicators of T cells, B cells, macrophages and NK cells. For qualitative and quantitative evaluation, we examined the cytokine expression levels, and directly measured the expression levels of cytokine-containing cells in peripheral blood, eliminating possible artificial factors that could arise from culturing in test tubes or changes in net value by catalyzation. To avoid any possible influence from the circadian rhythm, we obtained the whole blood from all donors at the same time.

In this investigation, we confirmed that FBT quantitatively and qualitatively regulated leukocytes, granulocytes, lymphocytes and their subsets. The increase of $CD2^+$, $CD4^+$, $CD8^+$, $CD11b^+$, $CD16^+$, $CD19^+$ and $CD56^+$ cell counts as well as the levels of IL-1$\beta$, IL-4 and IFN-$\gamma$ in blood cells suggested that hemopoitic formula might enhance the activities of humoral and cellular immunities, as well as NK cells. We also observed that levels of cytokine producing cells, in particular, increased rather than CD-positive lymphocytes, showing that FBT augmented lymphocyte production qualitatively than quantitatively. Moreover, FBT activated both CD11b cells and IL-1$\beta$ producing cells, suggesting the activation of phagocyte cells both in number and in function. Consequently, these data further demonstrated that FBT acted in macrophages in the same manner as *Mycobacterium tuberculosis* that had cell walls constructed of waxy substances which were famous for activating phagocytes in mammals [23]-[25].

In previous reports about hot-spring hydrotherapy and acupuncture, we had proposed that immune system regulation was an important factor for evaluating CAM. Since other substances, such as endotoxin and waxy substances from *Mycobacterium tuberculosis*, similar to Proplis, were known for augmenting host immune responses. This time, we decided to focus solely on Propolis. A possible explanation for immune enhancement could be the activation of the circular system and/or autonomic nervous system, although the details of the mechanism remained unclear. Further research regarding to the mechanism was necessary.

Abo *et al.* reported that granulocyte count was increased FBT. By the following conditions. the excitement of sympathetic nerve system directly regulated granulocytes in number and function,while lymphocyte count was regulated by parasympathetic nerve system [11] [26]-[29]. Our data also showed that granulocyte count was decreased in subjects with a high granulocyte count, while lymphocyte count was increased in the same subjects. The lymphocyte count, however, was decreased in subjects with a high lymphocyte level, while granulocyte count was

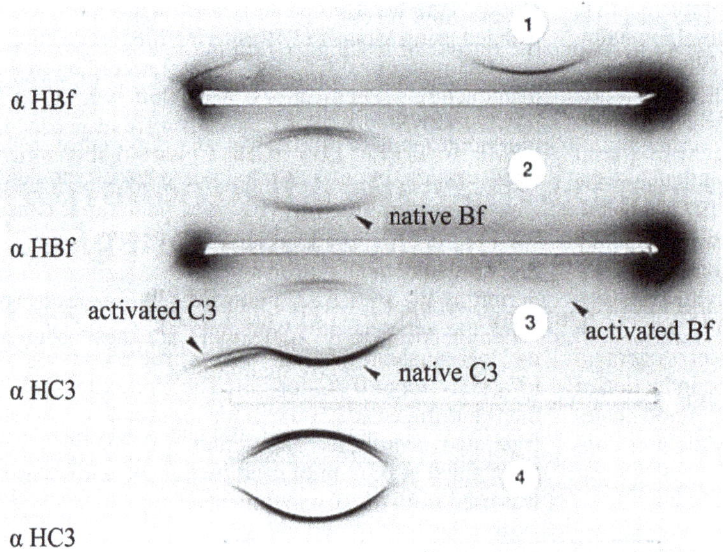


**Figure 5.** Immuno-electrophoretic demonstration of activated human complement components.

increased in the same subjects. In other words, the subjects dominated. The sympathetic nerve system could release stress, more over FBT could help these sympathetic neve system through the emotional hormones such as adrenalin and dopamine. The parasympathetic nerve might be excited by hemopoietic formula. This way, the cell counts appeared to converge at appropriate levels after hemopoietic formula. Finally, in order to determine whether the elevation of leukocyte counts resulted from an infection triggered by hemopoitic formula or not, the subjects were followed up for 8 days after the last administration of hemopoitic formula. During that period, we could not observe any infectious signs such as pyodermitis, fever, or enhancement of C-Reactive Protein (CRP). The value of CRP was 0.57 g/dl to 1.23 g/dl in our subjects, suggesting very mild inflammatory responses, which showed that hemopoitic formula did not cause infection. Since the meridian might influence cells throughout the body and might pass through every organ system, and hemopoitic formula stimulation might provide maximum benefits without side effects [30]-[35]. As an immunopotenciating agent, this FBT was an interesting material for regulate peripheral leukocyte number that suggesting one's constitution. FBT also regulated leukocyte subset, granulocyte and lymphocyte ratio concerning constitution, including QOL for all young to the senile.

## References


[1] Kitada, Y., Wan, W., Matsui, K., Matsui, K., Shimizu, S. and Yamaguchi, N. (2000) Regulation of Peripheral White Blood Cells in Numbers and Functions through Hot-Spring Bathing during a Short Term—Studies in Control Experiments. *Journal of Japanese Society Balneology Climatology Physiological Medicine*, **63**, 151-164.

[2] Yamaguchi, N., Takahashi, T., Sugita, T., Ichikawa, K., Sakaihara, S., Tsugiyasu Kanda, T., Arai, M. and Kawakita, K. (2007) Acupuncture Regulates Leukocyte Subpopulations in Human Peripheral Blood. *Evidence Based Complementary and Alternative Medicine*, **4** ,447-453

[3] Suzuki, S., Toyabe, S., Moroda, T., Tada, T., Tsukahara, A. and Iiai, T. (1997) Circadian Rhythm of Leukocytes and Lymphocytes Subsets and Its Possible Correlation with the Function of the Autonomic Nervous System. *Clinical Experimental Immunology*, **110**, 500-508.

[4] Yamaguchi, N., Kawada, N., Ja, X.-S., Okamoto, K., Okuzumi, K., Chen, R. and Takahashi, T. (2013) Overall Estimation of Anti-Oxidant Activity by Mammal Mammal Macrophage, *OJRA*, **4**, 13-21.

[5] Hamada, M. and Yamaguchi, N. (1988) Effect of Kanpo Medicine, Zyuzentaihoto, on the Immune Reactivity of Tumor-Bearing Mice. *Journal of Ethnopharmacology*, **24**, 311-320. http://dx.doi.org/10.1016/0378-8741(88)90160-2

[6] Tu, C.C., Li, C.S., Liu, C.M. and Liu, C.C. (2011) Comparative Use of Biomedicine and Chinese Medicine in Taiwan: Using the NHI Research Database. *Journal of Alternative and Complementary Medicine*, **17**, 339-346.

[7] Lin, M.H., Chou, M.Y., Liang, C.K., Peng, L.N. and Chen, L.K. (2010) Population Aging and Its Impacts: Strategies of the Health-Care System in Taipei. *Ageing Research Reviews*, **9**, S23-S27.

[8] Liao, H.L., Ma, T.C., Chiu, Y.L., Chen, J.T. and Chang, Y.S. (2008) Factors Influencing the Purchasing Behavior of TCM Outpatients in Taiwan. *Journal of Alternative and Complementary Medicine*, **14**, 741-748.

[9] Lin, Y.H. and Chiu, J.H. (2011) Use of Chinese Medicine by Women with Breast Cancer: A Nationwide Cross- Sectional Study in Taiwan. *Complementary Therapies in Medicine*, **19**, 137-143.

[10] Navo, M.A., Phan, J. and Vaughan, C. (2004) An Assessment of the Utilization of Complementary and Alternative Medication in Women with Gynecologic or Breast Malignancies. *Journal of Clinical Oncology*, **22**, 671-677.

[11] Liu, J.P., Yang, H., Xia, Y. and Cardini, F. (2009) Herbal Preparations for Uterine Fibroids. *Cochrane Database of Systematic Reviews*, **4**, Article ID: CD005292. http://dx.doi.org/10.1002/14651858.cd005292.pub2

[12] Murayama, T., Yamaguchi, N., Iwamoto, K. and Eizuru, Y. (2006) Inhibition of Ganciclovir-Resistant Human Cytomegalovirus Replication by Kampo (Japanese Herbal Medicine). *Antiviral Chemistry & Chemotherapy*, **17**, 11-16.

[13] Abo, T., Kawate, T., Itoh, K. and Kumagai, K. (1981) Studies on the Bioperiodicity of the Immune Response. 1. Circadian Rhythms of Human T, B and K Cell Traffic in the Peripheral Blood. *Journal of Immunology*, **126**, 1360-1363.

[14] Abo, T. and Kumagai, T. (1978) Studies of Surface Immunoglobulins on Human B Lymphocytes. Physiological Variations of Sig+ Cells in Peripheral Blood. *Clinical Experimental Immunology*, **33**, 441-452.

[15] Landmann, R.M.A., Muller, F.B., Perini, C., Wesp, M., Erne, P. and Buhler, F.R. (1984) Changes of Immunoregulatory Cells Induced by Psychological and Physical Stress: Relationship to Plasma Catecholamines. *Clinical Experimental Immunology*, **58**, 127-135.

[16] Iio, A., Ohguchi, K., Naruyama, H., Tazawa, S., Araki, Y., Ichihara, K., Nozawa, Y. and Ito, M. (2012) Ethanolic Extract of Brazilian Red Propolis ABC A1 Expression and Promote Cholesterol Efflux from THP-1 Macrophage. *Phytomedicine*, **19**, 383-388. http://dx.doi.org/10.1016/j.phymed.2011.10.007

[17] Kitada, Y., Okamoto, K., Takei, T., Jia, X.F., Chen, R., Yamaguchi, N., Tsubokawa, M., Wu, W.H., Murayama, T. and Kawakita, K. (2013) Hot Spring Hydro Therapy Regulate Peripheral Leukocyte Together with Emotional Hormone and Receptor Positive Lymphocytes According to Each Constitution/Condition. *Open Journal of Rheumatology and Autoimmune Diseases*, **3**, 140-153. http://dx.doi.org/10.4236/ojra.2013.33022

[18] Jerne, N.K. and Nordin, A.A. (1963) Plaque Formation in Agar by Single Antibody Producing Cells. *Science*, **140**, 405-408. http://dx.doi.org/10.1126/science.140.3565.405

[19] Jerne, N.K., Nordin, A.A. and Henry, C. (1963) The Agar Technique for Recognizing Antibody Producing Cells. In: Amons, B. and Kaprowski, H., Eds., *Cell-Bound Antibodies*, The Wistar Institute Press, Philadelphia, 109-125.

[20] Hamada, M. and Yamaguchi, N. (1988) Effect of Kanpo Medicine, Zyuzentaihoto, on the Immune Reactivity of Tumor-Bearing Mice. *Journal of Ethnopharmacology*, **24**, 311-320. http://dx.doi.org/10.1016/0378-8741(88)90160-2

[21] Shimizu, S., Kitada, H., Yokota, H., Yamakawa, J., Murayama, T., Sugiyama, K., Izumi, H. and Yamaguchi, N. (2002) Activation of the Alternative Complement Pathway by *Agaricus blazei* Murill. *Phytomedicine*, **9**, 536-545.

[22] Tu, C.C., Li, C.S., Liu, C.M. and Liu, C.C. (2011) Comparative Use of Biomedicine and Chinese Medicine in Taiwan: Using the NHI Research Database. *Journal of Alternative and Complementary Medicine*, **17**, 339-346. http://dx.doi.org/10.1089/acm.2010.0200

[23] Jong, M.S., Hwang, S.J., Chen, C., Chen, T.J., Chen, F.J. and Chen, F.P. (2010) Prescriptions of Chinese Herbal Medicine for Constipation under the National Health Insurance in Taiwan. *Journal of the Chinese Medical Association*, **73**, 375-383. http://dx.doi.org/10.1016/S1726-4901(10)70081-2

[24] Lin, Y.H. and Chiu, J.H. (2011) Use of Chinese Medicine by Women with Breast Cancer: A Nationwide Cross-Sectional Study in Taiwan. *Complementary Therapies in Medicine*, **19**, 137-143. http://dx.doi.org/10.1016/j.ctim.2011.04.001

[25] Yamaguchi, N., Ueyama, T., Amat, N., Yimit, D., Hoxur, P., Sakamoto, D., Katoh, Y., Watanabe, I. and Su, S.Y. (2015) Bi-Directional Regulation by Chinese Herbal Formulae to Host and Parasite for Multi-Drug Resistant *Staphylococcus aureus* in Humans and Rodents. *Open Journal of Immunology*, **5**, 18-32. http://dx.doi.org/10.4236/oji.2015.51003

[26] Jyumonji, N. and Fujii, Y. (1993) A New Assay for Delayed-Type Hypersensitivity *in Vitro* Detection FB, The Macrophage Migration by Boyden Chamber. *Journal of Kanazawa Medical University*, **18**, 198-203.

[27] Wan, W., Li, A.I., Izumi, H., Kawada, N., Arai, M., Takada, A., Taru, A., Hashimoto, H. and Yamaguchi, N. (2002) Effect of Acupuncture on Leukocyte and Lymphocyte Sub-Population in Human Peripheral Blood Qualitative Discussion. *The Journal of Japanese Association of Physical Medicine, Balneology and Climatology*, **65**, 207-211.

[28] Wang, X.X., Katoh, S. and Liu, B.X. (1998) Effect of Physical Exercise on Leukocyte and Lymphocyte Subpopulations in Human Peripheral Blood. *Cytometry Research*, **8**, 53-61.

[29] Kitada, Y., Wan, W., Matsui, K., Shimizu, S. and Yamaguchi, N. (2000) Regulation of Peripheral White Blood Cells in Numbers and Functions through Hot-Spring Bathing during a Short Term Studies in Control Experiments. *Journal of Japanese Society Balneology Climatology Physiological Medicine*, **63**, 151-164.

[30] Yamaguchi, N., Takahashi, T., Sugita, T., Ichikawa, K., Sakaihara, S., Kanda, T., Arai, M. and Kawakita, K. (2007) Acupuncture Regulates Leukocyte Subpopulations in Human Peripheral Blood. *eCAM*, **4**, 447-453.

[31] Yamaguchi, N., Shimizu, S. and Izumi, H. (2004) Hydrotherapy Can Modulate Peripheral Leukocytes: An Approach to Alternative Medicine, Complementary and Alternative Approaches to Biomedicine. Kluwer Academic/Plenum Publishers, New York, 239-251.

[32] Murayama, T., Yamaguchi, N., Matsuno, H. and Eizuru, Y. (2004) *In Vitro* Anti-Cytomegalovirus Activity of Kampo (Japanese Herbal) Medicine. *eCAM*, **1**, 285-289.

[33] Abe, S., Yamaguchi, N., Tansho, S. and Yamaguchi, H. (2005) Preventive Effects of Juzen-Taiho-to on Infectious Disease. Juzen-Taiho-to (Shi-Quan-Da-Bu-Tang) Scientific Evaluation and Clinical Applications: Traditional Herbal Medicines for Modern Times, Edited by Haruki Yamada, Ikuo Saiki.

[34] Yamaguchi, N., Ueyama, T., Amat, N., Yimit, D., Hoxur, P., Sakamoto, D., Katoh, Y., Watanabe, I. and Su, S.-Y. (2015) Bi-Directional Regulation by Chinese Herbal Formulae to Host and Parasite for Multi-Drug Resistant *Staphylococcus aureus* in Humans and Rodents. *Open Journal of Immunology*, **4**, 18-32.

[35] Yamaguchi, N., Araai, M. and Murayama, T. (2015) Aspect of QOL Assessment and Proposed New Scale for Evaluation. *Open Journal of Immunology*, **4**. (In Press)

## Abbreviations

CAM: Complementary and alternative medicine, beside the western medicine, there are many traditional medicine and/or health promoting menu all over the world.
CD: Cluster of differentiation. Each lymphocyte has name that expressed CD number, for example CD2, CD4, etc.
CBT: Conventional Black Turmeric before fermentation.
DM: Diabetes mellitus.
FBT: Fermented Black Turmeric, that had been depredated to micro fragment by Lactobacillus.
FCM: Flow Cytometry.
G-rich type: The individual that exhibit over 60% of granulocyte in peripheral blood, finding many in young gentleman.
L-rich type: The individual that exhibit over 40% of lymphocyte in peripheral blood, finding lot in ladies and senile.

# 10

# Functional Characterization of Porcine (*Sus scrofa*) BCL10

**Pellegrino Mazzone[1*], Ivan Scudiero[1*], Angela Ferravante[1], Marina Paolucci[2], Luca E. D'Andrea[1], Ettore Varricchio[2], Gianluca Telesio[1,3], Maddalena Pizzulo[1], Tiziana Zotti[1,2], Carla Reale[1], Pasquale Vito[1,2], Romania Stilo[1,2]**

[1]Laboratory of Immunogenetics, Biogem, Via Camporeale, Ariano Irpino, Italy
[2]Dipartimento di Scienze e Tecnologie, Università del Sannio, Benevento, Italy
[3]Dipartimento di Medicina molecolare Biotecnologie mediche, Università di Napoli "Federico II", Napoli, Italy
Email: vito@unisannio.it

## Abstract

**Human BCL10 (hBCL10) protein is a signal transduction molecule originally identified because of its direct involvement in a subset of mucosa-associated lymphoid tissue (MALT) lymphomas, and later recognized as a crucial factor in regulating activation of NF-kB transcription factor following antigen receptor stimulation on lymphocytes. In this study, we characterized the NF-kB inducing activity of porcine BCL10 (pBCL10). pBCL10 oligimerizes, binds to components of the CARMA/BCL10/MALT1 complex and forms cytoplasmic filaments. Functionally, in human cells pBCL10 is more effective in activating NF-kB compared to hBCL10, possibly due to the lack of carboxy-terminal inhibitory serine residues present in the human protein. Also, depletion experiments carried out through expression of short hairpin RNAs targeting hBCL10 indicate that pBcl10 can functionally replace the human protein and retains its higher NF-kB-inducing property in the absence of hBCL10. Our results contribute useful information on BCL10 protein in pigs, and may help the development of strategies based on the control of the immune response in pigs.**

## Keywords

**BCL10, CARMA, NF-kB, CARD**

## 1. Introduction

Human BCL10 (hBCL10) was originally identified because of its direct involvement in a subset of MALT B

[*]The first two authors contributed equally to this work.

cell lymphomas [1] [2]. As a result of the translocation t(1;14)(p22;q32), BCL10 is placed under the control of the immunoglobulin heavy chain enhancer, and is over expressed in these tumors [1] [2]. At the same time, BCL10 was identified in several other laboratories for the presence of a caspase recruitment domain (CARD) in its sequence [3]. Functionally, BCL10 regulates activation of NF-kB transcription factor, which transcribes genes that control both innate and acquired immune response and genes that play a positive effect on cell survival and proliferation [4] [5]. Genetic alteration of the BCL10 locus leads to immunodeficiency in mice, due to impaired NF-kB activation following antigen receptor stimulation in both T and B cells [6]. The biological activity of BCL10 is explicated through formation of the CBM complex, a molecular complex that comprises one of three members of the family of CARMA proteins and the protease MALT1 [7]. The three CARMA proteins constitute a family of proteins conserved across many species which are characterized by the presence of different functional domains shared by all members of the family [8]. Functionally, all three CARMA proteins are able to associate BCL10 through an homophilic interaction between the corresponding CARD domains, and to cooperate with it in inducing the transcriptional activity of NF-kB [8]. Thus, correct assembly of the CBM complex is an essential step in the NF-kB inducing pathway mediated by BCL10. Formation of this complex in fact triggers non-conventional ubiquitination events, which eventually result in recruitment and K63-linked ubiquitination of the noncatalytic IKKg/NEMO subunit of the I-kB kinase complex, responsible for NF-kB transcription factor activation [9]-[11].

Pork is the most highly consumed meat worldwide, and the related industry represents a crucial economical sector for many countries. Maintaining pork safety and minimizing production losses associated with diseases impacts profitability, food safety and animal health. As such, there is a major interest in characterizing aspects of the porcine immune response. A porcine homologue of hBCL10 was recently cloned [12]. pBCL10 mRNA is distributed in different tissue, and in cultured porcine cells its expression increases following treatments with lipopolysaccharide and polyriboinosinic-polyribocytidylic acid [12], two treatments that mimic bacteria and virus infections, respectively. In the present work, we have analyzed the NF-kB-inducing property of pBCL10.

## 2. Materials and Methods

### 2.1. RNA Extraction and Cloning of pBCL10 Full-Length cDNA

Spleen specimens were obtained from slaughtered Large White and Landrace hybrids F1 hybrids. Total RNA was extracted from the splenic tissue by using Trizol reagent as previously described [13], and 1 μg of total RNA was reverse-transcribed to generate a first-strand cDNA. The following primers were used to amplify pBCL10: forward 5'-ATGGAGCCCGCCGCGCC-3' and reverse 5'-TCATTGCCGCAAAAGAGCACG-3'. PCR conditions were as follows: 98˚C for 30 s, 30 cycles (98˚C/15s; 63˚C/22s; 72˚C/30s). The RT-PCR product of the expected size (702 bp, Genebank accession number FJ376731) was gel purified, cloned into HA- and FLAG-tagged expression vectors using standard methodologies and confirmed by sequencing.

### 2.2. Sequence Analysis

The BCL10 protein sequences were analyzed by using the BLAST algorithm at the NCBI web site (http://www.ncbi.nlm.nih.gov/blast).

### 2.3. Cell Culture and Transfection

HEK293 cells were obtained from ATCC and were maintained in Dulbecco's modified Eagle's medium (DMEM) supplemented with 10% FBS. The expression vectors used in transfection experiments for this study have been previously described [13]-[18]. DNA plasmids were transfected by standard calcium-phosphate method. Short hairpin RNAs targeting hBCL10 were the following: shBCL10 #3 5'-CCTTAAGATCACGTACTGTTTCTCGAGAAACAGTACGTGATCTTAAGG-3' and shBCL10 #5 5'-GTTGAATCTATTCGGCGAGAACTCGAGTTCTCGCCGAATAGATTCAAC-3' and have been already described [18]. Retroviral infections were carried out as previously described [19].

### 2.4. Immunoblot Analysis and Coprecipitation

Cell lysates were made in lysis buffer (150 mM NaCl, 20 mM Hepes, pH 7.4, 1% Triton X-100, 10% glycerol, and a mixture of protease inhibitors). Proteins were separated by SDS-PAGE, transferred onto nitrocellulose membrane, and incubated with primary antibodies followed by horseradish peroxidase-conjugated secondary antibodies (Amersham Biosciences, Piscataway, NJ). Blots were developed using the ECL system (Amersham Biosciences). For co-immunoprecipitation experiments, cells were lysed in lysis buffer and immune complexes were bound to protein A/G, resolved by SDS-PAGE, and analyzed by immunoblot assay. Sources of antisera and monoclonal antibodies were the following: anti-FLAG, anti-$\beta$-Actin, Sigma; anti-HA, anti-MALT1, anti-CARMA3 and anti-BCL10 (H-197 SC5611, generated against an epitope corresponding to amino acids 1-197 of human BCL10), Santa Cruz Biotechnology. The calf-intestinal alkaline phosphatase was purchased from Roche.

## 2.5. Luciferase Assay

To assess for NF-kB activation, HEK293 were transfected with plasmidic DNAs together with pNF-κB-luc (Clontech) in 6-well plates. After transfection and treatments, luciferase activity was determined with Luciferase Assay System (Promega). A plasmids expressing $\beta$-galactosidase was added to the transfection mixture in order to normalize for the efficiency of transfection.

## 2.6. Immunofluorescence

$1 \times 10^4$ HEK293 were grown and transfected in chamber slides. Sixteen hours after transfection, cells were fixed in 4% paraformaldehyde for 15 min at room temperature and then permeabilized in PBS/0.1% Triton X-100. Cells were incubated for 30 min in 5% FCS-PBS with anti-FLAG antibody (Sigma-Aldrich) followed by several washes with 5% FCS-PBS, and then incubating for 30 min with secondary antibody in 5% FCS-PBS. All steps were done at room temperature.

## 3. Results and Discussion

A cDNA corresponding to the porcine homologue of hBCL10 was successfully amplified by RT-PCR from porcine spleen tissue. Sequence analysis revealed that it corresponds to the sequence already deposited in Genebank with the accession number FJ376731 [12]. Both human and porcine BCL10 proteins consist of 233 amino acidic residues, only 17 of which are dissimilar (**Figure 1**).

Amino acidic differences are mainly distributed in the carboxy terminal portion of the protein, emphasizing the conservation of the card domain (aa 6 - 108), which is in fact perfectly conserved between the two species. Interestingly, some amino acidic substitutions concern serine residues present in the human protein, particularly S134 and S231, which in pBCL10 are replaced by a proline and leucine residue, respectively. This aspect is par-

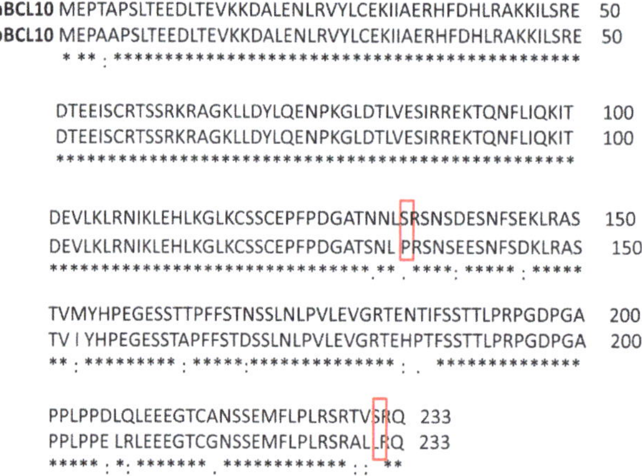


**Figure 1.** (*Alignment of human and porcine BCL*10) Alignment of hBCL10 (Gene Bank NP_003912) and pBCL10 (Gene Bank FJ-376731). Identical residues are indicated by stars, conservative and semi-conservative substitutions are indicated by double dot and single dot, respectively. Colored rectangles indicate serine residues which are not present in pBCL10.

ticularly important, because hBCL10 phosphorylation on serine residues, including S134, were shown to negatively regulate hBCL10-induced NF-kB activation [20].

When analyzed in immunoblot assay, pBCL10 expressed in mammalian cells migrates as a 37 kDa protein (**Figure 2(a)**), and is recognizes by a rabbit antisera raised against hBCL10 (**Figure 2(a)**, right panel). Similarly to hBCL10 [21] [22], pBCL10 migrates as a doublet on SDS-PAGE due to phosphorylation of the protein. In fact, the pBCL10 doublet resolves in a single band when cell lysates were treated with phosphatase prior to immunoblot analysis (**Figure 2(b)**).

BCL10 plays a crucial role in the signal transduction pathway that leads to activation of the transcription factor NF-kB [6] [7]. hBCL10-mediated activation of NF-kB requires oligomerization of hBCL10, assembly of the CBM complex and triggering of unconventional ubiquitination events, which eventually result in the recruitment of the IKK complex [7] [9]-[11]. Indeed, transfection experiments indicate that pBCL10 oligomerizes both with itself and with hBCL10 (**Figures 3(a)-(b)**). Furthermore, pBCL10 associates with human MALT1 (**Figure 3(c)**), with human CARMA2*sh* [14] (**Figure 3(d)**) and with human CARMA3 (**Figure 3(e)**).

Fluorescence microscopy experiments and structural studies have shown that the NF-kB-activity produced by hBCL10 is regulated through formation of cytosolic filamentous structures [23] [24]. We therefore verified whether also pBCL10 is able to form such structures. As shown in **Figure 4**, assembly of filamentous structures is readily visible following expression of pBCL10 in mammalian cells.

Next, we tested the NF-kB-inducing activity of pBCL10 using a luciferase-based reporter assay. The results of these experiments, shown in **Figure 5(a)**, indicate that pBCL10 is even more effective than hBCL10 in activating NF-kB in mammalian cells. In fact, while expression of hBCL10 produces a luciferase activity about 8-10-fold higher compared to the empty vector, the luciferase activity produced by pBCL10 expression was at least 4-fold higher than that produced by hBCL10. As for hBCL10 [11] [25] [26], pBCL10-induced NF-kB activation requires ubiquitination(s) events, since NF-kB activation is completely abrogated following co-expression of A20 de-ubiquitinase (**Figure 5(b)**).

To exclude the possibility that the higher NF-kB activation mediated by pBCL10 was due to its interaction and subsequent oligomerization of hBCL10, we abolished expression of hBCL10 in the human cell line HEK293 through retrovirus-mediated expression of short hairpin RNAs (shRNA) targeting hBCL10. As shown in **Figure 5(c)**, introduction of hBCL10sh#3 and hBCL10sh#5 in HEK293 cells results in a great reduction of hBCL10 expression. In fact, depletion of hBCL10 in these cells abrogates their ability to activate NF-kB following exposure to phorbol-12-myristate-13-acetate (PMA) (**Figure 5(c)**). However, introduction of pBCL10 in these hBCL10-depleted cells fully recovers their ability to activate NF-kB (**Figure 5(d)**). Thus, pBCL10 retains its higher NF-kB-inducing property even in the absence of hBCL10.

In recent years, there has been growing interest in the porcine immune system due to its potential as a model for the human immune system and because of the economic importance of pigs as livestock. Although great advances have been achieved in the field of porcine immunology, there are still some important issues that require more research and development. In the work here presented, we have analyzed the NF-kB-inducing property of

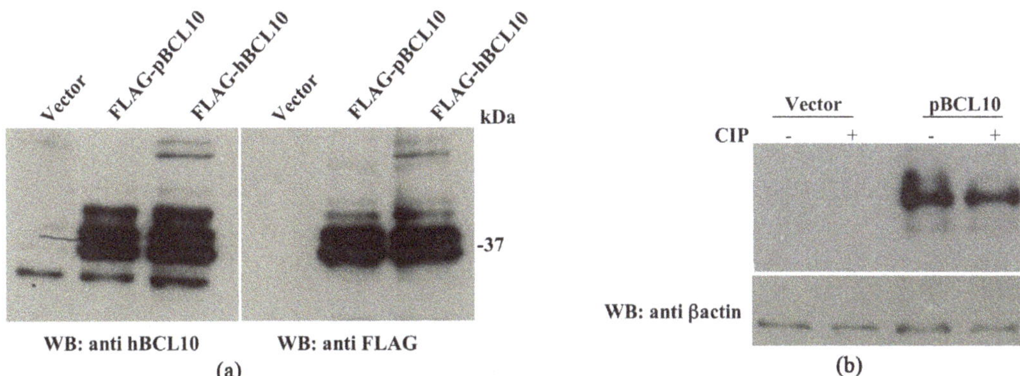


**Figure 2.** pBCL10 expression. (a)-(b) Immunoblot analysis of lysates from HEK293 cells transfected with the indicated expression vectors. Were indicated, prior to SDS-PAGE separation cell lysates were treated with 10 units of calf intestinal phosphatase (CIP) for 30 min at 37˚C.

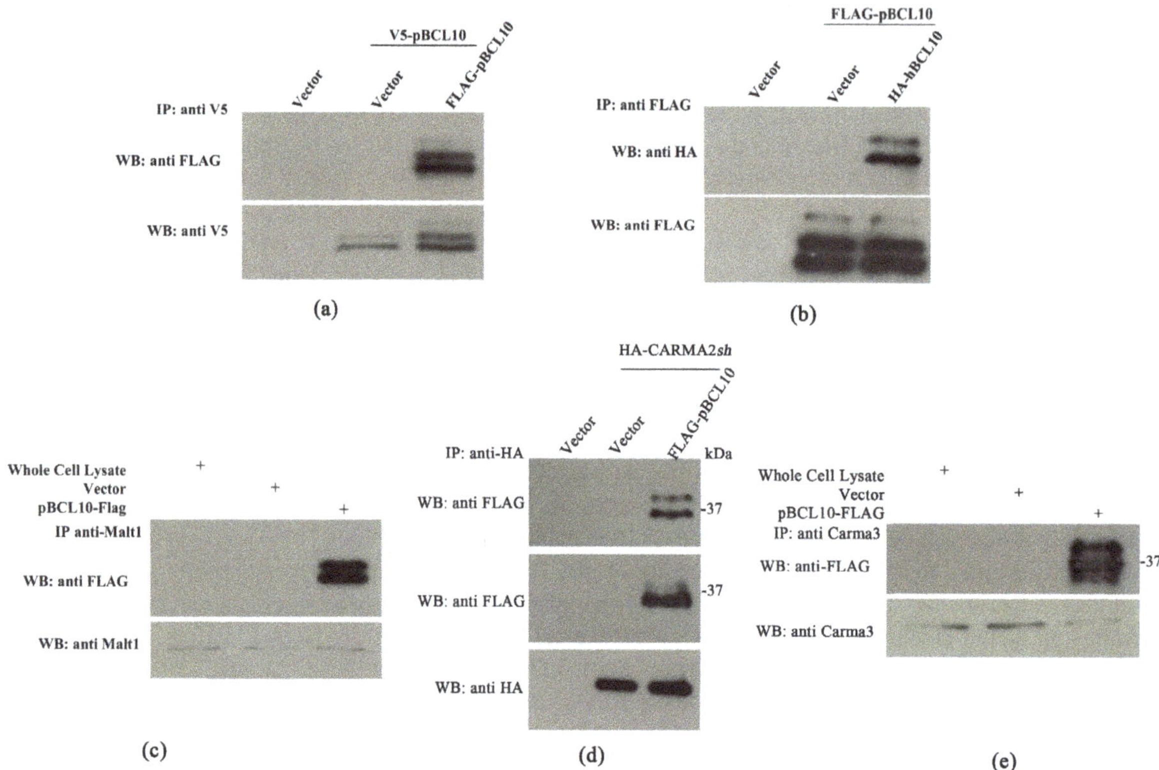


**Figure 3.** *pBCL10 olimerizes and binds to CBM proteins.* (a) HEK293 cells were transiently cotransfected with tagged versions of pBCL10 and hBCL10. 24 hrs later, cell lysates were prepared and immunoprecipitated with the indicated anti-tag mAb. Immuno complexes were separated by SDS-PAGE and transferred onto membranes subsequently assayed for associated (a) pBCL10; (b) hBCL10); (c) Malt1; (d) CARMA2*sh* and (e) CARMA3.

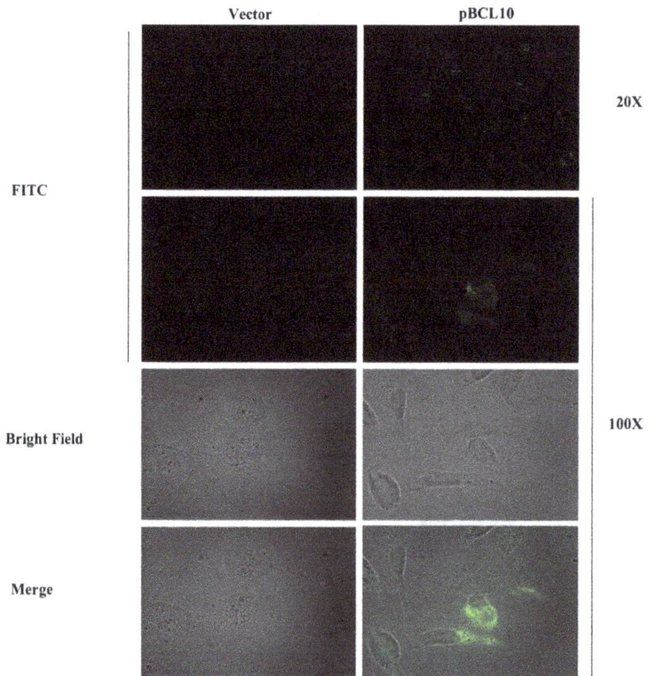


**Figure 4.** *Subcellular localization of pBCL10.* HEK-293 cells were transfected with mammalian FLAG-tagged vector, empty (vector) or expressing pBCL10. 16 hrs after transfection, cells were stained with anti-FLAG mAb, followed by FITC-conjugated anti-mouse IgG.

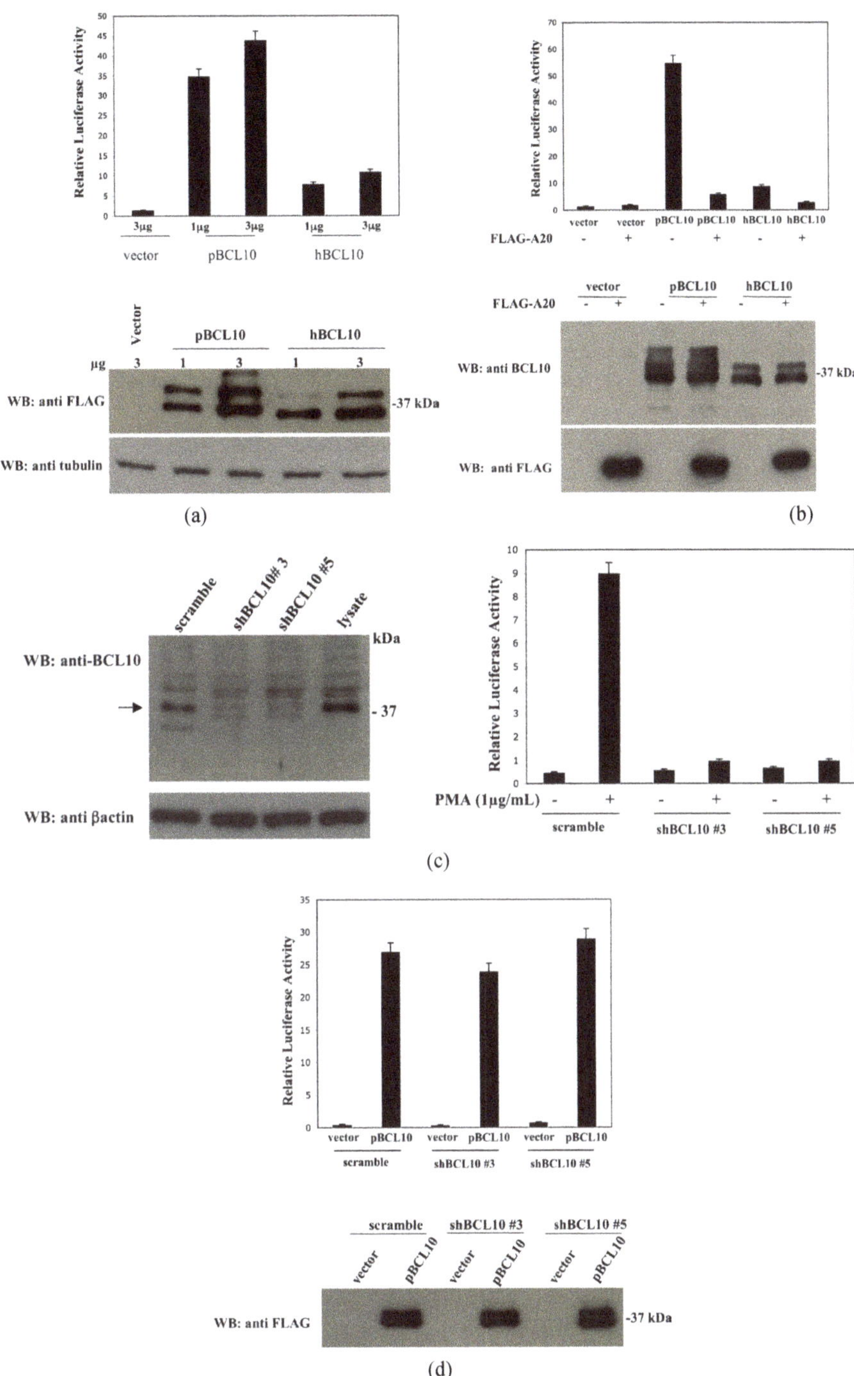

**Figure 5.** pBCL10 activates NF-κB (a)-(b) HEK293 cells were transiently cotransfected with expression vectors encoding for the indicated polypeptides, together with pNF-κB-luc and pRSV-$\beta$gal reporter vectors. The total amount of transfected plasmidic DNA was maintained constant by adding empty vector. 16 hrs after transfection, cell lysates were prepared and luciferase activity was measured. A fraction of the cell lystes were analyzed by immunoblot to monitor protein expression, shown in the lower panels. Data shown represents relative luciferase activity normalized on $\beta$-galactosidase activity and is representative of six independent experiments done in triplicate. (c) *Left panel* Cell lysates from HEK293 cells infected with retroviruses encoding for shRNAs targeting hBCL10 were monitored for hBCL10 expression by immunoblot assay; *Right panel* NF-κB-driven luciferase activity in HEK-293 cells silenced for hBCL10 and stimulated with PMA. (d) NF-κB-driven luciferase activity in HEK-293 cells silenced for hBCL10 and transfected with tBCL10. Data shown represent relative luciferase activity normalized on $\beta$-galactosidase activity and is representative of six independent experiments done in triplicate. A fraction of the cell lysates was analyzed by immunoblot to monitor protein expression.

pBCL10. We found that pBCL10 owns an higher NF-kB-inducing activity compared to the human protein, possibly because it lacks serine residues with inhibitory function present in hBCL10.

Given the importance of this transcription factor in regulating both normal immune response and autoimmune, immunoproliferative and tumoral disorders, and also considering the economic value of this organism, our results may benefit the development of strategies based on the control of the immune response in pigs.

## References


[1] Willis, T.G., Jadayel, D.M., Du, M.Q., Peng, H., Perry, A.R., *et al.* (1999) Bcl10 is Involved in t(1;14)(p22;q32) of MALT B Cell Lymphomas and Mutated in Multiple Tumor Types. *Cell*, **96**, 35-45 http://dx.doi.org/10.1016/S0092-8674(00)80957-5

[2] Zhang, Q., Siebert, R., Yan, M., Hinzmann, B., Cui, X., *et al.* (1999) Inactivating Mutation and BCL10, a Caspase Recruitment Domain-Containing Gene, in MALT Lymphoma with t(1;14)(p22;q32). *Nature Genetics* **22**, 63-68. http://dx.doi.org/10.1038/8767

[3] Vito, P. and Stilo, R. (2014) Fifteen Years of BCL10. *Immunology Letters*, **160**, 102-103. http://dx.doi.org/10.1016/j.imlet.2014.02.002

[4] Oeckinghaus, A., Hayden, M.S. and Ghosh, S. (2011) Crosstalk in NF-kappaB Signaling Pathways. *Nature Immunology*, **12**, 695-708. http://dx.doi.org/10.1038/ni.2065

[5] Vallabhapurapu, S. and Karin, M. (2009) Regulation and Function of NF-kappaB Transcription Factors in the Imune System. *Annual Review of Immunology*, **27**, 693-733.http://dx.doi.org/10.1146/annurev.immunol.021908.132641

[6] Ruland, J., Duncan, G.S., Elia, A., del Barco Barrantes, I., Nguyen, L., *et al.* (2001) Bcl10 is a Positive Regulator of Antigen Receptor-Induced Activation of NF-kappaB and Neural Tube Closure. *Cell*, **104**, 33-42. http://dx.doi.org/10.1016/S0092-8674(01)00189-1

[7] Thome, M., Charton, J.E., Pelzer, C. and Hailfinger, S. (2012) Antigen Receptor Signaling to NF-kB via CARMA1, BCL10, and MALT1. Cold Spring Harbor Perspectives in Biology, **2**, Article ID: a003004. http://dx.doi.org/10.1101/cshperspect.a003004

[8] Scudiero, I., Vito, P. and Stilo, R. (2014) The Three CARMA Sisters: So Different, So Similar. A Portrait of the Three CARMA Proteins and Their Involvement in Human Disorders. *Journal of Cellular Physiology*, **229**, 990-997. http://dx.doi.org/10.1002/jcp.24543

[9] Stilo, R., Liguoro, D., Di Jeso, B., *et al.* (2004) Physical and Functional Interaction of CARMA1 and CARMA3 with Ikappa Kinase Gamma-NF-kappaB Essential Modulator. *Journal of Biological Chemistry*, **279**, 34323-34331. http://dx.doi.org/10.1074/jbc.M402244200

[10] Sun, L., Deng, L., Ea, C.K., Xia, Z.P. and Chen, Z.J. (2004) The TRAF6 Ubiquitin Ligase and TAK1 Kinase Mediate IKK Activation by BCL10 and MALT1 in T lymphocytes. *Molecular Cell*, **14**, 289-301. http://dx.doi.org/10.1016/S1097-2765(04)00236-9

[11] Zhou, H.L., Wertz, I., O'Rourke, K., Ultsch, M., Seshagiri, S., *et al.* (2004) Bcl10 Activates the NF-κB Pathway through Ubiquitination of NEMO. *Nature*, **427**, 167-171. http://dx.doi.org/10.1038/nature02273

[12] Huang, J., Ma, G.-J., Sun, N.N., Wu, Z.F., Li X.Y. and Zhao, S.H. (2010) BCL10 as a New Candidate Gene for Immune Response in Pigs: Cloning, Expression and Association Analysis. *International Journal of Immunogenetics*, **37**, 103-110. http://dx.doi.org/10.1111/j.1744-313X.2010.00898.x

[13] Mazzone, P., Scudiero, I., Coccia, E., Ferravante, A., Paolucci, M., *et al.* (2015) Functional Characterization of a BCL10 Isoform in the Rainbow Trout *Oncorhynchus mykiss*. *FEBS Open Bio*, **5**, 175-181. http://dx.doi.org/10.1016/j.fob.2015.01.007

[14] Scudiero, I., Zotti, T., Ferravante, A., Vessichelli, M., Vito, P., *et al.* (2011) Alternative Splicing of CARMA2/CARD14 Transcripts Generates Protein Variants with Differential Effect on NF-κB Activation and Endoplasmic Reticulum Stress-Induced Cell Death. *Journal of Cellular Physiology*, **226**, 3121-3131. http://dx.doi.org/10.1002/jcp.22667

[15] Zotti, T., Uva, A., Ferravante, A., Vessichelli, M., Scudiero, I., *et al.* (2011) TRAF7 Protein Promotes Lys-29-Linked Polyubiquitination of IκB Kinase (IKKγ)/NF-κB Essential Modulator (NEMO) and p65/RelA Protein and Represses NF-κB Activation. *Journal of Biological Chemistry*, **286**, 22924-22933. http://dx.doi.org/10.1074/jbc.M110.215426

[16] Scudiero, I., Zotti, T., Ferravante, A., Vessichelli, M., Reale, C., *et al.* (2012) Tumor Necrosis Factor (TNF) Receptor-Associated Factor 7 Is Required for TNFα-Induced Jun NH2-Terminal Kinase Activation and Promotes Cell Death by Regulating Polyubiquitination and Lysosomal Degradation of c-FLIP Protein. *Journal of Biological Chemistry*, **287**, 6053-6061. http://dx.doi.org/10.1074/jbc.M111.300137

[17] Stilo, R., Liguoro, D., di Jeso, B., Leonardi, A. and Vito, P. (2003) The Alpha-Chain of the Nascent Polypeptide-Asso-

ciated Complex Binds to and Regulates FADD Function. *Biochemical and Biophysical Research Communications*, **303**, 1034-1041. http://dx.doi.org/10.1016/S0006-291X(03)00487-X

[18] Costanzo, A., Guet, C. and Vito, P. (1999) c-E10 Is a Caspase-Recruiting Domain-Containing Protein That Interacts with Components of Death Receptors Signaling Pathway and Activates Nuclear Factor-κB. *Journal of Biological Chemistry*, **274**, 20127-20132. http://dx.doi.org/10.1074/jbc.274.29.20127

[19] Guiet, C., Silvestri, E., De Smaele, E., Franzoso, G. and Vito, P. (2002) c-FLIP Efficiently Rescues TRAF-$2^{-/-}$ Cells from TNF-Induced Apoptosis. *Cell Death & Differentiation*, **9**, 138-144. http://dx.doi.org/10.1038/sj.cdd.4400947

[20] Wegener, E., Oeckinghaus, A., Papadopoulou, N., Lavitas, L., Schmidt-Supprian, M., *et al.* (2006) Essential Role for IκB Kinase Beta in Remodeling Carma1-Bcl10-Malt1 Complexes upon T Cell Activation. *Molecular Cell*, **23**, 13-23. http://dx.doi.org/10.1016/j.molcel.2006.05.027

[21] Yoneda, T., Imaizumi, K., Maeda, M., Yui, D., Manabe, T., *et al.* (2000) Regulatory Mechanisms of TRAF2-Mediated Signal Transduction by Bcl10, a MALT Lymphoma-Associated Protein. *Journal of Biological Chemistry*, **275**, 11114-11120. http://dx.doi.org/10.1074/jbc.275.15.11114

[22] Gaide, O., Martinon, F., Micheau, O., Bonnet, D., Thome, M., *et al.* (2001) Carmal, a CARD-Containing Binding Partner of Bcl10, Induces Bcl10 Phosphorylation and NF-κB Activation. *FEBS Letters*, **496**, 121-127. http://dx.doi.org/10.1016/S0014-5793(01)02414-0

[23] Qiao, Q., Yang, C.H., Zheng, C., Fontán, L., David, L., *et al.* (2013) Structural Architecture of the CARMA1/Bcl10/ MALT1 Signalosome: Nucleation Induced Filamentous Assembly. *Molecular Cell*, **51**, 766-779. http://dx.doi.org/10.1016/j.molcel.2013.08.032

[24] Guiet, C. and Vito, P. (2000) Caspase Recruitment Domain (CARD)-Dependent Cytoplasmic Filaments Mediate bcl10-Induced NF-kappaB Activation. *The Journal of Cell Biology*, **148**, 1131-40. http://dx.doi.org/10.1083/jcb.148.6.1131

[25] Stilo, R., Liguoro, D., Di Jeso, B., Baens, M., Kloo, B., *et al.* (2004) Physical and Functional Interaction of $CARMA_1$ and $CARMA_3$ with Iκ Kinase Gamma-NF-κB Essential Modulator. *Journal of Biological Chemistry*, **279**, 34323-34331. http://dx.doi.org/10.1074/jbc.M402244200

[26] Düwel, M., Welteke, V., Oeckinghaus, A., Baens, M., Kloo, B., *et al.* (2009) A20 Negatively Regulates T Cell Receptor Signaling to NF-κB by Cleaving Malt1 Ubiquitin Chains. *Journal of Immunology*, **182**, 7718-7728. http://dx.doi.org/10.4049/jimmunol.0803313

# 11

# B Cells with Regulatory Function in Animal Models of Autoimmune and Non-Autoimmune Diseases

**Mei Lin[1,2], Zuomin Wang[2*], Xiaozhe Han[1*]**

[1]Department of Immunology and Infectious Diseases, The Forsyth Institute, Cambridge, USA
[2]Department of Stomatology, Beijing Chao-Yang Hospital, Capital Medical University, Beijing, China
Email: *wzuomin@gmail.com, *xhan@forsyth.org

## Abstract

**Although the identification of B cell subsets with negative regulatory functions and the definition of their mechanisms of action are recent events, the important negative regulatory roles of B cells in immune responses are now broadly recognized. There is an emerging appreciation for the pivotal role played by B cells in several areas of human diseases including autoimmune diseases and non-autoimmune diseases such as parasite infections and cancer. The recent research advancement of regulatory B cells in human disease coincides with the vastly accelerated pace of research on the bridging of innate and adaptive immune system. Current study and our continued research may provide better understanding of the mechanisms that promote regulatory B10 cell function to counteract exaggerated immune activation in autoimmune as well as non-autoimmune conditions. This review is focused on the current knowledge of BREG functions studied in animal models of autoimmune and non-autoimmune diseases.**

## Keywords

**Bregs, Animal Models, IL-10, Autoimmune Disease, Immune Regulation**

## 1. Introduction

Historically, B cells have been characterized as positive regulators of humoral immune responses and are distinguished by their ability to terminally differentiate into antibody (Ab)-secreting plasma cells [1] [2] or serve as antigen (Ag)-presenting cells (APCs), for optimal Ag-specific $CD4^+$ T-cell expansion, memory formation, cytokine production [3]-[5] and positively regulate $CD8^+$ T-cell responses by expression of co-stimulatory molecules

*Corresponding authors.

[6]-[8].

Evidence for B-cell negative regulatory function has accumulated over the past 30 years. The hypothesis that suppressor or regulatory B (Bregs) cells orchestrate the immune system was originally proposed in the 1970s and maintains that the suppressive function of B cells was mainly restricted to their ability to produce "inhibitory" antibodies [9]. These initial findings were later followed by a flurry of seminal papers supporting a "suppressive framework" for B cells and a link with T-cell tolerance [10]-[13]. Later studies showed that a B-cell-restricted IL-10 deficiency had a similar exacerbating effect on EAE [14] [15] and rheumatoid arthritis [16], suggesting that activated B cells exerted regulatory activity that resolved the inflammation. From this, this term "regulatory B cell" was coined.

More recently, a relatively rare negative regulatory B-cell subset was identified that was predominantly contained within a phenotypically unique $CD1d^{hi}CD5^{+}CD19^{hi}$ subset in the spleens of naive wild-type mice [17]. This regulatory B-cell subset is Ag-specific and significantly influences T-cell activation and inflammatory responses through IL-10 production [17] [18]. Given that multiple regulatory B cell subsets are likely to exist, as now recognized for T cells, it has been specifically labeled this IL-10 competent $CD1d^{hi}CD5^{+}CD19^{hi}$ regulatory subset as B10 cells because they are responsible for most IL-10 production by B cells and they appear to only produce IL-10 [19].

Recently, many studies have used animal models of human diseases to demonstrate that B cells have regulatory functions *in vivo*, and most of them use B-cell-deficient μMT mice or the adoptive transfer of bulk B cells. In addition, multiple groups have identified IL-10-producing regulatory B cells of varying phenotypes in different disease models following diverse stimulation and culture protocols [14]-[16] [20]-[27].

## 2. Bregs in Autoimmune Diseases

### 2.1. Experimental Autoimmune Encephalomyelitis

B cells play a dual role in experimental autoimmune encephalomyelitis (EAE), which is the animal model of the human autoimmune disease multiple sclerosis (MS). The first one is contributing to the pathogenesis of EAE through the production of anti-myelin antibodies that contribute to demyelination. The other one is playing an essential role in the spontaneous recovery from EAE.

In 1996, Wolf found that B cells were not required for the onset of EAE, revealed that μMT mice failed to spontaneously recover from EAE [28]. This was the first indication in animal autoimmune models that B cells play a regulatory role in down-regulating inflammation. While in the later study, C57BL/6μMT mice were either not able to recover from EAE when an EAE induction protocol that allowed for recovery from EAE was used, which indicating that B cell production of IL-10 and expression of CD40 were requirements for their regulatory activity [14].

In regards to TLR signaling TLR2/4 ligands are present in the CFA adjuvant not only used to induce EAE but also induce the production of IL-10 by B cells [29]. Thereby, IL-10-producing regulatory B cells, most likely B10 cells, are important for controlling EAE severity and resolution. More specifically, Myd88 expression by B cells was required for recovery from EAE in MOG-peptide EAE [29].

The Tedder laboratory studied that both genetic disruption of CD19 and the transfer of $CD19^{-/-}$ B cells from MOG peptide-primed mice exacerbated EAE which demonstrated that signaling was important for regulatory B cell functions [30]. They analysed $CD19^{-/-}$ and human CD19 transgenic (hCD19tg) mice, with the later harboring hyperactive B cells, indicating that $CD19^{-/-}$ mice exhibit enhanced T cell-mediated inflammation (contact hypersensitivity (CHS)), and inflammation in hCD19tg mice was reduced [17].

The B cell regulatory effects were recently shown not to be IL-10 dependent [31]. On the contrary, the Tedder laboratory showed that the adoptive transfer of $CD1d^{hi}CD5^{+}$B cells from $CD19^{-/-}$ mice or from MOG-sensitized animals prior to EAE induction by MOG peptide attenuated EAE disease severity. Meanwhile, B cells from $IL\text{-}10^{-/-}$ mice did not reduce disease severity, indicating an IL-10-dependent mechanism [1]. B cell depletion therapy in early MS clinical trials with anti-CD20 showed remarkable efficacy in preventing disease progression [32] [33]. However, much still needs to be learned regarding how each B cell function can harnessed to either prevent or induce the recovery from MS.

### 2.2. Type 1 Diabetes

Studies on B10 cells and mouse models of diabetes are limited to the nonobese diabetic (NOD) mouse, a spontaneous model of type 1 diabetes in which autoimmune destruction of the insulin-producing pancreatic $\beta$ cells is primarily T cell mediated [34].

Although B cells play the pathogenic role in T1D initiation [35], B cells activated *in vitro* can maintain tolerance and transfer protection from T1D in NOD mice, both delay the onset and reduces the incidence of T1D. Protection from T1D is IL-10 dependent since the transfusion of activated NOD-IL-$10^{-/-}$ B cells does not confer protection from T1D or the severe insulitis observed in NOD recipients [36] [37]. In another study, LPS-activated B cells were transferred into prediabetic NOD mice and found that Fas ligand and secreted transforming growth factor-$\beta$ were upregulated, which were considered to contribute to inhibit autoimmunity [37].

Although the animal studies in TID have shed some light on the limitation of the rarity of circulating B10 cells, the possibility of therapeutic transfusion of autologous, IL-10-producing, BCR-activated B cells or B10 cells in order to protect human subjects at risk for T1D remains elusive.

## 2.3. Arthritis

CIA is a model for human rheumatoid arthritis that develops in susceptible mouse strains immunized with heterologous type II collagen emulsified in complete Freund's adjuvant [38] [39], which shares in common with rheumatoid arthritis having an association with a limited number of MHC-II haplotypes that determine disease susceptibility [40] [41].

B cells are important for initiating inflammation and arthritis [42]. By contrast, IL-10-producing B-cell subsets regulate inflammation during CIA. Activation of arthritogenic splenocytes with Ag and agonistic anti-CD40 mAb induces a B cell population that produces high levels of IL-10 and low levels of IFN$\gamma$ [16]. Specifically, multiple studies have tested whether the adoptive transfer of activated B cells could inhibit CIA. Mauri's lab injected CD40 mAb and collagen-activated B cells from the spleens of arthritogenic mice into recipient mice, observed that arthritis incidence (>50% reduction), disease severity (>90%), and Th1 cell differentiation are inhibited. Moreover, adoptive transfer of B cells also partially inhibits arthritis incidence and severity, even after disease initiation. However, the adoptive transfer of IL-$10^{-/-}$ B cells does not prevent arthritis in this model system [16]. Evans has tested the adoptive transfer of B cells into mice immunized with bovine collagen (type II collagen) inhibits TH1 responses, prevents arthritis development, and is effective in ameliorating established disease, while the adoptive transfer of $CD21^{hi}CD23^{+}IgM^{+}$ B cells from DBA/1 mice in the remission phase could prevents CIA and reduces disease severity through IL-10 secretion [22]; Gu also found a substantial reduction in the number of $T_{H17}$ cells [43]. Other studies administered apoptotic thymocytes to mice up to 1 month before the clinical onset of CIA is also protective for severe joint inflammation and bone destruction [23].

Collectively, activated spleen B cells responded directly to apoptotic cell treatment, increasing secretion of IL-10, which is important for inducing T-cell-derived IL-10. Moreover, the passive transfer of B cells from apoptotic cell-treated mice provided significant protection from arthritis.

## 2.4. Systemic Lupus Erythematosus

Studies in the NZB/W spontaneous lupus model therefore suggest that B10 cells have protective and potentially therapeutic effects. In wild type NZB/W mice, the $CD1d^{hi}CD5^{+}B220^{+}$ B cell subset, which is enriched in B10 cells, is increased 2.5-fold during the disease course, whereas $CD19^{-/-}$ NZB/W mice lack this $CD1d^{hi}CD5^{+}$ regulatory B cell subset [44]. Mature B cell depletion initiated in NZB/W F1 mice, hastens disease onset, which parallels depletion of B10 cells, suggesting that B cell-negative regulatory effects are important in NZB/ W mice [45]. Moreover, the potential therapeutic effect of B10 cells in lupus is highlighted by the prolonged survival of $CD19^{-/-}$ NZB/W recipients following the adoptive transfer of splenic $CD1d^{hi}CD5^{+}$ B cells from wildtype NZB/W mice [44]. However, in the MRL.Fas(lpr) mouse lupus model, B cell-derived IL-10 does not regulate spontaneous autoimmunity [46]. The study suggests fundamental differences in the pathogenesis and immune dysregulation in the NZB/W lupus model compared with the MRL.Fas(lpr) model.

## 2.5. Inflammatory Bowel Disease

Early studies showed that B cells and their autoantibody products suppress colitis in T cell receptor alpha chain-deficient mice that spontaneously develop chronic colitis, while B cells are not required for disease initiation [47].

Mizoguchi's group has subsequently demonstrated that B cells are the regulatory mediators and were the first to identify a B-cell subset with up regulated CD1d expression that is induced in the gut-associated lymphoid tissues of mice with intestinal inflammation, and they also suggested IL-10-producing B-cell subsets with varying phenotypes and origins regulate intestinal inflammation during inflammatory bowel disease [15] [48].

Dextran sulfate sodium-induced intestinal injury is more severe in $CD19^{-/-}$ mice where B10 cells are absent than in wild type mice [49], suggesting these inflammatory responses are negatively regulated by $CD1d^{hi}CD5^{+}$ B cells producing IL-10. Moreover the other study observed the adoptive transfer of mesenteric lymph node B cells also suppresses inflammatory bowel disease through a mechanism that correlates with an increase in regulatory T-cell subsets [50]. Thus, cytokine-producing B cells can regulate immune-mediated gut inflammation. B10 cells therefore emerge during chronic inflammation in mouse models of inflammatory bowel disease, where they suppress the progression of inflammatory responses and ameliorate disease manifestations.

## 3. Bregs in Parasitic Infection

The first clue for an anti-inflammatory role of Bregs in infections with parasites came from a study demonstrating a regulatory role of B cells during *Schistosoma mansoni* worm plus egg infection. Infection of μMT mice led to an enlargement of hepatic granuloma and a decreased lifespan [51] [52]. Recently, it has been demonstrated that B cells induced by *Schistosoma mansoni* worms is in an IL-10-dependent manner, which are responsible for protecting mice against fatal, experimentally induced anaphylaxis [53]. Breg cell function during different stages of natural *S. mansoni* infections and showed the existence of active regulatory mechanisms during chronic, but not acute infection [54]. A similar liver pathology was observed in schistosome-infected, Fcg-chain receptor knockout mice [52], suggesting that B-cell regulation is mediated either by the production of antibodies neutralizing egg-derived inflammatory molecules or by triggering the production of anti-inflammatory mediators from $FcR^{+}$ cells.

The concept that helminth-induced B cells can protect against allergic inflammation has been extended to other helminth infections that are natural for mice: in H polygyrus-infected mice, adoptive transfer of mesenteric lymph node B cells suppressed both DerP1-specific airway inflammation and EAE [55]. Interestingly, Breg cell development can also be seen during the infections caused by Leishmania major [56]; IL-10-producing B cells were critical for the development of unprotective TH2 responses and susceptibility to infection. In addition, murine cytomegalovirus has been shown to induce IL-10-producing Breg cells, resulting in decreased virus-specific CD81 T-cell responses and plasma cell expansion [57]. Other studies investigated the role that B cells play in infection with the nematode *Brugia pahangi*. Adoptively transferred peritoneal B cells, isolated from wild-type mice that had been immunized with *B. pahangi*, have been shown to protect athymic recipient mice against infection by *B. pahangi* infection [58].

In another study, the depletion of B cells from splenocytes of infected mice resulted in a reduced level of antigen-specific $CD4^{+}$ T-cell proliferation paralleled by a reduced level of CD80 and CD86. Similar results were obtained if IL-10 was neutralized at the time of infection, suggesting that B cells producing IL-10 might modulate immune response in filarial-infected mice, via the suppression of CD80 and CD86 expression on Bregs [59]. Taken together, these studies show that helminths can induce Breg cells that can protect against allergic diseases via the release of IL-10 and that this process is particularly active during the chronic stage of infection. Furthermore, it can be concluded that the suppressive ability of Breg cells is not restricted to TH1 immune responses associated with autoimmunity, and the effect that the humoral immune response and FcR interactions might play a major role in controlling.

## 4. Bregs in Cancer

Given that Bregs have been shown to suppress autoimmunity via the inhibition of autoreactive T cells, it might be anticipated that Bregs could also downregulate the protective cytotoxic T lymphocyte responses directed against tumor cells. Terabe found that enhanced antitumor immunity can be seen in B-cell-deficient mice and is associated with an increased activity of T and NK cells, both of which are important for the promotion of natural tumor surveillance [60]. Increased $CD4^{+}$ and $CD8^{+}$ T-cell responses to TS/A tumors are observed in μMT mice [61]. In B16 melanoma, mature B-cell depletion using CD20 mAb dramatically exacerbates tumor progression and metastasis, arguing that B cells primarily support antitumor immune responses in this model [1]. Thus, these results suggest that B cells can also negatively regulate tumor immunity.

Scott and colleagues have shown that the interaction between $CD40^L$ expressed on tumors and CD40 on B cells induces IL-10 production by B cells, indicating that the release of IL-10 is probably responsible for the diminished IFN$\gamma$ production by $CD8^+$ T and NK cells and the decreased $CD8^+$ T-cell memory development. However, there is some evidence to suggest that IL-10 can suppress angiogenesis and, thus, encourage tumor regression [62] [63]. Furthermore, the ubiquitous expression of CD40 *in vivo* will probably lead to a more complex cascade of anti- and pro-inflammatory cytokines, which might overcome the inhibitory effect of Bregs. But it remains to be formally proven whether or not administration of anti-CD40 can generate Bregs *in vivo*. Another study demonstrated an excessively zealous Breg population may promote tumor cell growth, as one of the mechanisms used by tumor cells to escape from the immune response consists in activation of Bregs that produce TGF-beta [64].

A role for B cells in the development of tumor immunity has been assessed using μMT mice given Friend murine leukemia virus gag-expressing mouse EL-4, D5 melanoma, or MCA304 sarcoma cells. Inoue and colleagues have tested wild-type mice were unable to control tumor progression, whereas EL-4 gag and D5 tumors (but not MCA304) were eliminated in μMT mice, which developed tumor-specific cytotoxic T lymphocytes after tumor challenge. Similar study suggested the growth of EL4 thymoma, MC38 colon carcinoma, and B16 melanoma was prevented or slowed in μMT mice in contrast to control mice [62] [65].

By contrast, B-cell depletion using CD20 mAb in a syngeneic lymphoma model dramatically enhances tumor clearance through B10-cell elimination. Thus, as in autoimmunity, B10 cells are likely to be involved in regulating antitumor immunity. However, this regulation will be significantly influenced by the immunogenicity of the tumor and the nature of the antitumor immune response [66].

## 5. Summary

Despite the extensive efforts on the characterization of BREG subtypes and their mechanism of action in different animal models, questions still exist to unravel the mechanisms underlying Bregs biology and function. The precise phenotype and characteristic markers of Bregs are still the subject of debate. It remains unclear whether Bregs require self-reactive BCRs for function. Are Breg cells a developmentally distinct B-cell subset? Do Breg cells display a specific transcriptional signature such as FoxP3 for regulatory T cells? Understanding these questions may open novel avenues for the treatment of inflammatory diseases such as allergy and autoimmunity.

## References

[1] DiLillo, D.J., Hamaguchi, Y., Ueda, Y., Yang, K., Uchida, J., Haas, K.M., Kelsoe, G. and Tedder, T.F. (2008) Maintenance of Long-Lived Plasma Cells and Serological Memory despite Mature and Memory B Cell Depletion during CD20 Immunotherapy in Mice. *Journal of Immunology*, **180**, 361-371. http://dx.doi.org/10.4049/jimmunol.180.1.361

[2] LeBien, T.W. and Tedder, T.F. (2008) B Lymphocytes: How They Develop and Function. *Blood*, **112**, 1570-1580. http://dx.doi.org/10.1182/blood-2008-02-078071

[3] Linton, P.J., Harbertson, J. and Bradley, L.M. (2000) A Critical Role for B Cells in the Development of Memory CD4 Cells. *Journal of Immunology*, **165**, 5558-5565. http://dx.doi.org/10.4049/jimmunol.165.10.5558

[4] Crawford, A., Macleod, M., Schumacher, T., Corlett, L. and Gray, D. (2006) Primary T Cell Expansion and Differentiation *in Vivo* Requires Antigen Presentation by B Cells. *Journal of Immunology*, **176**, 3498-3506. http://dx.doi.org/10.4049/jimmunol.176.6.3498

[5] Bouaziz, J.D., Yanaba, K., Venturi, G.M., Wang, Y., Tisch, R.M., Poe, J.C. and Tedder, T.F. (2007) Therapeutic B Cell Depletion Impairs Adaptive and Autoreactive CD4+ T Cell Activation in Mice. *Proceedings of the National Academy of Sciences of the United States of America*, **104**, 20878-20883. http://dx.doi.org/10.1073/pnas.0709205105

[6] Homann, D., Tishon, A., Berger, D.P., Weigle, W.O., von Herrath, M.G. and Oldstone, M.B. (1998) Evidence for an Underlying CD4 Helper and CD8 T-Cell Defect in B-Cell-Deficient Mice: Failure to Clear Persistent Virus Infection after Adoptive Immunotherapy with Virus-Specific Memory Cells from muMT/muMT Mice. *Journal of Virology*, **72**, 9208-9216.

[7] Bergmann, C.C., Ramakrishna, C., Kornacki, M. and Stohlman, S.A. (2001) Impaired T Cell Immunity in B Cell-Deficient Mice Following Viral Central Nervous System Infection. *Journal of Immunology*, **167**, 1575-1583. http://dx.doi.org/10.4049/jimmunol.167.3.1575

[8] O'Neill, S.K., Cao, Y., Hamel, K.M., Doodes, P.D., Hutas, G. and Finnegan, A. (2007) Expression of CD80/86 on B Cells Is Essential for Autoreactive T Cell Activation and the Development of Arthritis. *Journal of Immunology*, **179**, 5109-5116. http://dx.doi.org/10.4049/jimmunol.179.8.5109

[9] Morris, A. and Moller, G. (1968) Regulation of Cellular Antibody Synthesis Effect of Adoptively Transferred Antibody-Producing Spleen Cells on Cellular Antibody Synthesis. *Journal of Immunology*, **101**, 439-445.

[10] Shimamura, T., Hashimoto, K. and Sasaki, S. (1982) Feedback Suppression of the Immune Response *in Vivo*. I. Immune B Cells Induce Antigen-Specific Suppressor T Cells. *Cellular Immunology*, **68**, 104-113. http://dx.doi.org/10.1016/0008-8749(82)90093-4

[11] L'Age-Stehr, J., Teichmann, H., Gershon, R.K. and Cantor, H. (1980) Stimulation of Regulatory T Cell Circuits by Immunoglobulin-Dependent Structures on Activated B Cells. *European Journal of Immunology*, **10**, 21-26. http://dx.doi.org/10.1002/eji.1830100105

[12] Shimamura, T., Habu, S., Hashimoto, K. and Sasaki, S. (1984) Feedback Suppression of the Immune Response *in Vivo*. III. Lyt-$1^+$ B Cells Are Suppressor-Inducer Cells. *Cellular Immunology*, **83**, 221-224. http://dx.doi.org/10.1016/0008-8749(84)90242-9

[13] Kennedy, M.W. and Thomas, D.B. (1983) A Regulatory Role for the Memory B Cell as Suppressor-Inducer of Feedback Control. *The Journal of Experimental Medicine*, **157**, 547-558. http://dx.doi.org/10.1084/jem.157.2.547

[14] Fillatreau, S., Sweenie, C.H., McGeachy, M.J., Gray, D. and Anderton, S.M. (2002) B Cells Regulate Autoimmunity by Provision of IL-10. *Nature Immunology*, **3**, 944-950. http://dx.doi.org/10.1038/ni833

[15] Mizoguchi, A., Mizoguchi, E., Takedatsu, H., Blumberg, R.S. and Bhan, A.K. (2002) Chronic Intestinal Inflammatory Condition Generates IL-10-Producing Regulatory B Cell Subset Characterized by CD1d Upregulation. *Immunity*, **16**, 219-230. http://dx.doi.org/10.1016/S1074-7613(02)00274-1

[16] Mauri, C., Gray, D., Mushtaq, N. and Londei, M. (2003) Prevention of Arthritis by Interleukin 10-Producing B Cells. *The Journal of Experimental Medicine*, **197**, 489-501. http://dx.doi.org/10.1084/jem.20021293

[17] Yanaba, K., Bouaziz, J.D., Haas, K.M., Poe, J.C., Fujimoto, M. and Tedder, T.F. (2008) A Regulatory B Cell Subset with a Unique $CD1d^{hi}CD5^+$ Phenotype Controls T Cell-Dependent Inflammatory Responses. *Immunity*, **28**, 639-650. http://dx.doi.org/10.1016/j.immuni.2008.03.017

[18] Matsushita, T., Yanaba, K., Bouaziz, J.D., Fujimoto, M. and Tedder, T.F. (2008) Regulatory B Cells Inhibit EAE Initiation in Mice While Other B Cells Promote Disease Progression. *Journal of Clinical Investigation*, **118**, 3420-3430. http://dx.doi.org/10.1172/JCI36030

[19] Yanaba, K., Bouaziz, J.D., Matsushita, T., Tsubata, T. and Tedder, T.F. (2009) The Development and Function of Regulatory B Cells Expressing IL-10 (B10 Cells) Requires Antigen Receptor Diversity and TLR Signals. *The Journal of Immunology*, **182**, 7459-7472. http://dx.doi.org/10.4049/jimmunol.0900270

[20] Harris, D.P., Haynes, L., Sayles, P.C., Duso, D.K., Eaton, S.M., Lepak, N.M., Johnson, L.L., Swain, S.L. and Lund, F.E. (2000) Reciprocal Regulation of Polarized Cytokine Production by Effector B and T Cells. *Nature Immunology*, **1**, 475-482. http://dx.doi.org/10.1038/82717

[21] Brummel, R. and Lenert, P. (2005) Activation of Marginal Zone B Cells from Lupus Mice with Type A(D) CpG-Oligodeoxynucleotides. *The Journal of Immunology*, **174**, 2429-2434. http://dx.doi.org/10.4049/jimmunol.174.4.2429

[22] Evans, J.G., Chavez-Rueda, K.A., Eddaoudi, A., Meyer-Bahlburg, A., Rawlings, D.J., Ehrenstein, M.R. and Mauri, C. (2007) Novel Suppressive Function of Transitional 2 B Cells in Experimental Arthritis. *The Journal of Immunology*, **178**, 7868-7878. http://dx.doi.org/10.4049/jimmunol.178.12.7868

[23] Gray, M., Miles, K., Salter, D., Gray, D. and Savill, J. (2007) Apoptotic Cells Protect Mice from Autoimmune Inflammation by the Induction of Regulatory B Cells. *Proceedings of the National Academy of Sciences of the United States of America*, **104**, 14080-14085. http://dx.doi.org/10.1073/pnas.0700326104

[24] Burke, F., Stagg, A.J., Bedford, P.A., English, N. and Knight, S.C. (2004) IL-10-Producing $B220^+CD11c^-$ APC in Mouse Spleen. *The Journal of Immunology*, **173**, 2362-2372. http://dx.doi.org/10.4049/jimmunol.173.4.2362

[25] Spencer, N.F. and Daynes, R.A. (1997) IL-12 Directly Stimulates Expression of IL-10 by $CD5^+$ B Cells and IL-6 by Both $CD5^+$ and $CD5^-$ B Cells: Possible Involvement in Age-Associated Cytokine Dysregulation. *International Immunology*, **9**, 745-754. http://dx.doi.org/10.1093/intimm/9.5.745

[26] O'Garra, A., Stapleton, G., Dhar, V., Pearce, M., Schumacher, J., Rugo, H., Barbis, D., Stall, A., Cupp, J., Moore, K., *et al.* (1990) Production of Cytokines by Mouse B Cells: B Lymphomas and Normal B Cells Produce Interleukin 10. *International Immunology*, **2**, 821-832. http://dx.doi.org/10.1093/intimm/2.9.821

[27] Zhang, X., Deriaud, E., Jiao, X., Braun, D., Leclerc, C. and Lo-Man, R. (2007) Type I Interferons Protect Neonates from Acute Inflammation through Interleukin 10-Producing B Cells. *The Journal of Experimental Medicine*, **204**, 1107-1118. http://dx.doi.org/10.1084/jem.20062013

[28] Wolf, S.D., Dittel, B.N., Hardardottir, F. and Janeway Jr., C.A. (1996) Experimental Autoimmune Encephalomyelitis Induction in Genetically B Cell-Deficient Mice. *The Journal of Experimental Medicine*, **184**, 2271-2278. http://dx.doi.org/10.1084/jem.184.6.2271

[29] Lampropoulou, V., Hoehlig, K., Roch, T., Neves, P., Calderon Gomez, E., Sweenie, C.H., Hao, Y., Freitas, A.A., Steinhoff, U., Anderton, S.M. and Fillatreau, S. (2008) TLR-Activated B Cells Suppress T Cell-Mediated Autoimmunity. *The Journal of Immunology*, **180**, 4763-4773. http://dx.doi.org/10.4049/jimmunol.180.7.4763

[30] Matsushita, T., Fujimoto, M., Hasegawa, M., Komura, K., Takehara, K., Tedder, T.F. and Sato, S. (2006) Inhibitory Role of CD19 in the Progression of Experimental Autoimmune Encephalomyelitis by Regulating Cytokine Response. *American Journal of Pathology*, **168**, 812-821. http://dx.doi.org/10.2353/ajpath.2006.050923

[31] Ray, A., Basu, S., Williams, C.B., Salzman, N.H. and Dittel, B.N. (2012) A Novel IL-10-Independent Regulatory Role for B Cells in Suppressing Autoimmunity by Maintenance of Regulatory T Cells via GITR Ligand. *The Journal of Immunology*, **188**, 3188-3198. http://dx.doi.org/10.4049/jimmunol.1103354

[32] Hauser, S.L., Waubant, E., Arnold, D.L., Vollmer, T., Antel, J., Fox, R.J., Bar-Or, A., Panzara, M., Sarkar, N., Agarwal, S., Langer-Gould, A. and Smith, C.H. (2008) B-Cell Depletion with Rituximab in Relapsing-Remitting Multiple Sclerosis. *The New England Journal of Medicine*, **358**, 676-688. http://dx.doi.org/10.1056/NEJMoa0706383

[33] Bar-Or, A., Calabresi, P.A., Arnold, D., Markowitz, C., Shafer, S., Kasper, L.H., Waubant, E., Gazda, S., Fox, R.J., Panzara, M., Sarkar, N., Agarwal, S. and Smith, C.H. (2008) Rituximab in Relapsing-Remitting Multiple Sclerosis: A 72-Week, Open-Label, Phase I Trial. *Annals of Neurology*, **63**, 395-400. http://dx.doi.org/10.1002/ana.21363

[34] Anderson, M.S. and Bluestone, J.A. (2005) The NOD Mouse: A Model of Immune Dysregulation. *Annual Review of Immunology*, **23**, 447-485. http://dx.doi.org/10.1146/annurev.immunol.23.021704.115643

[35] Xiu, Y., Wong, C.P., Bouaziz, J.D., Hamaguchi, Y., Wang, Y., Pop, S.M., Tisch, R.M. and Tedder, T.F. (2008) B Lymphocyte Depletion by CD20 Monoclonal Antibody Prevents Diabetes in Nonobese Diabetic Mice Despite Isotype-Specific Differences in Fc Gamma R Effector Functions. *The Journal of Immunology*, **180**, 2863-2875. http://dx.doi.org/10.4049/jimmunol.180.5.2863

[36] Hussain, S. and Delovitch, T.L. (2007) Intravenous Transfusion of BCR-Activated B Cells Protects NOD Mice from Type 1 Diabetes in an IL-10-Dependent Manner. *The Journal of Immunology*, **179**, 7225-7232. http://dx.doi.org/10.4049/jimmunol.179.11.7225

[37] Tian, J., Zekzer, D., Hanssen, L., Lu, Y., Olcott, A. and Kaufman, D.L. (2001) Lipopolysaccharide-Activated B Cells Down-Regulate Th1 Immunity and Prevent Autoimmune Diabetes in Nonobese Diabetic Mice. *The Journal of Immunology*, **167**, 1081-1089. http://dx.doi.org/10.4049/jimmunol.167.2.1081

[38] Trentham, D.E., Townes, A.S. and Kang, A.H. (1977) Autoimmunity to Type II Collagen an Experimental Model of Arthritis. *The Journal of Experimental Medicine*, **146**, 857-868. http://dx.doi.org/10.1084/jem.146.3.857

[39] Courtenay, J.S., Dallman, M.J., Dayan, A.D., Martin, A. and Mosedale, B. (1980) Immunisation against Heterologous Type II Collagen Induces Arthritis in Mice. *Nature*, **283**, 666-668. http://dx.doi.org/10.1038/283666a0

[40] Wordsworth, B.P., Lanchbury, J.S., Sakkas, L.I., Welsh, K.I., Panayi, G.S. and Bell, J.I. (1989) HLA-DR4 Subtype Frequencies in Rheumatoid Arthritis Indicate That DRB1 Is the Major Susceptibility Locus within the HLA Class II Region. *Proceedings of the National Academy of Sciences of the United States of America*, **86**, 10049-10053. http://dx.doi.org/10.1073/pnas.86.24.10049

[41] Brunsberg, U., Gustafsson, K., Jansson, L., Michaelsson, E., Ahrlund-Richter, L., Pettersson, S., Mattsson, R. and Holmdahl, R. (1994) Expression of a Transgenic Class II Ab Gene Confers Susceptibility to Collagen-Induced Arthritis. *European Journal of Immunology*, **24**, 1698-1702. http://dx.doi.org/10.1002/eji.1830240736

[42] Yanaba, K., Hamaguchi, Y., Venturi, G.M., Steeber, D.A., St Clair, E.W. and Tedder, T.F. (2007) B Cell Depletion Delays Collagen-Induced Arthritis in Mice: Arthritis Induction Requires Synergy between Humoral and Cell-Mediated Immunity. *The Journal of Immunology*, **179**, 1369-1380. http://dx.doi.org/10.4049/jimmunol.179.2.1369

[43] Gu, Y., Yang, J., Ouyang, X., Liu, W., Li, H., Bromberg, J., Chen, S.H., Mayer, L., Unkeless, J.C. and Xiong, H. (2008) Interleukin 10 Suppresses Th17 Cytokines Secreted by Macrophages and T Cells. *European Journal of Immunology*, **38**, 1807-1813. http://dx.doi.org/10.1002/eji.200838331

[44] Watanabe, R., Ishiura, N., Nakashima, H., Kuwano, Y., Okochi, H., Tamaki, K., Sato, S., Tedder, T.F. and Fujimoto, M. (2010) Regulatory B Cells (B10 Cells) Have a Suppressive Role in Murine Lupus: CD19 and B10 Cell Deficiency Exacerbates Systemic Autoimmunity. *The Journal of Immunology*, **184**, 4801-4809. http://dx.doi.org/10.4049/jimmunol.0902385

[45] Haas, K.M., Watanabe, R., Matsushita, T., Nakashima, H., Ishiura, N., Okochi, H., Fujimoto, M. and Tedder, T.F. (2010) Protective and Pathogenic Roles for B Cells during Systemic Autoimmunity in NZB/W F1 Mice. *The Journal of Immunology*, **184**, 4789-4800. http://dx.doi.org/10.4049/jimmunol.0902391

[46] Teichmann, L.L., Kashgarian, M., Weaver, C.T., Roers, A., Muller, W. and Shlomchik, M.J. (2011) B Cell-Derived IL-10 Does Not Regulate Spontaneous Systemic Autoimmunity in MRL.*Fas*$^{lpr}$ Mice. *The Journal of Immunology*, **188**, 678-685. http://dx.doi.org/10.4049/jimmunol.1102456

[47] Mizoguchi, A., Mizoguchi, E., Smith, R.N., Preffer, F.I. and Bhan, A.K. (1997) Suppressive Role of B Cells in Chron-

ic Colitis of T Cell Receptor Alpha Mutant Mice. *The Journal of Experimental Medicine*, **186**, 1749-1756. http://dx.doi.org/10.1084/jem.186.10.1749

[48] Mizoguchi, A. and Bhan, A.K. (2006) A Case for Regulatory B Cells. *The Journal of Immunology*, **176**, 705-710. http://dx.doi.org/10.4049/jimmunol.176.2.705

[49] Yanaba, K., Yoshizaki, A., Asano, Y., Kadono, T., Tedder, T.F. and Sato, S. (2011) IL-10-Producing Regulatory B10 Cells Inhibit Intestinal Injury in a Mouse Model. *American Journal of Pathology*, **178**, 735-743. http://dx.doi.org/10.1016/j.ajpath.2010.10.022

[50] Wei, B., Velazquez, P., Turovskaya, O., Spricher, K., Aranda, R., Kronenberg, M., Birnbaumer, L. and Braun, J. (2005) Mesenteric B Cells Centrally Inhibit $CD4^+$ T Cell Colitis through Interaction with Regulatory T Cell Subsets. *Proceedings of the National Academy of Sciences of the United States of America*, **102**, 2010-2015. http://dx.doi.org/10.1073/pnas.0409449102

[51] Amu, S., Saunders, S.P., Kronenberg, M., Mangan, N.E., Atzberger, A. and Fallon, P.G. (2010) Regulatory B Cells Prevent and Reverse Allergic Airway Inflammation via FoxP3-Positive T Regulatory Cells in a Murine Model. *Journal of Allergy and Clinical Immunology*, **125**, 1114-1124. http://dx.doi.org/10.1016/j.jaci.2010.01.018

[52] Jankovic, D., Cheever, A.W., Kullberg, M.C., Wynn, T.A., Yap, G., Caspar, P., Lewis, F.A., Clynes, R., Ravetch, J.V. and Sher, A. (1998) $CD4^+$ T Cell-Mediated Granulomatous Pathology in Schistosomiasis Is Downregulated by a B Cell-Dependent Mechanism Requiring Fc Receptor Signaling. *The Journal of Experimental Medicine*, **187**, 619-629. http://dx.doi.org/10.1084/jem.187.4.619

[53] Mangan, N.E., Fallon, R.E., Smith, P., van Rooijen, N., McKenzie, A.N. and Fallon, P.G. (2004) Helminth Infection Protects Mice from Anaphylaxis via IL-10-Producing B Cells. *The Journal of Immunology*, **173**, 6346-6356. http://dx.doi.org/10.4049/jimmunol.173.10.6346

[54] Saaf, A.M., Halbleib, J.M., Chen, X., Yuen, S.T., Leung, S.Y., Nelson, W.J. and Brown, P.O. (2007) Parallels between Global Transcriptional Programs of Polarizing Caco-2 Intestinal Epithelial Cells *in Vitro* and Gene Expression Programs in Normal Colon and Colon Cancer. *Molecular Biology of the Cell*, **18**, 4245-4260. http://dx.doi.org/10.1091/mbc.E07-04-0309

[55] Wilson, M.S., Taylor, M.D., O'Gorman, M.T., Balic, A., Barr, T.A., Filbey, K., Anderton, S.M. and Maizels, R.M. (2010) Helminth-Induced $CD19^+CD23^{hi}$ B Cells Modulate Experimental Allergic and Autoimmune Inflammation. *European Journal of Immunology*, **40**, 1682-1696. http://dx.doi.org/10.1002/eji.200939721

[56] Ronet, C., Hauyon-La Torre, Y., Revaz-Breton, M., Mastelic, B., Tacchini-Cottier, F., Louis, J. and Launois, P. (2009) Regulatory B Cells Shape the Development of Th2 Immune Responses in BALB/c Mice Infected with Leishmania Major through IL-10 Production. *The Journal of Immunology*, **184**, 886-894. http://dx.doi.org/10.4049/jimmunol.0901114

[57] Madan, R., Demircik, F., Surianarayanan, S., Allen, J.L., Divanovic, S., Trompette, A., Yogev, N., Gu, Y., Khodoun, M., Hildeman, D., Boespflug, N., Fogolin, M.B., Grobe, L., Greweling, M., Finkelman, F.D., Cardin, R., Mohrs, M., Muller, W., Waisman, A., Roers, A. and Karp, C.L. (2009) Nonredundant Roles for B Cell-Derived IL-10 in Immune Counter-Regulation. *The Journal of Immunology*, **183**, 2312-2320. http://dx.doi.org/10.4049/jimmunol.0900185

[58] Paciorkowski, N., Shultz, L.D. and Rajan, T.V. (2003) Primed Peritoneal B Lymphocytes Are Sufficient to Transfer Protection against *Brugia pahangi* Infection in Mice. *Infection and Immunity*, **71**, 1370-1378. http://dx.doi.org/10.1128/IAI.71.3.1370-1378.2003

[59] Gillan, V., Lawrence, R.A. and Devaney, E. (2005) B Cells Play a Regulatory Role in Mice Infected with the L3 of *Brugia pahangi*. *International Immunology*, **17**, 373-382. http://dx.doi.org/10.1093/intimm/dxh217

[60] Terabe, M., Swann, J., Ambrosino, E., Sinha, P., Takaku, S., Hayakawa, Y., Godfrey, D.I., Ostrand-Rosenberg, S., Smyth, M.J. and Berzofsky, J.A. (2005) A Nonclassical Non-$V\alpha14J\alpha18$ CD1d-Restricted (Type II) NKT Cell Is Sufficient for Down-Regulation of Tumor Immunosurveillance. *The Journal of Experimental Medicine*, **202**, 1627-1633. http://dx.doi.org/10.1084/jem.20051381

[61] Qin, Z., Richter, G., Schuler, T., Ibe, S., Cao, X. and Blankenstein, T. (1998) B Cells Inhibit Induction of T Cell-Dependent Tumor Immunity. *Nature Medicine*, **4**, 627-630. http://dx.doi.org/10.1038/nm0598-627

[62] Inoue, S., Leitner, W.W., Golding, B. and Scott, D. (2006) Inhibitory Effects of B Cells on Antitumor Immunity. *Cancer Research*, **66**, 7741-7747. http://dx.doi.org/10.1158/0008-5472.CAN-05-3766

[63] Rowe, V., Banovic, T., MacDonald, K.P., Kuns, R., Don, A.L., Morris, E.S., Burman, A.C., Bofinger, H.M., Clouston, A.D. and Hill, G.R. (2006) Host B Cells Produce IL-10 Following TBI and Attenuate Acute GVHD after Allogeneic Bone Marrow Transplantation. *Blood*, **108**, 2485-2492. http://dx.doi.org/10.1182/blood-2006-04-016063

[64] Olkhanud, P.B., Damdinsuren, B., Bodogai, M., Gress, R.E., Sen, R., Wejksza, K., Malchinkhuu, E., Wersto, R.P. and Biragyn, A. (2011) Tumor-Evoked Regulatory B Cells Promote Breast Cancer Metastasis by Converting Resting $CD4^+$ T Cells to T-Regulatory Cells. *Cancer Research*, **71**, 3505-3515. http://dx.doi.org/10.1158/0008-5472.CAN-10-4316

[65] Shah, S., Divekar, A.A., Hilchey, S.P., Cho, H.M., Newman, C.L., Shin, S.U., Nechustan, H., Challita-Eid, P.M., Segal, B.M., Yi, K.H. and Rosenblatt, J.D. (2005) Increased Rejection of Primary Tumors in Mice Lacking B Cells: Inhibition of Anti-Tumor CTL and TH1 Cytokine Responses by B Cells. *International Journal of Cancer*, **117**, 574-586. http://dx.doi.org/10.1002/ijc.21177

[66] Minard-Colin, V., Xiu, Y., Poe, J.C., Horikawa, M., Magro, C.M., Hamaguchi, Y., Haas, K.M. and Tedder, T.F. (2008) Lymphoma Depletion during CD20 Immunotherapy in Mice Is Mediated by Macrophage FcγRI, FcγRIII, and FcγRIV. *Blood*, **112**, 1205-1213. http://dx.doi.org/10.1182/blood-2008-01-135160

12

# Hemopoietic Formulae Rearranged Leukocyte Subsets and Implication for Use against the Type of Constitution and Infectious Agent for Further Modification to Future

**Nobuo Yamaguchi[1,2*], Wataru Hiruma[3], Kohei Suruga[3], Nurmuhamamt Amat[4], Dilxat Yimit[4], Parida Hoxur[4,5], Daisuke Sakamoto[5], Kazuhiro Okamoto[6], Shan-Yu Su[7,8]**

[1]Department of Fundamental Research for CAM, Kanazawa Medical University, Ishikawa, Japan
[2]Ishikawa Natural Medicinal Products Research Center, Ishikawa, Japan
[3]International Operation Department (FM Center for R & D), Kibun Foods Inc., Tokyo, Japan
[4]Traditional Uighur Medicine Department, Xinjiang Medical University, Urumchi, China
[5]Traditional Chinese Medicine Hospital, Xinjiang Medical University, Urumchi, China
[6]Department of Otolaryngology, Kanazawa Medical University, Ishikawa, Japan
[7]Department of Chinese Medicine, China Medical University Hospital, Taiwan
[8]School of Post-Baccalaureate Chinese Medicine, College of Chinese Medicine, China Medicinal University, Taiwan
Email: *serumaya@kanazawa-med.ac.jp

## Abstract

**A hemopoietic formula (HF) in traditional Chinese medicine (TCM) usually consists of more than six single herbs. We seek to look into changes of immune-competent cells by two commonly utilized HF, including Shi-Quan-Da-Bu-Tang (SDT) and Bu-Zong-Ye-Qi-Tang (BYT). However, the effects of both formulae on levels of leukocyte subsets are not yet defied. After administration of immno-suppressant to animals, the effects by HFs on the augmentation for subsets of leukocytes, CD positive cell counts of lymphocytes, and the cytokine-producing cells are measured. Our results show that SDT augments the level of lymphocytes, while BYT increases the level of granulocytes. In our clinical study with 15 healthy volunteers, positive cells for CD2, CD11b, CD14, IL-4, IL-1$\beta$ and IFN-$\gamma$ in peripheral blood are increased significantly 15 days after the ingestion of HFs. In rodents, compromised host as well as normal animal is administered with cancer chemotherapeutic agent**

*Corresponding author.

**(Mytomycin-C). Our observations show that SDT regulates phagocyte activities of the immune system, introducing it against intracellular parasite, and that BYT augments intercellular pathogen through humoral immunity. We discuss the significance and mechanism of HFs on the level of leukocyte subsets in number and function that are considered to be potential indicators for the evaluation of TCM modalities. We also propose an idea that TCM exhibits tonic effects via enhancing the ability to fight against infection and bacteria, as well as turning the multi-drug resistant bacteria to the sensitive ones. Together with these evidences, we suggest an ideal remedy for the compromised to fight host against pathogens. Moreover, we try to modify these hemopoietic formulae to more digestive forms. This modification brings to the significant lifted up for antibody producing cells and anti-oxidative activity for phagocytic cells.**

## Keywords

**Traditional Chinese Medicine, Cancer Chemotherapeutic Agent, Compromised Host, Intracellular Infectious Agent, Intercellular Infectious agent**

## 1. Introduction

In recent years, complementary and alternative medicines (CAM) have achieved more and more attentions since they are able to treat many chronic illnesses, such as fatigue syndrome that plagues the industrialized world. The present team has reported that typical styles of CAM, *i.e.* TCM regulate functions of leukocytes in human immune system [1] [2]. Dietary and hemopoietic formula holds promise as strong inducers of acquired immunity. While the immune system is working against the local infection of pathogens, cytokine and immuno-competent cells react throughout the body in close connection to the brain, the endocrine and immune system [3]. In this study, we hypothesize that HF may influence immuno-competent cells qualitatively and quantitatively by targeting lymphocytes based on the constitution dependent manner. SDT and BYT have been employed as tonic agent and the implication has little been made on the characteristics of the levels of leukocyte subset, such as granulocytes and lymphocytes. In this report, we seek to focus on the identity of each HF formula, comparing to another herbal medicine. The influence of HF on leukocyte and/or lymphocyte subpopulations in human peripheral blood is also discussed. Moreover, some trials have been made for herbal formulae by Lactobacillus and by Yeast Fungus in order to use-up original materials other than traditional hot-water extraction [4].

## 2. Materials and Methods

### 2.1. Clinical Findings

#### 2.1.1. Volunteers and Evaluation Methods

Fifteen healthy volunteers aged from 19 to 59 years were recruited and were administered HF for 15 days. Fifteen milliliters of blood were drawn from the forearm vein one hour before the first administration of HF and 15 days after the last HF administration (day 30). All volunteers provided informed consent prior to participation for this trial. This study was approved by Ethics Committee of Kanazawa Medical University.

#### 2.1.2. Herbal Decoction and Assessment for Host Immune Factor

Dried haemopoietic formula SDT and BYT in granules were chosen as representatives of HF [5]-[12]. Dang-Gui-Liu-Huang-Tang (dRHT) and Syao-Chin-Rong-Tang (sCRT) were chosen as controls. A dose of 5.25 g dried powder of each formula (supplied by Tsumura Pharmaceutical Co. Ltd., Japan) was administered two times per day for 15 days. Physiological functions were checked and possible side effects of the drug were inquired for all the subjects to ensure the safety of the trial.

#### 2.1.3. Leukocyte Counts

The assessments including a total number of leukocytes was ordered to count with blood chemical test for the medical diagnosis of public institution (Ishikawa Preventive Medicine Association, Ishikawa, Japan). In the differential counting, 200 cells were counted on a May-Grünewald-Gimsa stained slide, and percentages of lymphocytes and granulocytes were determined.

#### 2.1.4. Leukocyte Subset Analyses

The assessments including a total number of leukocytes was ordered to count with blood chemical test for the medical diagnosis of public institution (Ishikawa Preventive Medicine Association, Ishikawa, Japan). In the differential counting, 200 cells were counted on a May-Grunewald-Gimsa stained slide, and percentages of lymphocytes and granulocytes were determined [13] [14].

#### 2.1.5. Lymphocyte Subset Analyses

The whole blood obtained from the subjects was washed twice in phosphate buffered saline (PBS). One hundred micro-liters of the suspensions were stained with 20 μl of fluorescent monoclonal antibodies (anti-human $CD2^+$, $CD4^+$, $CD8^+$, $CD11b^+$, $CD14^+$, $CD16^+$, $CD19^+$ and CD56; antibodies). About 10,000 stained cells were re-suspended in PBS, then surface markers were detected by flow cytometry (FACS Calibur; Becton Dickinson Immnocytometry Systems, CA, USA).

#### 2.1.6. Measurement of Cytokine Expression Levels in Blood Cells

To test whether HF affected the functional maturation of immunocytes within a short period of time, we examined the number of cytokine containing cells using FACS analysis. This method reveals cytokine producing cell by peering off the surface of lymphocyte, enable to assess the cells in a festival evening, compare than serum cytokine level that correspond to paper tips of post festival [15].

Blood cell suspensions were cultured in phorbol 12-myristate 13-acetate (PMA), ionomycin and bovine serum albumin (BSA) (Sigma CO. Ltd., Mo, USA) for 4 - 5 h at 37˚C. Subsequently, the cell suspensions were stained with monoclonal antibodies (Percp-CD3, Percp-CD45, FITC-interferon (IFN)-$\gamma$, PE-interleukin (IL)-4, FITC-IL-1$\beta$) and analyzed by flow cytometry. All antibodies used in this study were purchased from Becton Dickinson Immunocytometry System (CA, USA).

### 2.2. Animal Experiment

#### 2.2.1. Experimental Design for Bone Marrow Suppressed Immune-Compromised Mice

In the animal model of immuno-competency reduction, male C57BL/6J mice, aged 8 - 9 weeks, were injected with Mitomycin-C (MMC) (5 mg/kg) to inhibit the bone marrow. Then, HF extracts was administered orally at a dosage of 1 g/kg/day for five consecutive days. tRHT and sCRT were chosen as controls [16]-[24].

1) Recovery of Total Leukocytes and Subsets of Leukocytes

2) Recovery of White Blood Cell by HF

The bone marrow-suppressed mice were administered herbal decoction HF 1g/kg dairy for 5 days and after 1 week later, their blood were withdrawn from their tail vain. Then, the number of leukocytes was counted in Bürker-Türk solution.

3) A Recovery of leukocyte Subsets

Bone marrow-suppressed mice were administered with herbal decoction of dLHT (1g/kg/day) for five days. One week later, the blood from their tail vain was withdrawn. Then the granulocyte and lymphocyte subsets were counted in Bürker-Türk solution.

4) A Recovery of Macrophage Activity, Migration

Cells from peritoneal exudates were collect from the peritoneal cavity of bone marrow-suppressed mice. Phagocytes were purified using adherent technique to get cell suspensions which contained more than 95% of phagocytes. The purified cells were loaded to the upper room of Boyden chamber to test migration ability at a concentration of $1 \times 10^4$ cell/ml. Human serum treated at 56˚C for 30 min was for the chemo tactic agent of mouse phagocyte [25].

5) Recovery of Macrophage Activity, Phagocytosis

The same cells suspension was purified by adherent technique for phagocyte, which produces cells contained more than 95% of phagocytes. The purified cells were adjusted to $1 \times 10^4$ cell/cm$^2$ and mixed with latex beads that are 5 μm in granule with fluorescence isochianate. After 90 min of incubation, remained granule were washed out from the glass slide. Number of phagocytic cell and their ability to catch up the latex beads were automatically measured by ACAS system, which outputs the result in a digital form (Adeherent cell activity evaluating system; Shimazu, Kyoto, Japan).

6) Recovery of Macrophage Activity, Target Cell Killing

The same phagocyte suspension, which contained over 95% of phagocytes, was produced by adherent technique for phagocyte. The purified cells were adjusted to 1 × $10^5$ cell/ml to examine the macrophage activity of killing by the nitroblue tetrazolium (NBT) reduction test [15].

### 2.2.2. A Recovery of Lymphocyte Activity, Antibody Secreting Cell

The bone marrow suppressed mice were administered herbal decoction of HF (1g/kg/day) for 5 days. One week later, mice were immunized with sheep red blood cells, (2 × $10^8$/mouse) intraperitoneally. Five days later, their spleen cells were collected. Plague-forming cells (PFC) were developed, and the ability of IgM and IgG antibody production was tested by the method reported by Jerne and Nordin [19] [20].

### 2.2.3. CD Positive Lymphocyte Distribution by HF against Different Constitution

Whole blood obtained from the subjects was washed twice with PBS. One hundred micro-liters of the suspensions were stained with 20 μl of fluorescent monoclonal antibodies (anti-human $CD2^+$, $CD4^+$, $CD8^+$, $CD11b^+$, $CD14^+$, $CD16^+$, $CD19^+$ and $CD56^+$ antibodies). Ten thousands stained cells were re-suspended in PBS to detect surface markers by flow cytometry (FACS Calibur; Becton Dickinson Immnocytometry Systems, CA, USA).

### 2.2.4. Distribution of Cytokine Producing Lymphocytes in Different Constitution

The blood cell suspensions were cultured with PMA (phorbol 12-myristate 13-acetate), ionomycin and BSA (bovine serum albumin) for 4 - 5 hours at 37˚C. After that, the cell suspensions were stained using the monoclonal antibodies of PE-IL-4, FITC-IFN-$\gamma$ and FITC-IL-1$\beta$. Then they were analyzed by the FACScan (Becton Dickinson Co. Ltd. USA). The antibodies and reagents used in the test were purchased from Becton Dickinson Immunocytometry system (USA).

### 2.2.5. Estimation of Macrophage Activity by the Examination of Phagocytosis

The peritoneal exudates cells were collect from the peritoneal cavity of bone marrow-suppressed mice. Cell suspensions were purified by adherent technique for phagocyte, getting a suspension which contained over 95% of phagocytes. The purified cells were adjusted to 1 × $10^4$ cell/ml and loaded at the upper chamber of Boyden chamber for test migration. Human serum with treated at 56˚C for 30 min was for the chemotactic agent for mouse phagocyte.

Phagocytic activity and antibody production of macrophages were analyzed using a classical test that could test the total activity of the immune system by examine chemotaxis, phagocytosis and intracellular degradation of macrophage. For identifying antibody-forming cells, plaque-forming cells were detected using heterogeneous erythrocyte; sheep erythrocyte was a target antigen. Peritoneal macrophages were collected and purified in fetal calf serum (FCS)-coated petri-dishes. The cell population was approximately 97% uniform in function and morphology. These cells were applied to the nuclepore-membrane (pore size: 5 μm; Neuro Probe Co. Ltd., Cabin John MD, USA) with a chemotaxis chamber (Neuro Probe Co. Ltd.). After 90 minutes' incubation, the membrane was vigorously washed with saline (37˚C), fixed, and then stained with methylene blue dye. After counting under a microscope for the total field of the membrane, the average number of migrating cells was expressed as cell counts/$mm^2$.

### 2.2.6. Phagocytic Ability of Phagocyte

The same cells suspension was purified by adherent technique for phagocyte, which contained over 95% of phagocytes. The purified cells were adjusted to 1 × $10^4$ cell/$cm^2$ and mixed with latex beads that were 5 um in granule with fluorescence isochianate. After 90 min of incubation, the remained granule were washed out from the glass slide and counting automatically by ACAS system, which outputs digital presentation, for evaluating phagocytes in number and in their ability to catch up the latex beads (Adeherent cell activity evaluating system, Shimazu, Kyoto, Japan). Latex beads in 5 μm with fluorescence were used to test phagocytic activity and *Candida albicans* was cell killing activity. A macrophage-target cell ratio of 1:10 was considered to be optimum. Ten minutes after incubating phagocytes and target cells, intracellular *Candida* cells were cultured on an agar dish with conventional medium 1640 until the next day to perform the colony forming assay. In this way, the phagocytic ability of the macrophages was monitored. To document intracellular killing activity, the same procedures were performed excepting that the incubation time was changed to 90 minutes.

### 2.2.7. Antibody Forming Cell Study

Sheep erythrocyte (SRBC), a T-dependent antigen, was used for antibody formation cell study. Ten days after tumor transplantation, each antigen was intra-peritoneally injected. After four and six days, the antibody-forming cells were detected using localized hemolysis in an agar gel. Plaque-forming cells were developed by the method of Jerne and Nordin [19] [20].

### 2.2.8. Anti-Oxidative Evaluation

1) Animals

Eight week-old female C57BL/6 were purchased from Sankyo Laboratory Service Corporation (Shizuoka, Japan). All mice were kept under specific pathogen-free conditions. Mice food and distilled water were freely accessible for each mouse. Housing temperature and humidity were controlled 25˚C ± 1˚C and 60% (**Figure 1**).

2) Reagents

As for the basic medium, HEPES buffer (HEPES 17mM, NaCl 120mM, Glucose 5mM, KCl 5mM, $CaCl_2$ 1mM, $MgCl_2$ 1mM) was prepared and sterilized by filtration. Phorbol 12-myristate 13-acetate (PMA, Sigma, USA) was diluted to $10^{-6}$ M by dimethyl sulfoxide (DMSO, Sigma, USA) and used as a stimulant for super oxide anion generation for murine peritoneal exudates cells. Cytochrome-c (Sigma, USA) was diluted to 1mM by HEPES buffer. Since cytochrome-c reduced by super oxide showed maximum absorbance at 550 nm, we used cytochrome-c to measure the amount of super oxide anion generation through spectro-photometrical technique. Oyster Glycogen (type, Sigma, USA) was diluted in the purified water (10% w/v, Wako, Japan) and autoclaved at 120˚C for 20 min. This solution was used for intraperitoneal injection to mice in order to induce peripheral neutrophils into the abdominal cavity.

3) Modified TCM and Other Materials

*Agaricus* was purchased from Ohbiken Co. Ltd. (Yamanashi, Japan), *Chlorella* was purchased from Taiwan *Chlorella* Co. Ltd. (Taipei, Taiwan) and Propolis was purchased from Epimedix Co. Ltd. (Kanazawa, Japan). The herbal medicine (TCM), Shi-Quan-Da-Bu-Tang and Bu-Zong-Ye-Qi-Tang were purchased from Tsumura Co. Ltd. (Tokyo, Japan) and fermented at Ohbiken Co. Ltd. (Yamanashi, Japan). Propolis was also degradated at

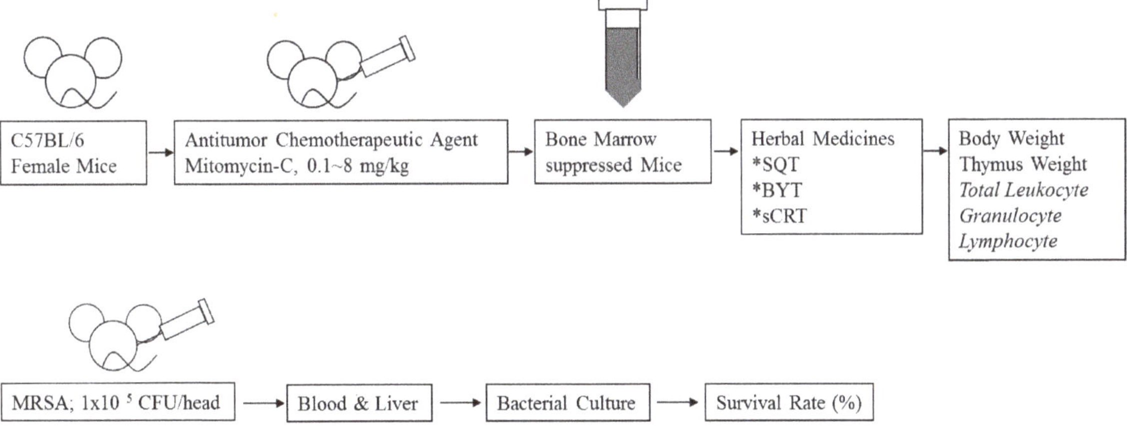


**Figure 1.** a) The effect on macrophage phagocytosis against latex beads by dHLT after administrating MMC. The procedure of treatment was the same in the text. The macrophage migration capacity was detected by computer analysis, ACAS. Data are expressed as the means ± SE. $^*P < 0.05$, MMC versus MMC + dRHT group; b) The effect on macrophage phagocytosis against latex beads by dHLT after administrating MMC. The procedure of treatment was the same in the text. The macrophage migration capacity was detected by computer analysis, ACAS. The data was shown from normal mice; c) The effect on macrophage phagocytosis against latex beads by dHLT after administrating MMC. The procedure of treatment was the same in the text. The macrophage migration capacity was detected by computer analysis, ACAS. The data was shown from MMC-treated mice. Data are expressed as the means ± SE. $^*P < 0.001$, MMC versus MMC + dRHT group; d) The effect on macrophage phagocytosis against latex beads by dHLT after administrating MMC. The procedure of treatment was the same in the text. The macrophage migration capacity was detected by computer analysis, ACAS. The data was shown from MMC-treated and dLHLT rescued mice.

Futaba Co. Ltd. (Shizuoka, Japan). Both micronized and not micronized Propolis, *i.e.* native Propolis were insoluble in water, so we used 10% DMSO as a solvent.

4) The Measuring the Amount of Super Oxide Anion Generated by Murine Peritoneal Exudates Cells

Each drug was orally administered to mice (500 mg/kg) for one week. Two milliliters of 10% Oyster glycogen was injected intraperitoneally 10 hours before the assay. Sufficient murine peritoneal exudative cells were induced ten hours after the stimulation. Mice were euthanized by cervical dislocation, murine peritoneal exudates cells (PEC) suspension was centrifuged twice for 5 minutes at 1500 rpm at 4˚C. Then PEC was prepared to $1 \times 10^6$ cells/ml of HEPES buffer. One hundred microliters of cytochrome-c and 10 µl of PMA were added to the cell suspension and this was incubated for 20 minutes at 37˚C. The reaction mixture was then centrifuged for 10 minutes at 1500 rpm, 4˚C. An OD of supernatant was measured at both 550 nm and 540 nm, the amount of generated super oxide anion was shown in the formula; increased absorbance at 550 nm $(\Delta A_{550\text{-}540})/19.1 \times 10^3$ (mmol/ml). In order to ensure if we really measured the amount of generated super oxide anion or not, we tried to add super oxide anion dismutase (SOD), an enzyme for its anti-oxidative effect, into our experimental system. The result was as expected that the reduction of cytochrome-c was inhibited after the addition of SOD (**Figure 2**). This showed us that our experimental system could be used properly for measuring the amount of generated super oxide anion.

#### 2.2.9. Statistical Analysis

Data are expressed as means ± standard deviations. The differences between HF-treated and non-treated conditions were compared using a one-tailed analysis of variance. A $P$ value < 0.05 was considered to be statistically significant.

## 3. Results

### 3.1. Clinical Findings

#### 3.1.1 Changes in Cell Number of Total Leukocyte and Subsets

Leukocyte numbers have been counted one hour before and 15 days after the treatment of hemopoitic formula. The cell number measured one hour before the administration was set as 100%. Relative percentage of cell number on the 15th day was calculated. No significant changes were observed in G-group after the administration of BYT. However, significant change was found in L-type group (**Table 1**).

#### 3.1.2. Dividing Subjects into Two Groups, G-Type and L-Type by Granulocyte and Lymphocyte Proportion

The volunteers were healthy subject, with no drastic change for the total number of leukocytes. However, we

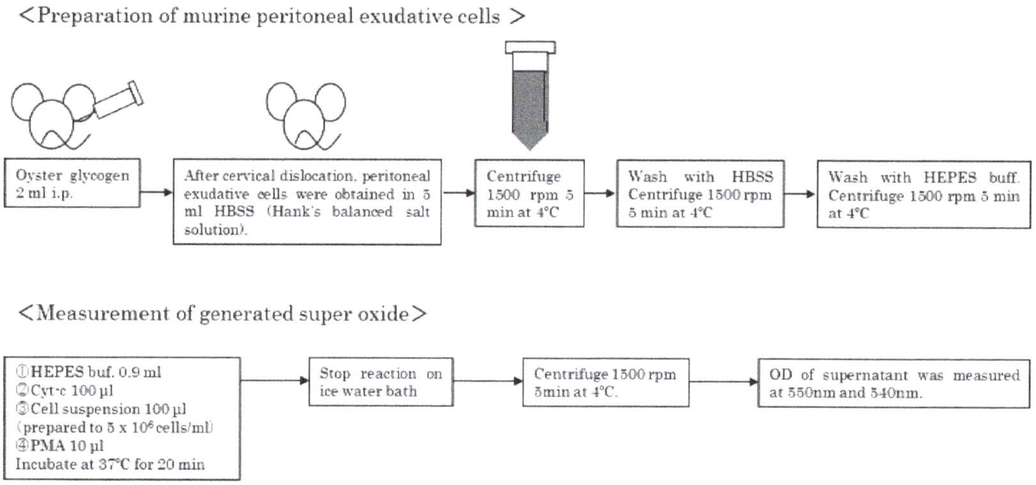

**Figure 2.** The effect on macrophage migration by dHLT after administrating MMC. The macrophage migration capacity was detected by millipore membrane method separated by 0.25 µm in diameter. Data are expressed as the means ± SE. $^*P < 0.05$, MMC versus MMC + dRHT group.

tried to check the regulative effect of herbal formulae for two different constitution, G-rich type and L-rich type. Analysis that mixed both groups together showed no significant differences in total leukocyte number except that for HF; in G-type group, total number of leukocytes was down regulated by SQT. This was a results of the down regulation of major group of leukocyte, granulocyte.

As for the L-type, no significant changes were found after the treatment of both HFs. In the L-type group, SQT, on the other hand, increased the tonal leukocyte and granulocyte in number, on the contrary to the down regulation for lymphocytes. To further clarify the influence of hemopoietic formula, we divided the subjects into two groups: the G-type group, who had a granulocyte count over 60%, and the L-type group, who had a lymphocyte count over 40%. In the L-type group, lymphocyte counts tended to decrease on day 15, accompanied by an increase in granulocyte numbers by SQT but not by BYT. On the contrary, the granulocyte counts of G-type group tended to decrease on day 15. The decrease of granulocyte count was raised by BYT, but not by SQT on day 15 (**Tables 1-3**).

### 3.1.3. Lymphocyte Subsets Showed Significant Variation

After HF treatment, cell counts of $CD2^+$, $CD4^+$, $CD8^+$, $CD11b^+$, $CD16^+$, $CD19^+$ and $CD56^+$ were tested to evaluate variations in T cells, B cells, macrophages and NK cells. These values were measured one hour before hemopoietic formula and 15 days thereafter. Our results showed that CD2 and CD4 cells were increased by both BYT and SQT. $CD11b^+$ and $CD14^+$ cell counts, which are closely associated with macrophage activity, increased by SDT in the L-type subjects. In particular, there was a remarkable increase in $CD11b^+$ cell number on day 15. T cell subsets that are closely associated with activity of immature T cells, ($CD2^+$, $CD4^+$ and $CD8^+$), the $CD2^+$ ($P < 0.05$) showed an increase with the treatment of BYT 15 days after administration. The number of

**Table 1.** Constitution dependent regulation of leukocyte by TCM.

| | G-type individual | | L-type individual | |
|---|---|---|---|---|
| | BYT | | SQT | |
| | Before | After | Before | After |
| Total WBC ($\times 10^3$ µl) | 6.95 | 5.88 | 3.82 | 5.04 |
| Lymphocyte (%) | 23.6 | 26.3 | 44.3 | 39.2 |
| Granulocyte (%) | 69.5 | 65.4 | 50.8 | 55.7 |
| Neutrophil (%) | 66.8 | 62.0 | 47.3 | 50.0 |
| Eosinophil (%) | 1.9 | 2.7 | 2.6 | 4.8 |
| Basophil (%) | 0.8 | 0.7 | 0.9 | 0.9 |

**Table 2.** Constitution dependent regulation of lymphocyte by TCM.

| CD | G-type individual | | L-type individual | |
|---|---|---|---|---|
| | BYT | | SQT | |
| | Before (%) | After (%) | Before (%) | After (%) |
| CD2 | 63.95 | 76.91 | 60.25 | 77.79 |
| CD4 | 19.75 | 28.53 | 31.05 | 45.14 |
| CD8 | 38.44 | 40.37 | 26.52 | 28.03 |
| CD11 | 73.54 | 70.36 | 63.37 | 70.78 |
| CD14 | 0.03 | 0.05 | 0.08 | 0.01 |
| CD16 | 66.93 | 58.02 | 54.00 | 41.23 |
| CD19 | 8.33 | 8.00 | 8.39 | 7.26 |
| CD56 | 1.68 | 1.74 | 1.96 | 2.41 |

**Table 3.** Constitution dependent regulation of cytokine producing cell by TCM.

| Cytokine | G-type individual | | L-type individual | |
|---|---|---|---|---|
| | BYT | | SQT | |
| | Before (%) | After (%) | Before (%) | After (%) |
| IFN-$\gamma$ | 6.95 | 5.88 | 3.82 | 5.04 |
| IL-4 | 1.9 | 2.7 | 2.6 | 4.8 |
| IL-1$\beta$ | 0.8 | 0.7 | 0.9 | 0.9 |

$CD19^+$ cells, which is closely associated with B cell activity, was not changed by both HF throughout the trial, neither were the numbers of $CD16^+$ and $CD56^+$ cells (**Table 2**).

#### 3.1.4. Cytokine Producing Cells

To test whether herbal decoction affected the functional maturation of immunocytes in a short time, we investigated the number of cytokine producing/containing cells by FACS analysis. This method reveals cytokine producing cell number by peering off the surface of lymphocyte, enable to express the number of cells in festival evening, compare than serum cytokine level that correspond to the paper tips of post festival. To determine whether HF influences functional maturation of immuno-competent cells, levels of IL-1$\beta$-, IL-4- and IFN-$\gamma$-expressed T cells were further examined using fluorescence-activated cell sorter analyses. There was a significant increase in the levels of IFN-$\gamma$ and IL-4 containing cells after administration of SQT. The result revealed that IFN-$\gamma$ expression, which increased highly on the 15th day after treatment, was different from the expression of IL-1$\beta$ and IL-4, those on the other hand, exponentially increased on day 15 after the administration of SQT. The augmentation of cytokine expression was confirmed by a classical method in the lymphoid organ, *i.e.* antibody-forming cells and plaque-forming cells. Both HFs down-regulated IL-1$\beta$ producing cells in both G-type and L-type groups (**Table 3**).

### 3.2. Animal Test

#### 3.2.1. Recovery of Whole Body Weight by HE

The body weight and thymus weight reduced in bone marrow-suppressed mice, resulting in the reduction of peripheral blood leukocyte to around 40%. After administered each herbal decoction 1 g/kg dairy for 5 days and after 1 week later, their blood were recovered to around 90% of normal value (**Figure 3**).

#### 3.2.2. Recovery of Thymus Weight

The bone marrow-suppressed mice were administered HF 1 g/kg dairy for 5 days, and one week later, their blood was withdrawn from their tail vein. The cell count of the peripheral blood is showed in **Figure 3** shows that the thymus weight decreased to half of normal control after 5 mg/kg of MMC was injected. However, all the three HFs recovered thymus weight to about 70% of the control.

#### 3.2.3. Recovery of $CD^+$ Cells and Cytokine Producing Cells

CD3, CD4 and CD19 cells of MMC treated mice were recovered to almost normal values after the administration of HFs. As for the functional recovery, IFN-$\gamma$ and IL-4 producing cells were also recovered by the all three decoction, including HFs and a functionally depressive agent of TCM. In cytokine producing cells, IFN-$r$ and IL-4 producing cell were recovered with HF. In all the three HFs tested, cytokine producing cells were recovered with HF and even by the formulae of sCRT (**Figure 4**).

#### 3.2.4. Recovery of Macrophage Activity, Phagocytosis by HF

**Figure 5** shows that MMC clearly suppressed the phagocytic activity of mice both in number and function. After the treatment of HF, the mice recovered their phagocytic activity to normal range. With a precise observation, the recovery activity was different between SQT and BYT. SQT was the strongest HF among the four formulae to augment in number and function of phagocytes. On the other hand, the augmentation by BYT was less than that by SQT (**Figures 5-9**).

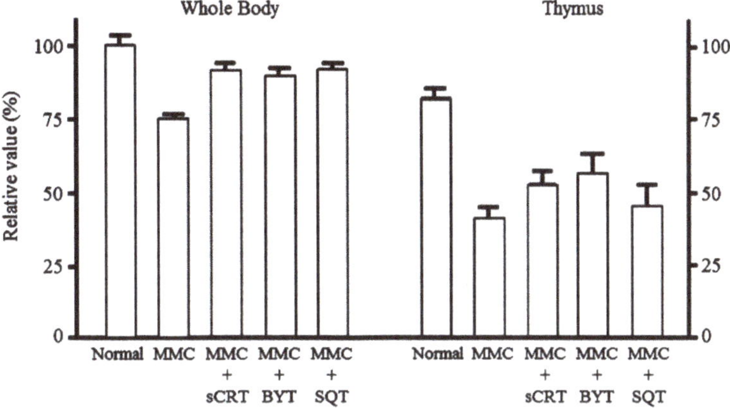


**Figure 3.** The effect on macrophage killing activity against revealed with NBT reduction by dHLT after administrating MMC. The procedure of treatment was the same in the text. The killing activity was detected by Nitro-blue Tetrazolium. Data are expressed as the means ± SE. $^{*}P < 0.001$, MMC versus MMC + dRHT group.

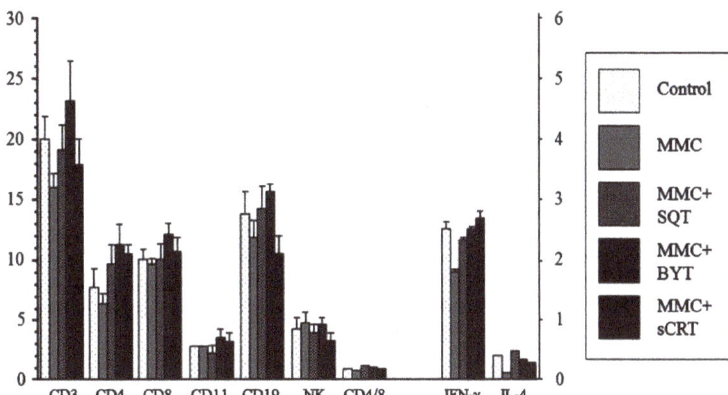


**Figure 4.** The experimental infection test were performed by the mice devided by 4 group. The groups were consisted by normal, MMC-treated, MMC-treated + dHLT, MMC-treated + dRHT plus chemotherapeutic agency vancomycin.

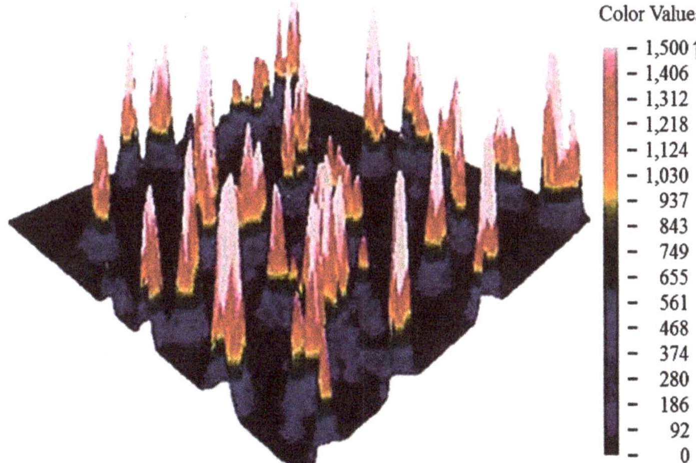


**Figure 5.** The number of MRSA counting in the organ that experimentally infected by $5 \times 10^6$ of microorganisms. Data are expressed as the means ± SE. $^{*}P < 0.001$, MMC versus MMC + dRHT group.

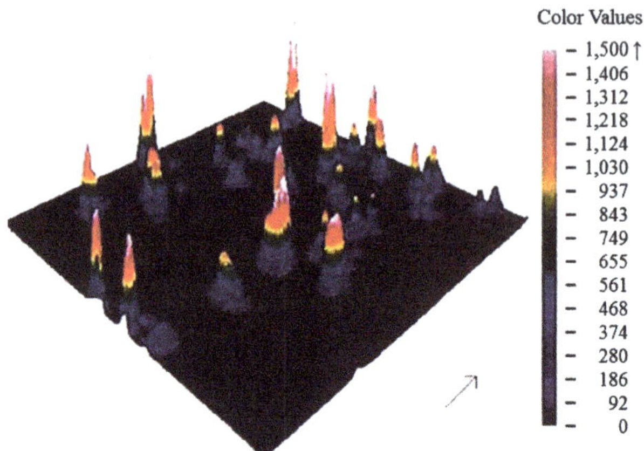


**Figure 6**. The site analysis that augmented by dHLT after inhibited by MMC. A granulocyte and lymphocyte were separate and adoptively transferred to MMC treated recipient mice. Then 5 × 1 MRSA were challenged and followed up their survival rate.

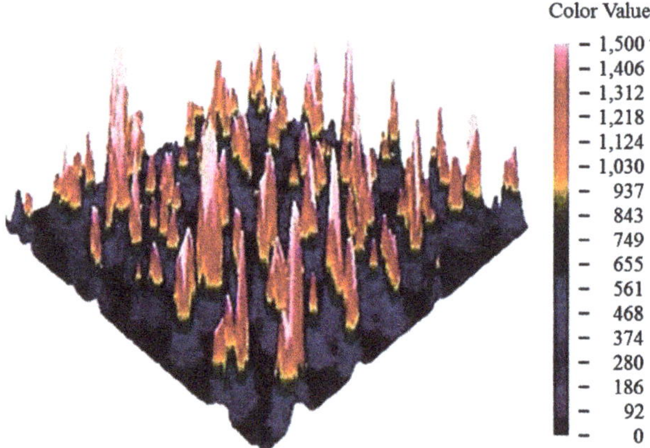


**Figure 7**. Human bed side test was done for stroke and/or heart infarction patient by dRHT. The herbal decoction, 8 g/head of dRHT was administered daily for at least one month. Then MRSA were chased by collecting sputa from the patient. The blood chemical data were shown in the figure.

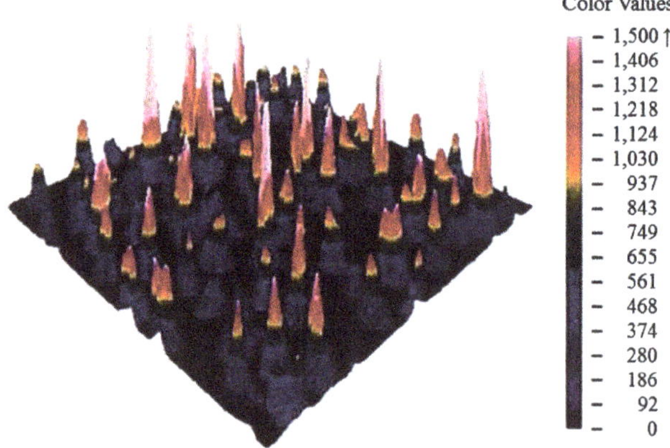


**Figure 8**. Human bed side test was done for the patient who were suffering heat infarction positive with administrating dRHT. The herbal decoction, 8 g/head of dRHT was administered daily for at least one month. Then MRSA were chased by collecting sputa from the patient. The MRSA containing from the patient sample were shown in the figure.

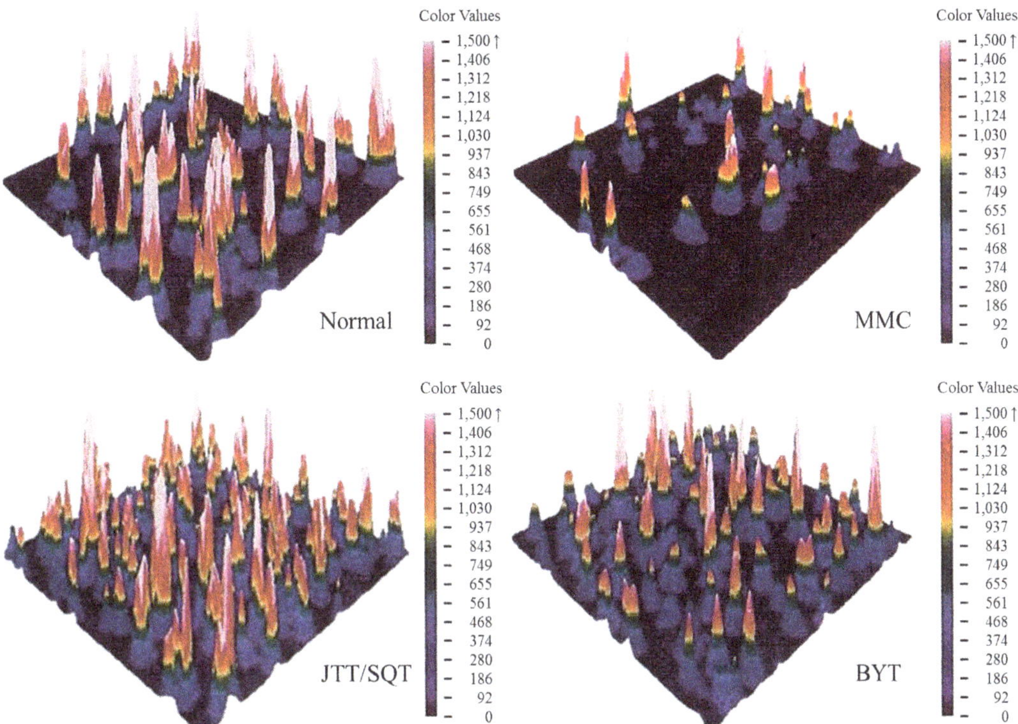


**Figure 9.** The clinical strain of multi-drug resistant bacteria were collected and incubated by various dose of sterile dRHT. After incubationg overnight, each bacteria was tested their drug sensitivity. The strains of clinical origin were *H. influluenzae* I-105, *H. influluenzae* I-147, *E. coli* ML 4901/Rms212, *E. coli* ML 4901/Rms213, *E. coli* ML 4901/Rte16, *E. coli* ML. 4901/Rms149, and *P. aeruginosa* PAO 0214/pMG26.

### 3.2.5. Recovery of Lymphocyte Activity, Antibody Secreting Cell

The bone marrow-suppressed mice were administered herbal decoction HF for five days. One week later, mice were immunized with sheep red blood cells, ($2 \times 10^8$/mouse) intraperitoneally. Four and six days later, their plague-forming cells (PFC) were developed. The ability of IgM and IgG antibody production was tested by the method reported by Jerne and Nordin [19] [20]. In this mouse model, MMC did not reduce the antibody forming cells significantly but the tendency was the same as shown in the former section. In this test, B was the most effective than that of A. BYT was the strongest material to augment antibody secreting cell among the four formulae (**Figure 10**).

### 3.2.6. Phagocytic Activity of Macrophage

So as to detect the supportive effect and important immunological stimulation by tonic agent, Bu-Ji, we traced the augmentation pattern of each remedy. As results of this trial, the phagocytic patterns by tonic agents, Bu-Ji, were clearly different from MMC-treated mice. Moreover, augmentation of phagocytes were different between each HF. SDT was prominent in activating phagocytes quantitatively and qualitatively compared to BYT.

We showed the diversity in the recovery pattern of HFs. Famous tonic remedies in China and Japan, SDT, strongly recovered phagocytic activity in compromised hosts, but the recovery by BYT was much less than that by SDT. The recovery level of phagocytic activity by sCRT was between SDT and BYT (**Figures 5-9**, **Table 4**).

### 3.2.7. The Amount of Generated Super Oxide Anion

The amount of generated super oxide anion was calculated in the formula shown above. The generated super oxide anion after one week administration of *Agaricus* and *Chlorella* were 2.64 and $1.95 \times 10^{-5}$ mmol/ml, respectively, whereas that was $2.85 \times 10^{-5}$ mmol/ml in control group. The generated super oxide anion after one week administration of herbal medicine, SDT, BYT and sCRT were 1.24, 1.25 and $2.88 \times 10^{-5}$ mmol/ml, respectively. The generated super oxide anion after one week administration of Propolis was $2.55 \times 10^{-5}$ mmol/ml. All these drugs, except for sCRT, decreased super oxide anion generation after administration for one week in

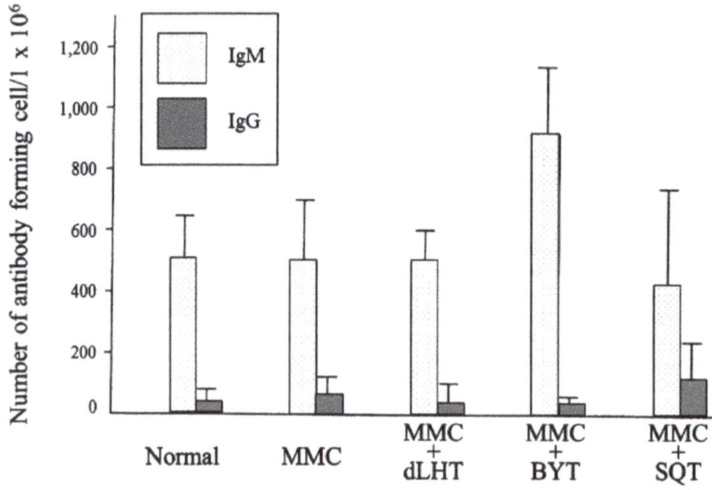


**Figure 10.** Recovery of antibody secreting cell.

**Table 4.** Relative activities of macrophage phagocytosis.

| | Phagocytosi | |
|---|---|---|
| | Positive Cells/10$^6$ cells | |
| | **Law active (%)** | **High active (%)** |
| Normal | 52 (100) | 45 (100) |
| MMC | 34 (65) | 5 (11) |
| MMC + SQT | 108 (207) | 59 (131) |
| MMC + BYT | 93 (178) | 12 (26) |
| MMC + GNT | 81 (155) | 46 (102) |
| MMC + dLHT | 73 (140) | 43 (95) |

mice (**Figure 11**).

### 3.2.8. The Comparison of Generated Super Oxide Anion between the Fermented and Not Fermented Herbal Medicine

Since the antioxidative effects of herbal medicine were demonstrated, we investigated the way to reinforce this effect. The fermentation is one of the possibilities. Since the fermentation is preceded by bacterial digestion and degradation, less efficient constituents would be lost than commonly used extraction by hot water. Therefore, we decided to ferment the herbal medicine by yeast (*Saccharomyces cerevisiae*), expecting the enhancement of its antioxidative effects. The generated super oxide anion after one week administration of fermented herbal medicine TCM, SDT, BYT and sCRT were 0.62, 0.84 and 1.50 × $10^{-5}$ mmol/ml, respectively. All the fermented herbal medicine decreased super oxide anion generation in compare with their corresponding unfermented ones (**Figure 12**, **Table 5**).

### 3.2.9. The Comparison of Generated Super Oxide Anion between the Pharmented and Original Propolis

The antioxidative activity of Propoils has been demonstrated, however, the particle of native Propolis was seen to be gross. In order to reinforce its antioxidative activity from physical constructive view point, we tried to micrified Propolis into 0.5 μm, expecting enlarged attachment area with reaction mixture. The generated super oxide anion after one week administration of micrified Propolis was 2.52 ×$10^{-5}$ mmol/ml, whereas that of non-micrified Propolis was 2.55 × $10^{-5}$mmol/ml. The antioxidative activity was slightly enhanced by micrifying the drug (**Figure 11**, **Table 6**).

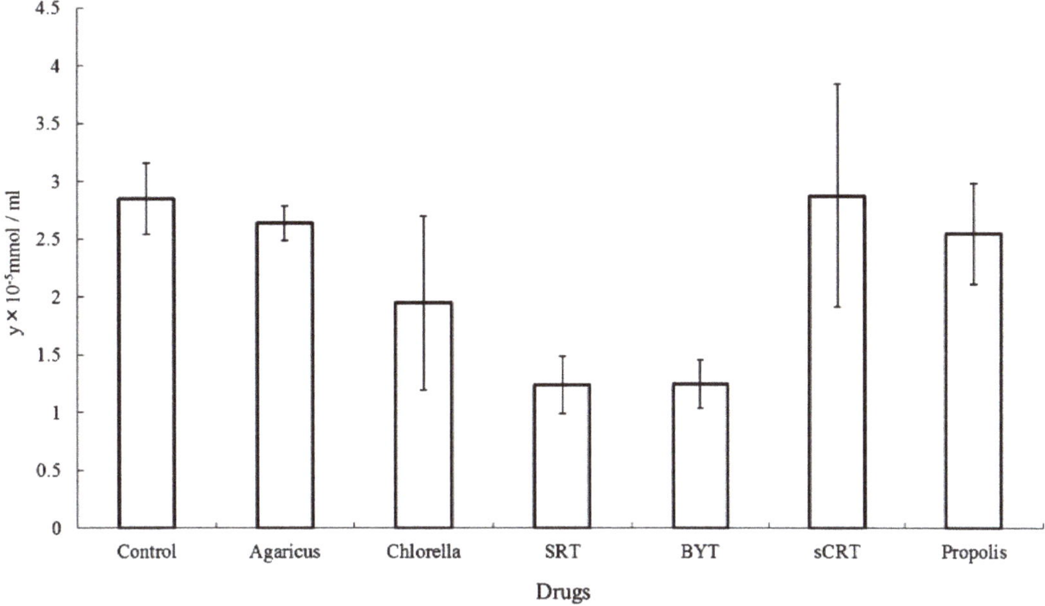


**Figure 11.** Anti-oxidative activity accessed by peritoneal macrophage.

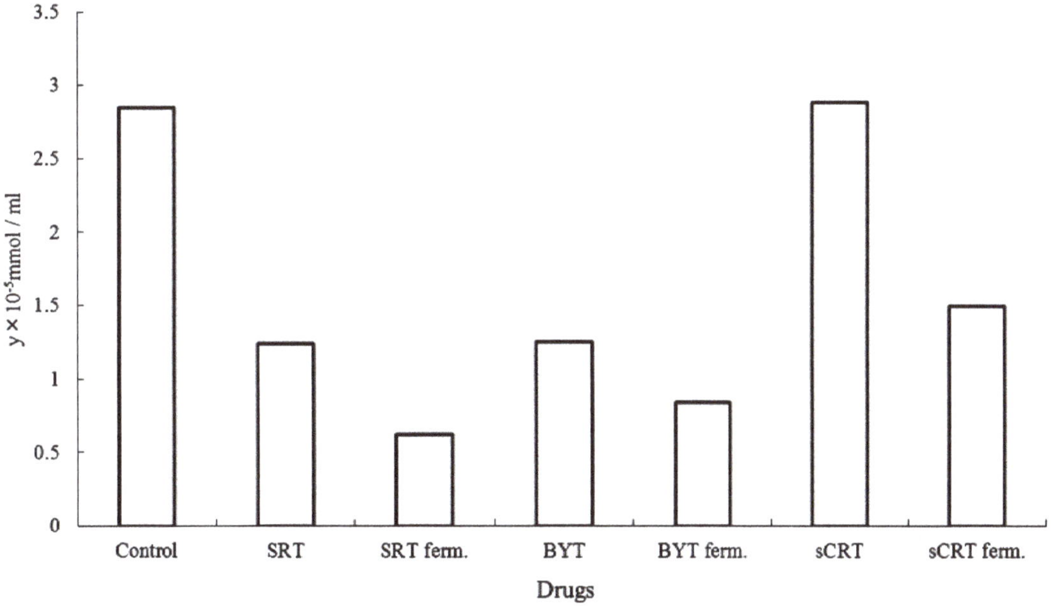


**Figure 12.** Effect of anti-oxidative activity on fermentation by yeast.

**Table 5.** Anti-oxidative activity by macrophages.

| Materials | Generated $O_2^-$ (×10$^5$ mmol/ml) |
|---|---|
| *Agaricus burazei* | 2.64 |
| *Chlorella pirenoidosa* | 1.95 |
| SQT | 1.24 |
| BYT | 1.25 |
| sCRT | 2.88 |
| Propolis | 2.55 |
| Control | 2.85 |

**Table 6.** Plaque forming/antibody secreting cell.

| Group Number | PFC/$10^6$ Spleen Cells |
|---|---|
| 1 Normal Mice | 543 ± 36 |
| 2 MMC Control | 203 ± 84 |
| 3 MMC + SQT | 486 ± 83* |
| MMC + fSQT | 656 ± 72** |
| 4 MMC + BYT | 553 ± 62* |
| MMC + fBYT | 776 ± 84** |
| 5 MMC + dLHT | 486 ± 55* |
| 6 MMC + sCRT | 352 ± 46* |

*$p < 0.01$ comparing to MMC control. **$p < 0.05$ comparing to non-fermented formulae.

### 3.2.10. Antibody Forming Cell Study by Parented TCM

Sheep erythrocyte (SRBC), a T-dependent antigen, was used for antibody formation cell study. Ten days after tumor transplantation, each antigen was intra-peritoneally injected. After four and six days, the antibody-forming cells were detected using localized hemolysis in an agar gel. Plaque-forming cells were developed by the method of Jerne and Nordin [19] [20].

The fermentation is preceded by bacterial digestion and degradation, less of the efficient constituents would be lost than commonly used extraction by hot water. Therefore we decided to ferment the herbal medicine by yeast (*Saccharomyces cerevisiae*), expecting the enhancement of lymphocyte activating effects through antibody forming cells. The antibody forming cells after one week's administration of fermented SQT and BYT were 135% and 140%, respectively. All the fermented herbal medicines from HF increased PFC (**Table 6**).

## 4. Discussion

Our investigation clarified how hemopoitic formula, also known as tonic agent and Bu-Ji, influenced the immune system (e.g. leukocyte, granulocyte and lymphocyte subsets in particular).

We quantified CD positive cell counts as indicators of T cells, B cells, macrophages and NK cells. For qualitative and quantitative evaluation, we examined the cytokine expression levels, and directly measured the expression levels of cytokine-containing cells in peripheral blood, eliminating possible artificial factors that could arise from culturing in test tubes or changes in net value by catalyzation. To avoid any possible influence from the circadian rhythm, we obtained the whole blood from all donors at the same time.

In this investigation, we confirmed that HF quantitatively and qualitatively regulated leukocytes, granulocytes, lymphocytes and their subsets. The increase of $CD2^+$, $CD4^+$, $CD8^+$, $CD11b^+$, $CD16^+$, $CD19^+$ and $CD56^+$ cell counts as well as the levels of IL-1$\beta$, IL-4 and IFN-$\gamma$ in blood cells suggested that hemopoitic formula might enhance the activities of humoral and cellular immunities, as well as NK cells. We also observed that levels of cytokine producing cells, in particular, increased rather than CD-positive lymphocytes, showing that HF augmented lymphocyte production qualitatively than quantitatively. Moreover, HF activated both CD11b cells and IL-1$\beta$ producing cells, suggesting the activation of phagocyte cells both in number and in function. Consequently, these data further demonstrated that HF acted in macrophages in the same manner as *Mycobacterium tuberculosis* that had cell walls constructed of waxy substances [13].

In previous reported about hot-spring hydrotherapy and acupuncture, we had proposed that immune system regulation was an important factor for evaluating CAM. Since other substances, such as endotoxin and waxy substances from *Mycobacterium tuberculosis*, similar to Proplis, were known for augmenting host immune responses. This time, we decided to focus solely on Propolis. A possible explanation for immune enhancement could be the activation of the circular system and/or autonomic nervous system, although the details of the mechanism remained unclear. Further research regarding to the mechanism was necessary.

Abo *et al.* reported that granulocyte count was increased by the excitation of the sympathetic nervous system, while lymphocyte count was increased by excitation of parasympathetic nervous system [14]-[18]. Our data also showed that granulocyte count was decreased in subjects with a high granulocyte count, while lymphocyte count was increased in the same subjects. The lymphocyte count, however, was decreased in subjects with a high lymphocyte level, while granulocyte count was increase in the same subjects. In other words, the subjects dominated by the sympathetic nerve could release stress, whereas the sympathetic activity of subjects who were dominated by the parasympathetic nerve might be excited by hemopoietic formula. This way, the cell counts appeared to converge at appropriate levels after hemopoietic formula. Finally, in order to determine whether the elevation of leukocyte counts resulted from an infection triggered by hemopoitic formula or not, the subjects were followed up for 8 days after the last administration of hemopoitic formula. During that period, we could not observe any infectious signs such as pyodermitis, fever, or enhancement of C-Reactive Protein (CRP). The value of CRP was 0.57 g/dl to 1.23 g/dl in our subjects, suggesting very mild inflammatory responses, which showed that hemopoitic formula did not cause infection. Since the meridian may influence cells throughout the body and may pass through every organ system, hemopoitic formula stimulation might provide maximum benefits without harmful side effects [21]-[25]. As an immune-enhancer, hemopoitic formula merits further investigation as a possible treatment for acquired immunodeficiency syndrome, chronic fatigue syndrome and other disorders that have been concerned throughout the world [26]-[28].

## References


[1] Blalock, J.E. (1989) A Molecular Basis for Bidirectional Communication between the Immune and Neuroendocrine Systems. *Physiological Reviews*, **69**, 1-32.

[2] Kitada, Y., Wan, W., Matsui, K., Matsui, K., Shimizu, S. and Yamaguchi, N. (2000) Regulation of Peripheral White Blood Cells in Numbers and Functions through Hot-Spring Bathing during a Short Term-Studies in Control Experiments. *Journal of Japanese Society Balneology Climatology Physiological Medicine*, **63**, 151-164.

[3] Yamaguchi, N., Takahashi, T., Sugita, T., Ichikawa, K., Sakaihara, S., Kanda, T., Arai, M. and Kawakita, K. (2007) Acupuncture Regulates Leukocyte Subpopulations in Human Peripheral Blood. *Evidence-Based Complementary and Alternative Medicine*, **4**, 447-453. http://dx.doi.org/10.1093/ecam/nel107

[4] Suzuki, S., Toyabe, S., Moroda, T., Tada, T., Tsukahara, A. and Iiai, T. (1997) Circadian Rhythm of Leukocytes and Lymphocytes Subsets and Its Possible Correlation with the Function of the Autonomic Nervous System. *Clinical Experimental Immunology*, **110**, 500-508. http://dx.doi.org/10.1046/j.1365-2249.1997.4411460.x

[5] Yamaguchi, N., Kawada, N., Ja, X.-S., Okamoto, K., Okuzumi, K., Chen, R. and Takahashi, T. (2013) Overall Estimation of Anti-oxidant Activity by Mammal Macrophage. *Open Journal of Rheumatology and Autoimmune Diseases*, **4**, Article ID: 42339.

[6] Hamada, M. and Yamaguchi, N. (1988) Effect of Kanpo Medicine, Zyuzentaihoto, on the Immune Reactivity of Tumor-Bearing Mice. *Journal of Ethnopharmacology*, **24**, 311-320.

[7] Tu, C.C., Li, C.S., Liu, C.M. and Liu, C.C. (2011) Comparative Use of Biomedicine and Chinese Medicine in Taiwan: Using the NHI Research Database. *Journal of Alternative and Complementary Medicine*, **17**, 339-346. http://dx.doi.org/10.1089/acm.2010.0200

[8] Jong, M.S., Hwang, S.J., Chen, C., Chen, T.J., Chen, F.J. and Chen, F.P. (2010) Prescriptions of Chinese Herbal Medicine for Constipation under the National Health Insurance in Taiwan. *Journal of the Chinese Medical Association*, **73**, 375-383. http://dx.doi.org/10.1016/S1726-4901(10)70081-2

[9] Lin, Y.H. and Chiu, J.H. (2011) Use of Chinese Medicine by Women with Breast Cancer: A Nationwide Cross-Sectional Study in Taiwan. *Complementary Therapies in Medicine*, **19**, 137-143. http://dx.doi.org/10.1016/j.ctim.2011.04.001

[10] Yamaguchi, N., Ueyama, T., Amat, N., Yimit, D., Hoxur, P., Sakamoto, D., Katoh, Y., Watanabe, I. and Su, S.Y. (2015) Bi-Directional Regulation by Chinese Herbal Formulae to Host and Parasite for Multi-Drug Resistant *Staphylococcus aureus* in Humans and Rodents. *Open Journal of Immunology*, **5**, 18-32. http://dx.doi.org/10.4236/oji.2015.51003

[11] Liu, J.P., Yang, H., Xia, Y. and Cardini, F. (2009) Herbal Preparations for Uterine Fibroids. *Cochrane Database of Systematic Reviews*, **4**, Article No. CD005292. http://dx.doi.org/10.1002/14651858.cd005292.pub2

[12] Murayama, T., Yamaguchi, N., Iwamoto, K. and Eizuru, Y. (2006) Inhibition of Ganciclovir-Resistant Human Cytomegalovirus Replication by Kampo (Japanese Herbal Medicine). *Antiviral Chemistry & Chemotherapy*, **17**, 11-16. http://dx.doi.org/10.1177/095632020601700102

[13] Abo, T., Kawate, T., Itoh, K. and Kumagai, K. (1981) Studies on the Bioperiodicity of the Immune Response. I. Circadian Rhythms of Human T, B and K Cell Traffic in the Peripheral Blood. *Journal of Immunology*, **126**, 1360-1363.

[14] Abo, T. and Kumagai, T. (1978) Studies of Surface Immunoglobulins on Human B Lymphocytes. Physiological Variations of Sig+ Cells in Peripheral Blood. *Clinical Experimental Immunology*, **33**, 441-452.

[15] Landmann, R.M., Muller, F.B., Perini, C., Wesp, M., Erne, P. and Buhler, F.R. (1984) Changes of Immunoregulatory Cells Induced by Psychological and Physical Stress: Relationship to Plasma Catecholamines. *Clinical Experimental Immunology*, **58**, 127-135.

[16] Iio, A., Ohguchi, K., Naruyama, H., Tazawa, S., Araki, Y., Ichihara, K., Nozawa, Y. and Ito, M. (2012) Ethanolic Extract of Brazilian Red Propolis ABCA1 Expression and Promote Cholesterol Effulux from THP-1 Macrophage. *Phytomedicine*, **19**, 383-388. http://dx.doi.org/10.1016/j.phymed.2011.10.007

[17] Kitada, Y., Okamoto, K., Takei, T., Jia, X.F., Chen, R., Yamaguchi, N., Tsubokawa, M., Wu, W.H., Murayama, T. and Kawakita, K. (2013) Hot Spring Hydro Therapy Regulate Peripheral Leukocyte Together with Emotional Hormone and Receptor Positive Lymphocytes According to Each Constitution/Condition. *Open Journal of Rheumatology and Autoimmune Diseases*, **3**, 140-153. http://dx.doi.org/10.4236/ojra.2013.33022

[18] Jerne, N.K. and Nordin, A.A. (1963) Plaque Formation in Agar by Single Antibody Producing Cells. *Science*, **140**, 405-408. http://dx.doi.org/10.1126/science.140.3565.405

[19] Jerne, N.K., Nordin, A.A. and Henry, C. (1963) The Agar Technique for Recognizing Antibody Producing Cells. In: Amons, B. and Kaprowski, H., Eds., *Cell-Bound Antibodies*, Wistar Institute Press, Philadelphia, USA, 109-125.

[20] Shih, C.C., Liao, C.C., Su, Y.C., Tsai, C.C. and Lin, J.G. (2008) Gender Differences in Traditional Chinese Medicine Use among Adults in Taiwan. *PLoS ONE Safety*, **17**, 609-619.

[21] Navo, M.A., Phan, J., Vaughan, C., Palmar, J.L., Michaud, L., Jones, K.L., Bodurka, D.C., Basen-Engguist, K., Hortobagyi, G.N., Kavanagh, J.J. and Smith, J.A. (2004) An Assessment of the Utilization of Complementary and Alternative Medication in Women with Gynecologic or Breast Malignancies. *Journal of Clinical Oncology*, **22**, 671-677. http://dx.doi.org/10.1200/JCO.2004.04.162

[22] Jyumonji, N. and Fujii, Y. (1993) A New Assay for Delayed-Type Hypersensitivity *in Vitro* Detection by the Macrophage Migration by Boyden Chamber. *Journal of Kanazawa Medical University*, **18**, 198-203.

[23] Wan, W., Li, A.L., Izumi, H., Kawada, N., Arai, M., Takada, A., Taru, A., Hashimoto, H. and Yamaguchi, N. (2002) Effect of Acupuncture on Leukocyte and Lymphocyte Sub-Population in Human Peripheral Blood Qualitative Discussion. *The Journal of Japanese Association of Physical Medicine, Balneology and Climatology*, **65**, 207-211

[24] Wang, X.X., Katoh, S. and Liu, B.X. (1998) Effect of Physical Exercise on Leukocyte and Lymphocyte Subpopulations in Human Peripheral Blood. *Cytometry Research*, **8**, 53-61.

[25] Yamaguchi, N., Takahashi, T., Sugita, T., Ichikawa, K., Sakaihara, S., Kanda, T., Arai, M. and Kawakita, K. (2007) Acupuncture Regulates Leukocyte Subpopulations in Human Peripheral Blood. *Evidence-Based Complementary and Alternative Medicine*, **4**, 447-453. http://dx.doi.org/10.1093/ecam/nel107

[26] Yamaguchi, N., Shimizu, S. and Izumi, H. (2004) Hydrotherapy Can Modulate Peripheral Leukocytes: An Approach to Alternative Medicine, Complementary and Alternative Approaches to Biomedicine. *Advances in Experimental Medicine and Biology*, **546**, 239-251. http://dx.doi.org/10.1007/978-1-4757-4820-8_18

[27] Murayama, T., Yamaguchi, N., Matsuno, H. and Eizuru, Y. (2004) *In Vitro* Anti-Cytomegalovirus Activity of Kampo (Japanese Herbal) Medicine. *Evidence-Based Complementary and Alternative Medicine*, **1**, 285-289.

[28] Abe, S., Yamaguchi, N., Tansho, S. and Yamaguchi, H. (2005) Preventive Effects of Juzen-taiho-to on Infectious Disease. In: Yamada, H. and Saiki, I., Eds., *Juzen-taiho-to* (*Shi-Quan-Da-Bu-Tang*): *Scientific Evaluation and Clinical Applications*, Traditional Herbal Medicines for Modern Times, CRC Press, Boca Raton, 18-22.

## Abbreviations

BYT; Bu-Zong-Ye-Qi-Tang: a famous TCM formula for augment blood cell in number and function.

CAM: Complementary and alternative medicine, beside the western medicine, there are many traditional medicine and/or health promoting menu all over the world.

CD; Cluster of differentiation. Each lymphocyte has name that expressed CD number, for example CD2, CD4, etc.

FCM; Flow Cytometry

G-rich type; The individual that exhibit over 60% of granulocyte in peripheral blood, finding many in young gentleman.

L-rich type; The individual that exhibit over 40% of lymphocyte in peripheral blood, finding lot in ladies and senile

SDT; Shi-Quan-Da-Bu-Tang: a famous TCM formula for augment blood cell in number and function.

sCRT; Shao-Chin-Rong-Tang: a famous TCM formula for allergic syndrome, suppressing lymphocyte in number and function

13

# Genetic Association of Interferon Gamma Induced Protein-10 (IP-10), *CXCL*-10 Gene Polymorphisms with TB Pleurisy Susceptibility in South Indian Population


**Ghousunnissa Sheikh[1], Venkata Sanjeev Kumar Neela[1], Satya Sudheer Pydi[1], Naveen Chandra Suryadevara[1], Ramulu Gaddam[2], Suman Latha Gaddam[3,4], Sai Kumar Auzumeedi[2], Vijaya Lakshmi Valluri[1,3*]**

[1]LEPRA-India, Blue Peter Public Health & Research Centre, Hyderabad, India
[2]Government Chest & General Hospital, Hyderabad, India
[3]Bhagwan Mahavir Medical Research Centre, Hyderabad, India
[4]Osmania University, Hyderabad, India
Email: *vijayavalluri@gmail.com, *vijayavalluri@leprahealthinaction.in



## Abstract

**_CXCL_-10 known as Interferon gamma-induced protein 10 (IP-10) or small-inducible cytokine 10 is a 8.7 kDa protein, which is secreted in response to IFN-$\gamma$ by monocytes, endothelial cells and fibroblasts. It has chemo-attraction for monocytes/macrophages, T cells, NK cells and dendritic cells in promotion of T cell adhesion to endothelial cells. In the present study, we investigated whether polymorphisms in _CXCL_-10 _gene_ have any role in the manifestation of Tuberculous (TB) pleurisy. Two SNPs in _CXCL_-10 promoter region (−1447A > G and −135G > A) were genotyped in patients with TB Pleurisy (n = 186), Pulmonary TB patients (n = 159) and healthy controls (n = 205) by PCR-RFLP. Disease associations were statistically analyzed by Fisher exact test. At the −135G > A position, the frequencies of genotype GA and allele G were significantly high in TB pleurisy patients compared to healthy controls. While the frequencies of genotype AA and allele A were significantly low in TB pleurisy patients compared to healthy controls. The frequency of haplotype A-G with the combination of 1447A > G and −135G > A was significantly high in TB pleurisy. Our results reveal that genotype GA and allele G at −135G > A position were strongly associated with susceptibility to tuberculous pleurisy. The GA genotype may be a useful genetic marker for early detection of the disease in high risk individuals.**



*Corresponding author.

## Keywords

***CXCL*-10, Polymorphism, Haplotype, Susceptibility, Tuberculous Pleurisy**

## 1. Introduction

Tuberculosis (TB) is a major global public health problem in developing countries with an estimated 1.4 million deaths and 8.7 million new cases reported in 2011 [1]. Pulmonary TB is the most common form of TB, with extra-pulmonary tuberculosis accounting for ~25% of adult cases, but this estimate increases to ~50% in high HIV prevalence settings [2]. Tuberculous (TB) pleurisy is the second most common form of extra-pulmonary tuberculosis after lymph node TB.

The occurrence of TB pleurisy is less than 1% of total exudative effusions in western countries out of which 3% - 5% corresponds to tuberculosis patients. However, in India, it is accountable for 30% - 80% of all pleural effusions encountered and may complicate tuberculosis in 31% of all cases [3] [4]. The first cells to encounter organisms invading the pleural space are mesothelial cells, which produce chemotactic molecules called chemokines, which are responsible for leukocyte activation and trafficking of cells for initiating inflammatory responses. Chemokines are low-molecular-weight chemotactic cytokines (8 - 14 kDa) that act through interactions with a subset of seven-transmembrane domain and G1protein-coupled receptors. There are 40 human chemokines, the majority of which are categorized as either C-X-C or C-C chemokines based on the arrangement of the two N-terminal conserved cysteine residues in mammalian genomes [5]-[7]. C-X-C motif chemokine 10 (*CXCL*-10) also known as Interferon gamma-induced protein 10 (IP-10) or small-inducible cytokine 10 is a 8.7 kDa protein and located on human chromosome 4 in a cluster among several other CXC chemokines [8]. In response to IFN-$\gamma$ *CXCL*-10 is secreted by monocytes, endothelial cells and fibroblasts. The principal function of *CXCL*-10 is chemoattraction of monocytes/macrophages, NK cells, T cells and dendritic cells. It also helps in promoting T cell adhesion to endothelial cells, antitumor activity, and angiogenesis [9] [10]. Earlier studies have revealed the association of gene polymorphisms with host susceptibility to various infectious diseases including TB [11]-[13]. Likewise the polymorphisms in chemokine genes were found to be associated with several autoimmune, infectious diseases including tuberculosis [14] [15].

*CXCL*-10 gene has been reported to play important role in the immune response to hepatitis and the innate immune response to respiratory tract pathogens including SARS, coronavirus and TB [16]-[18]. Recent studies have showed that chemokines are important as an early inflammatory mediator which determines the host immune response after exposure to pathogens. Tang *et al.* reported that polymorphism in the promoter region of *CXCL*-10 at −135G/A position was moderately associated with tuberculosis in Chinese population. The same variant was suggested to contribute to *CXCL*-10 *gene* expression by NF-κB transactivation [18]. Hence, we used a genetic association approach to study whether the variations in the promoter regions of *CXCL*-10 were associated with tuberculosis. The aim of the study was to investigate the association of *CXCL*-10 gene polymorphism (−1447 and −135) with PTB and TB pleurisy.

## 2. Subjects and Methods

### 2.1. Study Subjects

A total of 345 patients of which 159 had pulmonary TB (PTB), 186 with TB pleurisy and 205 healthy ethnically matched, un-related controls of South Indian population were included in the study. Pulmonary Tuberculosis (mean age ± SD: 43.8 ± 6.99) patients were registered at the Directly Observed Treatment Short course (DOTS) Clinics under the Revised National Tuberculosis Control program (RNTCP) centers at Bhagwan Mahavir Hospital & Research Centre, Blue Peter Public Health and Research Center (BPHRC) India. Tuberculous pleurisy subjects (mean age ± SD: 35.76 ± 15.10) were registered at Government General and Chest Hospital, Hyderabad, India. Healthy, asymptomatic subjects (mean age ± SD: 42.36 ± 20.14) with no familial history of TB were included as controls for this study.

### 2.2. Inclusion Criteria

Newly diagnosed patients with no past history of TB or anti-tuberculosis treatment were enrolled. PTB patients were clinically confirmed by sputum smear acid-fast bacilli (AFB) staining and chest X-ray (CXR) and TB pleurisy patients were diagnosed based on Adenosine Deaminase (ADA) levels with a cut off >40, biopsy and fine-needle aspiration cytology (FNAC), protein RBS, radiological chest X Ray (CXR) and non-positivity in acid-fast bacilli (AFB) staining [19]. Healthy controls were asymptomatic individuals without any past history of TB or any other major illness. Peripheral blood was collected from the subjects after obtaining written informed consent and ethical guidelines practiced at the Chest hospital, Mahavir Hospital & Research Centre and Blue Peter Research Centre (BPHRC). The study was approved by institutional ethical and biosafety committee.

### 2.3. DNA Isolation

DNA was extracted from whole blood using Flexigene DNA kit (cat no # 51206) according to the manufacturer instructions (QIAGEN, Hilden, Germany). DNA concentrations were quantitated using nanodrop (ND-1000) spectrophotometer (Thermo scientifics, Wilmington, DE).

### 2.4. Genotyping of *CXCL*-10 (IP-10) Gene

Polymerase chain reaction (PCR) based restriction fragment length polymorphism (PCR-RFLP) was used for genotyping. Briefly, the reaction contained 100 ng of genomic DNA, 10 pM of specific primer along with 1x of Taq Master Mix (New England Biolabs) and adjusting the total volume to 25 µl PCR reaction mixtures with water. The PCR was set in a programmable thermal cycler (Bio-Rad Thermo scientific CA). PCR conditions were: initial denaturation at 95˚C for 5 min followed by 35 PCR cycles [95˚C for 30 sec, 60˚ for 45sec, 72˚C for 45 sec] and final extension at 72˚C for 10 min. The PCR product was used to perform the restriction enzyme digestion for 3 hrs with 1 unit of respective restriction enzymes (New England Biolabs, Inc, Ipswich, USA) at 37˚C and the digested product was subjected to electrophoresis on 3% agarose gel for 45 min at 80 V. The genotypes were determined based on product sizes compared to a 50 bp ladder. The primer sequences, annealing temperatures for PCR, restriction enzymes and the restriction digestion patterns are mentioned in **Table 1**.

### 2.5. Statistical Analysis

The results were analyzed utilizing Open Epi Open Source Epidemiologic Statistics for Public Health software (version 2.2.1, Emory University and Rollins School of Public Health, GA). Disease associations were examined by uncorrected chi square ($\chi^2$) and Fisher exact test. To determine Odds ratios (OR) with 95% confidence interval the 2 × 2 cross-tabulation method was used. Hardy Weinberg equilibrium (HWE) testing was done using SNP stats online software and haplotyping was performed using the Haploview software (version 4.2). A p value of ≤0.05 was considered statistically significant.

## 3. Results

### 3.1. Single Nucleotide Polymorphisms IP-10-1447 Position

The frequency of the homozygous GG genotype at −1447 position was significantly low in both PTB (p = 0.04, OR: 0.33, CI: 0.07 - 1.05) and in TB pleurisy (p = 0.007, OR: 0.21, CI: 0.03 - 0.75) compared to healthy con-

**Table 1.** Primer sequences, PCR product and RFLP patterns for IP-10 genes.

| polymorphisms *CXCL*-10 | Sequences of the primers (5'-3'orientation) | PCR product (bp) | RE enzymes | Annealing temp | RFLP pattern |
|---|---|---|---|---|---|
| −1447 A/G (rs4508917) | F-TTGGTCAGGGAATGGAAAAG<br>R-CGGTTTCCCACAGCTAATTC | 290 | SacI | 60 | AA-290<br>AG-290 + 145<br>GG-145 |
| −135 G/A (rs56061981) | F-CCGTTCATGTTTTGGAAAGTGA<br>R-GGGAAGTCCCATGTTGCAGATT | 123 | BstBI. | 60 | GG-123<br>GA-123 + 100<br>AA-100 |

Nelsons tang *et al.* 2009.

trols representing a negative association. The distribution of other homozygous AA, heterozygous AG genotypes, alleles A and G were similar in PTB and TB pleurisy groups compared to the healthy controls (**Table 2**).

## 3.2. Single Nucleotide Polymorphisms IP-10-135 Position

The frequency of the heterozygous GA genotype at −135 position was significantly high in both PTB (p = 0.0000001, OR: 3.48, CI: 2.18 - 5.56) and TB pleurisy (p = 0.0000004, OR: 2.86, CI: 1.85 - 4.42) compared to healthy controls indicating a positive association. The homozygous AA genotype was significantly low in both TB pleurisy (p < 0.0000001, OR: 0.20, CI: 0.11 - 0.37) and PTB (p = 0.0000001, OR: 0.10, CI: 0.04 - 0.22) compared to healthy controls respectively, indicating a negative association. The frequency of allele G was significantly high in PTB (p = 0.0001, OR: 1.79, CI: 1.32 - 2.43) and TB pleurisy (p = 0.0009884, OR: 1.60, CI: 1.12 - 2.2) compared to healthy controls indicating a positive association, while the frequency of allele A was significantly low in PTB (p = 0.0001, OR: 0.56, CI: 0.41 - 0.76) and in TB pleurisy (p = 0.0009, OR: 0.62, CI: 0.46 - 0.83) compared to healthy controls indicating a negative association (**Table 3**).

## 3.3. Haplotype of IP-10 (−1447 and −135 Position) Gene

On haplotype analysis (−1447 and −135 polymorphisms) four combinations were observed. The frequency of haplotype with A-G combination was significantly high (p = 0.003, p = 0.000006) in PTB and TB pleurisy; similarly the frequency of haplotype with A-A combination was significantly low (p = 0.001, p = 0.02) in both PTB and TB pleurisy respectively. The haplotype combination G-G frequency was significantly high (p = 0.02) in PTB alone whereas the frequency of haplotype combination G-A was significantly low (p = 0.02) in TB pleurisy respectively.

We observed that the frequency of A-G haplotype combination was over-representing in active pulmonary TB and TB pleurisy groups indicating their association with increased risk of developing these clinical forms of TB. The frequency of haplotype A-A combination appeared to be associated with resistance to pulmonary TB and TB pleurisy (**Table 4**).

## 3.4. Hardy-Weinberg Equilibrium

When the Hardy-Weinberg (HW) equilibrium test was performed, distribution of all genotypes in the healthy

**Table 2.** Frequency distribution of IP-10 (−1447 position) genotype. Genotype and allele frequencies of IP-10 (−1447 position) gene polymorphisms.

| Genotype distribution | AA vs other | | | AG vs others | | | GG vs others | | |
|---|---|---|---|---|---|---|---|---|---|
| **1447A/G** | **n (%)** | **p value** | **OR (CI)** | **n (%)** | **p value** | **OR (CI)** | **n (%)** | **p value** | **OR (CI)** |
| HC (205) | 90 (43.9) | - | - | 100 (48.7) | - | - | 15 (7.3) | - | - |
| TBpleurisy (186) | 90 (48.4) | 0.43 | 1.19 (0.78 - 1.82) | 93 (50) | 0.88 | 1.05 (0.69 - 1.59) | 3 (1.6) | 0.01 | 0.21 (0.03 - 0.75) |
| PTB(159) | 62 (39.0) | 0.40 | 0.81 (0.52 - 1.27) | 93 (58.4) | 0.08 | 1.48 (0.95 - 2.29) | 4 (2.5) | **0.04** | **0.33 (0.07 - 1.05)** |
| EPTB VS PTB | - | 0.08 | 1.47 (0.93 - 2.30) | - | 0.11 | 0.71 (0.45 - 1.11) | - | 0.55 | 0.63 (0.09 - 3.82) |
| **Allele distribution** | **A (%)** | **p value** | **OR (CI)** | **G (%)** | **p value** | **OR (CI)** | | | |
| HC (410) | 280 (68.3) | - | - | 130 (31.7) | - | - | | | |
| TB pleurisy (372) | 273 (73.4) | 0.13 | 1.28 (0.92 - 1.77) | 99 (26.6) | 0.12 | 0.78 (0.56 - 1.08) | | | |
| PTB(318) | 217 (68.2) | 0.99 | 0.99 (0.72 - 1.38) | 101 (31.8) | 0.99 | 1.0 (0.72 - 1.39) | | | |
| EPTB VS PTB | - | 0.14 | 1.3 (0.91 - 1.8) | - | 0.14 | 0.78 (0.55 - 1.1) | | | |

All the comparisons are with Healthy control vs. Pulmonary and Pleurisy patients. Values are represented in (n). p value calculated by Chi-Square and value ≤ 0.05 was considered significant. OR: odds ratio, CI: class intervals. HC: Healthy Controls, PTB: Pulmonary Tuberculosis, TBP: Tuberculous pleurisy.

**Table 3.** Frequency distribution of IP-10 (−135 position) genotype. Allele and genotype frequencies of IP-10 (−135 position) gene polymorphisms.

| Genotype distribution | GG vs others | | | GA vs others | | | AA vs others | | |
|---|---|---|---|---|---|---|---|---|---|
| **135 G/A** | **n (%)** | **p value** | **OR (CI)** | **n (%)** | **p value** | **OR (CI)** | **n (%)** | **p value** | **OR (CI)** |
| HC (205) | 47 (22.9) | - | - | 88 (42.9) | - | - | 70 (34.1) | - | - |
| TB pleurisy (186) | 41 (22) | 0.93 | 0.95 (0.57 - 1.57) | 127 (68.2) | **0.0000007** | **2.86 (1.85 - 4.42)** | 18 (9.6) | **<0.0000001** | **0.20 (0.11 - 0.37)** |
| PTB (159) | 36 (22.6) | 0.99 | 0.98 (0.58 - 1.65) | 115 (72.3) | **<0.0000001** | **3.48 (2.18 - 5.56)** | 8 (5) | **<0.0000001** | **0.10 (0.04 - 0.22)** |
| TBP VS PTB | - | 0.89 | 0.96 (0.56 - 1.66) | - | 0.4 | 0.82 (0.50 - 1.34) | | 0.1 | 2.02 (0.80 - 5.52) |
| **Allele distribution** | **G (%)** | **p value** | **OR (CI)** | **A (%)** | **p value** | **OR (CI)** | | | |
| HC (410) | 182 (44.4) | - | - | 228 (55.6) | | - | | | |
| TB pleurisy (372) | 209 (56.18) | **0.001** | **1.60 (1.19 - 2.15)** | 163 (43.81) | **0.001** | **0.62 (0.46 - 0.83)** | | | |
| PTB (318) | 187 (58.8) | **0.0001** | **1.79 (1.31 - 2.43)** | 131 (41.19) | **0.0001** | **0.55 (0.41 - 0.76)** | | | |
| TBP VS PTB | | 0.49 | 0.89 (0.66 - 1.23) | | 0.49 | 1.11 (0.81 - 1.52) | | | |

All the comparisons are with Healthy control vs. Pulmonary and Pleurisy patients. Values are represented in (n). p value calculated by Chi-Square and value ≤ 0.05 was considered significant. OR: odds ratio, CI: class intervals. HC: Healthy Controls, PTB: Pulmonary Tuberculosis, TBP: Tuberculous pleurisy.

**Table 4.** Haplotype combinations for IP-10 (−1447 and −135 position) polymorphisms. Haplotype frequencies of IP-10 gene polymorphisms in TB pleurisy and pulmonary TB. (a) TB pleurisy; (b) Pulmonary TB (PTB).

(a)

| TB pleurisy IP 10 | | | | |
|---|---|---|---|---|
| **Haplotype** | **Frequency** | **Case ctrl ratio** | **Chi square** | **p value** |
| A - G | 0.358 | 0.421, 0.302 | 11.84 | 0.0006 |
| A - A | 0.355 | 0.314, 0.392 | 5.086 | 0.024 |
| G - A | 0.159 | 0.128, 0.187 | 4.91 | 0.026 |
| G - G | 0.128 | 0.137, 0.120 | 0.517 | 0.472 |

(b)

| TB IP 10 | | | | |
|---|---|---|---|---|
| **Haplotype** | **Frequency** | **Case ctrl ratio** | **Chi square** | **p value** |
| A - A | 0.345 | 0.275, 0.395 | 10.76 | 0.001 |
| A - G | 0.344 | 0.406, 0.299 | 8.703 | 0.003 |
| G - A | 0.164 | 0.136, 0.184 | 2.859 | 0.090 |
| G - G | 0.148 | 0.183, 0.123 | 4.878 | 0.027 |

p-value calculated by Chi-Square and value ≤ 0.05 was considered significant. OR: odds ratio, CI: class intervals. PTB: Pulmonary Tuberculosis, TBP: Tuberculous pleurisy.

controls followed HW equilibrium ($p < 0.05$). The p value for the position −1447 is $p = 0.07$ and for −135 is $p = 0.06$.

## 4. Discussion

Host genetic factors influence an individual response to infection with M. *tuberculosis.* These factors can possibly explain the susceptibility/resistance to the disease. Recent studies have shown that chemokines in addition to cytokines are crucial in mediating early inflammation which determines the host response after exposure to M. *tuberculosis* [20]. Since the polymorphisms studied (−1447 & −135) in *CXCL*-10 gene are located in promoter region they may affect the gene expression or its function leading to impaired signaling which may further cause susceptibility to tuberculosis.

Our data suggests the homozygous genotype GG at −1447 position renders resistance to both PTB and TB pleurisy respectively. Contrastingly Tang *et al.* reported no association of −1447 loci with tuberculosis in Chinese population [18]. The disparity in association may be due to difference in ethnic groups and the complex etiology of the disease.

Our data indicates that the heterozygous GA genotype at −135 position may render susceptibility while homozygous AA genotype was offering resistance to both PTB and TB pleurisy respectively unlike, Tang *et al.*'s report that homozygous GA genotype and allele A was offering protection to TB in Chinese population [18]. Also allele G was rendering susceptibility to both PTB & TB pleurisy which is in concordance with Deng *et al.* explaining allele G susceptibility to Hepatitis B virus infection [16].

The SNP-135 position is located 14 base pairs upstream of *CXCL*-10 gene, which has a binding site to *NF-kB* and may also affect the transactivation effect of *NF-kB* on *CXCL*-10 expression [18]. Therefore the genotype GA may play a crucial role in the genetic susceptibility to TB. Hence we conclude that individuals with GA genotype or G allele (−135 position) and GG genotype (−1447 position) may be vulnerable to PTB/TB pleurisy. Functional work based on allelic variants at these positions may provide further information on the mechanisms lying behind the susceptibility/disease progression which was one of the limitations of this study.

Our data reveals that the haplotype A-G, (−1447, −135) might render susceptibility while A-A, G-A may offer resistance to TB pleurisy. While haplotype A-G, G-G may confer susceptibility and A-A may offer resistance to PTB respectively. Contrarily Nelson Tang *et al* reported haplotype G-A-G at −1447, −872, −135 positions to offer resistance with the disease [18]. To best of our knowledge, this is the first study to report *CXCL*-10 (IP-10) genotype and haplotype association with tuberculous pleurisy in south Indian population.

## 5. Conclusion

We demonstrate that the promoter polymorphisms (−1447, −135) in *CXCL*-10 gene are associated with susceptibility to PTB and tuberculous pleurisy. The susceptible genotype GA, allele G and haplotype A-G and G-G could be used as genetic marker to identify high risk individuals. However, there is a need to validate the results in larger cohort and in other populations.

## Acknowledgements

The authors are thankful to The Department of Biotechnology (DBT), Government of India (BT/01/COE/07/02) for funding the project and LEPRA INDIA, Blue Peter public health & Research Centre for providing facility and support. Also to R.S.S. Sharada and D.K. Prudhula for their valuable suggestions in manuscript preparation and all the participants in the study.

## Ethical Approval

The study was approved by Institutional Ethical Committee (IEC).

## Funding

Department of Biotechnology (DBT), Government of India (Grant No: BT/01/COE/07/02).

## Conflict of Interest

The authors declare no conflict of interest. The funding agency had no role in the design of the study, collection and analysis of the data, or in the preparation of the manuscript.

## References


[1] World Health Organization (2012) WHO: Global Tuberculosis Report. WHO, Geneva, 100.

[2] Light, R.W. (2010) Update on Tuberculous Pleural Effusion. *Respirology*, **15**, 451-458. http://dx.doi.org/10.1111/j.1440-1843.2010.01723.x

[3] Sharma, S.K. and Mohan, A. (2004) Extrapulmonary Tuberculosis. *Indian Journal of Medical Research*, **120**, 316-353.

[4] Udwadia, Z.F. and Sen, T. (2010) Pleural Tuberculosis: An Update. *Current Opinion in Pulmonary Medicine*, **16**, 399-406.

[5] Yoshie, O., Imai, T. and Nomiyama, H. (2001) Chemokines in Immunity. *Advances in Immunology*, **78**, 57-110.

[6] Murdoch, C. and Finn, A. (2000) Chemokine Receptors and Their Role in Inflammation and Infectious Diseases. *Blood*, **95**, 3032.

[7] Zlotnik, A. and Yoshie, O. (2000) Chemokines: A New Classification System and Their Role in Immunity. *Immunity*, **12**, 121. http://dx.doi.org/10.1016/S1074-7613(00)80165-X

[8] O'Donovan, N., Galvin, M. and Morgan, J.G. (1999) Physical Mapping of the CXC Chemokine Locus on Human Chromosome 4. *Cytogenetic and Genome Research*, **84**, 39-42. http://dx.doi.org/10.1159/000015209

[9] Dufour, J.H., Dziejman, M., Liu, M.T., Leung, J.H., Lane, T.E. and Luster, A.D. (2002) IFN-Gamma-Inducible Protein 10 (IP-10; CXCL10)-Deficient Mice Reveal a Role for IP-10 in Effector T Cell Generation and Trafficking. *Journal of Immunology*, **168**, 3195-3204. http://dx.doi.org/10.4049/jimmunol.168.7.3195

[10] Angiolillo, A.L., Sgadari, C., Taub, D.D., Liao, F., Farber, J.M., Maheshwari, S., Kleinman, H.K., Reaman, G.H. and Tosato, G. (1995) Human Interferon-Inducible Protein 10 Is a Potent Inhibitor of Angiogenesis *in Vivo*. *Journal of Experimental Medicine*, **182**, 155-162. http://dx.doi.org/10.1084/jem.182.1.155

[11] Hill, A.V. (2001) The Genomics and Genetics of Human Infectious Disease Susceptibility. *Annual Review of Genomics and Human Genetics*, **2**, 373-400. http://dx.doi.org/10.1146/annurev.genom.2.1.373

[12] Hill, A.V. (2006) Aspects of Genetic Susceptibility to Human Infectious Diseases. *Annual Review of Genetics*, **40**, 469-486. http://dx.doi.org/10.1146/annurev.genet.40.110405.090546

[13] Bellamy, R. (2006) Genome-Wide Approaches to Identifying Genetic Factors in Host Susceptibility to Tuberculosis. *Microbes Infect*, **8**, 1119-1123. http://dx.doi.org/10.1016/j.micinf.2005.10.025

[14] Navratilova, Z. (2006) Polymorphisms in CCL2 & CCL5 Chemokines/Chemokine Receptors Genes and Their Association with Diseases. *Biomedical Papers*, **150**, 191-204. http://dx.doi.org/10.5507/bp.2006.028

[15] Smith, M.W., Dean, M., Carrington, M., *et al.* (1997) Contrasting Genetic Influence of CCR2 and CCR5 Variants on HIV-1 Infection and Disease Progression: Hemophilia Growth and Development Study (HGDS), Multicenter AIDS Cohort Study (MACS), Multicenter Hemophilia Cohort Study (MHCS), San Francisco City Cohort (SFCC), ALIVE Study. *Science*, **277**, 959-965. http://dx.doi.org/10.1126/science.277.5328.959

[16] Deng, G., Zhou, G., Zhang, R., *et al.* (2008) Regulatory Polymorphisms in the Promoter of CXCL10 Gene and Disease Progression in Male Hepatitis B Virus Carriers. *Gastroenterology*, **134**, 716-726. http://dx.doi.org/10.1053/j.gastro.2007.12.044

[17] Tang, N.L., Chan, P.K., Wong, C.K., *et al.* (2005) Early Enhanced Expression of Interferon-Inducible Protein-10 [*CXCL*-10] and Other Chemokines Predict Adverse Outcome in Severe Acute Respiratory Syndrome. *Clinical Chemistry*, **51**, 2333-2340. http://dx.doi.org/10.1373/clinchem.2005.054460

[18] Tang, N.L., Fan, H.P., Chang, K.C., *et al.* (2009) Genetic Association between a Chemokines Gene *CXCL*-10 (IP-10, Interferon Gamma Inducible Protein 10) and Susceptibility to Tuberculosis. *Clinica Chimica Acta*, **406**, 98-102. http://dx.doi.org/10.1016/j.cca.2009.06.006

[19] Gupta, B.K., Bharat, V. and Bandyopadhyay, D. (2010) Sensitivity, Specificity, Negative and Positive Predictive Values of Adenosine Deaminase in Patients of Tubercular and Non-Tubercular Serosal Effusion in India. *Journal of Clinical Medicine Research*, **2**, 121-126. http://dx.doi.org/10.4021/jocmr2010.05.289w

[20] Moller, M. and Hoal, E.G. (2010) Current Findings, Challenges and Novel Approaches in Human Genetic Susceptibility to Tuberculosis. *Tuberculosis* (*Edinb*), **90**, 71-83. http://dx.doi.org/10.1016/j.tube.2010.02.002

14

# Clinico-Radiological Correlation in Children with Ataxia Telangiectasia in Qatar

**Mohammad Ehlayel[1,2*], Mahmoud F. Elsaid[1,3], Rana Shami[3], Khalid Salem[4], Abdulbari Bener[5,6]**

[1]Weill Cornell Medical College, Doha, Qatar
[2]Section of Pediatric Allergy-Immunology, Department of Pediatrics, Hamad Medical Corporation, Doha, Qatar
[3]Section of Pediatric Neurology, Department of Pediatrics, Hamad Medical Corporation, Doha, Qatar
[4]Department of Radiology, Hamad Medical Corporation, Doha, Qatar
[5]Deptartment of Biostatistics & Medical Informatics, Cerrahpaşa Faculty of Medicine, Istanbul University, Istanbul, Turkey
[6]Department Evidence for Population Health Unit, School of Epidemiology and Health Sciences, The University of Manchester, Manchester, UK
Email: *mehlaye@gmail.com, *mehlayel@hmc.org.qa

## Abstract

**Introduction: Ataxia telangiectasia (AT) is a rare disease characterized by immunodeficiency and neurological manifestations. Ataxia, resulting from cerebella atrophy, runs a progressive incapacitating course. Clinical monitoring of the disease course is mandatory for early treatment. Aim: To study clinical severity of AT and correlate it with the degree of cerebellar atrophy. Patients and Methods: We retrospectively studied all children (less than 14 years) with AT seen at Hamad General Hospital Clinics between 1998-2013. We collected basic demographic data, parental consanguinity, family history, AT clinical severity scores, and reviewed CBC with differential counts; alpha-fetoprotein, serum immunoglobulins and lymphocyte subsets. Cranial MRI scans of each subject were reviewed by a neuroradiologist. Cerebellar atrophy was visually and semi-quantitatively scored. Results: We analyzed data on 18 AT children (10 males and 8 females), mean age of 76.9 months. 77.8% had a positive family history of AT and 41.7% parental consanguinity. Lymphopenia was observed in 77.8% and high serum alpha-fetoprotein in 87.5% of children. Clinical severity of ataxia was 17.1 ± 8.4 (mean ± SD); 86.7% of patients were moderate-severe. MRI cerebellar atrophy score was 1.9 ± 1.3 (mean ± SD), and moderate in 51% of patients. AT clinical severity score correlated (coefficient r = 0.566) but not statistically significant p = 0.088) with MRI cerebellar atrophy scores. Conclusions: Moderate to severe ataxia and marked cerebellar atrophy are quite common in AT children. There is a correlation between AT clinical severity and cerebellar**

*Corresponding author.

**atrophy. Larger prospective studies might further determine the significance of our observations and help practicing practitioners monitor the progression of the disease.**

## Keywords

**Ataxia Telangiectasia, Cerebellar Atrophy, MRI, Clinical Severity, Children**

## 1. Introduction

Ataxia telangiectasia (AT) is one of the rare, genetic, primary immunodeficiency diseases [1]. It is mainly characterized by immunodeficiency and neurological manifestations, with increased risk of infections, autoimmunity and malignancy [2]. It is caused by mutations involving ATM (ataxia telangiectasia, mutated) gene [3]. The ATM gene encodes for production of "serine/threonine kinase", an enzyme that has multiple important functions that lead to tumor suppression and DNA repair [4]. Mutations of ATM make cells prone to degenerative changes, most important of which neurodenegation. Studies of lymphoblastoid cell lines form AT patients revealed correlation between ATM mutations and clinical phenotype of the disease in these patients [5] [6]. Furthermore, the degree of ATM kinase activity determined the clinical severity of the disease [7].

Neurologic abnormalities of AT include truncal and limbs ataxia, dysarthria, swallowing incoordination, masked faces, ophthalmoplegia, and others such as delayed peripheral and movement disorders [2]. Although severe immunodeficiency may not be apparent in some patients [8], neurological features are constant and start in the first few years of life. Patients become wheelchair-dependent by early adolescence. Cerebellar atrophy, the hallmark of the disease, is related to neurodegenerative changes involving Purkinje cells [4] [9]. Head CT scanning was used in some studies, and MRI imaging is currently used for evaluation of cerebellar atrophy in AT patients [10]-[12]. Positron emission tomography has been utilized to study the functional aspects of the brain in these cases [13]. There are no studies trying to correlate the clinical severity of AT with that of cerebellar atrophy in either children or adults with the disease.

## 2. Objectives

In this study, we tried to categorize clinical severity of disease among AT children, score degree of cerebellar atrophy, and determine if there is any correlation between the clinical severity and degree of cerebellar atrophy.

## 3. Methods and Patients

In this retrospective cross-sectional study, we reviewed the medical records of all children, younger than 14 years, who were diagnosed (by ME, MFO) to have ataxia telangiectasia at Ped Allergy-Immunology and Ped Neurology Clinics at Hamad General Hospital between 1998 and 2013.

Each case record of AT children was reviewed, and data collected on a standard form, included patient's age, sex, nationality, parental consanguinity, and family history of AT.

Scale for assessment and rating of ataxia (SARA) was used with adaptation to be more practical for young ages [14]. Children were considered to be normal if AT Clinical severity score = 0, mild disease if score = 1 - 10, moderate if score = 11 - 20, severe if score = 21 - 30.

Laboratory workup included CBC with differential counts; alpha fetoprotein,; and immunological tests (serum IgG, IgA, IgM, IgE, IgG-subclasses, and lymphocyte subpopulations of T-cell subsets (CD3, CD4, CD8), B cell (CD19) and natural killer cell (CD56/16). Patient's age at time of head MRI was also noted.

Head MRI scan were independently reviewed by a senior experienced neuroradiologist (KS) who for cerebellar atrophy, brain stem, basal ganglia, cerebra, and thoracic spine. Cerebellar atrophy was visually and semi-quantitatively scored and graded into 4 Cerebellar Atrophy Severity Grades (CASG): a) normal CASG = 0, no abnormalities noticed; b) mild CASG = 1, mild, widening of few folia; c) moderate CASG = 2, where several sulci and cisterni are wide and fourth ventricle is prominent; and d) severe CASG = 3, where all sulci and cisterni are markedly wide. Other radiological abnormalities were observed. The Research Ethics Committee at Hamad General Hospital of Hamad Medical Corporation approved this study.

## 4. Statistical Analysis

Data was analyzed using Statistical Package for Social Sciences (SPSS version 21). Student-t test was used to ascertain the significance of differences between mean values of two continuous variables and confirmed by non-parametric Mann-Whitney test. Spearman's non-parametric correlation coefficient was used for determine the association between the two different scores. The level $p < 0.05$ was considered as the cut-off value for significance.

## 5. Results

A total of 18 patients with AT were seen during 1998-2013. **Table 1** demonstrates their basic characteristics. They were born to 12 families: 8 (44.4%) children were born to 5 (41.7%, of 12 families) consanguineous families, and 10 (55.6%) children belonged to non-consanguineous marriages. Having a high rate of positive family history of AT in the cohort helped diagnosing 8 patients (44.4%) before age of 5 years and 3 of them were less than 24 months. Elevated serum alpha-fetoprotein was demonstrated in 14 patients (16 of patients tested, 87.5%), and lymphopenia (defined by the presence of <3000 cells/μL of lymphocytes in peripheral blood in infants younger than 24 months, and <1500 cells/μL in older children) was observed in 14 (77.8%) patients. We utilized high alpha-fetoprotein and lymphopenia in presence of family history as laboratory markers on possibility of AT diagnosis even before clinical neurological or immunological abnormalities detected.

The median AT clinical severity score was 16, close to the average of 17.1. There was complete data of AT clinical score in 15 patients: 2 patients (11.1%) had mild ataxia, 9 patients (50%) moderate and 4 patients (22.2%) severe. Head MRI was done in 13 patients (72.2%). The average age of patients for head MRI scanning 102 ± 61.8 months (median = 102 months). The average grade of cerebellar atrophy on head MRI was 1.9 ± 1.3 (mean ± SD), median 2.0. Moderate cerebellar atrophy was noticed in 51% of patients. Sinusitis was incidentally observed in head MRI in 7 patients (38.9%).

Correlation of AT clinical severity score and MRI grade of cerebellar atrophy are shown in **Figure 1**. Ten patients had data on both AT clinical severity score and MRI cerebellar atrophy grades, and revealed correlation (coefficient $r = 0.566$) but it was not statistically significant ($p = 0.088$, 95% CI for $r = -0.2790$ to 0.8321).

**Table 1.** The demographic and laboratory characteristics of children with AT.

| Variable | N = 18 patients |
|---|---|
| Age (months, mean ± SD) | 76.9 ± 39.3 |
| Sex: | |
| Male | 10 |
| Females | 8 |
| M/F ratio | 1.25/1.0 |
| No. of families | 6 |
| Family history of AT | |
| Positive | 14 (77.78%) |
| Negative | 4 (22.2%) |
| White blood cells ($\times 10^3$ cells/μL)* | 5180 ± 1593 |
| Absolute lymphocyte count | 1894.0 ± 1093 |
| Alpha-fetoprotein (mg/L, mean ± SD) | 104.1 ± 91.7 |
| AT clinical severity score: | |
| Average (mean ± SD) | 17.1 ± 8.4 |
| Median | 16 |
| Mild | 2 (11.1%) |
| Moderate | 9 (50%) |
| Severe | 4 (22.2%) |
| No data | 3 (16.7%) |

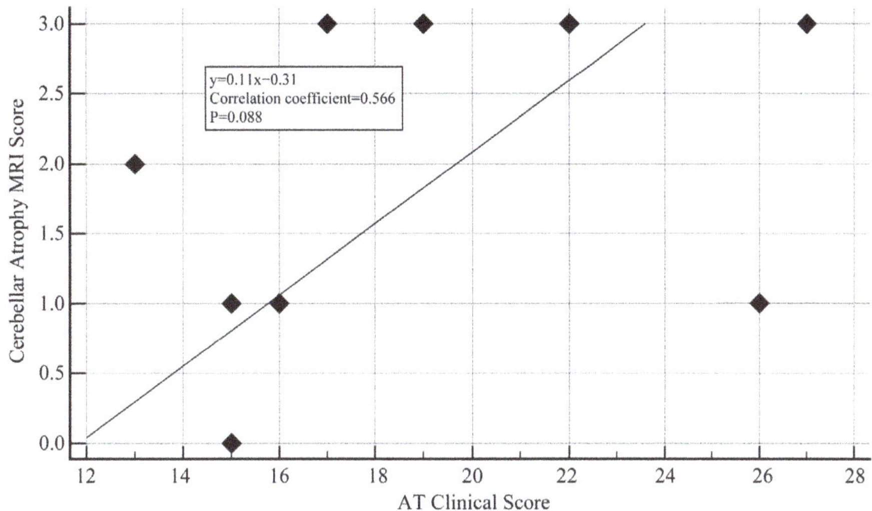


**Figure 1.** Correlation between clinical severity score AT and MRI cerebellar atrophy in children with AT.

## 6. Discussion

Among children or adults with AT, there are no studies on distribution of AT according to clinical severity, or any literature trying to correlate clinical severity with cerebellar atrophy. This study, to the best of our knowledge, is the first to describe how common the cerebellar atrophy, and objectively attempt to correlate the AT clinical severity with MRI imaging in this disease among children. More than 80% of our patients had moderate to severe AT, 85% had cerebellar atrophy, 62% of which was moderate to severe.

Medical literature is deficient on distribution of AT according to clinical severity. This could be attributable to lack of simple, quick, and reliable, age-dependent, clinical toolkits. Various studies indicate that clinical severity of AT is determined by type and severity of ATM mutations (e.g. null, missense, or specific types of mutations) affecting level or function of ATM protein [5]. This effect seems to be in a dose-dependent manner where milder phenotypes were reported late and in adults [7] [15] [16]. Different types of clinical severity scales (e.g. A-T Neuro Examination Scale Toolkit, International Cooperative Ataxia Rating Scale, Brief Ataxia Rating Scale) are used to evaluate or monitor the severity of adults-variants AT and other types of ataxias such as (Friedreich spinocerebellar ataxia) [17]-[22]. Validity and reliability of these scales in children with ataxia has recently been determined [23]. They are influenced by child's age [23]. This seems to be a factor that limits their routine clinical use in monitoring progression of AT in children. In our study, majority of patients had moderate-to-severe AT.

The fact that our study revealed a clinical but non-significant correlation between AT clinical score and severity of cerebellar atrophy could be attributed to some factors such as sample size and nature of study. A larger sample and prospective cohort study with serial AT clinical scores simultaneous with MRI scores done at specific age of each child might have increased the significance of the association.

Use of clinical score, as a clinical tool surrogate to MRI neuroimaging, for monitoring AT progression is important. MRI is used as the safe instrument to evaluate cerebellar atrophy in AT [24]. In our cohort, 85% our patients had cerebellar atrophy and correlated, though not statically significant, with clinical severity. The newer MRI-based newer techniques [25]-[27], such proton spectroscopy, functional MR imaging, and various diffusion-related imaging recently used in evaluating progressive ataxia may not be readily available to patients and in a cost-effective manner. Thus development of useful clinical toolkits sensitive to evaluate AT are essential.

Our study has some limitations, the foremost is the small sample size but this is inevitable. In 2014, the total of Qatar population reached 2,123,160 of whom 302,313 are children younger than 14 years [28]. The frequency of AT in Qatar is estimated to be 1 per 16,796 live births, still higher than reported in other regions of the world (in 40,000 to 100,000 people worldwide) [29], and due to high consanguinity rate among primary immunodeficiency diseases in Qatar [30]. Although our study revealed a correlation between clinical severity scales and cerebellar atrophy scores, a larger sample size most likely would have shown a statistical significance. Other limitations include the retrospective and cross-sectional nature of the study.

## 7. Conclusion

In summary, this study suggests that the majority of children with AT have moderate to severe clinical disease and high rates of cerebellar atrophy. Additionally, our data revealed correlation between clinical severity of the disease and that of cerebellar atrophy, and its statistical non-significance was most likely a result of sample size. Future studies of a larger population with a prospective designs comparing clinical severity with cerebellar structural and/ or functional abnormalities will further determine the significance of our observation. In addition, they would help practicing practitioners utilize clinical scales as a reliable clinical tool in monitoring the disease progression in AT children.

## Acknowledgements

The authors would like to thank Hamad Medical Corporation for their support and ethical approval (HMC Research Protocol No. 10078/10).

## Authors Contribution

The study proposal was prepared by Ehlayel, and data was collected by Ehlayel, Elsaid, Shami and Salem, analyzed by Bener. The manuscript was drafted, reviewed and approved by all authors.

## References

[1] Rezaei, N., Bonilla, F.A., Sullivan, K.E., de Vries, E. and Orange, J.S. (2008) Chapter 1. An Introduction to Primary Immunodeficiency Diseases. In: Rezaei, N., Aghamohammadi, A. and Notarangelo, L.D., Eds., *Primary Immunodeficiency Diseases, Definition Diagnosis and Management*, Springer-Verlag, Berlin, 1-38. http://dx.doi.org/10.1007/978-3-540-78936-9_1

[2] (2013) OMIM ATM: 208900. http://www.omim.org/entry/208900

[3] Savitsky, K., Bar-Shira, A., Gilad, S., Rotman, G., Ziv, Y., Vanagaite, L., Tagle, D.A., Smith, S., Uziel, T., Sfez, S., Ashkenazi, M., Pecker, I., Frydman, M., Harnik, R., Patanjali, S.R., Simmons, A., Clines, G.A., Sartiel, A., Gatti, R.A., Chessa, L., Sanal, O., Lavin, M.F., Jaspers, N.G., Taylor, A.M., Arlett, C.F., Miki, T., Weissman, S.M., Lovett, M., Collins, F.S. and Shiloh, Y. (1995) A Single Ataxia Telangiectasia Gene with a Product Similar to PI-3 Kinase. *Science*, **268**, 1749-1753. http://dx.doi.org/10.1126/science.7792600

[4] Hoche, F., Seidel, K., Theis, M., Vlaho, S., Schubert, R., Zielen, S. and Kieslich, M. (2012) Neurodegeneration in Ataxia Telangiectasia: What Is New? What Is Evident? *Neuropediatrics*, **43**, 119-129. http://dx.doi.org/10.1055/s-0032-1313915

[5] Gilad, S., Chessa, L., Khosravi, R., Russell, P., Galanty, Y., Piane, M., Gatti, R.A., Jorgensen, T.J., Shiloh, Y. and Bar-Shira, A. (1998) Genotype-Phenotype Relationships in Ataxia-Telangiectasia and Variants. *American Journal of Human Genetics*, **62**, 551-561. http://dx.doi.org/10.1086/301755

[6] Becker-Catania, S.G., Chen, G., Hwang, M.J., Wang, Z., Sun, X., Sanal, O., Bernatowska-Matuszkiewicz, E., Chessa, L., Lee, E.Y. and Gatti, R.A. (2000) Ataxia-Telangiectasia: Phenotype/Genotype Studies of ATM Protein Expression, Mutations, and Radiosensitivity. *Molecular Genetics and Metabolism*, **70**, 122-133. http://dx.doi.org/10.1006/mgme.2000.2998

[7] Verhagen, M.M., Last, J.I., Hogervorst, F.B., Smeets, D.F., Roeleveld, N., Verheijen, F., Catsman-Berrevoets, C.E., Wulffraat, N.M., Cobben, J.M., Hiel, J., Brunt, E.R., Peeters, E.A., Gomez Garcia, E.B., van der Knaap, M.S., Lincke, C.R., Laan, L.A., Tijssen, M.A., van Rijn, M.A., Majoor-Krakauer, D., Visser, M., van't Veer, L.J., Kleijer, W.J., van de Warrenburg, B.P., Warris, A., de Groot, I.J., de Groot, R., Broeks, A., Preijers, F., Kremer, B.H., Weemaes, C.M., Taylor, M.A., van Deuren, M. and Willemsen, M.A. (2012) Presence of ATM Protein and Residual Kinase Activity Correlates with the Phenotype in Ataxia-Telangiectasia: A Genotype-Phenotype Study. *Human Mutation*, **33**, 561-571. http://dx.doi.org/10.1002/humu.22016

[8] Spacey, S.D., Gatti, R.A. and Bebb, G. (2000) The Molecular Basis and Clinical Management of Ataxia Telangiectasia. *Canadian Journal of Neurological Sciences*, **27**, 184-191. http://dx.doi.org/10.1017/S0317167100000822

[9] Fatterpekar, G., Naidich, T.P. and Som, P.M. (2012) The Teaching Files: Brain and Spine Imaging. Elsevier Health Sciences, 102-103.

[10] Meshram, C.M., Sawhney, I.M.S., Prabhakar, S. and Chopra, J.S. (1986) Ataxia Telangiectasia in Identical Twins: Unusual Features. *Journal of Neurology*, **233**, 304-305. http://dx.doi.org/10.1007/BF00314163

[11] Lin, D.D.M., Barker, P.B., Lederman, H.M. and Crawford, T.O. (2014) Cerebral Abnormalities in Adults with Ataxia-Telangiectasia. *American Journal of Neuroradiology*, **35**, 119-123. http://dx.doi.org/10.3174/ajnr.A3646

[12] Sahama, I., Sinclair, K., Pannek, K., Lavin, M. and Rose, S. (2014) Radiological Imaging in Ataxia Telangiectasia: A Review. *The Cerebellum*, **13**, 521-530. http://dx.doi.org/10.1007/s12311-014-0557-4

[13] Volkow, N.D., Tomasi, D., Wang, G.J., Studentsova, Y., Margus, B. and Crawford, T.O. (2014) Brain Glucose Metabolism in Adults with Ataxia-Telangiectasia and Their Asymptomatic Relatives. *Brain*, **137**, 1753-1761. http://dx.doi.org/10.1093/brain/awu092

[14] Schmitz-Hubsch, T., du Montcel, S.T., Baliko, L., Berciano, J., Boesch, S., Depondt, C., Giunti, P., Globas, C., Infante, J., Kang, J.S., Kremer, B., Mariotti, C., Melegh, B., Pandolfo, M., Rakowicz, M., Ribai, P., Rola, R., Schols, L., Szymanski, S., van de Warrenburg, B.P., Durr, A., Klockgether, T. and Fancellu, R. (2006) Scale for the Assessment and Rating of Ataxia: Development of a New Clinical Scale. *Neurology*, **66**, 1717-1720. http://dx.doi.org/10.1212/01.wnl.0000219042.60538.92

[15] Saviozzi, S., Saluto, A., Taylor, A.M., Last, J.I., Trebini, F., Paradiso, M.C., Grosso, E., Funaro, A., Ponzio, G., Migone, N. and Brusco, A. (2002) A Late Onset Variant of Ataxia-Telangiectasia with a Compound Heterozygous Genotype, A8030G/7481insA. *Journal of Medical Genetics*, **39**, 57-61. http://dx.doi.org/10.1136/jmg.39.1.57

[16] Sutton, I.J., Last, J.I., Ritchie, S.J., Harrington, H.J., Byrd, P.J. and Taylor, A.M. (2004) Adult-Onset Ataxia Telangiectasia Due to ATM 5762ins137 Mutation Homozygosity. *Annals of Neurology*, **55**, 891-895. http://dx.doi.org/10.1002/ana.20139

[17] Burk, K., Schulz, S.R. and Schulz, J.B. (2013) Monitoring Progression in Friedreich Ataxia (FRDA): The Use of Clinical Scales. *Journal of Neurochemistry*, **126**, 118-124. http://dx.doi.org/10.1111/jnc.12318

[18] Crawford, T.O., Mandir, A.S., Lefton-Greif, M.A., Goodman, S.N., Goodman, B.K., Sengul, H. and Lederman, H.M. (2000) Quantitative Neurologic Assessment of Ataxia-Telangiectasia. *Neurology*, **54**, 1505-1509. http://dx.doi.org/10.1212/WNL.54.7.1505

[19] Schmitz-Hubsch, T., Tezenas du Montcel, S., Baliko, L., Boesch, S., Bonato, S., Fancellu, R., Giunti, P., Globas, C., Kang, J.S., Kremer, B., Mariotti, C., Melegh, B., Rakowicz, M., Rola, R., Romano, S., Schols, L., Szymanski, S., van de Warrenburg, B.P., Zdzienicka, E., Durr, A. and Klockgether, T. (2006) Reliability and Validity of the International Cooperative Ataxia Rating Scale: A Study in 156 Spinocerebellar Ataxia Patients. *Movement Disorders*, **21**, 699-704. http://dx.doi.org/10.1002/mds.20781

[20] International Cooperative Ataxia Rating Scale. http://checkyone.bplaced.net/dokus/ICARS.pdf

[21] Saute, J.A., Donis, K.C., Serrano-Munuera, C., Genis, D., Ramirez, L.T., Mazzetti, P., Perez, L.V., Latorre, P., Sequeiros, J., Matilla-Duenas, A. and Jardim, L.B. (2012) Ataxia Rating Scales—Psychometric Profiles, Natural History and Their Application in Clinical Trials. *The Cerebellum*, **11**, 488-504. http://dx.doi.org/10.1007/s12311-011-0316-8

[22] Schmahmann, J.D., Gardner, R., MacMore, J. and Vangel, M.G. (2009) Development of a Brief Ataxia Rating Scale (BARS) Based on a Modified Form of the ICARS. *Movement Disorders*, **24**, 1820-1828. http://dx.doi.org/10.1002/mds.22681

[23] Brandsma, R., Spits, A.H., Kuiper, M.J., Lunsing, R.J., Burger, H., Kremer, H.P. and Sival, D.A. (2014) Ataxia Rating Scales Are Age-Dependent in Healthy Children. *Developmental Medicine & Child Neurology*, **56**, 556-563. http://dx.doi.org/10.1111/dmcn.12369

[24] Sardanelli, F., Parodi, R.C., Ottonello, C., Renzetti, P., Saitta, S., Lignana, E. and Mancardi, G.L. (1995) Cranial MRI in Ataxia-Telangiectasia. *Neuroradiology*, **37**, 77-82. http://dx.doi.org/10.1007/BF00588526

[25] Currie, S., Hadjivassiliou, M., Craven, I.J., Wilkinson, I.D., Griffiths, P.D. and Hoggard, N. (2013) Magnetic Resonance Imaging Biomarkers in Patients with Progressive Ataxia: Current Status and Future Direction. *The Cerebellum*, **12**, 245-266. http://dx.doi.org/10.1007/s12311-012-0405-3

[26] Baldarcara, L., Currie, S., Hadjivassiliou, M., Hoggard, N., Jack, A., Jackowski, A.P., Mascalchi, M., Parazzini, C., Reetz, K., Righini, A., Schulz, J.B., Vella, A., Webb, S.J. and Habas, C. (2014) Consensus Paper: Radiological Biomarkers of Cerebellar Diseases. *Cerebellum*, **14**, 175-196.

[27] Wallis, L.I., Griffiths, P.D., Ritchie, S.J., Romanowski, C.A., Darwent, G. and Wilkinson, I.D. (2007) Proton Spectroscopy and Imaging at 3T in Ataxia-Telangiectasia. *American Journal of Neuroradiology*, **28**, 79-83.

[28] Ministry of Development, Planning, and Statistics (2013) Qatar Information Exchange. http://www.qsa.gov.qa/eng/index.htm

[29] Genetics Home Reference (2014) Ataxia-Telangiectasia. http://ghr.nlm.nih.gov/condition/ataxia-telangiectasia

[30] Ehlayel, M., Bener, A. and Abu Laban, M. (2013) Effects of Family History and Consanguinity in Primary Immunodeficiency Diseases in Children in Qatar. *Open Journal of Immunology*, **3**, 47-53. http://dx.doi.org/10.4236/oji.2013.32008

15

# A New Activated Water Charged by Electrophoresis, Effect on the Experimentally Immuno-Suppressed Animal and Their Anti-Oxidative Activity

**Yasuteru Eguchi[1*], Nobuo Yamaguchi[1,2], Nurmuhamamt Amat[3], Dilxat Yimit[3], Parida Hoxur[4], Kei Yokokawa[1]**

[1]Ishikawa Natural Medicinal Products Research Center, Ishikawa, Japan
[2]Department of Fundament Research for CAM, Kanazawa Medical University, Ishikawa, Japan
[3]Traditional Uighur Medicine Department, Xinjiang Medical University, Urumqi, China
[4]Traditional Chinese Medicine Hospital, Xinjiang Medical University, Urumqi, China
Email: [*]yas-tel@zpost.plala.or.jp

## Abstract

**Every individuals expose to the lisk of conventional immunodeficiency in daily life with both internal and externals. In a series of investigation, we have been assessed the various health promoting menu such as hot spring hydrotherapy, acupuncture & moxibution, light excurse, evidenced Control water western medicine technique. In this report, we try to investigate the regulatory effect of hydrotherapy by activated water molecule as our representative menu under the influence of hypothalamus system. We set up both animal and human model for assessment of hydrotherapy. Before starting experimental assessment, six males and females seven-week-old ddY mice, are used for the acute oral toxicity study. There is no sign for toxicity as judged by body weight, organ inspection by veterinary doctor. Next, young ddY mice are experimentally induced diabetes and immune-deficient status by administrating cancer chemotherapeutic agent, Streptzotosin. *Charged Water* was evident to control the blood sugar level compared to the *Control Water* group together with conventional control group. Both experimental group of mice wear statistically significant for recovery from blood sugar level and antibody secreting cell both IgM and IgG plaque-forming cell. We confirm also activated water group delivered the granulocyte that slow down the oxidative stress by super oxide.**

## Keywords

**New *Charged Water*, Hydrotherapy, Peripheral Leukocyte, Leukocyte Subsets Ratio, Diabetes**

[*]Corresponding author.

**Meritesanti-Oxidative Activity, CAM**

## 1. Introduction

In Japan, around 25% of the population is over 60 year old people. In aged people, diabetes meritus and acquired immune-deficiency brought depressive and reduction in Quality of Life (QOL). Any trials have been made as health prompting menu. The water itself has been known elsewhere in the world and served as historically and regionally. However, almost all of them are provided as non-data based manner. Here we try to show the special charged water with some evidence-based manner by the western medicine. This water is specially charged by magnetic resonance system, and has been taking for a therapeutic treatment of the health promoting supplement. However, induced the well known adverse reactions such as hypertension and other syndrome such in senile have been popular in world-wide. Therefore, we need safer supplement that are allowed to use for long-term therapy without any adverse reactions in digestive organs. Then, development of a new type of a health supplement that consists of foods and produces anti-oxidative and analgesic activities will be requested. The authors have already developed a new health water supplement, SRE. In this report, we would like to present the efficacy of *Charged Water* as health supplement in order to know the clinical efficacy (blood sugar level and anti-oxidative activity) of *Charged Water*. It is assessed by giving to normal animal as well human subjects as health promoting supplemental water. As a result, *Charged Water* promotes regulative activity for leukocyte subsets in number, blood sugar level and anti-oxidative activities. The popularity of complementary and alternative medicine (CAM) is an international trend in cancer therapy. Due to the severe side effects and limitation of their therapeutic efficacy of anticancer chemotherapeutic agents in the conventional cancer treatment, CAM will be expected to be able to improve clinical outcome and to reduce adverse reaction of anticancer drugs. The World Health Organization says that an estimated 80% of people worldwide are interested in traditional medicine.

It is well known in natural defense system, there are two primary systems: innate and adaptive. The innate and adoptive do not seem to guard or even prevent the development of one internal threat to survival, but direct sometimes to autoimmunity accompanying hypersensitivity. However, every individuals in the world expose to the lisk of immunodeficiency in daily life with both internal and externals. The factors that influence the acquired immune activity are systemic metabolic disorder such in diabetes meritus, malnutrition, extreme stress, senile and side effect by cellular activity in cancer cell [1]-[12]. So we have to select appropriate menu to regulate immune function through leukocyte storage. The menu has been summarized and listed as CAM: complementary and alternative medicine [13]-[18].

Throughout the world, the phenomenon of the natural hot hydro therapy spawns in the central Asia and East Asia and Europe. Mongolia has a long history of so-called immersion therapy recorded in Chinese or Mongolian medical works. In Gallo-Roman France, a most important number of documents, coins, various china, and votive stones survive from the province of Aquitaine. Even after two thousand years the therapeutic qualities of several mineral hot waters springs of that era are still recognized. This impressive history expands up into Germany, the Netherlands and through the whole of middle and Eastern Europe, extending as far as the well-known bathing centers and customs of Turkey. Japanese geological position on the edge of the Pacific Plate has given it volatile underpinnings, and are always changing and bursting forth in volcanic and earthquake activity. The legacy of this activity is the plethora of hot springs scattered all through its abundant islands. For centuries, these hot springs have been therapeutic destinations for the islands' inhabitants.

Traditionally, such in CAM has its own character and efficacy for various complaints. Through the years, each water source was evaluated for its specific properties and with the advent of better transportation in our mountainous land, even remote springs in the mountains were visited for their specific medicinal effect. For example, the hot spring of Fukatani, which is located just below our research facility, was known all over the area to cure hemorrhoids. However, almost all the judgments of efficacy are VAS (visual analog scale). The proprietors of the hot spring inns say that many of the guests came to cure that sort of ailment since about 20 years ago. Now in Japan, hot spring hydrotherapy is often used as a supplementary therapy for many diseases [19]-[21]. It has shown to reduce surgical complaints such as shoulder pain, amyloidosis and various rheumatic problems. It can also lighten the burden to the heart and improve the condition of patients who suffer from emphysema as well as other respiratory ailments. Hot springs have also traditionally functioned as places to relax and enjoy oneself, even though resort-type hot springs always exist along with those for illnesses. In recent years, trends have been seen that even remote hot springs, such as the one below our facility, transform into fashionable resorts for the healthy to visit for relaxation and stress release. It is interesting to note that this historical duplicity encompassed by hot springs has also entered the world of Western medicine as the release of mental stress and physical fatigue has been shown to be essential for good health. Put into other words: the relaxation side of the hot spring promotes prevention, including health enhancement, and the medicinal side, the treatment of illness. In our investigation, we measured the number of leukocyte subsets, granulocyte and lymphocytes regulated before and after hot spring hydrotherapy. Moreover, every individual expose to the lisk of immunodeficiency in daily life with both internal and externals stimuli. In this report, we tried to report the suitable menu for regulate the immune system modulate and discuss how we can compare and select each menu by evidence-based manner more than VAS.

The major purpose of this script is concern with the following issues. One is to confirm the effect of hot spring hydrotherapy within a short time is crucial or not. In other words, the reputational results are possible or not. The regulation was constitution/condition dependent manner and regulate the ideal value to each individual from the condition before the menu. The second was that this regulatory bias was coincides with other factors influenced by pituitary nervous system, such as emotional hormone and the hormone receptor positive lymphocyte. The third one was reputational effect can express linear function and could compared each other with the value of slope. We tried to discuss more, the possibility of the exhibition and comparison between, each menu and established medicine in East and West. The results showed that these subsets could reflect the number and function of immuno-competent cells. For example, in an individual with a low granulocyte number, the number increased after treatment, while it decreased in another individual with a higher cell number. Our results led us to believe that leukocyte subsets could be an interesting indicator for the evaluation of alternative therapies. Many systems are in place to evaluate Western therapies that aim at healing the symptoms of an illness. However, when the purpose of a therapy is to enhance the QOL of healthy people, such as some alternative medical therapies, it is not widely-accepted. Evaluation system has been established. To fill this lack, we would like to propose the umber and functions of leukocyte subsets as indicators for the evaluation of alternative therapies.

## 2. Subjects and Methods

### 2.1. Single and Multiple Dose Toxicity Study

Ten female seven-week-old ddY mice, were used for the acute oral toxicity study. The tests were carried out according to Ethics of the Organization for Economic Co-operation and Development (OECD) Test Guideline 401. The mice were housed at 24˚C ± 1˚C, 50% relative humidity. Both *Conventional* and *Charged Water* were suspended in sterile and administered to mice in free supplemental system, calculating daily consumption. Mice were weighted at 0 - 7 days after administration, and clinical observations were made once a day. Necropsy was performed on all mice seven days after administration.

### 2.2. Experimental Design for Bone Marrow Suppressed Immune-Compromised Mice

In the animal model of immuno-competency reduction, male C57BL/6J mice, aged 8 - 9 weeks, were injected with Mitomycin-C (MMC) (5 mg/kg) to inhibit the bone marrow. Then, *Charged Water* was administered orally and the *Conventional Water* was set up as control [22] (**Figure 1**, **Figure 2**).

### 2.3. Regulation of Total Leukocytes Number

The bone marrow-suppressed mice were administered herbal decoction FBT 1g/kg dairy for 5 days and after 1 week later, their blood were withdrawn from their tail vain. Then, the number of leukocytes was counted in Bürker-Türk solution.

#### 2.3.1. Regulation of Leukocyte Subsets

Bone marrow-suppressed mice were administered with *Conventional Water* and *Charged Water* for 30 days. One week later, the blood from their tail vain was withdrawn. Then the granulocyte and lymphocyte subsets were counted in Bürker-Türk solution.

#### 2.3.2. Regulation of CD Positive Cells

Cells from peritoneal exudates were collect from the peritoneal cavity of bone marrow-suppressed mice. Phagocytes were purified using adherent technique to get cell suspensions which contained more than 95% of phagocytes. The purified cells were loaded to the upper room of Boyden chamber to test migration ability at a concentration of $1 \times 10^4$ cell/ml. Human serum treated at 56˚C for 30 min was for the chemo tactic agent of mouse phagocyte [23].

#### 2.3.3. Regulation of Cytokine Producing Cells

The same cells suspension was purified by adherent technique for phagocyte, which produces cells contained more than 95% of phagocytes. The purified cells were adjusted to $1 \times 10^4$ cell/cm$^2$ and mixed with latex beads that are 5 μm in granule with fluorescence isocyanate. After 90 min of incubation, remained granule were washed out from the glass slide. Number of phagocytic cell and their ability to catch up the latex beads were automatically measured by ACAS system, which outputs the result in a digital form (Adeherent cell activity evaluating system; Shimazu, Kyoto, Japan).

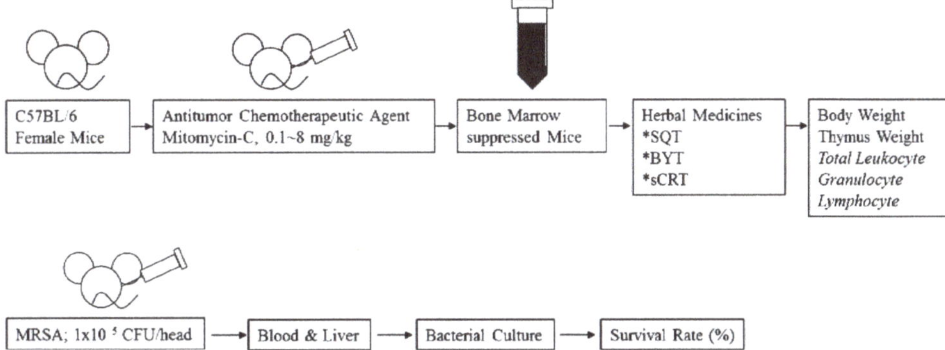


**Figure 1.** Experimental design for access the *Charged Water* for Immuno Compromised host in Mice. We sampled peripheral blood from the 12 volunteers before and after hot hydro therapy, at the same time on each day, in accordance with the consideration of circadian rhythm of leukocyte. The spring quality is a weak sodium chloride with sodium carbohydrate of the water temperature 40 ± 1C. During the night and in the morning of the next day, they had a bath in the hot spring two or three times, for 20 - 30 minutes each time. Time interval of blood sampling between before and after hot-spring hydrotherapy was approximately 24 hours. The total and differential leukocyte counts were measured control water he automated hematology analyzer.

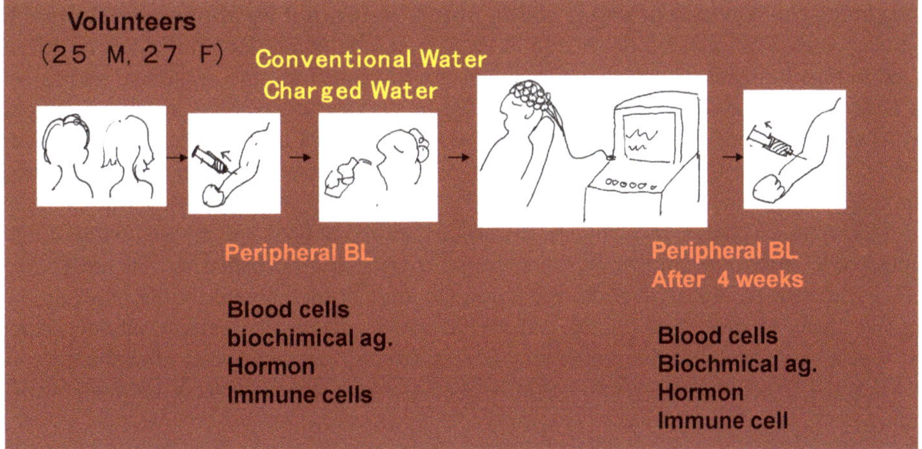


**Figure 2.** Experimental design for access the *Charged Water* for Immuno Compromised host in Human. We tried to express the effect of peripheral total leukocyte number by individual level of change and plot in the x-axis as in each age. Variations in leukocyte subpopulations in the peripheral blood before and after hot spring hydrotherapy.

### 2.3.4. Regulation of Lymphocyte Activity, Antibody Secreting Cell

The bone marrow suppressed mice were administered herbal decoction of FBT (1 g/kg/day) for 5 days. One-week later, mice were immunized with sheep red blood cells, (2 × $10^8$/mouse) intraperitoneally. Five days later, their spleen cells were collected. Plague-forming cells (PFC) were developed, and the ability of IgM and IgG antibody production was tested *Charged Water*, method reported by Jerne and Nordin [24].

### 2.3.5. Regulation of CD Positive Lymphocyte Distribution by *Charged Water* against Different Constitution

Whole blood obtained from the subjects was washed twice with PBS. One hundred micro-liters of the suspensions were stained with 20 μl of fluorescent monoclonal antibodies (anti-human $CD2^+$, $CD4^+$, $CD8^+$, $CD11b^+$, $CD14^+$, $CD16^+$, $CD19^+$ and $CD56^+$ antibodies). Ten thousands stained cells were re-suspended in PBS to detect surface markers by flow cytometry (FACS Calibur; Becton Dickinson Immnocytometry Systems, CA, USA).

### 2.3.6. Distribution of Cytokine Producing Lymphocytes in Different Constitution

The blood cell suspensions were cultured with PMA (phorbol 12-myristate 13-acetate), ionomycin and BSA (bovine serum albumin) for 4 - 5 hours at 37˚C. After that, the cell suspensions were stained using the monoclonal antibodies of PE-IL-4, FITC-IFN-$\gamma$ and FITC-IL-1$\beta$. Then they were analyzed by The FACScan (Becton Dickinson Co. Ltd. U.S.A.). The antibodies and reagents used in the test were purchased from Becton Dickinson Immunocytometry system (USA).

## 2.4. Animals

Eight week-old female C57BL/6 were purchased from Sankyo Laboratory Service Corporation (Shizuoka, Japan). All mice were kept under specific pathogen-free conditions. Mice food and distilled water were freely accessible for each mouse. Housing temperature and humidity were controlled 25˚C ± 1˚C and 60%.

### 2.4.1. Reagents

As for the basic medium, HEPES buffer (HEPES 17 mM, NaCl 120 mM, Glucose 5 mM, KCl 5mM, $CaCl_2$ 1 mM, $MgCl_2$ 1 mM) was prepared and sterilized by filtration. Phorbol 12-myristate 13-acetate (PMA, Sigma, USA) was diluted to $10^{-6}$ M by dimethyl sulfoxide DMSO, Sigma, USA) and used as a stimulant for super oxide anion generation for murine peritoneal exudates cells. Cytochrome-c (Sigma, USA) was diluted to 1 mM by HEPES buffer. Since cytochrome-c reduced by super oxide showed maximum absorbance at 550 nm, we used cytochrome-c to measure the amount of super oxide anion generation through spectro-photometrical technique. Oyster glycogen (type Ⅱ, Sigma, USA) was diluted in the purified water (10% w/v, Wako, Japan) and autoclaved at 120˚C for 20 mins. This solution was used for intraperitoneal injection to mice in order to induce peripheral neutrophils into the abdominal cavity [25].

### 2.4.2. Measuring the Amount of Super Oxide Anion Generated by Murine Peritoneal Exudates Cells

Each drug was orally administered to mice (500 mg/kg) for one week. Two milliliters of 10% Oyster glycogen was injected intraperitoneally 10 hours before the assay. Sufficient murine peritoneal xadate cells were induced ten hours after the stimulation. Mice were euthanized by cervical dislocation, murine peritoneal exudates cells (PEC) suspension was centrifuged twice for 5 minutes at 1500 rpm at 4˚C. Then PEC was prepared to 1 × $10^6$ cells/ml of HEPES buffer. One hundred microliters of cytochrome-c and 10 μl of PMA were added to the cell suspension and this was incubated for 20 minutes at 37˚C. The reaction mixture was then centrifuged for 10 minutes at 1500 rpm, 4˚C. An OD of supernatant was measured at both 550 nm and 540 nm, the amount of generated super oxide anion was shown in the formula; increased absorbance at 550 nm $(\Delta A_{550-540})/19.1 \times 10^3$ (mmol/ml). In order to ensure if we really measured the amount of generated super oxide anion or not, we tried to add super oxide anion dismutase (SOD), an enzyme for its anti-oxidative effect, into our experimental system. The result was as expected that the reduction of Cytochrome-c was inhibited after the addition of SOD. This showed us that our experimental system could be used properly for measuring the amount of generated super oxide anion.

## 2.5. Statistical Analysis

Data are expressed as means ± standard deviations. The differences between FBT-treated and non-treated conditions were compared using a one-tailed analysis of variance. A $P$ value < 0.05 was considered to be statistically significant.

## 3. Results

### 3.1. Mice System

#### 3.1.1. Single Dose and Multiple Dose Toxicity Study of *Conventional Water* and *Charged Water*

No deaths or abnormalities of body weight, water and food consumption, or coat condition were observed in the treated mice. Necropsy evaluation of the mice did not reveal any significant differences in thymus, liver, spleen, kidney, adrenal gland and testicle weights between the control group and both control water and charged and activated water.

#### 3.1.2. A Measuring the Amount of Super Oxide Anion Generated by Murine Peritoneal Macrophage

Each group of mice was orally administered freely from administrating bottle for one month. At the day for assay, two ml of 10% Oyster glycogen was injected intraperitonealy about 10 hours before the assay. Sufficient murine peritoneal exudate cells were induced ten hours after the stimulation (data not shown). Mice were euthanized by cervical dislocation, murine peritoneal exudate cells (PEC) suspension was centrifuged twice for 5 minutes at 1500 rpm, 4˚C. Then PEC was prepared to $1 \times 10^6$ cells/ml of HEPES buffer. One hundred μl cytochrome-c and 10 μl PMA were added to the cell suspension and this was incubated for 20 minutes at 37˚C. The reaction mixture was then centrifuged for 10 minutes at 1500 rpm, 4˚C. OD of supernatant was measured at both 550 nm and 540 nm, the amount of generated super oxide anion was shown in the formula; increased absorbance at 550 nm $(\Delta A_{550\text{-}540})/19.1 \times 10^3$ (mmol/ml) [25] (**Figure 3**, **Figure 4**).

#### 3.1.3. Experimental Model for Diabetes Meritus and the Effect of Hydrotherapy

Each group of ddY mice (female 8w-old) were administered Streptozotosin (STZ) in order to induced experimental diabetes meritus. Then each mice was orally administered freely for one mon The rate of diabetes model mice acquisition which can be used for an examination is about 50%.

Tail vein injection of STZ containing physiological saline solution was carried out at the control group.

STZ-Sterilization distilled water is given to a contrast group.

The influence of hydrotherapy was tested by employing the glucose tolerance-ability with orally loading (**Table 1**, **Table 2**).

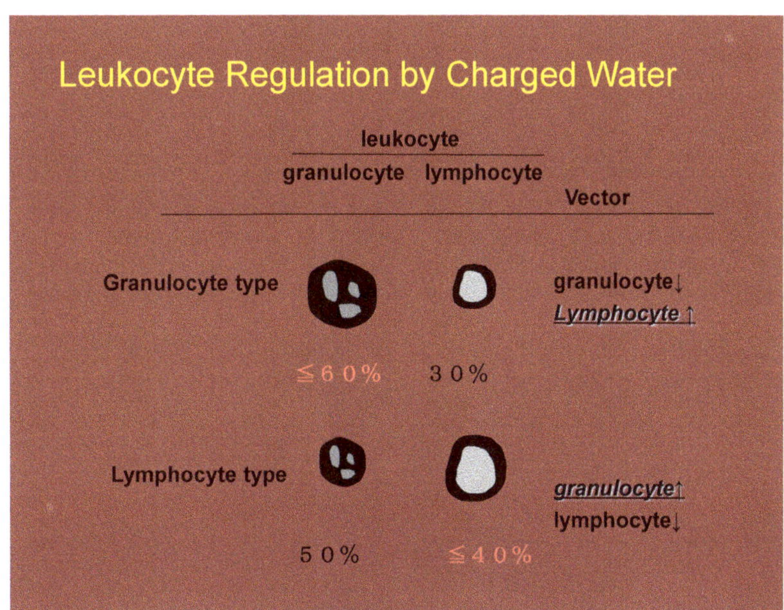


**Figure 3.** Leukocyte Regulation by *Charged Water*. We sampled peripheral blood from the 12 volunteers before and after hot spring hydrotherapy, at the same time on each day, in accordance with the consideration of circadian rhythm of leukocyte in this figure, we tried to show the date simply pooled and make mean, then compared.

### 3.1.4. Changes in Cell Number of Total Leukocyte and Subsets

Leukocyte numbers have been counted one hour before and 15 days after the treatment of hemopoietic formula. The cell number measured one hour before the administration was set as 100%. Relative percentage of cell number on the 15th day was calculated. No significant changes were observed in G-group after the administration of control water. However, significant change was found in L-type group (**Table 1**).

## 3.2. Dividing Subjects into Two Groups, G-Type and L-Type by Granulocyte and Lymphocyte Proportion

The volunteers were healthy subject, with no drastic change for the total number of leukocytes. However, we tried to check the regulative effect of herbal formulae for two different constitution, G-rich type and L-rich type. Analysis that mixed both groups together showed no significant differences in total leukocyte number except that for HF; in G-type group, total number of leukocytes was down regulated by *Charged water*. This was a results of the down regulation of major group of leukocyte, granulocyte.

As for the L-type, no significant changes were found after the treatment of both HFs. In the L-type group, *Charged Water*, on the other hand, increased the tonal leukocyte and granulocyte in number, on the contrary to the down regulation for lymphocytes. To further clarify the influence of hemopoietic formula, we divided the subjects into two groups: the G-type group, who had a granulocyte count over 60%, and the L-type group, who

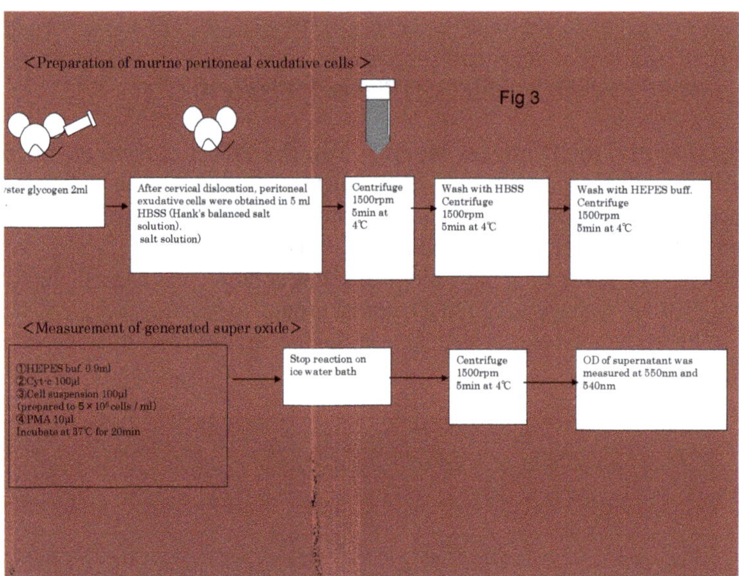


**Figure 4.** Protocol for Assessing the Effect by *Charged Water* for Anti-oxidative Activity in Macrophage. Each spot were obtained from the calculation comparing relative value from before and after levels in the serum, catecholamines levels in the peripheral blood. The constitution dependent analysis, the detail change and vector of each change could find from individual data, showing higher value volunteer down regulated much more than lower leveled one.

**Table 1.** Constitution dependent regulation of leukocyte *Charged Water*.

| | **G-type individual** | | **L-type individual** | |
|---|---|---|---|---|
| | ***Conv. Water*** | | ***Charged Water*** | |
| | **Before** | **After** | **Before** | **After** |
| Total WBC ($\times10^3$ μl) | 6.26 | 5.79 | 3.45 | 5.67 |
| Lymphocyte (%) | 23.7 | 25.8 | 43.1 | 42.5 |
| Granulocyte (%) | 65.5 | 65.7 | 56.7 | 57.8 |
| Neutrophil (%) | 64.6 | 52.4 | 45.7 | 51.3 |

had a lymphocyte count over 40%. In the L-type group, lymphocyte counts tended to decrease on day 15, accompanied by an increase in granulocyte numbers by *Charged Water* but not by *Conventional Water*. On the contrary, the granulocyte counts of G type group tended to decrease on day 15. The decrease of granulocyte count was raised by *Conventional Water* but not by *Charged Water* on day 15.

### 3.3. Lymphocyte Subsets Showed Significant Variation

After HF treatment, cell counts of $CD2^+$, $CD4^+$, $CD8^+$, $CD11b^+$, $CD16^+$, $CD19^+$ and $CD56^+$ were tested to evaluate variations in T cells, B cells, macrophages and NK cells. These values were measured one hour before hemopoietic formula and 15 days thereafter. Our results showed that CD2 and CD4 cells were increased by both *Conventional Water* and *Charged Water* $CD11b^+$ and $CD14^+$ cell counts, which are closely associated with macrophage activity, increased by *Conventional Water* in the L-type subjects. In particular, there was a remarkable increase in $CD11b^+$ cell number on day 15. T cell subsets that are closely associated with activity of immature T cells, ($CD2^+$, $CD4^+$ and $CD8^+$), the $CD2^+$ ($P < 0.05$) showed an increase with the treatment of *Conventional Water* and *Charged Water* 15 days after administration. The number of $CD19^+$ cells, which is closely associated with B cell activity, was not changed by both HF throughout the trial, neither were the numbers of $CD16^+$ and $CD56^+$ cells (**Table 2**).

### 3.4. Cytokine Producing Cells

To test whether herbal decoction affected the functional maturation of immunocytes in a short time, we investigated the number of cytokine producing/containing cells by FACS analysis. This method reveals cytokine producing cell number by peering off the surface of lymphocyte, enable to express the number of cells in festival evening, compare than serum cytokine level that correspond to the paper tips of post festival. To determine whether HF influences functional maturation of immuno-competent cells, levels of IL-1$\beta$-, IL-4- and IFN-$\gamma$-expressed T cells were further examined using fluorescence-activated cell sorter analyses. There was a significant increase in the levels of IFN-$\gamma$ and IL-4 containing cells after administration of *Charged Water*. The result revealed that IFN-$\gamma$ expression, which increased highly on the 15th day after treatment, was different from the expression of IL-1$\beta$ and IL-4, those on the other hand, exponentially increased on day 15 after the administration of *Charged Water*. The augmentation of cytokine expression was confirmed by a classical method in the lymphoid organ, *i.e.* antibody-forming cells and plaque-forming cells. Both HFs down-regulated IL-1$\beta$ producing cells in both G-type and L-type groups (**Table 3**).

### 3.5. Antibody Forming Cell Study by Parented *Charged Water*

Sheep erythrocyte (SRBC), a T-dependent antigen, was used for antibody formation cell study. Ten days after

**Table 2.** Constitution dependent regulation of CD Positive Cell by *Charged Water*.

| CD | G-type individual | | L-type individual | |
|---|---|---|---|---|
| | *Conv. Water* | | *Charged Water* | |
| | Before (%) | After (%) | Before (%) | After (%) |
| CD2 | 62.67 | 74.76 | 62.25 | 78.56 |
| CD4 | 20.34 | 29.87 | 32.34 | 46.56 |
| CD8 | 39.68 | 41.57 | 24.21 | 28.76 |
| CD11 | 73.54 | 71.77 | 63.65 | 73.57 |
| CD14 | 0.04 | 0.07 | 0.06 | 0.07 |
| CD16 | 64.44 | 57.56 | 55.65 | 50.76 |
| CD19 | 8.56 | 8.98 | 8.45 | 7.99 |
| CD56 | 1.76 | 1.77 | 1.67 | 2.65 |

tumor transplantation, each antigen was intra-peritoneally injected. After four and six days, the antibody-forming cells were detected using localized hemolysis in an agar gel. Plaque-forming cells were developed by the method of Jerne and Nordin [24].

The fermentation is proceeded by bacterial digestion and degradation, less of the efficient constituents would be lost than commonly used extraction by hot water. Therefore we decided to ferment the herbal medicine by yeast (*Saccharomyces cerevisiae*), expecting the enhancement of lymphocyte activating effects through antibody forming cells. The antibody forming cells after one week's administration of fermented *Conventional Water* and *Charged Water* were 135% and 140%, respectively. All the fermented herbal medicines from HF increased PFC (**Table 4**).

## 4. Discussion

Every creature in the world including human exposes to the lisk of immunodeficiency in daily life [26]. The factors that influence the acquired immune activity are systemic metabolic disorder such in diabetes meritus, malnutrition, extreme stress, senile and side effect by cellular activity in cancer cell. So we have to select daily an appropriate menu to regulate immune function through leukocyte storage. The menu has been summarized and listed as CAM: complementary and alternative medicine. One of the major menu is *Charged Water* in western medicine world, some trying o integrate Western Medicine and Eastern Medicine.

We have been trying to regulate the immune responsiveness through much mature for fragile daily condition from circumstance stress and so on. The main menu is acupuncture, hotspring hydrotherapy, light exercise etc. In this article, we would like to show the regulatory mechanism of the hot spring hydrotherapy. The circumstance, the balneotherapy using the effectiveness of the hydrotherapy, except for cases of contraindication, has been medically useful approved to be effective in many stress-related disorders and the improvement of dysfunction of the biological rhythm disturbance as well as chronic disease. The mechanism of effects has been reported in many studies, but many things are still unclear. Balneotherapy needs to be treated in general a period of time, but the effectiveness has been suggested even if the short duration hot-springs hydrotherapy. We examine the effect of hot spring hydrotherapy for a short duration on immune system and report about the quantitative and qualitative variation of immuno-competent cells [27]. The mechanism is suggested the association with an autonomic nervous system and the endocrine system. Hot spring hydrotherapy for a short duration is expected to stimulate sympathetic nerve or parasympathetic nerve and to change the levels of catecholamines (adrenalin, noradrenaline, and dopamine), which are neurotransmitters and hormones, as well as the number and function of immune cells.

**Table 3.** Constitution dependent regulation of Cytokine Producing Cell by *Charged Water*.

| Cytokine | G type individual | | L type individual | |
|---|---|---|---|---|
| | *Conv. Water* | | *Charged Water* | |
| | Before (%) | After (%) | Before (%) | After(%) |
| IFN-$\gamma$ | 6.87 | 5.33 | 3.46 | 5.45 |
| IL-4 | 1.6 | 1.7 | 2.8 | 3.8 |
| IL-1$\beta$ | 0.9 | 0.7 | 0.8 | 1.3 |

**Table 4.** Plaque Forming/Antibody Secreting Cell.

| Group Number | PFC/10$^6$ Spleen Cells |
|---|---|
| 1 Normal Mice | 348 ± 461 |
| 2 MMC Control | 58 ± 54 |
| 3 MMC + *Conventional Water* | 71 ± 21 |
| 4 MMC + *Charged Water* | 296 ± 55* |

*$p < 0.05$ comparing to MMC control.

Our results showed that within 24 hours after hot spring hydrotherapy, the white blood cells in peripheral blood had changed significantly, not only in cell count but also cell function. We hoped that our work would attract more attention to the mechanisms of which hot spring hydrotherapy regulates the human immune system. Abo reported that according to the lymphocyte subset content, lymphocyte rich type showed over 40% on the other hand granulocyte rich type show over 60% of granulocyte [17]-[30]. Each type exhibited different character even in the same age, sexuality and each age. In the figure, within the same age and the sex, even in mankind could sort out as G-rich type (granulocyte 60%), and L-rich type (lymphocyte 40%). On the other hand, as a stand point of sex difference, the ladies belonged to L-rich type but the man belonged to G-rich type. According to the age-related change, G-rich type of man changed to L-rich type within the same sex.

## References

[1] Kurashige, S., Yoshida, T. and Mitsuhashi, S. (1980) Immune Response in Sarcoma 10-Bearing Mice. *Annual Report of Gunnma University*, **1**, 36-44.

[2] Miyazaki, S. (1977) Immunodificiency in Clinical Origin. *Clinical Pediatrics*, 1001-1006.

[3] Kishida, K., Miyazaku, S., Take, H., Fujimoto, T., Shi, H., Sasaki, K. and Goya, N. (1978) Granial Irradiation and Lymphocyte Subpopulation in Acute Lymphatic Leukemia. *Journal of Pediatrics*, **92**, 785-786. http://dx.doi.org/10.1016/S0022-3476(78)80155-3

[4] Yamaguchi, N., Takei, T., Chen, R., Wushuer, P. and Wu, H.W. (2013) Maternal Bias of Immunity to Her Offspring: Possibility of an Autoimmunity Twist out from Maternal Immunity to Her Young. *Open Journal of Rheumatology and Autoimmune Diseases*, **3**, 40-55. http://dx.doi.org/10.4236/ojra.2013.31008

[5] Murgita, R.A. and Tomasi Jr., T.B. (1975) Suppression of the Immune Response by Alpha-Fetoprotein. *The Journal of Experimental Medicine*, **141**, 269-286. http://dx.doi.org/10.1084/jem.141.2.269

[6] Paul, G., Margaret, S., Liew, Y.F. and Allan, M.M. (1995) $CD^{4+}$ But Not $CD^{8+}$ T Cells Are Required for the Induction of Oral Tolerance. *International Immunology*, **7**, 501-504. http://dx.doi.org/10.1093/intimm/7.3.501

[7] Koshimo, H., Miyazawa, H.Y., Shimizu, Y. and Yamaguchi, N. (1989) Maternal Antigenic Stimulation Actively Produces Suppressor Activity in Offspring. *Developmental & Comparative Immunology*, **13**, 79-85. http://dx.doi.org/10.1016/0145-305X(89)90020-7

[8] Zoeller, M. (1988) Tolerization during Pregnancy: Impact on the Development of Antigen-Specific Help and Suppression. *European Journal of Immunology*, **18**, 1937-1943. http://dx.doi.org/10.1002/eji.1830181211

[9] Auerback, R. and Clark, S. (1975) Immunological Tolerance: Transmission from Mother to Offspring. *Science*, **189**, 811-813. http://dx.doi.org/10.1126/science.1162355

[10] Shinka, S., Dohi, Y., Komatsu, T., Natarajan, R. and Amano, T. (1974) Immunological Unresponsiveness in Mice. I. Immunological Unresponsiveness Induced in Embryonic Mice by Maternofetal Transfer of Human-Globulin. *Biken Journal*, **17**, 59-72.

[11] Aase, J.M., Noren, G.R., Reddy, D.V. and Geme Jr., J.W. (1972) Mumps-Virus Infection in Pregnant Women and the Immunologic Response of Their Offspring. *The New England Journal of Medicine*, **286**, 1379-1382. http://dx.doi.org/10.1056/NEJM197206292862603

[12] Cramer, D.V., Kunz, H.W. and Gill III, T.J. (1974) Immunologic Sensitization Prior to Birth. *American Journal of Obstetrics & Gynecology*, **120**, 431-439.

[13] Yamaguchi, N., Hashimoto, H., Arai, M., Takada, S., Kawada, N., Taru, A., Li, A.-L., Izumi, H. and Sugiyama, K. (2002) Effect of Acupuncture on Leukocyte and Lymphocyte Subpopulation in Human Peripheral Blood-Quantitative discussion. *The Journal of Japanese Association of Physical Medicine, Balneology and Climatology*, **65**, 199-206.

[14] Wan, W., Li, A.-L., Izumi, H., Kawada, N., Arai, M., Takada, A., Taru, A., Hashimoto, H. and Yamaguchi, N. (2002) Effect of Acupuncture on Leukocyte and Lymphocyte Subpopulation in Human Peripheral Blood Qualitative discussion. *The Journal of Japanese Association of Physical Medicine, Balneology and Climatology*, **65**, 207-211.

[15] Wang, X.-X., Katoh, S. and Liu, B.-X. (1998) Effect of Physical Exercise on Leukocyte and Lymphocytes Subpopulations in Human Peripheral Blood. *Cytometry Research*, **8**, 53-61.

[16] Kitada, Y., Wan, W., Matsui, K., Matsui, K., Shimizu, S. and Yamaguchi, N. (2000) Regulation of Peripheral White Blood Cells in Numbers and Functions through Hot-Spring Bathing during a Short Term—Studies in Control Experiments. *Journal of Japanese Society Balneology Climatology Physiological Medicine*, **63**, 151-164.

[17] Bylund, D.B., Eikenberg, D.C., Hieble, J.P., Langer, S.Z., Lefkowitz, R.J. and Minneman, K.P. (1994) Intenational union of Pharmacology Nomenclature of Adrenoceptors. *Pharmacological Review*, **46**, 121-136.

[18] Dulis, B.H. and Wilson, I.B. (1980) The $\beta$-Adrenergic Receptor of Live Human Polymorphonuclear Leukocytes.

*Journal of Biological and Chemistry*, **255**, 1043-1048.

[19] Ostberg, J.R., Patel, R. and Repasky, E.A. (2000) Regulation of Immune Activity by Mild (Fever-Range) Whole Body Hyperthermia: Effect on Epidermal Langerhans Cells. *Cell Stress Chaperones*, **5**, 458-461. http://dx.doi.org/10.1379/1466-1268(2000)005<0458:ROIABM>2.0.CO;2

[20] Huang, Y.H., Haegerstrand, A. and Frostegard, J. (1996) Effect of *in Vitro* Hyperthermia on Proliferative Responses and Lymphocyte Activity. *Clinical Experimental Immunology*, **103**, 61-66. http://dx.doi.org/10.1046/j.1365-2249.1996.00932.x

[21] Mats, H., Orion, E. and Wolf, R. (2003) Balneotherapy in Dermatology. *Dermatological Therapy*, **16**, 132-140.

[22] Elenkov, I.J. and Chrousos, G.P. (1999) Stress Hormones, Th1/Th2 Patterns, Pro/Anti-Inflammatory Cytokines and Susceptibility to Disease. *Trends in Endocrinology and Metabolism*, **10**, 359-368.

[23] Abo, T. and Kumagai, K. (1978) Studies of Surface Immunoglobulins on Human B Lymphocytes. III. Physiological Variations of Sig$^{+}$ Cells in Peripheral Blood. *Clinical Experimental Immunology*, **33**, 441-452.

[24] Landmann, R.M.A., Muller, F.B., Perini, C., Wesp, M., Erne, P. and Buhler, F.R. (1954) Changes of Immunoregulatory Cells Induced by Psychological and Physical Stress: Relationship to Plasma Catecholamines. *Clinical Experimental Immunology*, **58**, 127-135.

[25] Yamaguchi, N., Araai, M. and Murayama, T. (2015) Aspect of QOL Assessment and Proposed New Scale for Evaluation. *Open Journal of Immunology*, in press.

[26] Yamaguchi, N., Kawada, N., Ja, X.-S., Okamoto, K., Okuzumi, K., Chen, R. and Takahashi, T. (2014) Overall Estimation of Anti-Oxidant Activity by Mammal Macrophage. *Open Journal of Rheumatology and Autoimmune Diseases*, **4**, 13-21.

[27] Abo, T., Kawate, T., Itoh, K. and Kumagai, K. (1981) Studies on the Bioperiodicity of the Immune Response. 1. Circadian Rhythms of Human T, B and K Cell Traffic in the Peripheral Blood. *Journal of Immunology*, **126**, 1360-1363.

[28] Jerne, N.K. and Nordin, A.A. (1963) Plaque Formation in Agar by Single Antibody Producing Cells. *Science*, **140**, 405-408.

[29] Maisel, A.S., Harris, T., Rearden, C.A. and Michel, M.C. (1990) Beta-Adrenergic Receptors in Lymphocyte Subsets after Exercise. Alterations in Normal Individuals and Patients with Congestive Heart Failure. *Circulation*, **82**, 2003-2010. http://dx.doi.org/10.1161/01.CIR.82.6.2003

[30] Suzuki, S., Toyabe, S., Moroda, T., Tada, T., Tsukahara, A. and Iiai, T. (1997) Circadian Rhythm of Leukocytes and Lymphocytes Subsets and Its Possible Correlation with the Function of the Autonomic Nervous System. *Clinical Experimental Immunology*, **110**, 500-508. http://dx.doi.org/10.1046/j.1365-2249.1997.4411460.x

## Abbreviations

CAM: Complementary and alternative medicine, beside the western medicine, there are many traditional medicine and/or health promoting menu all over the world

CD: Cluster of differentiation. Each lymphocyte has name that expressed CD number, for example CD2, CD4, etc.

FCM: Flow cytometry.

G-rich type: The individual that exhibit over 60% of granulocyte in peripheral blood, finding many in young gentleman.

L-rich type: The individual that exhibit over 40% of lymphocyte in peripheral blood, finding lot in ladies and senile.

*Charged Water*: *Conventional Water* was electrophoretically separated by direct current. Then *Charged Water* were obtained by both anode side and cathode site.. In this experiment cathode side of water was served as *Charged Water*.

QOL: Quality of life.

VAS: Visual analog scale.

16

# Antitumor Effects and Acute Oral Toxicity Studies of a Plant Extract Mixture Containing *Rhus verniciflua* and Some Other Herbs

**Wataru Hiruma[1,2], Kohei Suruga[1*], Kazunari Kadokura[1], Tsuyoshi Tomita[1], Ayaka Miyata[1], Yoshihiro Sekino[1], Masahiko Kimura[2], Nobuo Yamaguchi[3,4], Yasuhiro Komatsu[5,6], C. A. Tony Buffington[7], Nobufumi Ono[2]**

[1]International Operation Department (FM Center for R & D), Kibun Foods Inc., Tokyo, Japan
[2]Faculty of Pharmaceutical Sciences, Fukuoka University, Fukuoka, Japan
[3]Ishikawa Natural Medicinal Products Research Center, Ishikawa, Japan
[4]Department of Fundamental Research for CAM, Kanazawa Medical University, Ishikawa, Japan
[5]Kitasato Institution for Life Science, Kitasato University, Tokyo, Japan
[6]Sun R & D Institute for Natural Medicines Co. Inc., Tokyo, Japan
[7]Department of Veterinary Clinical Sciences, The Ohio State University College of Veterinary Medicine, Columbus, USA
Email: [*]kouhei_suruga@kibun.co.jp

## Abstract

**A novel antitumor agent was developed from six kinds of herbs containing *Rhus verniciflua* (Rv-PEM01). The components were traditionally established for each formula for traditional medicine. The formula was designed to affect antitumor effect as well as maintain host immune functions. First, we investigated the antiproliferative activities of Rv-PEM01 on human and canine tumor cell lines *in vitro*, and on antitumor effects using BALB/cAJcl-nu/nu mice *in vivo*. Acute oral toxicity of Rv-PEM01 was also investigated *in vivo* in ddY mice. Rv-PEM01 exhibited antiproliferative activities against PC-3 ($IC_{50}$: 0.328 ± 0.081 mg/ml), A549 ($IC_{50}$: 0.520 ± 0.070 mg/ml), D-17 ($IC_{50}$: 0.124 ± 0.037 mg/ml) and MRC-5 ($IC_{50}$: 0.505 ± 0.058 mg/ml) cells. Luteolin 7-$\beta$-D-glucopyranoside and apigenin 7-$\beta$-D-glucopyranoside were identified as the main active compounds in Rv-PEM01 by HPLC analysis. The single dose toxicity study of Rv-PEM01 did not result in any deaths or abnormalities in daily behavior, body weight gain, or anatomical observations at necropsy. Thus, so we could not calculate the 50% lethal dose ($LD_{50}$) in mice, but it would be higher than 5.0 g/kg. Treatment with Rv-PEM01 at a dose of 2.5 g/kg tended to show antitumor activities on mice bearing Colon26 tumors compared with the control group. It was concluded that the formula was a safe**

[*]Corresponding author.

**antitumor agent with no side effects on mouse physiological function as judged by survival and organ weight.**

## Keywords

***Rhus verniciflua*, Antitumor, Antiproliferation, Acute Toxicity**

## 1. Introduction

Many phytochemicals from fruits, vegetables, and herbs which have antitumor activities may represent promising therapeutic and prophylactic treatment approaches against different types of cancers. The effects of phytochemicals on inhibition of tumor growth are well demonstrated both *in vitro* and *in vivo*. Many of these compounds, such as vinca alkaloids, have been reported to kill cancer cells [1].

The antitumor properties of medicinal herbs may be attributed to their antioxidant [2], anti-inflammatory [2], and immunomodulatory [3] properties. Many herbal extracts or their components also have been reported to induce apoptosis in cancer cells [4], so apoptosis-inducing activity of anticancer herbs may play an important role in tumor suppression.

The popularity of complementary and alternative medicine (CAM) is an international trend in cancer therapy. Due to the severe side effects and limited therapeutic efficacy of cancer chemotherapeutic agents used in conventional cancer treatment, CAM might improve clinical outcome and reduce adverse reactions to anticancer drugs. The World Health Organization has estimated that 80% of people worldwide are interested in traditional medicine [2]. Several Kampo (traditional Chinese or Japanese herbal) medicines, such as Keishi-ka-kei-to, Juzen-taiho-to, Shimotsu-to, Unsei-in, Hochu-ekki-to, Shosaiko-to and Shichimotsu-koka-to, have been reported to exhibit an antimetastatic effect, and among them, Keishi-ka-kei-to, Juzen-taiho-to, Shosaiko-to and Shichimotsu-koka-to also exert antiproliferative activity on cancer cell lines [5]. Tien-Hsien liquid (THL) is a Chinese herbal mixture consisting of extracts from 14 Chinese medicinal herbs that has been used as an anticancer dietary supplement for more than 20 years. THL is reported to have potent immunomodulatory effects [6] and antiproliferative activity [7].

We have been analyzing the antitumor activity of plant extracts, as well as their ability to maintain host immune capacity. *Rhus verniciflua* (*R. verniciflua*) is commonly known as the lacquer tree. The sap of this tree, which is collected by scratching the bark of the tree, has been used as a natural coating substance for wood carvings for several thousand years. In Korea, the bark, branch and stem of the tree are eaten with chicken and duck soups [8]. Urushiols, the major compounds of lacquer tree sap, have antioxidant and cytotoxic effects [9]. We recently reported that two novel urushiol derivatives, 1,2-dihydroxyphenyl-3-pentadeca-7′(*E*),9′(*Z*),11′(*Z*)-trien-14′-ol and 1,2-dihydroxyphenyl-3-pentadeca-8′(*Z*),10′(*E*),12′(*E*)-trien-14′-ol, isolated from the extract of leaves of *R. verniciflua* for the first time, showed inhibition of HIV-1 reverse transcriptase (RT) [10]. In our previous papers, we reported the anti-cell-proliferative activities of a plant extract mixture from six kinds of herbs containing *R. verniciflua* (Rv-PEM01) *in vitro*. Rv-PEM01 had an inhibitory effect on the proliferation of both human and mouse tumor cell lines, and we speculated that it might induce to apoptosis against these tumor cell lines [11]. However, toxicity studies and antitumor effects *in vivo* of Rv-PEM01 have not been investigated so far. In this paper, we report the antiproliferative activities of Rv-PEM01 on human and canine tumor cell lines *in vitro*, acute oral toxicity study using ddY mice, and antitumor effects using BALB/cAJcl-nu/nu mice *in vivo*.

## 2. Materials and Methods

### 2.1. Preparation of Rv-PEM01

Rv-PEM01 was prepared using method of Hiruma W., *et al.* [11]; the six herbs for preparation of Rv-PEM01 are shown in **Table 1**. The leaves of *R. verniciflua* were collected from Guizhou, China, in June 2002, and identified by Prof. Zhu Shougian, College of Forestry of Guizhou University. The *Ulmus hollandica* (*U. hollandica*) were collected from Amsterdam, The Netherlands. The *Polygonatum sibiricum*, *Lycium chinense*, *Ganoderma japonicum* and *Panax ginseng* were purchased from Oofuna-Kanpodo Pharmacy (Kanagawa, Japan). Each of the six herbs was ground and mixed to one powder (total volume is 230 g), which was extracted with 10 vol of 70%

**Table 1.** Extraction of Rv-PEM01 from six herbs [11].

| Herbs | Amount of herbs used for extraction (g) |
|---|---|
| *Rhus verniciflua* | 90 |
| *Ulmus hollandica* | 60 |
| *Polygonatum sibiricum* | 50 |
| *Lycium chinense* | 10 |
| *Ganoderma japonicum* | 10 |
| *Panax ginseng* | 10 |
| Total | 230 |

The extract of Rv-PEM01 was prepared as follows. Each of the six herbs was ground and mixed to one powder (total volume is 230 g), which was extracted with 10 vol of 70% ethanol in water at room temperature. The extracted solutions were filtered, and the solvents were evaporated, filtered and lyophilized, yielding 60 g of lyophilized Rv-PEM01 from 230 g of herb powder.

ethanol in water at room temperature. The extracted solution was filtered and the solvent evaporated, after which the extract was lyophilized, yielding approximately 60 g of lyophilized Rv-PEM01. Urushiols were not detected in Rv-PEM01 by HPLC analysis (**Figure 1**).

## 2.2. Cell Culture and Treatment

Human prostate adenocarcinoma cell line PC-3, human lung adenocarcinoma cell line A549, and human normal lung fibroblast cell line MRC-5 were obtained from Health Science Research Resources Bank (Osaka, Japan). The canine osteosarcoma cell line D-17 was purchased from American Type Culture Collection (Virginia, USA). The PC-3 cell line was maintained in RPMI1640 medium containing 10% fetal bovine serum (FBS), penicillin (100 U/ml), and streptomycin (100 μg/ml). The A549, MRC-5 and D-17 cell lines were maintained in Dulbecco's Modified Eagle medium (DMEM) containing 10% FBS, penicillin (100 U/ml), streptomycin (100 μg/ml), D-glucose (1 mg/ml), and sodium pyruvate (110 μg/ml). All cells were maintained in a humidified incubator containing 5% carbon dioxide at 37˚C and cultured with various concentration of Rv-PEM01 for 72 hs.

## 2.3. Analysis of Cell Viability

Analysis of tumor cell growth *in vitro* was carried out using 2-(4-iodophenyl)-3-(4-nitrophenyl)-5-(2,4-disulfophenyl)-2H-tetrazolium, monosodium salt (WST-1, DOJINDO, Kumamoto, Japan) and 1-methoxy-5-methylphenazinium methylsulfate (1-Methoxy PMS, DOJINDO, Kumamoto, Japan) colorimetric assay [12]. Cells were seeded onto 96 well microtiter culture plates at densities of 1000 cells per well (volume, 50 μl/well). After 16 hs, 50 μl of RPMI1640 medium or DMEM containing 1% ethanol (control wells), or various concentrations of Rv-PEM01 were added and the cells were incubated for 72 hs at 37˚C. The incubation was terminated using WST-1 and 1-Methoxy PMS mixture 10 μl per a well, after which absorbance was recorded on BIO-RAD Benchmark microplate reader at 450 nm/655 nm wavelength. The $IC_{50}$ values were determined from Rv-PEM01 dose versus control growth curves.

## 2.4. HPLC Analysis

The Rv-PEM01 was analyzed by HPLC using a Shimadzu LC6A system (Kyoto, Japan) equipped with a SPD-6AV UV-visible spectrophotometric detector and TSK gel ODS-80TM (7.8 i.d. × 300 mm) column (Tosoh, Tokyo, Japan). The mobile phase consisted of 50% methanol, and flow rate was 0.8 ml/min with UV detection at 254 nm. Measurement of urushiols was performed using the method of Du Y., *et al.* [13] with some modification. The urushiols were measured using Develosil ODS-5 (4.6 i.d. × 250 mm) column (Nomura Chemical, Aichi, Japan). The mobile phase consisted of acetonitrile (90:10) containing 2% acetic acid, and flow rate was 1 ml/min with UV detection at 272 nm.

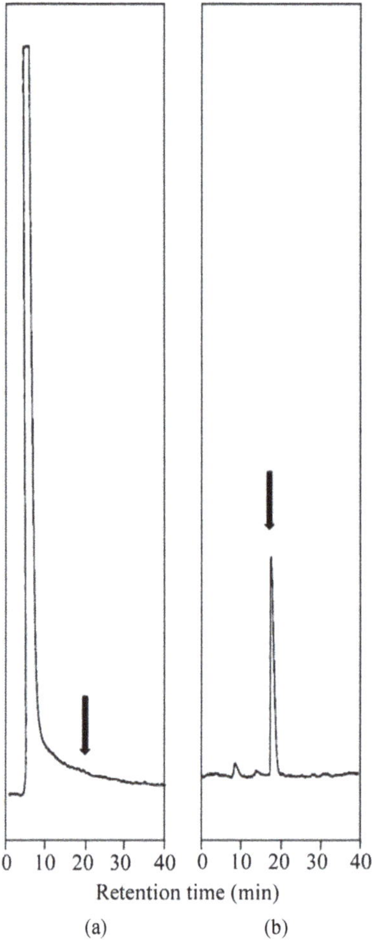


**Figure 1.** HPLC chromatogram of Rv-PEM01. (a) 10 mg/ml of Rv-PEM01 (20 µl injection); (b) 1 mg/ml urushiol (5 µl injection). Urushiols were measured using develosil ODS-5 (4.6 i.d. × 250 mm) column (Nomura Chemical, Aichi, Japan). The mobile phase consisted of acetonitrile (90:10) containing 2% acetic acid, and flow rate was 1 ml/min with UV detection at 272 nm. Arrows indicate the peak for urushiol.

## 2.5. Single Dose Toxicity Study

Six male and female seven-week-old ddY mice, were used for the acute oral toxicity study [14]. The tests were carried out according to Ethics of the Organization for Economic Co-operation and Development (OECD) Test Guideline 401. The mice were housed at 24°C ± 2°C, 50% relative humidity. The Rv-PEM01 was suspended in sterile water and administered to mice in single oral doses of 2 and 5 g/kg body weight. Mice were weighted at 0 - 7 days after administration, and clinical observations were made once a day. Necropsy was performed on all mice seven days after administration.

## 2.6. Antitumor Activity Test *in Vivo*

BALB/cAJcl-nu/nu mice were used to investigate the antitumor effects of Rv-PEM01 *in vivo* using the method of Kiyama S., *et al.* [15]. Mouse colorectal tumor cell line (Colon26; $1 \times 10^6$ cells in 0.1 ml of PBS) was injected into the right flank of six-week-old male BALB/cAJcl-nu/nu mice (CLEA Japan Inc., Tokyo, Japan). After ten days of tumor cell inoculation, the mice were treated with Rv-PEM01 for twenty eight days at a dose 0.0025 g/kg and 2.5 g/kg body weight per day and tumor size was measured daily. Tumor volumes were calculated by the formula of [$1/2 \times$ longest dimension $\times$ (shortest dimension)$^2$].

## 2.7. Statistical Analyses

The data are expressed as the mean ± standard deviation (SD.). The significance of differences between groups was assessed using the Student's $t$-test. $P < 0.05$ was considered to indicate statistical significance.

# 3. Results

## 3.1. Antiproliferative Activity of Rv-PEM01 on Tumor Cell Proliferation

The Rv-PEM01 treatment resulted in a dose-dependent decrease in cell growth in all cell lines (**Figure 2**). Calculated $IC_{50}$ values for each cell line were 0.328 ± 0.081, 0.520 ± 0.070, 0.124 ± 0.037 mg/ml, and 0.505 ± 0.058 mg/ml for PC-3, A549, D-17 and MRC-5, respectively (**Table 2**). The antiproliferative activity data of Rv-PEM01 against the other eight tumor cell lines presented in **Table 2** (MOLT-3, KG-1, HeLa, DLD-1, MCF-7, K-562, Colon26 and B16) were reported in our previous paper [11]. The antiproliferative activities of Rv-PEM01 in 12 different cell lines are presented in **Figure 3**. The values are calculated as follows: log ($IC_{50}$ each cell line)-log ($IC_{50}$ average) [16]. Negative values showed that the cell line was more sensitive than the average. Positive values showed that the cell line was more resistant than the average. HeLa, DLD-1, MCF-7, K-562, B16, A549 and MRC-5 were more resistant, and MOLT-3, KG-1, Colon26, PC-3 and D-17 were sensitive to Rv-PEM01 than other cell lines.

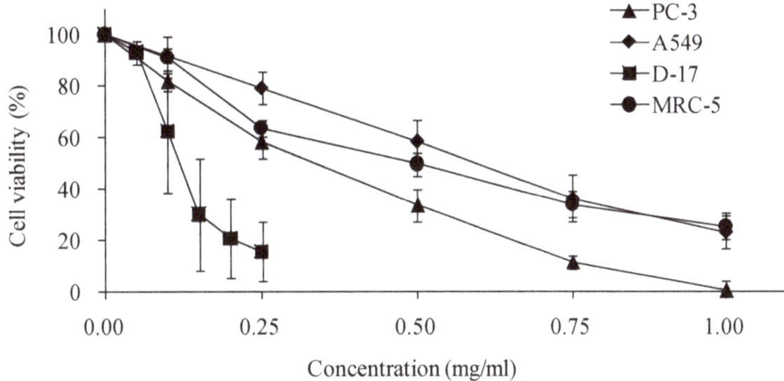


**Figure 2.** Dose dependent inhibitory effects of Rv-PEM01on PC-3 (triangles), A549 (diamonds), D-17 (squares) and MRC-5 (circles). Results are means ± SD. (n = 3).

**Table 2.** Antiproliferative activity of Rv-PEM01 in human, mouse and canine tumor cell lines.

| Cell lines | $IC_{50}$ (mg/ml)* | Cell origin | Reference |
|---|---|---|---|
| MOLT-3 | 0.208 ± 0.022 | Human tumor cell | Hiruma, *et al.* [11] |
| KG-1 | 0.293 ± 0.007 | Human tumor cell | Hiruma, *et al.* [11] |
| HeLa | 0.433 ± 0.043 | Human tumor cell | Hiruma, *et al.* [11] |
| DLD-1 | 0.510 ± 0.030 | Human tumor cell | Hiruma, *et al.* [11] |
| MCF-7 | 0.580 ± 0.054 | Human tumor cell | Hiruma, *et al.* [11] |
| K-562 | 0.610 ± 0.141 | Human tumor cell | Hiruma, *et al.* [11] |
| Colon26 | 0.389 ± 0.093 | Mouse tumor cell | Hiruma, *et al.* [11] |
| B16 | 0.565 ± 0.028 | Mouse tumor cell | Hiruma, *et al.* [11] |
| PC-3 | 0.328 ± 0.081 | Human tumor cell | This work |
| A549 | 0.520 ± 0.070 | Human tumor cell | This work |
| D-17 | 0.124 ± 0.037 | Canine tumor cell | This work |
| MRC-5 | 0.505 ± 0.058 | Human normal diploid fibroblast cell | This work |

*Results are means ± SD. (n = 3).

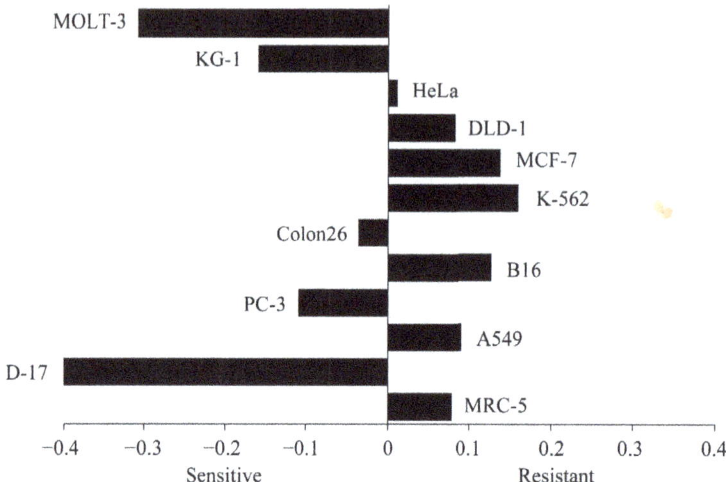


**Figure 3.** Antiproliferative activity of Rv-PEM01 in human, mouse and canine tumor cell lines. The values are calculated as follows: log ($IC_{50}$ each cell line)-log ($IC_{50}$ average) [16]. Negative values showed that the cell line was more sensitive than the average. Positive values showed that the cell line was more resistant than the average.

### 3.2. Identification of Active Compounds Contained in Rv-PEM01

The HPLC chromatogram of Rv-PEM01 is illustrated in **Figure 4**. Among the five peaks observed in the chromatogram, peaks 2 and 4 showed antiproliferative activity against MOLT-3, KG-1, Colon26, PC-3 and D-17 cell lines (**Figure 4**, **Table 3**). Peaks 2 and 4 were identified as luteolin 7-$\beta$-D-glucopyranoside and apigenin 7-$\beta$-D-glucopyranoside, respectively.

### 3.3. Single Dose Toxicity Study of Rv-PEM01

No deaths or abnormalities of body weight, water and food consumption, or coat condition were observed in the treated mice. Necropsy evaluation of the mice did not reveal any significant differences in thymus, liver, spleen, kidney, adrenal gland and testicle weights between the control group and the Rv-PEM01 treatment groups, or between males and females (**Table 4**).

### 3.4. *In Vivo* Antitumor Effects of Rv-PEM01 on Nude Mice

No deaths or significant differences in the body weight gain, tumor volume, or tumor size were observed between the control group and Rv-PEM01 treatment group (**Figure 5**). The Rv-PEM01 treatment at dose of 2.5 g/kg tended to have antitumor activities compared with the control group, but the difference did not reach statistical significance. Additional studies of antitumor effects of Rv-PEM01 *in vivo* are currently under investigation.

## 4. Discussion

In this study, Rv-PEM01 exhibited antitumor activities against human, canine and mouse tumor cell lines *in vitro*. These results confirmed our previous data, which suggested the main active herb in Rv-PEM01 was *R. verniciflua*. The branches and the sap from *R. verniciflua* contain active compounds such as urushiol, fustin, quercetin, butein and sulfuretin, and the antioxidant [17] [18], antitumorigenic [19] and cytotoxic [20] effects of these compounds have been reported. Urushiols, which are mixture of olefinic catechols with alkyl side chain [21], are characteristic compounds in *R. verniciflua* branches and sap. These compounds have shown the biological activities including cytotoxic effects on human cancer cell lines [22] and antioxidant properties [23]. Recently, two novel urushiol derivatives, 1,2-dihydroxyphenyl-3-pentadeca-7′(*E*),9′(*Z*),11′(*Z*)-trien-14′-ol and 1,2-dihydroxyphenyl-3-pentadeca-8′(*Z*),10′(*E*),12′(*E*)-trien-14′-ol, were isolated from leaves of *R. verniciflua*, and shown to inhibit HIV-1 RT [10]. In addition to these activities of *R. verniciflua*, urushiol compounds are well known as allergenic compounds that can induce contact dermatitis [24]. Therefore, urushiols and their deri-

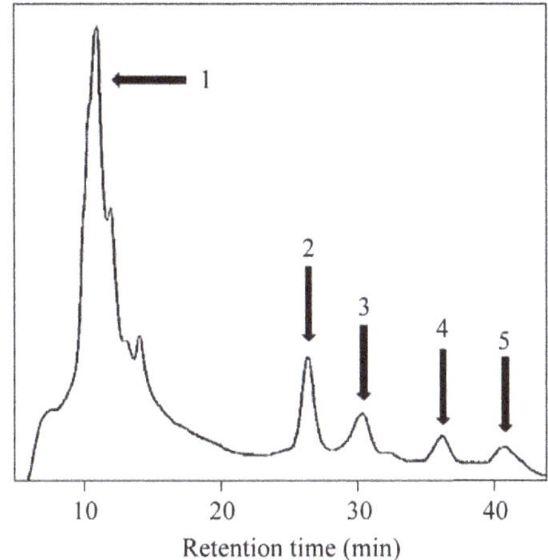


**Figure 4.** HPLC chromatogram of Rv-PEM01. Rv-PEM01 was analyzed by HPLC using Shimadzu LC6A system (Kyoto, Japan) equipped with a TSK gel ODS-80TM (7.8 i.d. × 300 mm) column (Tosoh, Tokyo, Japan) and a SPD-6AV UV-visible spectrophotometric detector. The mobile phase consisted of 50% methanol, and flow rate was 0.8 ml/min with UV detection at 254 nm.

**Table 3.** Antiproliferative activity of fraction No.1-5 from Rv-PEM01 in human, mouse and canine tumor cell lines.

| Peak No. | MOLT-3 $IC_{50}$ (mg/ml) | KG-1 $IC_{50}$ (mg/ml) | Colon26 $IC_{50}$ (mg/ml) | PC-3 $IC_{50}$ (mg/ml) | D-17 $IC_{50}$ (mg/ml) |
|---|---|---|---|---|---|
| 1 | 0.035 ± 0.009 | >0.750 | >0.750 | >0.750 | >0.750 |
| 2 | 0.010 ± 0.001 | 0.022 ± 0.003 | 0.030 ± 0.005 | 0.023 ± 0.004 | 0.011 ± 0.004 |
| 3 | 0.063 ± 0.025 | 0.089 ± 0.032 | 0.184 ± 0.025 | 0.182 ± 0.034 | 0.162 ± 0.028 |
| 4 | 0.013 ± 0.005 | 0.007 ± 0.003 | 0.013 ± 0.002 | 0.011 ± 0.003 | 0.009 ± 0.004 |
| 5 | 0.055 ± 0.012 | 0.046 ± 0.014 | 0.127 ± 0.030 | 0.073 ± 0.011 | 0.096 ± 0.033 |

*Results are means ± SD. (n = 3).

**Table 4.** Absolute organ weights of mice after 7 days oral administration of Rv-PEM01.

| Dose (g/kg) | Male (n = 6) | | | Female (n = 6) | | |
|---|---|---|---|---|---|---|
| | 0 | 2.5 | 5.0 | 0 | 2.5 | 5.0 |
| Body weight (g) | 38.0 ± 1.0 | 38.0 ± 1.7 | 38.0 ± 0.9 | 30.3 ± 0.4 | 31.3 ± 1.1 | 30.8 ± 0.5 |
| Thymus (mg) | 59.8 ± 13.0 | 68.0 ± 17.4 | 66.7 ± 21.1 | 82.6 ± 20.6 | 78.3 ± 6.7 | 81.2 ± 15.6 |
| Liver (g) | 2.1 ± 0.3 | 1.9 ± 0.2 | 2.0 ± 0.2 | 1.6 ± 0.1 | 1.6 ± 0.2 | 1.6 ± 0.1 |
| Spleen (mg) | 135.0 ± 15.3 | 159.4 ± 12.6 | 161.7 ± 31.9 | 147.1 ± 28.8 | 170.3 ± 23.2 | 154.6 ± 17.8 |
| Left kidney (mg) | 335.1 ± 76.9 | 338.1 ± 41.5 | 333.7 ± 28.2 | 227.0 ± 42.6 | 219.9 ± 23.9 | 206.6 ± 18.7 |
| Right kidney (mg) | 280.7 ± 21.0 | 310.6 ± 42.8 | 340.3 ± 52.5 | 227.0 ± 42.6 | 210.1 ± 20.6 | 205.8 ± 18.9 |
| Adrenal gland (mg) | 17.4 ± 6.2 | 18.7 ± 6.3 | 15.6 ± 4.3 | 19.7 ± 2.7 | 21.3 ± 3.0 | 20.6 ± 1.5 |
| Testicles (mg) | 264.6 ± 25.1 | 273.2 ± 16.3 | 281.5 ± 18.3 | 33.8 ± 12.2 | 41.9 ± 13.2 | 36.7 ± 6.9 |

*Results are means ± SD. (n = 6).

vatives from *R. verniciflua* were not contained in Rv-PEM01 (**Figure 1**), and antiproliferative activities of these on human and mouse tumor cell lines were investigated in previous our paper [11]. In the present study, the antiproliferative activity of Rv-PEM01 was evaluated in human and canine tumor cell lines that were different from the previous tumor cell lines used *in vitro*.

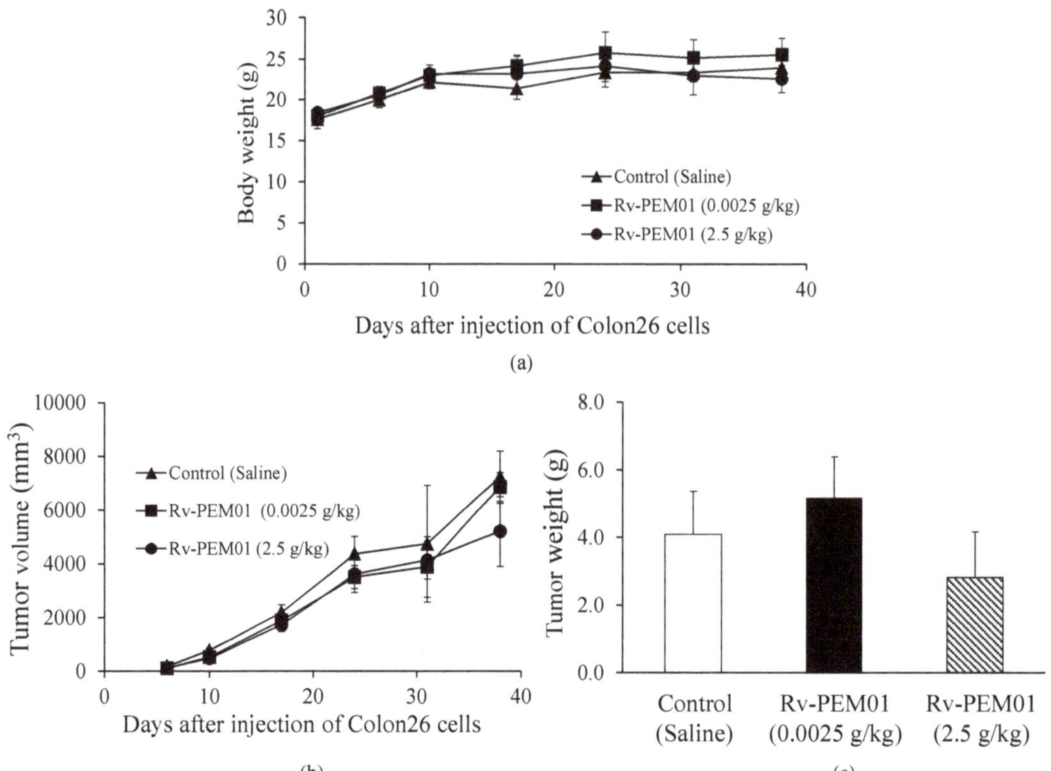


**Figure 5.** Effects of Rv-PEM01 on BALB/cAJcl-nu/nu mice bearing Colon26 tumor cells. Mouse colorectal tumor cell line (Colon26; $1 \times 10^6$ cells in 0.1 ml of PBS) was injected into the right flank of six-week-old male BALB/cAJcl-nu/nu mice. After 10 days of inoculation, the mice were treated with Rv-PEM01 for 28 days. (a) Change of body weight (g); (b) Change in tumor volume ($mm^3$); (c) Tumor weight (g) after 38 days. Results are means ± SD. (n = 5).

Rv-PEM01 had antiproliferative activities on PC-3, A549, D-17 and MRC-5 cell lines (**Figure 2**, **Table 2**). Evaluation of the antiproliferative activities of Rv-PEM01 in 12 different cell lines, indicated that HeLa, DLD-1, MCF-7, K-562, B16, A549 and MRC-5 were more resistant to Rv-PEM01, whereas MOLT-3, KG-1, Colon26, PC-3 and D-17 were more sensitive to it (**Figure 3**). The antiproliferative activity of Rv-PEM01 was more potent on D-17 than on any of the other tumor cell lines. Our previous investigation found that Rv-PEM01 induced apoptosis in MOLT-3, KG-1 and K-562 leukemia cell lines by measurement of DNA fragmentation and caspase-3 and caspase-9 activities [11]. The mechanisms of Rv-PEM01's antiproliferative effects on Colon26, PC-3 and D-17 are still unclear, but it may induce apoptosis on these tumor cell lines as it did in the leukemia cell lines in our previous report. Spontaneous canine tumors show many clinical and molecular similarities to human tumors, and such offer an attractive model for preclinical investigations [25]. This study is the first to our knowledge to evaluate the effects of Rv-PEM01 on canine tumor cell lines. Additional investigations of the effectiveness of Rv-PEM01 on canine tumor cell lines are indicated.

HPLC analysis showed five major peaks (**Figure 4**). The antiproliferative activity of peaks 2 and 4 on MOLT-3, KG-1, Colon26, PC-3 and D-17 cell lines were more potent than that of other peaks (**Table 3**). Peaks 2 and 4 were identified as luteolin 7-$\beta$-D-glucopyranoside and apigenin 7-$\beta$-D-glucopyranoside, respectively. Rashed KN., *et al.* recently reported that a hydromethanolic extract of *Sapindus saponaria* showed cytotoxicity against human carcinoma cell lines, and that the active compounds were luteolin 8-*C*-$\beta$-glucoside, luteolin 6-*C*-$\beta$-glucoside, luteolin 7-*O*-$\beta$-glucuronide, and rutin [26]. Nakazaki E., *et al.* found that the apigenin 7-glucoside inhibited HL-60 leukemia cell line [27]. Kim S., *et al.* reported that extraction of *R. verniciflua* leaf with 70% methanol showed the neuroprotective effects, and that the active compounds were fisetin, sulfuretin, quercetin and butein [28]. There was a report that mansonone E and F, which were extracted with 80% ethanol from *Ulmus pumila*, showed potent antiproliferative effects on human tumor cell lines [29]. Ahn MJ., *et al.* also reported that neosibiricoside A-D isolated from the rhizomes of *Polygonatum sibiricum* had cytotoxic activity on MCF-7 breast cancer cells [30]. From these reports, we expected that antitumor effects of the Rv-PEM01 may be related to the luteolin 7-$\beta$-D-glucopyranoside, apigenin 7-$\beta$-D-glucopyranoside and some other compounds such as fisetin, sulfuretin, quercetin, butein, mansonone species and neosibiricoside species that are contained in the extract.

In the acute oral toxicity study, there were no changes attributable to Rv-PEM01 administration at doses of 2.5 or 5.0 g/kg. The 50% mortality rate $LD_{50}$ could not be calculated, but must be higher than 5.0 g/kg. In the chronic study, we found no adverse effects of Rv-PEM01 at the doses used, suggesting longer-term safety at these doses. Unfortunately, no statistically significant difference of antitumor efficacy from the control group was found, although Rv-PEM01 treatment at dose of 2.5 g/kg resulted in a trend toward antitumor activity compared with control. Additional studies, using different doses and model systems, as well as a study of potential prophylactic antitumor effects of Rv-PEM01 *in vivo* currently are in progress.

## 5. Conclusion

Biological activities of Rv-PEM01, as well as its antitumor effects, safety, and toxicity, were investigated. Rv-PEM01 exhibited antiproliferative activities against PC-3, A549, D-17 and MRC-5 *in vitro*, and tendency toward tumor growth inhibition *in vivo*. The main active compounds of Rv-PEM01 were luteolin 7-$\beta$-D-glucopyranoside and apigenin 7-$\beta$-D-glucopyranoside. The safety studies did not identify any adverse reactions in mice. Therefore, it could be useful as a novel functional food material and/or nutritional supplement. Additional studies of the antitumor effects of Rv-PEM01 *in vivo* are needed.

## Acknowledgements

We are grateful to Chairman and C.E.O. Masahito Hoashi, Kibun Foods Inc., for supporting the present work.

## References

[1] Cherng, J.M., Shieh, D.E., Chiang, W., Chang, M.Y. and Chiang, L.C. (2007) Chemopreventive Effects of Minor Dietary Constituents in Common Foods on Human Cancer Cells. *Bioscience, Biotechnology, and Biochemistry*, **71**, 1500-1504. http://dx.doi.org/10.1271/bbb.70008

[2] Sharma, N., Samarakoon, K.W., Gyawali, R., Park, Y.H., Lee, S.J., Oh, S.J., Lee, T.H. and Jeong, D.K. (2014) Evaluation of the Antioxidant, Anti-Inflammatory, and Anticancer Activities of *Euphorbia hirta* Ethanolic Extract. *Molecules*, **19**, 14567-14581. http://dx.doi.org/10.3390/molecules190914567

[3] Yu, T., Moh, S.H., Kim, S.B., Yang, Y., Kim, E., Lee, Y.W., Cho, C.K., Kim, K.H., Yoo, B.C., Cho, J.Y. and Yoo, H.S. (2013) HangAmDan-B, an Ethnomedicinal Herbal Mixture, Suppresses Inflammatory Responses by Inhibiting Syk/NF-kB and JNK/ATF-2 Pathways. *Journal of Medicinal Food*, **16**, 56-65. http://dx.doi.org/10.1089/jmf.2012.2374

[4] Eo, H.J., Park, J.H., Park, G.H., Lee, M.H., Lee, J.R., Koo, J.S. and Jeong, J.B. (2014) Anti-Inflammatory and Anti-Cancer Activity of Mulberry (*Morus alba L.*) Root Bark. *BMC Complementary and Alternative Medicine*, **14**, 200. http://dx.doi.org/10.1186/1472-6882-14-200

[5] Ohno, T., Inoue, M. and Ogihara, Y. (2002) Suppressive Effect of Shichimotsu-Koka-To (Kampo Medicine) on Pulmonary Metastasis of B16 Melanoma Cells. *Biological and Pharmaceutical Bulletin*, **25**, 880-884. http://dx.doi.org/10.1248/bpb.25.880

[6] Sun, A., Chia, J.S., Wang, W.B. and Chiang, C.P. (2004) Immunomodulating Effects of "*Tien-Hsien* Liquid" on Peripheral Blood Mononuclear Cells and T Lymphocytes from Patients with Recurrent Aphthous Ulcerations. *American Journal of Chinese Medicine*, **32**, 221-234. http://dx.doi.org/10.1142/S0192415X04001886

[7] Sun, A., Chia, J.S., Chiang, C.P., Hsuen, S.P., Du, J.L., Wu, C.W. and Wang, W.B. (2005) The Chinese Herbal Medicine *Tien-Hsien* Liquid Inhibits Cell Growth and Induces Apoptosis in a Wide Variety of Human Cancer Cells. *Journal of Alternative and Complementary Medicine*, **11**, 245-256. http://dx.doi.org/10.1089/acm.2005.11.245

[8] Kim, J.S. and Kim, M.J. (2011) Anti-Oxidant Activity of *Rhus verniciflua* Stokes by Extract Conditions. *Journal of Medicinal Plants Research*, **5**, 2617-2623.

[9] Rayne, S. and Mazza, G. (2007) Biological Activities of Extracts from Sumac (*Rhus* spp.): A Review. *Plant Foods for Human Nutrition*, **62**, 165-175. http://dx.doi.org/10.1007/s11130-007-0058-4

[10] Kadokura, K., Suruga, K., Tomita, T., Hiruma, W., Yamada, M., Kobayashi, A., Takatsuki, A., Nishio, T., Oku, T. and Sekino, Y. (2015) Novel Urushiols with Human Immunodeficiency Virus Type 1 Reverse Transcriptase Inhibitory Activity from the Leaves of *Rhus verniciflua*. *Journal of Natural Medicines*, **69**, 148-153. http://dx.doi.org/10.1007/s11418-014-0871-7

[11] Hiruma, W., Suruga, K., Kadokura, K., Tomita, T., Sekino, Y., Komatsu, Y., Kimura, M. and Ono, N. (2013) The Antitumor Effects of a Plant Extract Mixture. *Yakugaku Zasshi*, **133**, 487-491. http://dx.doi.org/10.1248/yakushi.12-00278-1

[12] Cory, A.H., Owen, T.C., Barltrop, J.A. and Cory, J.G. (1991) Use of an Aqueous Soluble Tetrazolium/Formazan Assay for Cell Growth Assays in Culture. *Cancer Communications*, **3**, 207-212.

[13] Du, Y. and Oshima, R. (1984) Reversed-Phase Liquid Chromatographic Separation and Identification of Constituents of Urushiol in the Sap of the Lac Tree *Rhus vernicifera*. *Journal of Chromatography A*, **284**, 463-473. http://dx.doi.org/10.1016/S0021-9673(01)87848-1

[14] Sano, Y., Satoh, H., Chiba, M., Okamoto, M., Serizawa, K., Nakashima, H. and Omae, K. (2005) Oral Toxicity of Bismuth in Rat: Single and 28-Day Repeated Administration Studies. *Journal of Occupational Health*, **47**, 293-298. http://dx.doi.org/10.1539/joh.47.293

[15] Kiyama, S. (1995) Effect of Growth Hormone on Cancerous Cachexia in Mice Bearing Colon 26 Tumor. *Journal of Tokyo Women's Medical University*, **65**, 873-882.

[16] Poindessous, V., Koeppel, F., Raymond, E., Comisso, M., Waters, S.J. and Larsen, A.K. (2003) Marked Activity of Irofulven toward Human Carcinoma Cells: Comparison with Cisplatin and Ecteinascidin. *Clinical Cancer Research*, **9**, 2817-2825.

[17] Lee, J.C., Kim, J., Lim, K.T., Yang, M.S. and Jang, Y.S. (2001) Ethanol Eluted Extract of *Rhus verniciflua* Stokes Showed both Antioxidant and Cytotoxic Effects on Mouse Thymocytes Depending on the Dose and Time of the Treatment. *Journal of Biochemistry and Molecular Biology*, **34**, 250-258.

[18] Lee, J.C., Lim, J. and Jang, Y.S. (2002) Identification of *Rhus verniciflua* Stokes Compounds That Exhibit Free Radical Scavenging and Anti-Apoptotic Properties. *Biochimica et Biophysica Acta*, **1570**, 181-191. http://dx.doi.org/10.1016/S0304-4165(02)00196-4

[19] Lee, J.C., Lee, K.Y., Kim, J., Na, C.S., Jung, N.C., Chung, G.H. and Jang, Y.S. (2004) Extract from *Rhus verniciflua* Stokes Is Capable of Inhibiting the Growth of Human Lymphoma Cells. *Food and Chemical Toxicology*, **42**, 1383-1388. http://dx.doi.org/10.1016/j.fct.2004.03.012

[20] Kitts, D.D. and Lim, K.T. (2001) Antitumorigenic and Cytotoxic Properties of an Ethanol Extract Derived from *Rhus verniciflua* Stokes (RVS). *Journal of Toxicology and Environmental Health, Part A*, **64**, 357-371.

[21] Watson, E.S., Murphy, J.C., Wirth, P.W., Waller, C.W. and Elsohly, M.A. (1981) Immunologic Studies of Poisonous Anacardiaceae: I. Production of Tolerance and Desensitization to Poison Ivy and Oak Urushiols Using Esterified Urushiol Derivatives in Guinea Pigs. *Journal of Investigative Dermatology*, **76**, 164-170. http://dx.doi.org/10.1111/1523-1747.ep12525589

[22] Hong, D.H., Han, S.B., Lee, C.W., Park, S.H., Jeon, Y.J., Kim, M.J., Kwak, S.S. and Kim, H.M. (1999) Cytotoxicity of Urushiols Isolated from Sap of Korean Lacquer Tree (*Rhus vernicifera* Stokes). *Archives of Pharmacal Research*, **22**, 638-641. http://dx.doi.org/10.1007/BF02975339

[23] Kim, M.J., Choi, Y.H., Kim, W.G. and Kwak, S.S. (1997) Antioxidative Activity of Urushiol Derivatives from the Sap of Lacquer Tree (*Rhus vernicifera* Stokes). *Korean Journal of Plant Resources*, **10**, 227-230.

[24] Johnson, R.A., Baer, H., Kirkpatrick, C.H., Dawson, C.R. and Khurana, R.G. (1972) Comparison of the Contact Allergenicity of the Four Pentadecylcatechols Derived from Poison Ivy Urushiol in Human Subjects. *Journal of Allergy and Clinical Immunology*, **49**, 27-35. http://dx.doi.org/10.1016/0091-6749(72)90120-0

[25] London, C.A., Bernabe, L.F., Barnard, S., Kisseberth, W.C., Borgatti, A., Henson, M., Wilson, H., Jensen, K., Ito, D., Modiano, J.F., Bear, M.D., Pennell, M.L., Saint-Nartin, J.R., Mccauley, D., Kauffman, M. and Shacham, S. (2014) Preclinical Evaluation of the Novel, Orally Bioavailable Selective Inhibitor of Nuclear Export (SINE) KPT-335 in Spontaneous Canine Cancer: Results of a Phase I Study. *PLoS ONE*, **9**, e87585. http://dx.doi.org/10.1371/journal.pone.0087585

[26] Rashed, K.N., Ciric, A., Glamoclija, J., Calhelha, R.C., Ferreira, I.C.F.R. and Sokovic, M. (2013) Antimicrobial Activity, Growth Inhibition of Human Tumour Cell Lines, and Phytochemical Characterization of the Hydromethanolic Extract Obtained from *Sapindus saponaria* L. Aerial Parts. *BioMed Research International*, **2013**, Article ID: 659183. http://dx.doi.org/10.1155/2013/659183

[27] Nakazaki, E., Tsolmon, S., Han, J. and Isoda, H. (2013) Proteomic Study of Granulocytic Differentiation Induced by Apigenin 7-Glucoside in Human Promyelocytic Leukemia HL-60 Cells. *European Journal of Nutrition*, **52**, 25-35. http://dx.doi.org/10.1007/s00394-011-0282-4

[28] Kim, S., Park, S.E., Sapkota, K., Kim, M.K. and Kim, S.J. (2011) Leaf Extract of *Rhus verniciflua* Stokes Protects Dopaminergic Neuronal Cells in a Rotenone Model of Parkinson's Disease. *Journal of Pharmacy and Pharmacology*, **63**, 1358-1367. http://dx.doi.org/10.1111/j.2042-7158.2011.01342.x

[29] Wang, D., Xia, M.Y., Cui, Z., Tashiro, S., Onodera, S. and Ikejima, T. (2004) Cytotoxic Effects of Mansonone E and F

Isolated from *Ulmus pumila*. *Biological and Pharmaceutical Bulletin*, **27**, 1025-1030. http://dx.doi.org/10.1248/bpb.27.1025

[30] Ahn, M.J., Kim, C.Y., Yoon, K.D., Ryu, M.Y., Cheong, J.H., Chin, Y.W. and Kim, J. (2006) Steroidal Saponins from the Rhizomes of *Polygonatum sibiricum*. *Journal of Natural Products*, **69**, 360-364. http://dx.doi.org/10.1021/np050394d

17

# Is There a Relation between Adenosine and Caffeines' Mechanisms of Action and Toll-Like Receptor-4 (TLR-4)?

**Sarah Moodad[1], Nayla Al-Akl[1], Joseph Simaan[2], Alexander M. Abdelnoor[1*]**

[1]Department of Experimental Pathology, Immunology and Microbiology, Faculty of Medicine, American University of Beirut, Beirut, Lebanon

[2]Department of Pharmacology and Toxicology, Faculty of Medicine, American University of Beirut, Beirut, Lebanon

Email: [*]aanoor@aub.edu.lb

## Abstract

**Previous studies showed that endogenous adenosine, an anti-inflammatory agent, was released at sites of injury and inflammation thereby decreasing the excessive production of pro-inflammatory cytokines. Caffeine, a non-specific adenosine blocker, has been reported in several studies to have opposing immune-modulatory effects. In this study, the effects of caffeine and adenosine on TLR-4 in promoting or decreasing the production of TNF-$\alpha$ and IL-12 by LPS-stimulated monocytes were investigated. Monocytes were isolated using Pluribead® kit from pooled blood obtained from ten volunteers. The monocytes were then incubated for 24 hours with Lipopolysaccharide (pLPS) extracted from *Escherichia coli* (aTLR-4 ligand activator), adenosine, caffeine and LPS extracted from *Rhodobacter sphaeroides* (LPS-RS, a TLR-4 ligand blocker), each alone or in different combinations. Later, the levels of pro-inflammatory cytokines TNF$\alpha$ and IL-12 were assessed in supernatants using an Enzyme Linked Immuno Assay (ELISA). Caffeine and adenosine significantly reduced the amount of TNF$\alpha$ and IL-12 produced by LPS-stimulated monocytes. Regarding non-stimulated and LPS-RS blocked monocytes, the presence of adenosine and caffeine significantly decreased TNF$\alpha$ levels produced by these cells but had little or non-significant effect on the levels of IL-12. In conclusion, both caffeine and adenosine blocked the production of the pro-inflammatory cytokines by pLPS-stimulated-monocytes. TLR-4 did not appear to be involved in the signaling pathway of caffeine and adenosine since blocking of TLR-4 did not abolish the effects of adenosine and caffeine on production of cytokines, in particular TNF-$\alpha$.**

## Keywords

**TLR-4, Adenosine, Caffeine, LPS-RS, Cytokines**

[*]Corresponding author.

# 1. Introduction

Pathogenic Lipopolysaccharide (pLPS) containing six fatty acyl groups is a constituent of the cell wall of pathogenic Gram-negative bacteria such as *Escherichia coli* [1] [2]. Binding of pLPS to Toll-Like Receptor-4 (TLR-4), results in the activation of two signaling pathways that lead to the production of pro-inflammatory cytokines, such as IL-12 and TNF-$\alpha$. Cytokine release results in the initiation of an inflammatory cascade aimed at elimination of the invading pathogen [3]-[5]. On the other hand, LPS containing 4 or 5 fatty acyl groups such as the LPS of the photosynthetic bacterium, *Rhodobacter sphaeroides* (LPS-RS), which binds to TLR-4, does not activate the signaling pathways and block pLPS from doing so [6] [7].

Adenosine, an endogenous anti-inflammatory agent, is normally present at low concentrations in the body as it is produced by almost all cells as a by-product of metabolism [8]. However, during inflammation, stress, or tissue injury, adenosine is released in high amounts reaching 10 - 100 folds in an attempt to control the inflammatory response [8]. Referred to as "retaliatory metabolite", adenosine exerts its anti-inflammatory role by binding to its receptors (A1, A2A, A2B, and A3) present on different immune cells [9]. While the activation of different adenosine receptors results in opposing immune-modulatory effects, it is shown that during stress, adenosine binds and activates A2A receptors which are anti-inflammatory in nature [8]. Previous studies demonstrated that binding of adenosine to its A2A receptors specifically, decreased TNF-$\alpha$ and IL-12 production in pLPS-stimulated monocytes and neutrophils, and thus suppressed inflammation [10]-[12].

On the other hand, caffeine, the widely consumed psychostimulant, is a non-specific adenosine antagonist which blocks all adenosine receptors [13]. Despite being a weak phosphor-diesterase (PDE) blocker, it is believed that at normal physiological concentrations the major effects of caffeine are exerted via adenosine receptors inhibition and not PDE blockage [13]. Being a blocker of an anti-inflammatory molecule, the role of caffeine on immunity had been assessed before. However, previous studies concerning caffeine and immunity had been controversial; while most studies showed that caffeine decreased cytokines production during inflammation and tissue injury [14] [15], other studies showed that caffeine either worsens inflammation or plays no significant role at all [16]-[18]. One of the previous studies indicating a possible anti-inflammatory role of caffeine suggested that caffeine reduced cytokine levels by increasing endogenous cAMP levels [14] [15]. However, other studies argued that the elevation in cAMP was due to phosphor-diesterase (PDE) inhibition which was unlikely to occur at normal physiological concentrations of caffeine [13]. Another study by Verani *et al.* reported that caffeine upregulated the anti-inflammatory A2A receptors and thus decreased inflammation [19].

The aims of this study are to determine the effect of both caffeine and adenosine on pLPS-stimulated monocytes and to assess whether TLR-4, the LPS receptor, is implicated in the signaling of either adenosine or caffeine.

# 2. Materials and Methods

## 2.1. Reagents

LPS extracted from *Escherichia coli* 111:B4 strain (Invivogen 3950 sorrento Valley Blvd., San Diego CA-92121-USA), adenosine (Sigma, 3050 Spruce Street, Saint Louis, USA), caffeine (Sigma, 3050 Spruce Street, Saint Louis, USA), and LPS extracted from *Rhodobacter sphaeroides* (Invivogen, 3950 Sorrento Valley Blvd., San Diego CA-92121-USA).

## 2.2. Blood Specimens and Isolation of Monocytes

Human monocytes were isolated from blood withdrawn from 10 informed healthy volunteers (age > 18 years old) using vacutainers containing an anticoagulant. Blood specimens were pooled and monocytes were separated using the PluriBeads® M-kit (PluriSelect Life Science, Leipzig, Germany) (viability, >95%). Collected cells were then cultured in 0.5 ml RPMI medium containing 1% pen-strep, 1% L-glutamine, and 10% heat-inactivated FBS at a concentration of $2 \times 10^5$ cells/ml.

Recruitment of volunteers was approved by the Institutional Review Board of American University of Beirut (IRB-AUB). Volunteers refrained from caffeine consumption for at least 48 hours before blood withdrawal to insure that previous high plasma caffeine levels could not interfere with the purpose of the study.

## 2.3. Culture of Monocytes

Monocyte culture was performed in a 48 well plate. Cells were incubated with the different reagents at 37°C and

5% $CO_2$ for 24 hours according to the protocol indicated in **Table 1**. Each well contained 2 × $10^5$ monocytes/ml and were incubated with 2 µl of 0.1 µg/ml pLPS extracted from *Escherichia coli* 111:B4 strain, 381 µl of 100M adenosine, 121 µl of 100 M caffeine and 10 µl of 1 µg/ml LPS-RS extracted from *Rhodobacter sphaeroides*, each alone or in different combinations in 0.5 ml culture media (**Table 1**). LPS-RS (TLR-4 antagonist) and caffeine (adenosine antagonist) were added to the cells before the other reagents at time t = −2 hours and t = −1 hour respectively. Following incubation for 24 hours, cytokine levels in supernatants were determined.

### 2.4. TNF-*α* and IL-12 Levels

TNF-*α* and IL-12, in supernatants were determined using ELISA (Abcam TNF alpha Human ELISA kit (Ab46087) and Abcam IL-12 human ELISA kit; (Abcam company, Moscow, Russia) according to the manufacturer's instructions.

### 2.5. Statistical Analysis

The unpaired student T-test was implemented to assess the sample variations between groups using the Graphpad online software. Results were considered to be statistically significant when p value was $<0.05$.

## 3. Results

### 3.1. Effect of Adenosine on pLPS-Stimulated Monocytes

The addition of adenosine to pLPS-stimulated monocytes resulted in a significant six fold decrease in the level of TNF-*α* (p = 0.0024) and one-and-a-half fold decrease in IL-12 (p = 0.023) levels as compared to LPS-stimulated monocytes alone (**Figure 1** and **Figure 2**).

### 3.2. Effect of Adenosine on TLR-4

To assess the effect of adenosine on TLR-4, adenosine was added to non-stimulated monocytes and to LPS-RS blocked monocytes. This resulted in a significant decrease in TNF-*α* levels by four folds (p = 0.0003) and two-and-half fold (0.0011) as compared to non-stimulated monocytes and LPS-RS blocked monocytes respectively. However, no significant reduction in IL-12 levels was observed ($p > 0.05$) (**Figure 1** and **Figure 2**).

**Table 1.** Culture and treatment of monocytes.

| Wells | Monocytes 2 × $10^5$ cells/ml in 0.5 ml culture media | | | |
|---|---|---|---|---|
| | pLPS (0.01 µg/ml*) T = 0 hr | LPS-RS (0.1 µg/ml) T = −2 hr | Adenosine (100 M) T = 0 hr | Caffeine (100 M) T = −1 hr |
| Well 1 | -- | -- | -- | -- |
| Well 2 | + | -- | -- | -- |
| Well 3 | -- | + | -- | -- |
| Well 4 | + | + | -- | -- |
| Well 5 | -- | -- | + | -- |
| Well 6 | -- | -- | + | -- |
| Well 7 | -- | -- | + | + |
| Well 8 | + | -- | -- | + |
| Well 9 | + | -- | + | -- |
| Well 10 | + | -- | + | + |
| Well 11 | -- | + | -- | + |
| Well 12 | -- | + | + | -- |
| Well 13 | -- | + | + | + |

*Concentrations used were: 2 µl of 0.1 µg/ml pLPS extracted from *Escherichia coli* 111:B4 strain, 381 µl of 100 M adenosine, 121 µl of 100 M caffeine and 10 µl of 1 µg/ml LPS-RS extracted from *Rhodobacter sphaeroides*.

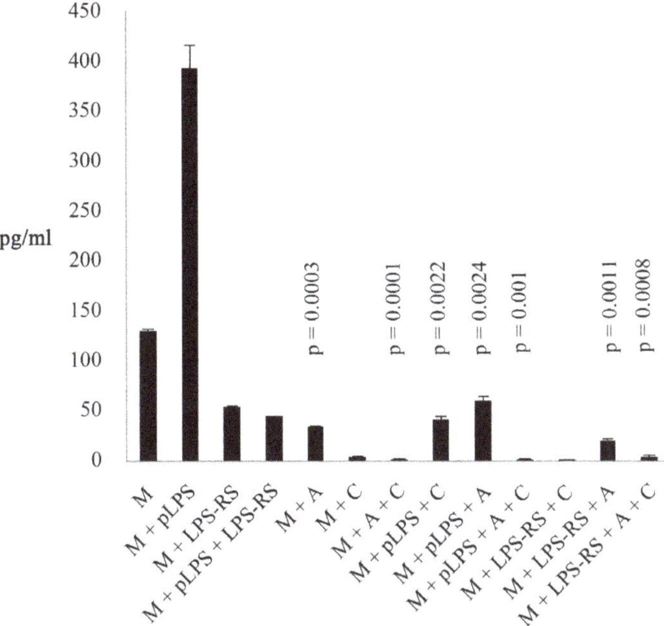


**Figure 1.** TNF-*α* levels in supernatants determined by ELISA. Results after 24 hrs incubation of monocytes with the presence or absence of 2 μl of 0.1 μg/ml pLPS extracted from *Escherichia coli* 111:B4 strain, 381 μl of 100 M adenosine, 121 μl of 100 M caffeine and 10 μl of 1 μg/ml LPS-RS extracted from *Rhodobacter sphaeroides*. After incubation, supernatant was used to assess the TNF-*α* level in each well. M = monocytes, pLPS = *E. coli* Lipopolysaccharide, LPS-RS = *Rh. sphaeroides* Lipopolysaccharide, A = adenosine and C = caffeine. Only significant p values (<0.5) are displayed on figure.

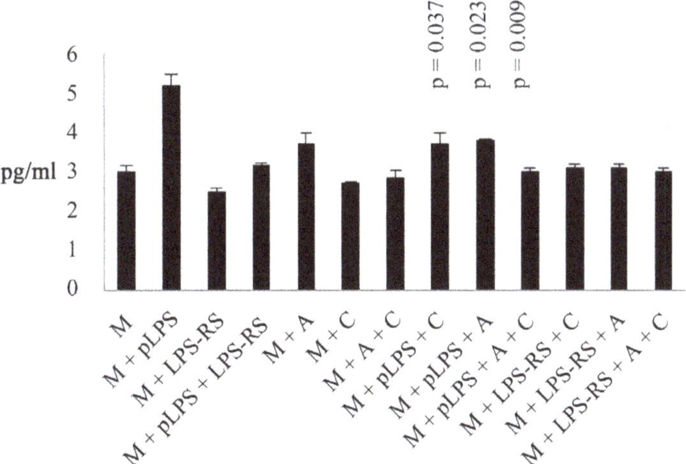


**Figure 2.** IL-12 levels in supernatants determined by ELISA. Results after 24 hrs incubation of Monocytes with the presence or absence of 2 μl of 0.1 μg/ml pLPS extracted from *Escherichia coli* 111:B4 strain, 381 μl of 100 M adenosine, 121 μl of 100 M caffeine and 10 μl of 1 μg/ ml LPS-RS extracted from *Rhodobacter sphaeroides*. After incubation, supernatant was used to assess the TNF-*α* level in each well. M = monocytes, pLPS = *E. coli* Lipopolysaccharide, LPS-RS = *Rh. sphaeroides* Lipopolysaccharide, A = adenosine and C = caffeine. Only significant p values (<0.5) are displayed on figure.

### 3.3. Effect of Caffeine on pLPS Stimulated Monocytes

This resulted in a significant nine fold decrease in the level of TNF-$\alpha$ ($p = 0.0022$) and a significant one-and-a-half fold decrease in the level of IL-12 ($p = 0.037$) as compared to LPS-stimulated monocytes alone.

### 3.4. Effect of Caffeine on TLR-4

When caffeine was added to non-stimulated monocytes or LPS-RS blocked monocytes, it resulted in a significant decrease in the levels of TNF-$\alpha$ by twenty nine fold and fifty fold respectively ($p = 0.0001$, and $p = 0.0001$ respectively) but IL-12 levels were not affected significantly ($p > 0.05$). Moreover, it is worth noting that in all scenarios caffeine was decreasing TNF-$\alpha$ levels more than adenosine.

### 3.5. Effect of the Combination of Adenosine and Caffeine; (Figure 1 and Figure 2)

- On pLPS-stimulated monocytes; significantly decreased TNF-$\alpha$ levels by three hundred fold ($p = 0.001$) and IL-12 levels by about 2 fold ($p = 0.0097$).
- On non-stimulated monocytes; significantly decreased TNF-$\alpha$ by fifty folds ($p = 0.0001$). Had no significant effect on IL-12 levels ($p > 0.05$).
- On LPS-RS blocked monocytes; significantly decreased TNF-$\alpha$ by thirteen fold ($p = 0.0008$). Had no significant effect on IL-12 levels ($p > 0.05$).
- It is worth noting that the combination of adenosine and caffeine decreased TNF-$\alpha$ levels more than when each reagent was used alone.

## 4. Discussion

In the presence of Gram negative bacteria, TLR-4 recognizes pLPS and initiates an inflammatory response in an attempt to eliminate these bacteria. While inflammation is usually beneficial, excessive inflammation can result in tissue injury or sepsis. To control the inflammatory response, adenosine is released at sites of tissue injury and inflammation where it acts as an endogenous anti-inflammatory agent [8]. It has been reported that adenosine decreases TNF-$\alpha$ and IL-12 production in LPS-stimulated monocytes and thus suppresses inflammation [10]-[12].

Our results indicated that when adenosine was added to pLPS-stimulated monocytes, a significant decrease in both cytokines, IL-12 and TNF$\alpha$, was observed. These results are consistent with previous studies demonstrating that adenosine decreases the production of pro-inflammatory cytokines in pLPS-stimulated monocytes [10] [11]. On the other hand, the addition of adenosine to LPS-RS blocked monocytes or to non-stimulated monocytes significantly decreased TNF$\alpha$ levels but had little effect on the levels of IL-12 released by these cells. Such results suggest that TLR-4 is probably not implicated in the signaling of adenosine since the blockage of TLR-4 by LPS-RS or the lack of its stimulation in non-stimulated monocytes did not prevent adenosine from exerting its anti-inflammatory role and decreasing TNF$\alpha$ levels mainly.

Caffeine, a popular psychostimulant, belongs to the methyl xanthine family of drugs [13]. It is a non-specific adenosine blocker that antagonizes all adenosine receptors. Previous studies investigating the role of caffeine in immunity were controversial. While most studies agreed that caffeine decreases inflammation [14]-[16], other studies presented evidence on caffeine increasing tissue injury, inflammation, or even playing no significant role in immunity [14] [18]. Thus, the aim was to assess the role of caffeine in promoting or decreasing inflammation in pLPS stimulated monocytes. Moreover, knowing that caffeine has no identified receptors yet, we investigated the role of TLR-4 in caffeine signaling. The results indicated that caffeine significantly decreased the levels of both TNF$\alpha$ and IL-12 produced by pLPS stimulated monocytes. These findings are in agreement with previous studies suggesting that caffeine decreases cytokines production in pLPS-stimulated monocytes and might play an anti-inflammatory role [14] [15]. The addition of caffeine to LPS-RS blocked monocytes and to non-stimulated monocytes resulted in a significant decrease in TNF$\alpha$ levels but had a little effect on the levels of IL-12 released by these cells. These results again indicate that TLR-4 might not be involved in the signaling of caffeine since a significant decrease in cytokines, in particular TNF$\alpha$, was still observed when TLR-4 receptor was not stimulated or blocked. It is worth noting that in all cases the decreased TNF$\alpha$ level caused by caffeine was greater than that caused by adenosine. This reinforces the possibility that caffeine is an immune-modulatory molecule.

This result concurs with the report of Verani *et al.* who showed that caffeine had an anti-inflammatory effect [19]. They suggested that caffeine upregulated the adenosine anti-inflammatory $A_{2a}$ receptors. Thus, despite previous data stating that the major effects of caffeine are due to adenosine antagonism, caffeine does not seem to block the anti-inflammatory adenosine receptors present on monocytes.

It had been noted that in LPS-RS blocked monocytes and non-stimulated monocytes, the addition of adenosine, caffeine, or both reagents decreased TNF$\alpha$ levels significantly but did not result in significant changes in IL-12 levels. This different effect can be due to the fact that TNF-$\alpha$ is usually produced in higher levels than IL-12 and thus we expect that the decrease in TNF-$\alpha$ levels, upon blockage of TLR-4 in LPS-RS blocked monocytes or the lack of its stimulation in monocytes alone, will be more pronounced than that of IL-12. Another possible explanation is that the production of IL-12 is regulated by different mechanism than that of TNF-$\alpha$ [20].

## 5. Conclusion

In conclusion, both caffeine and adenosine blocked the production of the pro-inflammatory cytokines by pLPS-stimulated monocytes. TLR-4 did not appear to be involved in the signaling pathway of caffeine and adenosine since blocking of TLR-4 did not abolish the effects of adenosine and caffeine on production of cytokines, in particular TNF-$\alpha$.

## References


[1] Alexander, C. and Rietschel, E.T. (2001) Invited Review: Bacterial Lipopolysaccharides and Innate Immunity. *Journal of Endotoxin Research*, 7, 167-202. http://dx.doi.org/10.1177/09680519010070030101

[2] Fujihara, M., Muroi, M., Tanamoto, K.I., Suzuki, T., Azuma, H. and Ikeda, H. (2003) Molecular Mechanisms of Macrophage Activation and Deactivation by Lipopolysaccharide: Roles of the Receptor Complex. *Pharmacology & Therapeutics*, **100**, 171-194. http://dx.doi.org/10.1016/j.pharmthera.2003.08.003

[3] Park, B.S. and Lee, J.O. (2013) Recognition of Lipopolysaccharide Pattern by TLR4 Complexes. *Experimental & Molecular Medicine*, **45**, e66. http://dx.doi.org/10.1038/emm.2013.97

[4] Bryant, C.E., Spring, D.R., Gangloff, M. and Gay, N.J. (2010) The Molecular Basis of the Host Response to Lipopolysaccharide. *Nature Reviews Microbiology*, **8**, 8-14.

[5] Liaunardy-Jopeace, A. and Gay, N.J. (2014) Molecular and Cellular Regulation of Toll-Like Receptor-4 Activity Induced by Lipopolysaccharide Ligands. *Frontiers in Immunology*, **5**, 473. http://dx.doi.org/10.3389/fimmu.2014.00473

[6] Teghanemt, A., Zhang, D., Levis, E.N., Weiss, J.P. and Gioannini, T.L. (2005) Molecular Basis of Reduced Potency of Underacylated Endotoxins. *The Journal of Immunology*, **175**, 4669-4676. http://dx.doi.org/10.4049/jimmunol.175.7.4669

[7] Coats, S.R., Pham, T.T.T., Bainbridge, B.W., Reife, R.A. and Darveau, R.P. (2005) MD-2 Mediates the Ability of Tetra-Acylated and Penta-Acylated Lipopolysaccharides to Antagonize *Escherichia coli* Lipopolysaccharide at the TLR4 Signaling Complex. *The Journal of Immunology*, **175**, 4490-4498. http://dx.doi.org/10.4049/jimmunol.175.7.4490

[8] Haskó, G. and Cronstein, B.N. (2004) Adenosine: An Endogenous Regulator of Innate Immunity. *Trends in Immunology*, **25**, 33-39. http://dx.doi.org/10.1016/j.it.2003.11.003

[9] Haskó, G., Linden, J., Cronstein, B. and Pacher, P. (2008) Adenosine Receptors: Therapeutic Aspects for Inflammatory and Immune Diseases. *Nature Reviews Drug Discovery*, **7**, 759-770. http://dx.doi.org/10.1038/nrd2638

[10] McNeill, B.W. (2004) Adenosine Receptor Mediated Inhibition of Tumor Necrosis Factor Alpha in Human Monocytic Cells. Doctoral Dissertation, University of Georgia.

[11] McColl, S.R., St-Onge, M., Dussault, A.A., Laflamme, C., Bouchard, L., Boulanger, J. and Pouliot, M. (2006) Immunomodulatory Impact of the $A_{2A}$ Adenosine Receptor on the Profile of Chemokines Produced by Neutrophils. *The FASEB Journal*, **20**, 187-189.

[12] Hamano, R., Takahashi, H.K., Iwagaki, H., Kanke, T., Liu, K., Yoshino, T. and Tanaka, N. (2008) Stimulation of Adenosine $A_{2A}$ Receptor Inhibits LPS-Induced Expression of Intercellular Adhesion Molecule 1 and Production of TNF-$\alpha$ in Human Peripheral Blood Mononuclear Cells. *Shock*, **29**, 154-159. http://dx.doi.org/10.1097/shk.0b013e31812385da

[13] Horrigan, L.A., Kelly, J.P. and Connor, T.J. (2006) Immunomodulatory Effects of Caffeine: Friend or Foe? *Pharmacology & Therapeutics*, **111**, 877-892. http://dx.doi.org/10.1016/j.pharmthera.2006.02.002

[14] Horrigan, L.A., Kelly, J.P. and Connor, T.J. (2004) Caffeine Suppresses TNF-$\alpha$ Production via Activation of the Cyclic AMP/Protein Kinase A Pathway. *International Immunopharmacology*, **4**, 1409-1417. http://dx.doi.org/10.1016/j.intimp.2004.06.005

[15] Deree, J., Martins, J.O., Melbostad, H., Loomis, W.H. and Coimbra, R. (2008) Insights into the Regulation of TNF-$\alpha$ Production in Human Mononuclear Cells: The Effects of Non-Specific Phosphodiesterase Inhibition. *Clinics*, **63**, 321-328. http://dx.doi.org/10.1590/S1807-59322008000300006

[16] Ramakers, B.P., Riksen, N.P., van den Broek, P., Franke, B., Peters, W.H., van der Hoeven, J.G. and Pickkers, P. (2011) Circulating Adenosine Increases during Human Experimental Endotoxemia but Blockade of Its Receptor Does Not Influence the Immune Response and Subsequent Organ Injury. *Critical Care*, **15**, R3. http://dx.doi.org/10.1186/cc9400

[17] Ohta, A., Lukashev, D., Jackson, E.K., Fredholm, B.B. and Sitkovsky, M. (2007) 1, 3, 7-Trimethylxanthine (Caffeine) May Exacerbate Acute Inflammatory Liver Injury by Weakening the Physiological Immunosuppressive Mechanism. *The Journal of Immunology*, **179**, 7431-7438. http://dx.doi.org/10.4049/jimmunol.179.11.7431

[18] Meiners, I., Hauschildt, S., Nieber, K. and Münch, G. (2004) Pentoxyphylline and Propentophylline Are Inhibitors of TNF-$\alpha$ Release in Monocytes Activated by Advanced Glycation Endproducts. *Journal of Neural Transmission*, **111**, 441-444. http://dx.doi.org/10.1007/s00702-003-0066-y

[19] Varani, K., Portaluppi, F., Gessi, S., Merighi, S., Vincenzi, F., Cattabriga, E. and Borea, P.A. (2005) Caffeine Intake Induces an Alteration in Human Neutrophil $A_{2A}$ Adenosine Receptors. *Cellular and Molecular Life Sciences CMLS*, **62**, 2350-2358. http://dx.doi.org/10.1007/s00018-005-5312-z

[20] Aste-Amezaga, M., Ma, X., Sartori, A. and Trinchieri, G. (1998) Molecular Mechanisms of the Induction of IL-12 and Its Inhibition by IL-10. *The Journal of Immunology*, **160**, 5936-5944.

18

# Fyn Expression Predicates Both Protective Immunity and Onset of Autoimmunity

**Behrouz Moemeni[1,2], Nathalie Vacaresse[1], Marina Vainder[1], Michael E. Wortzman[2], Tania H. Watts[2], André Veillette[3], Thomas F. Gajewski[4], Michael Julius[1,2]**

[1]Sunnybrook Research Institute, Toronto, Canada
[2]Department of Immunology, University of Toronto, Toronto, Canada
[3]Laboratory of Molecular Oncology, Clinical Research Institute of Montreal, Montreal, Canada
[4]Department of Pathology, University of Chicago, Chicago, IL, USA
Email: michael.julius@sri.utoronto.ca

## Abstract

**Genomic disruption of Fyn has not been associated with an immune-deficient phenotype, notwithstanding the profound impairment in IL-2 production by T cells derived from Fyn-deficient animals observed *in vitro*. The results presented demonstrate that Fyn deficient animals succumb to influenza infection ahead of the protective expansion of lung infiltrating T cells and viral clearance observed in wild-type hosts. Formal proof that Fyn-dependent IL-2 production mediates T cell expansion *in vivo* is provided using a model of T cell induced enteropathy. Specifically, Fyn deficient naïve T cells do not induce colitis in SCID animals due to their lack of expansion, and Fyn re-expression rescues both IL-2 production and its capacity to support *in vivo* expansion leading to colitis. These results reconcile the obligatory role of Fyn in T cell activation and autocrine IL-2 supported growth; and underscore the mechanism through which its function is integrated with and regulated by Lck.**

## Keywords

**Fyn, Lck, TcR Signaling, Immunity, Autoimmunity**

## 1. Introduction

FynT is the T cell specific form of Fyn, a Src Family Tyrosine Kinase involved in intracellular signal transduction [1] [2]. The role of Fyn in mediating the most proximal signals emanating from the T cell antigen receptor complex [TcR/CD3] in support of cellular activation and IL-2 mediated T cell expansion remains enigmatic. The two studies in which Fyn deficient animals were prepared and T cell signaling characterized revealed that TcR-induced IL-2 production, calcium flux, and proliferation assessed *in vitro*, were profoundly impaired [1] [2]. Further, Fyn deficient mice contain comparable numbers of peripheral T cells of both lineages [1]-[3], their T cell repertoire appears unperturbed [1]-[3] and they contain a normal complement of Tregs [3]. The only lesion described to date is absence of NK T cells [4]. The lack of an overt phenotype attributed to Fyn deficiency has supported the conclusion that Lck and Fyn are at least in part, redundant.

However, accumulating evidence supports the inter-related yet unique functions of Lck and Fyn in supporting TcR induced IL-2 production. Ordered lipid microdomains (LR) function to segregate Lck and Fyn and regulate the temporal and spatial coordination of their activation [5] [6]. Specifically, TcR-CD4 co-aggregation induces Lck activation outside LR, followed by the translocation of activated Lck into LR where it physically associates with and activates LR-resident Fyn [6] [7].

In the present study, the essential role of Fyn in TcR-mediated IL-2 production in primary T cells was formally demonstrated using an adenoviral gene delivery system. Next, the role of IL-2 in the impaired expansion of Fyn deficient T cells *in vivo* was formally established using a model of experimental colitis [8]-[10]. Specifically, the environmental antigen driven expansion of Fyn deficient CD45RB$^{hi}$ CD4$^{+}$ T "inducer" cells in the large bowel of SCID recipients was virtually ablated, and rescued, along with the capacity to induce disease, upon re-expression of Fyn. Further, the capacity of anti-IL-2 to inhibit the initial expansion of colitis inducing T cells *in vivo* mechanistically tethers the role of Fyn in supporting TcR mediated IL-2 production *in vitro* with the inefficient IL-2 dependent expansion of Fyn deficient T cells *in vivo* and their failure to induce enteropathy.

The consequences of impaired expansion of Fyn-deficient T cells *in vivo* extend to profoundly impaired protective immunity. The immune-competence of Fyn-deficient animals was assessed using a flu infection model [11] [12]. Both wild-type and Fyn deficient hosts exhibited chronic inflammatory peribronchiolitis at day 6 and contained comparable numbers of lung infiltrating T cells of both lineages. The infection was cleared in wild-type hosts over the next 3 days and correlated with a 10 - 20-fold increase in infiltrating T cells, while Fyn deficient hosts succumbed to respiratory death due to pulmonary consolidation.

These results are first to demonstrate that the genomic disruption of *fyn* has profound consequences on T cell function *in vivo*; demonstrating the essential role of Fyn in TcR signaling in support of IL-2 mediated T cell expansion *in vivo*; and they provide the mechanistic basis underpinning the unique, yet inter-dependent roles of Lck and Fyn in the regulation of T cell homeostasis.

## 2. Materials and Methods

### 2.1. Mice

WT (C57BL/6), SCID, and Fyn$^{-/-}$ [2] were purchased from Jackson Laboratories. Fyn$^{-/-}$ mice were bred to CARΔ1 [13] (here referred to as CAR$^{+}$ mice) in our animal facility to develop Fyn$^{-/-}$CAR$^{+}$ mice. All mice, including SCID recipients, were kept in specified pathogen-free conditions prior to adoptive cell transfers. All experiments were approved by Sunnybrook Research Institute Animal Care Committee and followed guidelines set by the Canadian Council on Animal Care.

### 2.2. Flu-Infection Model

Five week old (20 grams) male mice were infected with the influenza virus A/PR8 (PR8, H1N1) through intranasal administration with either $10^5$ or $10^4$ $TCID_{50}$ in PBS as indicated. For survival experiments, following the procedure the mice were monitored daily and sacrificed when the body temperature had dropped below 32 degrees C, they had lost >30% of total body weight, or appeared moribund. Otherwise, the mice were sacrificed at specific time points post infection.

### 2.3. Viral Clearance Assay

For viral clearance assays, lungs were excised from the animal at 3, 6, and 9 days post intranasal infection with influenza A/PR8. After weighing, lungs were homogenized in RPMI 1640 medium (1 g of lung tissue/10 ml). Supernatant was obtained and stored at −70˚C after centrifugation at 1200 × *g* for 20 min at 4˚C. $TCID_{50}$ was determined by the MDCK assay with the Reed and Muench technique as previously described [14]. The infected lungs and sacrificed mice were disposed of in accordance with Sunnybrook Research Institute Animal Care

Committee and followed guidelines set by the Canadian Council on Animal Care.

## 2.4. Antibodies, Cytokines and Reagents

Polyclonal anti-Lck and anti-Fyn antibodies have been previously described [5]. Anti-phosphotyrosine (4G10) and anti-actin antibodies were purchased from Upstate, anti-Fyb from Lifespan Bio, anti-SLP-76 (clone AS55) from Millipore, anti-CD3$\varepsilon$ (145-2C11), anti-CD4 (GK1.5), anti-TcRC$\beta$ (H57), anti-CD69 (H1.2F3), anti-CD45RB (C363.16A), anti-IL-4 (11B11), anti-IFN-$\gamma$ (R4-6A2), mouse recombinant IL-6 and recombinant human TGF-$\beta$1 from eBiocience. Murine recombinant IL-7 was purchased from Peprotech. Anti-CAR (RmcB), anti-IL-2 (S4B6), and anti-IL-2 isotype control (rat IgG2) were isolated from their respective hybridomas cultured in our laboratory. Brij-58, Cholera toxin B-HRP (CT-HRP) and Streptavidin were purchased from Sigma-Aldrich.

## 2.5. Cell Sorting, Cell Transfer and Isolation of Lamina Propria Lymphocytes

Splenic CAR$^+$ CD4$^+$ CD45RB$^{hi}$ or CD45RB$^{lo}$ T cells [11] were sorted using BDAria cell sorter and $2.5 \times 10^6$ cells were injected iv into each SCID recipient. After cell transfer, SCID recipients were fed non-sterile food and water and kept in cages in the absence of filter tops. Recipients were monitored and sacrificed when bloody diarrhea and/or rectal prolapse was evident. To determine the number of infiltrating donor cells, Lamina Propria lymphocytes were isolated from the large gut of recipients as described [15], stained using fluorochrome labeled anti-CD4 and anti-CAR and the number of donor cells was determined using percentage of CD4$^+$CAR$^+$ assessed flow cytometrically using a BD FACSCalibur.

## 2.6. *In Vivo* CFSE Dilution Assay

Sorted splenic CAR$^+$ CD4$^+$ CD45RB$^{hi}$ T cells were CFSE labeled [16] and $2.5 \times 10^6$ cells were injected iv into each SCID recipient on day zero. Recipients also received daily intraperitoneal injections of 0.5 mg of S4B6, 0.5 mg of isotype control, or PBS in a total volume of 200 µL, starting on day zero, for seven days. Recipients were sacrificed on day seven, and donor CAR$^+$CD4$^+$ T cells in spleen and lymph nodes were analyzed for CFSE expression flow cytometrically [16].

## 2.7. Shuttle Vector Design

The shuttle vector (pENTR-UbC) was designed by cloning human Ubiquitin C promoter [13] followed by a multiple cloning site (MCS) and a region containing the simian virus 40 late polyadenylation sequence [13] using pENTR (Invitrogen) as the vector backbone. emGFP (Invitrogen) and wild type murine FynT (WT-Fyn) [5] cDNAs were cloned into the MCS of pENTR-UbC.

## 2.8. Adenoviral Constructs, Purification, Titration

Adenoviral constructs were created using Clonase-mediated recombination between pENTR-UbC-emGFP or pENTR-UbC-WT-Fyn with pAd/PL-DEST (Invitrogen), followed by preparation of amplified adenoviral stocks according to the manufacturer's recommendations. Adenoviral stocks were purified using Adeno-X Maxi purification kits from Clontech and titered using plaque formation assays in 293A cells (Invitrogen) and Quantum's AdEasy $TCID_{50}$ protocol.

## 2.9. Adenoviral Transduction

Primary T cells were suspended at a concentration of $1 \times 10^6$ cells/100 µL in serum free medium [17] in the presence of adenoviral particles at a multiplicity of infection (MOI) of 10 for one hour at 37°C. The cells were then washed and cultured in serum free medium in the presence of 10 ng/ml of IL-7 for 24 hours prior to IL-2 and IL-17A assays or for 72 hours prior to cell transfer experiments.

## 2.10. Isolation of CD4+ T Cells, *in Vitro* CD4/TcR Coaggregation, Immunoprecipitation, Immunoblotting and Immune Complex Kinase Assay

Splenic CD4$^+$ T cells were isolated using EasySep negative selection kit from STEMCELL Technologies. $10^6$

$CD4^+$ T cells were labeled with biotinylated H57 and/or biotinylated GK1.5 and CD4/TcR coaggregation was achieved using streptavidin as previously described [6]. The cells were lysed and subjected to immunoprecipitation (IP) using anti-Lck [6]. The IP samples were subjected to immune complex kinase assay [6] and probed for Lck. For Fyb IPs, $10^7$ $CD4^+$ T cells were lysed and subjected to IP using anti-Fyb. The IP samples were equally divided and probed for phosphotyrosine, Fyb, SLP-76, and Fyn.

### 2.11. IL-2 and IL-17A ELISA

For IL-2, $5 \times 10^4$ $CD4^+$ T cells were cultured in 200 μL of serum free medium [17] per well of a 96-well plate (Corning Costar) previously coated with H57 (0.5 μg/ml), GK1.5 (10 μg/ml), or both, in triplicates, for 48 hours. The level of IL-2 was determined using an IL-2 specific ELISA kit (eBioscience). For IL-17A, the cells were cultured in the presence of anti-IL-4 (10 μg/ml), anti-IFN-$\gamma$ (10 μg/ml), IL-6 (10 ng/ml) and TGF-$\beta$1 (5 ng/ml) in 96-well plates (Corning Costar) previously coated with H57 (1.5 μg/ml), GK1.5 (30 μg/ml), or both, in triplicates, for 72 hours. The level of IL-17A was determined using an IL-17A specific ELISA kit (eBioscience).

### 2.12. Lipid Raft Isolation

Lipid rafts (LR) were isolated from $10^6$ cells, as previously described [17], and 40 μL of each fraction was probed for GM1 ganglioside as a marker for lipid rafts using CT-HRP. LR distributions of Lck and Fyn were determined by immunoblotting 40 μL of each fraction using anti-Lck and anti-Fyn antibodies respectively.

### 2.13. Densitometry

Densitometric analysis was performed using GS-800 densitometer and Quantity One software from Bio-Rad Laboratories on non-saturated signals.

### 2.14. H & E and Immunofluorescence

Large intestine from SCID recipients was collected, washed with PBS, cut longitudinally, wrapped to form a roll before being frozen in OCT (Electron Microscopy Sciences), and 8 μm sections were stained with hematoxylin and eosin. Pictures were taken using a DFC300 FX Digital Color Camera and the Application Suite software, both from Leica. For immunofluorescent microscopy the sections were fixed in ice-cold acetone for 10 min and air-dried at room temperature for 30 min, blocked in PBS plus 5% normal goat serum for 30 min followed by incubation in anti-CD3$\varepsilon$ diluted in PBS plus 5% normal goat serum. Lastly, the sections were probed using Cy5 conjugated secondary antibody (goat anti-Armenian Hamster IgG (H $^+$ L), Jackson ImmunoResearch Laboratories) as well as 4′,6-Diamidino-2-phenylindole dihydrochloride (DAPI, Sigma-Aldrich). Images were captured using a Zeiss microscope (Carl Zeiss) and analyzed using the AxioVision software (Carl Zeiss). Same time of exposure during the acquisition and same values during processing were applied to each image.

### 2.15. Statistical Analysis

*P* values among experimental groups were determined by the unpaired Student's *t*-test.

## 3. Results

### 3.1. Fyn Expression Predicates Antigen Receptor Induced IL-2 Production in $CD4^+$ T Cells

An *in vitro* assay involving antibody-mediated co-aggregation of CD4 and associated Lck with the TcR/CD3 complex was employed. $CD4^+$ T cells were cultured in plates pre-coated with anti-CD4, anti-TcRC$\beta$, or both and IL-2 production was assessed at 48 hours. As has been previously described [1] [2], IL-2 production by $Fyn^{-/-}$ T cells was profoundly impaired, giving rise to <10% of the IL-2 produced by WT $CD4^+$ T cells (**Figure 1**).

Formal proof of the role of Fyn underpinning this defect was achieved through ectopic expression of *fyn* in primary resting T cells using an adenoviral gene delivery system. As mice do not express an adenovirus receptor, WT and $Fyn^{-/-}$ mice were mated with those transgenic for the coxsackie/adenoviral receptor (CAR) [13]. CAR transgenic mice have been constructed to express the coxsackie/adenoviral receptor using a T cell specific pro-

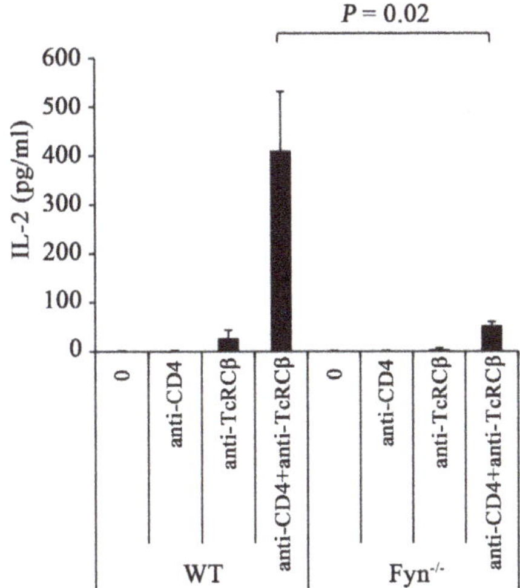


**Figure 1.** Profound impairment in CD4/TcR-induced IL-2 production in primary Fyn$^{-/-}$ CD4$^{+}$ T cells. IL-2 ELISA of supernatants from primary WT or Fyn$^{-/-}$ T cell cultures stimulated with plate-bound anti-CD4, anti-TcRC$\beta$ or both for 48 hours. Data (mean and s.d.) represent mean values from three independent experiments.

moter to allow for the expression of CAR specifically on T cells. CAR expression in these transgenic mice is mainly restricted to T cells, and these animals exhibit normal T cell development and T cells expressing CAR allow for the efficient transfer of any gene of interest into primary resting T cells [13].

The efficacy of adenoviral transduction is illustrated in **Figure 2**. Specifically, transduction of WT CAR$^{+}$ CD4$^{+}$ T cells with GFP containing virus (Ad/GFP) resulted in ~90% GFP$^{+}$ cells within 24 hours (**Figure 2(a)**). **Figure 2(b)** illustrates the kinetics of ectopic expression of Fyn in CD4$^{+}$Fyn$^{-/-}$CAR$^{+}$ primary T cells. Further, the levels of ectopic Fyn expression achieved in these circumstances were comparable to WT levels of endogenous Fyn expression, and there were no detectable alterations in the levels of endogenous Lck expression (**Figure 2(c)**). As illustrated in **Figure 2(d)**, the cellular localization of ectopically expressed Fyn was identical to that observed for endogenous Fyn in WT cells with >90% localizing to LR [6].

As illustrated in **Figure 3**, Ad/WT-Fyn transduction of Fyn$^{-/-}$ CD4$^{+}$ primary T cells rescued levels of IL-2 production upon co-aggregation of TcR and CD4 comparable to those observed in WT CD4$^{+}$ T cells. Ad/GFP transduction of either WT or Fyn$^{-/-}$ T cells had no significant effect (**Figure 3**).

Previous reports have demonstrated that the activities of Lck and Fyn are reciprocally regulated [18] [19]. It is therefore possible that the impaired TcR/CD4 induced IL-2 production observed in Fyn$^{-/-}$ T cells is not due to the absence of Fyn *per se*, rather, impaired function of Lck in Fyn$^{-/-}$ T cells. To investigate this possibility, the activity of Lck was assessed subsequent to TcR-CD4 co-aggregation in each of three CAR$^{+}$CD4$^{+}$ T cell populations: WT or Fyn$^{-/-}$ transduced with Ad/GFP and Fyn$^{-/-}$ transduced with Ad/WT-Fyn. As illustrated in **Figure 4(a)**, both aggregation of CD4 and co-aggregation of CD4-TcR resulted in a robust and comparable induction of Lck kinase activity, in each of the three T cell populations, as assessed by levels of phosphorylation of substrate enolase. Hence, the capacity to activate Lck is not impaired in the absence of Fyn, and therefore, taken together, these results formally prove that Fyn predicates TcR induction of IL-2 production *in vitro*.

We next sought to characterize the signalling defect underpinning compromised IL-2 production in Fyn$^{-/-}$ T cells. Fyb is a specific Fyn substrate and it has been reported that it is not tyrosine phosphorylated in Fyn$^{-/-}$ T cells [20]. As illustrated in **Figure 4(b)**, the basal level of tyrosine phosphorylation of Fyb is indeed reduced in Fyn$^{-/-}$ T cells and is restored in primary resting CD4$^{+}$ T cells transduced with Ad/WT-Fyn (**Figure 4(b)**). However, and of note, is that notwithstanding the reduced level of PY-Fyb in Fyn$^{-/-}$ T cells, anti-Fyb co-immunoprecipitated SLP-76 from Fyn$^{-/-}$ T cells as efficiently as it did from WT T cells (**Figure 4(b)**). Upon TcR-mediated cellular activation, levels of P-Y Fyb and P-Y SLP-76 increase in both WT CD4$^{+}$ T cells and Fyn$^{-/-}$ CD4$^{+}$ T cells transduced with Ad/WT-Fyn, but not in Fyn$^{-/-}$ CD4$^{+}$ T cells transduced with Ad/GFP (**Figure 4(b)**). These results confirm that Fyb is a direct Fyn substrate and also reveal the presence of a tri-molecular complex of Fyb-SLP-76-Fyn in WT and Fyn$^{-/-}$ T cells transduced with Ad/WT-Fyn in resting T cells. Further, that TcR mediated activation results in the parallel and Fyn-dependent increases in P-Y of both Fyb and SLP-76.

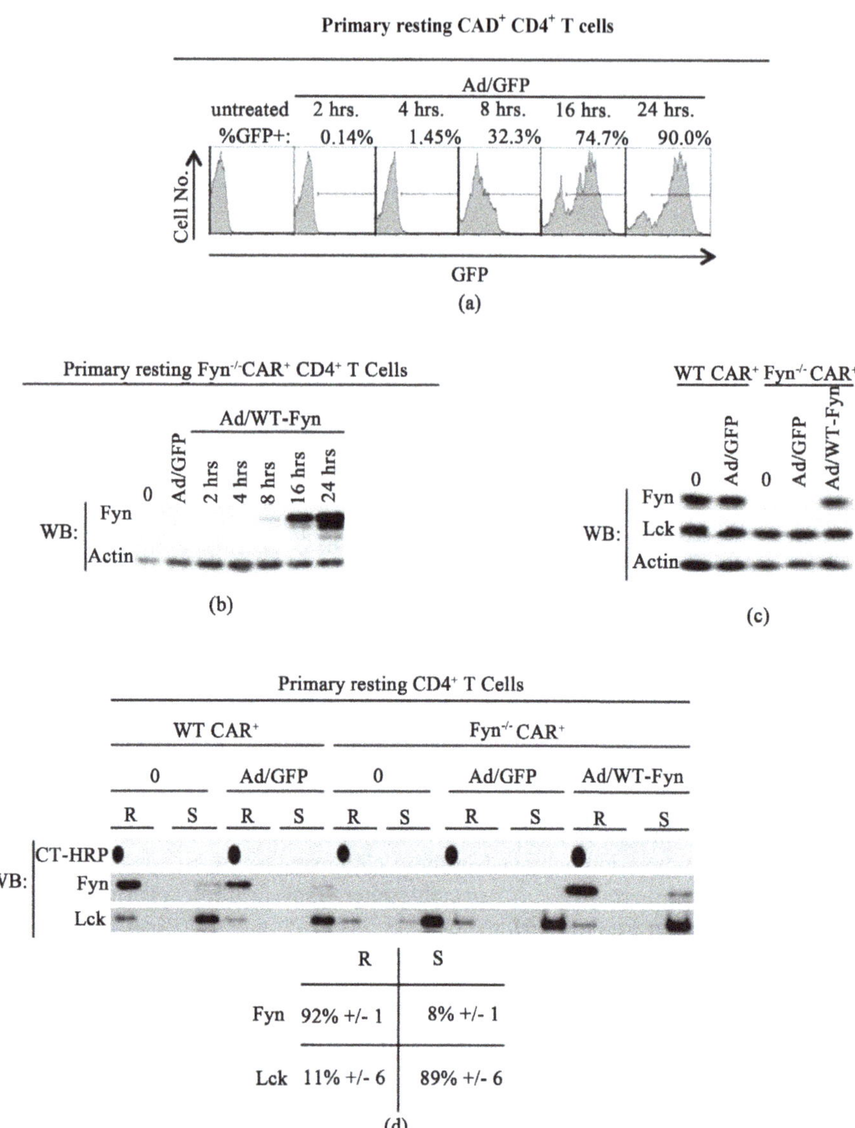


**Figure 2.** Efficient gene expression in primary resting T cells through adenoviral-mediated transduction. (a) Flow cytometric analysis of primary resting WT CAR$^+$ CD4$^+$ T cells transduced with adenoviral particles encoding GFP. The percentage of GFP$^+$ cells in each sample, at the indicated time points, is shown above each histogram; (b) Western blot analysis, over the indicated time points, of primary resting Fyn$^{-/-}$ CAR$^+$ CD4$^+$ T cells transduced with adenoviral particles encoding WT-Fyn. Levels of Fyn (top) and Actin (bottom) are shown; (c) Western blot analysis of WT and Fyn$^{-/-}$ primary resting CAR$^+$ CD4$^+$ T cells untreated or transduced with either Ad/GFP, or Ad/WT-Fyn. Presented are levels of Fyn (top), Lck (middle), and Actin (bottom), in each sample, 48 hours post transduction; (d) Western blot analysis of sucrose gradient fractions derived from WT and Fyn$^{-/-}$ primary resting CAR$^+$ CD4$^+$ T cells that were untreated or transduced with either Ad/GFP, or Ad/WT-Fyn. Lipid raft (R) and soluble (S) fractions from each sample were probed with cholera toxin B-HRP (CT-HRP) (top), anti-Fyn (middle) and anti-Lck (bottom). The numbers represent the mean distribution of Fyn and Lck in R vs. S fractions across all samples.

## 3.2. Impaired *in Vivo* T Cell Expansion and Disease Onset in the Absence of Fyn

Towards mechanistically tethering the observed impairment in IL-2 production *in vitro* by CD4$^+$Fyn$^{-/-}$ T cells with a phenotype attributable to Fyn deficiency in an *in vivo* setting, we sought a model system whose endpoint was predicated by T cell expansion. The T cell-induced colitis model is suitable in this regard. Briefly, reconsti-

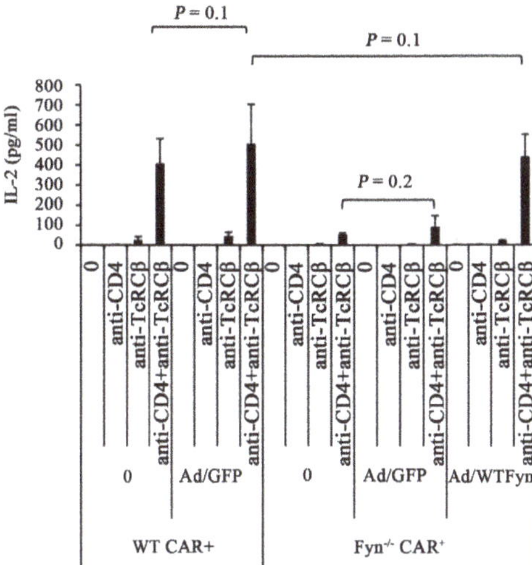


**Figure 3.** Fyn expression in Fyn$^{-/-}$ CD4$^{+}$ T cells rescues CD4/TcR induced IL-2 production. IL-2 ELISA of supernatants from primary CD4$^{+}$ CAR$^{+}$ WT or Fyn$^{-/-}$ T cell cultures untreated or transduced with either Ad/GFP, or Ad/WT-Fyn and stimulated with plate-bound anti-CD4, anti-TcRC$\beta$ or both, for 48 hours. Data (mean and s.d.) represent mean values from three independent experiments.

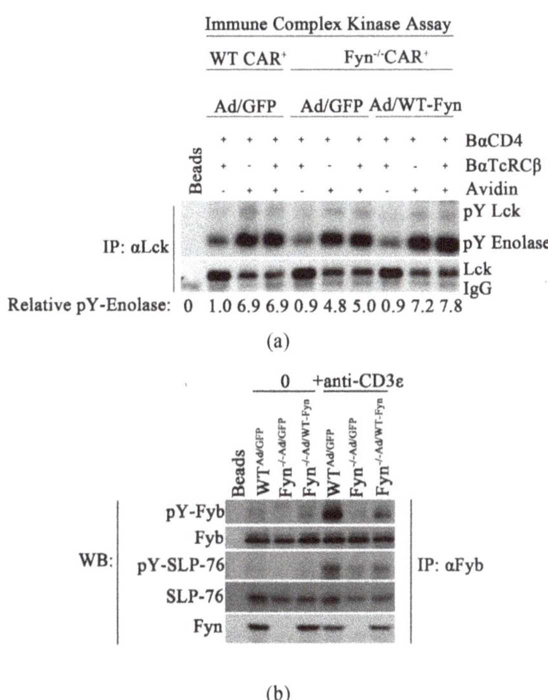


**Figure 4.** Fyn is not required for Lck activation but predicates tyrosine phophorylation of Fyb and SLP-76. (a) Immune complex kinase assay analysis of Lck from primary CD4$^{+}$ CAR$^{+}$ WT or Fyn$^{-/-}$ T cells transduced with either Ad/GFP, or Ad/WT-Fyn. Cells were pre-coated with either biotinylated anti-CD4, biotinylated anti-TcRC$\beta$ or both, followed by addition of streptavidin or not ("+" or "–" signs respectively) for 30 seconds. Cells were lysed and Lck immunoprecipitated (IP). The top panel indicates the levels of phosphorylated Lck (pY-Lck) and phosphorylated enolase (pY-Enolase), revealed using radiolabelled $\gamma$-32P ATP. The bottom panel indicates levels of Lck from each sample assessed by western blot. Relative pY-Enolase, normalized to levels of Lck, indicates Lck kinase activity in each sample, quantified by densitometric analysis, and is represented as fold activity over background, assigned a value of 1.0; (b) Immunoprecipitation (IP) and western blot (WB) analysis of WT and Fyn$^{-/-}$ primary resting CAR$^{+}$ CD4$^{+}$ T cells transduced with either Ad/GFP or Ad/WT-Fyn. Resting cells or cells activated for 1.5 minutes using 1 μg/ml of anti-CD3ε (145-2C11) followed by 10 μg/ml of anti-Armenian Hamster IgG antibody were lysed and Fyb immunoprecipitated. Fyb immunoprecipitates were probed using anti-phosphotyrosine, anti-Fyb, anti-SLP-76, and anti-Fyn antibodies, as indicated.

tution of severe combined immune deficient (SCID) mice with WT CD4$^+$ CD45RB$^{hi}$ T cells has been shown to cause colitis due to expansion of the injected T cells in the large intestine [8]-[10].

To determine whether CD4$^+$ Fyn$^{-/-}$CD45RB$^{hi}$ T cells were impaired inducers of disease, groups of SCID recipients were injected with either WT CD4$^+$ CD45RB$^{hi}$ T cells, or the same phenotypic subset derived from Fyn$^{-/-}$ animals. As illustrated in **Figure 5(a)**, SCID recipients of WT naïve inducer T cells developed colitis starting at 6 weeks post injection. By 13 weeks, 100% of the recipients of WT inducer T cells had succumbed to enteropathy. In striking contrast, recipients of Fyn deficient inducer T cells remained symptom free for the duration of the 16-week observation period (**Figure 5(a)**).

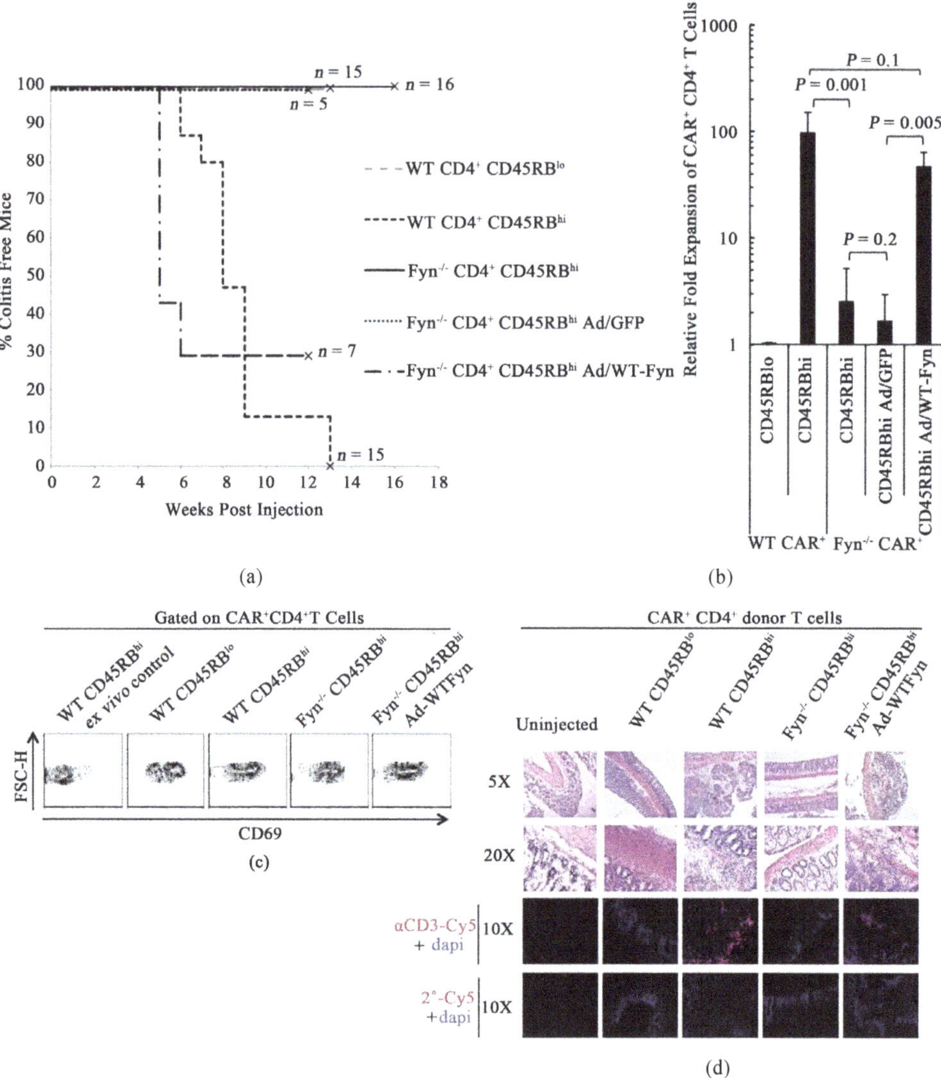


**Figure 5.** Impaired colitogenic capacity and *in vivo* T cell expansion in the absence of Fyn. (a) SCID mice were injected intravenously (iv) with CAR$^+$CD4$^+$ CD45RB$^{hi}$ T cells from the indicated donors. Recipients were followed over time for symptoms of colitis, including bloody stool and/or rectal prolapse, and sacrificed. The graph shows the percentage of colitis free mice in each group over the indicated time period. Time of injection is indicated as week 0, "n" represents the number of animals per group, and "x" indicates the end point; (b) SCID mice injected iv with either of the indicated T cell populations were sacrificed at specific time points post injection, and Lamina Propria T cells were isolated from the large intestine. The number of donor T cells was calculated based on CAR expression. The bar graph indicates the fold expansion of the injected cells relative to the WT CD45RB$^{lo}$ population that was assigned a value of 1; (c) Flow cytometric analysis of CD69 expression by donor cells obtained in (b); (d) H&E staining (top two panels) and immunofluorescence staining (bottom two panels) of large intestine sections from SCID mice injected with the indicated cell populations. Data (mean and s.d.) are mean values (b), or representative ((c) and (d)) of four to seven animals per group obtained from four independent experiments.

Towards formally demonstrating that Fyn deficiency was at the root of impaired disease induction by CAR$^+$CD4$^+$ Fyn$^{-/-}$CD45RB$^{hi}$ T cells, the latter were transduced with either Ad/GFP or Ad/WT-Fyn and their colitogenic capacity assessed. As illustrated in **Figure 5**, Fyn transduction restored the disease inducing capacity of Fyn$^{-/-}$ cells.

The symptoms correlated with profound expansion of inducer T cells rescued in the Lamina Propria of the large bowel of SCID recipients. As illustrated in **Figure 5(b)**, colitogenic WT CD4$^+$ CD45RB$^{hi}$ T cells expanded ~100-fold over the course of the assay, in contrast to the ~2-fold expansion of Fyn$^{-/-}$ CD4$^+$ CD45RB$^{hi}$ T cells. Notwithstanding the lack of expansion of Fyn$^{-/-}$ T cells, their upregulated expression of CD69 was comparable to that observed in WT inducer T cell populations, evidence that they were indeed engaging environmental antigens in the gut (**Figure 5(c)**). **Figure 5(d)** illustrates the characteristic histology and gut pathology induced by the WT colitigenic T cells, with flattening of the villi and T cell infiltration, not observed in recipients of their Fyn$^{-/-}$ counterparts. Importantly, these characteristic indicators were rescued upon ectopic expression of Fyn (**Figure 5(b)** and **Figure 5(d)**), formally demonstrating that Fyn predicated the disease inducing capacity of CD4$^+$CD45RB$^{hi}$ T cells (**Figure 5(a)**).

The obligate role of Fyn in supporting colitogenic T cells *in vivo* appears directly related to its role in supporting IL-2 production. As illustrated in **Figure 6(a)** and **Figure 6(b)**, of the 22 cytokines assessed subsequent to TcR/CD4 co-aggregation of CD4$^+$ primary T cells derived from either WT or Fyn$^{-/-}$ animals, only IL-2 production was significantly affected. Further, as illustrated in **Figure 6(c)**, IL-17 production by Fyn$^{-/-}$ T cells was within 2-fold of levels derived from WT T cells when cytokine induction was assessed in circumstances known to skew CD4$^+$ responders towards Th17 cells [21] [22].

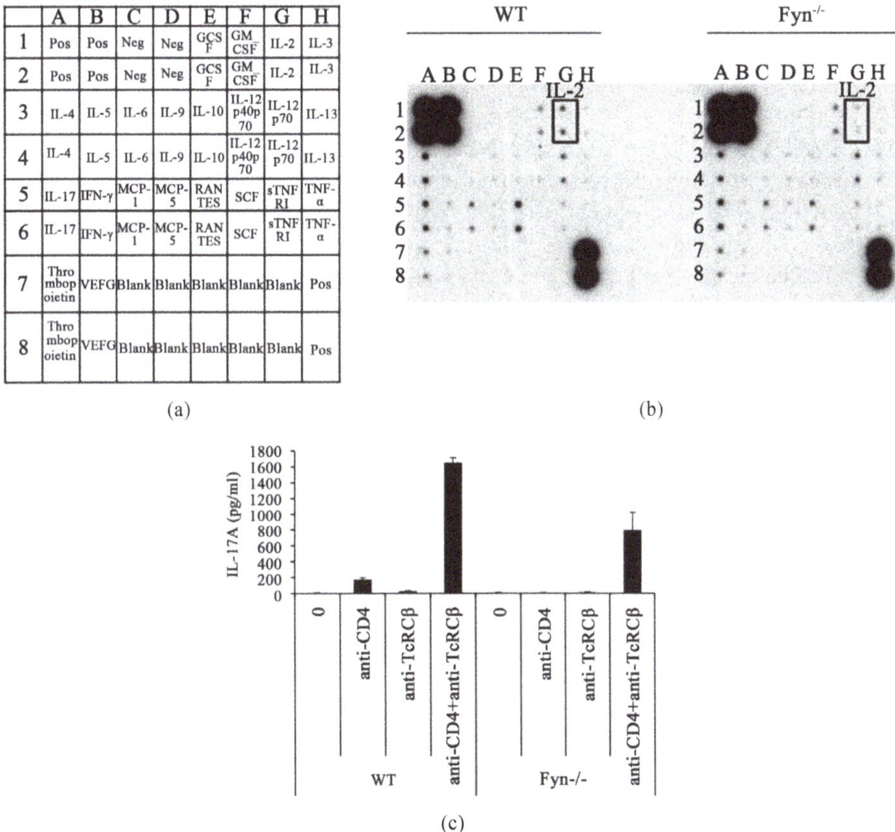

| | A | B | C | D | E | F | G | H |
|---|---|---|---|---|---|---|---|---|
| 1 | Pos | Pos | Neg | Neg | GCSF | GM CSF | IL-2 | IL-3 |
| 2 | Pos | Pos | Neg | Neg | GCSF | GM CSF | IL-2 | IL-3 |
| 3 | IL-4 | IL-5 | IL-6 | IL-9 | IL-10 | IL-12 p40p70 | IL-12 p70 | IL-13 |
| 4 | IL-4 | IL-5 | IL-6 | IL-9 | IL-10 | IL-12 p40p70 | IL-12 p70 | IL-13 |
| 5 | IL-17 | IFN-γ | MCP-1 | MCP-5 | RANTES | SCF | sTNFRI | TNF-α |
| 6 | IL-17 | IFN-γ | MCP-1 | MCP-5 | RANTES | SCF | sTNFRI | TNF-α |
| 7 | Thrombopoietin | VEFG | Blank | Blank | Blank | Blank | Blank | Pos |
| 8 | Thrombopoietin | VEFG | Blank | Blank | Blank | Blank | Blank | Pos |



**Figure 6.** Role of Fyn in CD4/TcR induced cytokine production is specific to IL-2. (a) Matrix identifying the cytokines detected in cytokine array used in (b); (b) Cytokine array analysis of supernatants from primary CD4$^+$ WT or Fyn$^{-/-}$ T cell cultures stimulated with plate-bound anti-CD4 and anti-TcRC$\beta$ for 48 hours. Only cytokines at levels > 5 fold different from those derived from WT T cells, as assessed densitometrically, are boxed; (c) IL-17A ELISA of supernatants from primary CD4$^+$ WT or Fyn$^{-/-}$ T cell stimulated with either anti-CD4, anti-TcRC$\beta$ or both in the presence of IL-6, TGF-$\beta$1, anti-IL-4 and anti-IFN-$\gamma$ for 72 hours. Data (mean and s.d.) are representative of two independent experiments.

### 3.3. Fyn-Dependent IL-2 Mediated Expansion of CD4+CD45RBhi T Cells *in Vivo*

IL-2 mediated expansion of CAR$^+$ CD4$^+$ CD45RB$^{hi}$ T cells was directly assessed by treating SCID recipients with 6 daily injections of PBS, mAb specific for IL-2 (S4B6), or its isotype control. As illustrated in **Figure 7**, ~10% of donor WT CD4$^+$ CD45RB$^{hi}$ T cells rescued in the spleen and lymph nodes of these recipients had divided less than 6 times at day 7 post injection in SCID recipients treated with either PBS or isotype control. In contrast, in recipients treated with S4B6 the proportion of cells that had divided less than 6 times increased ~3-4 fold (**Figure 7**).

Analysis of Fyn$^{-/-}$ CAR$^+$ CD4$^+$ CD45RB$^{hi}$ T cells in this assay revealed that ~35% of cells divided less than 6 times, consistent with their impaired expansion in comparison to WT cells (**Figure 5(b)** and **Figure 7**). Further, anti-IL2 treatment increased the proportion of cells dividing less than 6 times to >90% at day 7 (**Figure 6**). These results support the conclusion that autocrine IL-2 mediates the expansion of both WT and Fyn$^{-/-}$ CD4$^+$T cells *in vivo* and provides the mechanistic basis for the non-colitogenic capacity of Fyn$^{-/-}$ CD4$^+$ CD45RB$^{hi}$ T cells.

### 3.4. Fyn Deficient Animals Fail to Mount a Protective Immune Response to Flu

Fyn deficiency has not been previously associated with compromised immunity. As Fyn-dependent IL-2 production and T cell expansion was profoundly impaired in Fyn deficient T cells, we next sought to examine the impact of Fyn deficiency on immunocompetency of Fyn deficient mice *in vivo*, noting that IL-2, likely produced by CD4$^+$ T cells, is the key cytokine involved in the early programming of naïve CD8$^+$ T cell effector and memory differentiation [23]-[25] in circumstances of viral infection.

A flu-infection model [11] [12] was used to directly assess the immune-competence of Fyn-deficient animals. As illustrated in **Figure 8(a)**, >90% of Fyn-deficient hosts succumbed 7 - 8 days post infection with either dose of A/PR-8 (H1N1) used, exhibiting up to 30% loss of body weight within the first week. In contrast, 60% of wild-type (WT) hosts survived at the higher dose and 80% at a 10-fold lower dose of flu virus (**Figure 8(a)**).

**Figure 8(b)** illustrates lung pathology of uninfected WT; and WT and Fyn-deficient hosts at day 6 after PR-8 infection. Both WT and Fyn-deficient hosts exhibited chronic inflammatory peribronchiolitis. The WT hosts presented with minimal alveolar involvement, characterized by vascular congestion and focal inflammatory cell infiltration. In contrast, the Fyn-deficient hosts exhibited extensive and severe alveolar congestion with infiltrating blood and polymorphonuclear leukocytes; and succumbed to respiratory failure due to pulmonary consolidation (**Figure 8(b)**).

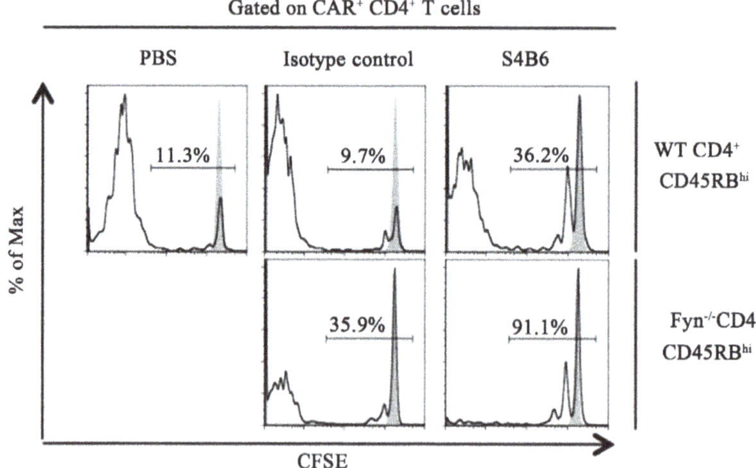


**Figure 7.** Fyn-dependent expansion of CAR$^+$ CD4$^+$CD45RB$^{hi}$ T cells is mediated by IL-2 *in vivo*. Spleens and lymph nodes of SCID recipients of 2.5 × 10$^6$ CSFE-labelled donor cells were harvested on day 7. Groups of recipients received daily injections of PBS, or 0.5 mg of either anti-IL-2 mAb S4B6 or isotype control. CSFE labeling of donor cells derived from recipients treated as indicated was assessed flow cytometrically on day 7. Numbers represent percentage of cells that had undergone 0 - 5 divisions. Grey histograms indicate CSFE levels of non-stimulated cells after overnight incubation at 37°C. Data are representative of three mice per group.

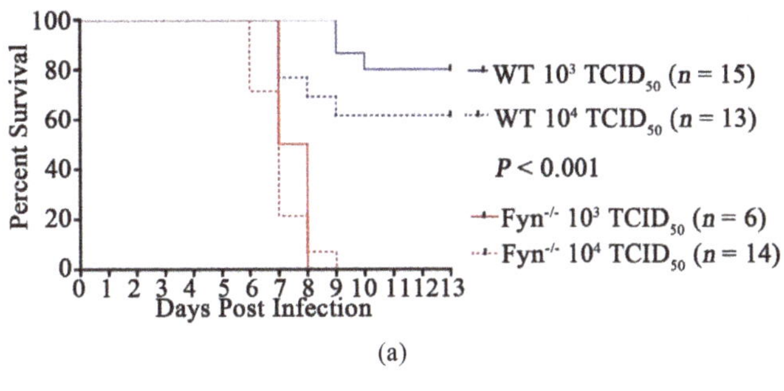


(a)

Lymphocyte Infiltration of the Lung

| | WT-PBS | WT-PR8 | Fyn$^{-/-}$-PR8 |
|---|---|---|---|
| H & E 50 X | | | |
| H & E 200 X | | | |

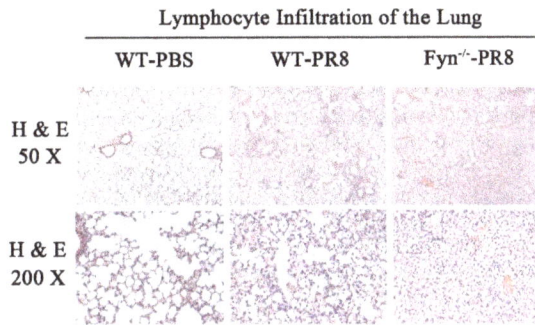

(b)

Number of Infiltrating T Cells (× $10^4$)

| WT | | | | | | Fyn$^{-/-}$ | | |
|---|---|---|---|---|---|---|---|---|
| Day 6 | | | Day 9 | | | Day 6 | | |
| CD4 | CD8 | Tet-I | CD4 | CD8 | Tet-I | CD4 | CD8 | Tet-I |
| 0.23 +/-0.072 | 0.47 +/-0.074 | 0.052 +/-0.023 | 5.2 +/-1.3 | 4.2 +/-0.73 | 1.1 +/-0.31 | 0.34 +/-0.025 | 0.50 +/-0.035 | 0.062 +/-0.024 |

(c)

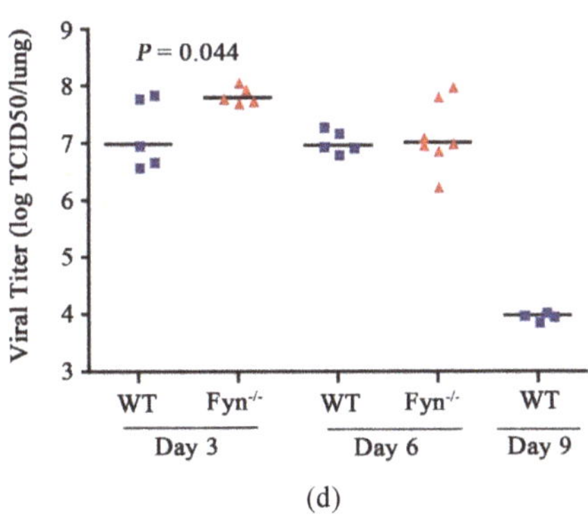


(d)

**Figure 8.** Fyn deficient animals fail to mount a protective immune response to flu. (a) Survival analysis of WT and Fyn$^{-/-}$ mice following intranasal infection with the influenza virus A/PR8 (PR8, H1N1) at the indicated $TCID_{50}$. "n" represents the number of animals per group; (b) Immunohistochemistry analysis of lung sections from flu infected WT and Fyn$^{-/-}$ mice ($10^4$ $TCID_{50}$) using H&E staining at day 6 post infection. Data are representative of 4 animals per group; (c) Number of infiltrating T cells post flu infection. Lungs were analyzed flow cytometrically for the presence of CD8$\alpha^+$ CD90$^+$, CD4$^+$CD90$^+$, and CD8$\alpha^+$PR8-specific tetramer $D^b/NP_{366\text{-}374}{}^+$ T cells before and after flu infection at the indicated time points. The number of cells was calculated based on flow cytometric analysis and total viable lymphocyte cell counts. Data are representative of 3 animals per group; (d) Lung viral titer analysis of WT and Fyn$^{-/-}$ flu infected mice ($10^4$ $TCID_{50}$) at indicated time points. Each square or triangle represents the value for each WT and Fyn$^{-/-}$ mouse, respectively, and the horizontal line represents the mean value.

The primary immune response to PR-8 infection is known to involve both T-cell lineages as well as B-cells, all of which localize to the lung toward resolving infection [26]. Day 6 is the inflection point in the primary response reported herein. As illustrated in **Figure 8(c)**, the number of $CD4^+$ and $CD8^+$ T cells localized to the lungs of infected WT and Fyn-deficient hosts is comparable at day 6 post infection; as is the frequency of contained PR8-specific $CD8^+$ T cells (**Figure 8(c)**). It merits comment that flu-specific T cells of both lineages were assessed and while enumeration of $CD8^+$ flu-specific T cells binding the dominant MHC Class I binding PR8-derived peptide was reproducible, results assessing binding of one of many MHC Class II PR8-derived peptides were not (data not shown). Notwithstanding, these results support the conclusion that neither the T cell repertoire [1]-[3] nor T cell homing capacity is compromised in the absence of Fyn.

As illustrated in **Figure 8(c)**, the survival of WT hosts correlated with a 20-fold and 9-fold increase in the number of lung infiltrating $CD4^+$ and $CD8^+$ T cells, respectively, at day 9 post infection, and a concomitant 20-fold increase in the number of contained flu-specific $CD8^+$ T cells (**Figure 8(c)**). Viral titers assessed over the course of PR8 infection in both WT and Fyn-deficient hosts mirrored the physiological outcome of infection. Specifically, while there was a significant difference in viral titers observed at day 3 post-infection, possibly due to Fyn-dependent differences in an innate component of the immune response [4], the viral titers at day 6 post-infection were comparable in WT and Fyn-deficient hosts (**Figure 8(d)**). The Fyn-deficient animals were moribund at this time point and succumbed shortly thereafter, while the primary adaptive immune response in the WT animals [26], as expected, increased over the following 3 days and resolved the viral burden (**Figure 8(c)** and **Figure 8(d)**).

These results provide the first physiological evidence that Fyn deficient animals are profoundly immune-compromised. As formal proof of Fyn-dependent IL-2 production underpinning *in vivo* $CD4^+$ T cell expansion was demonstrated in the colitis model system reported herein, a rational hypothesis underlying the observation that Fyn-deficient animals succumb to PR8 infection is that Fyn-deficient PR-8 specific T cells fail to sufficiently expand at the critical inflection point of the adaptive immune response; that in turn would suggest a central role for Fyn in T cell homeostasis.

## 4. Discussion

The results presented are the first to establish that the genomic disruption of Fyn results in immunodeficiency. They mechanistically tether the *in vitro* observations of profoundly impaired IL-2 production in Fyn deficient T cells with *in vivo* correlates of both protective immunity and the capacity of T cells to induce autoimmunity. Specifically, Fyn engagement in the earliest signalling sequelae initiated upon TcR/CD3 engagement predicates robust IL-2 production, which in turn limits T cell expansion *in vivo* and hence effective T cell immunity.

In the original studies [2], it was reported that $Fyn^{-/-}$ T cells did not produce detectable IL-2 in response to TcR/CD3 engagement. In the present study $Fyn^{-/-}$ T cells were observed to produce 5% - 10% the levels produced by WT T cells *in vitro*. Importantly, this result is consistent with and rationalizes the observation that $Fyn^{-/-}$ animals contain a normal complement of Tregs [3]. Further, and in this regard, it has been reported that proliferation of T cells from $Fyn^{-/-}$ animals transgenic for a pathogen specific TcR was as robust as for T cells from WT TcR transgenic mice, both *in vitro* and *in vivo* [3]. In circumstances where every T cell is antigen specific, the cumulative IL-2 produced in support of T cell expansion could be above threshold, masking the compromised IL-2 production by each T cell, and sufficient to support T cell function in the reported assays [3]. Hence the latter study is not at odds with results presented herein.

In contrast, as demonstrated in the present study using two model systems, notwithstanding the diverse repertoire of $Fyn^{-/-}$ T cells, Fyn deficient animals are unable to support effective T cell function. In the flu-infection model, protective T cell immunity cannot be mounted as infected host succumbs to virus mediated pulmonary consolidation ahead of the required and protective expansion virus specific T cells that have homed to the lung. Similarly, in the SCID model of enteropathy, while Fyn deficient T cells home to the gut and recognize environmental antigens as efficiently as WT T cells as assessed by levels of CD69 expression, expansion is also profoundly impaired and as a consequence inflammation does not ensue. And importantly this model enabled the formal proof that impaired IL-2 production by $Fyn^{-/-}$ T cells limits *in vivo* expansion and in turn an effective physiological response.

This conclusion derives from two convergent results. The first is that ectopic expression of Fyn in non-colitogenic $Fyn^{-/-}$ $CD4^+$ $CD45RB^{hi}$ T cells rescues both levels of expansion in the large bowel comparable to those achieved by WT $CD4^+$ $CD45RB^{hi}$ T cells, and the onset of colitis. The second is that the impaired expansion of

$Fyn^{-/-}$ $CD4^+$ $CD45RB^{hi}$ T cells *in vivo* is coupled with the significantly enhanced efficiency with which anti-IL-2 inhibited expansion. This is likely if the IL-2 supporting expansion is endogenous, as the efficacy of anti-IL-2 mediated neutralization would be directly related to levels of IL-2 produced.

Since its discovery, IL-2 has been accepted as a major T cell growth factor [27] [28], *in vitro* [29], and *in vivo* [30]. The characterization of IL-2 and IL-2R deficient animals, however, renewed attention to the role of IL-2 in T cell growth, differentiation and function *in vivo*, some aspects of which merit discussion in the context of results presented herein.

Both $IL\text{-}2^{-/-}$ and $IL\text{-}2R^{-/-}$ mice, unable to produce or utilize IL-2, respectively, develop autoimmune diseases, including colitis, due to T cell expansion in the large bowel [31] [32]. Two lesions contribute to disease onset in these animals. It has been demonstrated that while thymus-derived T cell development proceeds in these deficient strains at virtually normal levels [32] [33], intra-intestinal T cell development is ablated [15]. These observations led to studies that demonstrated the IL-10-dependent anti-inflammatory role of some subsets of gut-derived intra-epithelial T cells [34]. The second lesion evident in the absence of either IL-2 or the capacity to utilize it is the absence of Tregs [35].

At apparent odds with results reported herein is that $Fyn^{-/-}$ T cells fail to induce enteropathy due to the absence of IL-2-dependent expansion *in vivo*. A fundamental difference in these and previous analyses of disease onset in $IL\text{-}2^{-/-}$ and $IL\text{-}2R^{-/-}$ deficient animals is the ongoing production and export of T cells from the thymus in the latter circumstances. In the present study, the colitogenic T cells are limiting, and hence dependence on IL-2 mediated expansion *in vivo* predicates the generation of sufficient T cells to initiate and maintain localized inflammation in the large bowel. In support of this conclusion is the observation that limiting numbers of $IL\text{-}2^{-/-}$ $CD4^+CD45RB^{hi}$ T cells transferred to $RAG\text{-}2^{-/-}$ mice were unable to cause disease [36].

The role of Fyn in specifically regulating IL-2 production is rationalized based on the signalling cascade initiated upon TcR engagement. Some Fyn associated proteins and substrates, and in turn their downstream signalling partners have been characterized, including SAP [37], Pyk2 [38], and Fyb [20]. As IL-2 production is unimpaired in T cells from $SAP^{-/-}$ animals [39], and T cells from $Pyk2^{-/-}$ animals produce WT levels of IL-2 when optimally stimulated [40], Fyb and its binding partner, SLP-76 [41], were the focus of biochemical analyses.

Primary T cells from $Fyb^{-/-}$ animals exhibit impaired TcR induced IL-2 production [42], comparable to that observed in $Fyn^{-/-}$ T cells and consistent with the obligate role of the Fyn-Fyb pathway in the IL-2 defect observed in $Fyn^{-/-}$ T cells. Fyn is shown to support the parallel increase in levels of tyrosine phosphorylation of both Fyb and SLP-76 upon TcR mediated cellular activation. It is of note that anti-CD3, albeit infrequently, induced marginal increases in levels of P-Y-Fyb in $Fyn^{-/-}$ T cells, however it did not correlate with increased IL-2 production. As this sequelae predicts, in the absence of Fyn-dependent Fyb phosphorylation the increased phosphorylation of SLP-76 is ablated, as is its role as a docking site for PLC$\gamma$ [43]. As a consequence, hydrolysis of $PIP_2$ [44] production of $IP_3$ and the rise in $[Ca^{2+}]_i$ is impaired [1] [2]. As activation requirements for calcineurin are then impeded, the activation and translocation of NFAT that predicates the initiation of *de novo* transcription of the IL-2 gene [45] is compromised.

The results presented also establish the obligate, independent, yet interrelated roles of Lck and Fyn subsequent to TcR/CD3 engagement. Specifically, Lck and Fyn reside in distinct subcellular locations in primary resting $CD4^+$ T cells, with >90% of CD4-associated Lck residing outside of LR, while >95% of Fyn is LR-resident [6]. Upon TcR/CD4 engagement, Lck is activated and functions as a mobile signaling element, translocating into LR, where it physically associates with and is critical for Fyn activation [6] [7].

Elucidation of the functional consequences of the temporal and spatial regulation of these two kinases proffers the opportunity not only to design molecules that either promote or impede their interactions, enhancing or ablating T cell activation and expansion, respectively; it provides a framework to model mechanisms that regulate the involvement of multiple *src* family tyrosine kinases functioning in a variety of receptor-mediated signaling pathways.

## Acknowledgements

We gratefully acknowledge the expert technical assistance of Gisele Knowles, Manager, Scanning Microscopy and Flow Cytometry Facility and Kirishanthy Kathirkamathamby, Manager of the Antibody Core Facility at the Sunnybrook Research Institute; the assessment of the histopathology of lung sections by Professor Sylvia L. Asa Department of Laboratory Medicine & Pathobiology, University of Toronto; and the NIH Tetramer Facility for the flu-specific tetramers.

## Authorship Contributions

B.M. is the primary researcher having designed and executed the experiments, and prepared the manuscript. N.V. provided technical assistance with *in vivo* experiments, immunohistochemistry and immunofluorescence. M.V. provided technical assistance with *in vivo* experiments, flow cytometry, immunohistochemistry and immunofluorescence. M.W. and T.W. provided technical support with the influenza mouse model. A.V. provided anti-Lck and anti-Fyn antibodies and expert technical advice. T.F.G. provided $CAR^+$ mice. M.J. supervised the study and provided final draft of manuscript.

## Disclosure of Conflict of Interest

The authors declare no competing financial interests.

## References

[1] Appleby, M.W., Gross, J.A., Cooke, M.P., Levin, S.D., Qian, X. and Perlmutter, R.M. (1992) Defective T Cell Receptor Signaling in Mice Lacking the Thymic Isoform of p59fyn. *Cell*, **70**, 751-763. http://dx.doi.org/10.1016/0092-8674(92)90309-Z

[2] Stein, P.L., Lee, H., Rich, S. and Soriano, P. (1992) $pp59^{fyn}$ Mutant Mice Display Differential Signaling in Thymocytes and Peripheral T Cells. *Cell*, **70**, 741-750. http://dx.doi.org/10.1016/0092-8674(92)90308-Y

[3] Mamchak, A.A., Sullivan, B.M., Hou, B., Lee, L.M., Gilden, J.K., Krummel, M.F., Locksley, R.M. and DeFranco, A.L. (2008) Normal Development and Activation but Altered Cytokine Production of Fyn-Deficient $CD4^+$ T Cells. *The Journal of Immunology*, **181**, 5374-5385. http://dx.doi.org/10.4049/jimmunol.181.8.5374

[4] Eberl, G., Lowin-Kropf, B. and MacDonald, H.R. (1999) Cutting Edge: NKT cell Development Is Selectively Impaired in Fyn-Deficient Mice. *The Journal of Immunology*, **163**, 4091-4094.

[5] Filipp, D., Leung, B.L., Zhang, J., Veillette, A. and Julius, M. (2004) Enrichment of LCK in Lipid Rafts Regulates Colocalized Fyn Activation and the Initiation of Proximal Signals through TCR Alpha Beta. *The Journal of Immunology*, **172**, 4266-4274. http://dx.doi.org/10.4049/jimmunol.172.7.4266

[6] Filipp, D., Zhang, J., Leung, B.L., Shaw, A., Levin, S.D., Veillette, A. and Julius, M. (2003) Regulation of Fyn through Translocation of Activated LCK into Lipid Rafts. *The Journal of Experimental Medicine*, **197**, 1221-1227. http://dx.doi.org/10.1084/jem.20022112

[7] Filipp, D., Moemeni, B., Ferzoco, A., Kathirkamathamby, K., Zhang, J., Ballek, O., Davidson, D., Veillette, A. and Julius, M. (2008) Lck-Dependent Fyn Activation Requires C-Terminus-Dependent Targeting of Kinase-Active Lck to Lipid Rafts. *Journal of Biological Chemistry*, **283**, 26409-26422. http://dx.doi.org/10.1074/jbc.M710372200

[8] Leach, M.W., Bean, A.G., Mauze, S., Coffman, R.L. and Powrie, F. (1996) Inflammatory Bowel Disease in C.B-17 Scid Mice Reconstituted with the CD45RB High Subset of $CD4^+$ T Cells. *American Journal of Pathology*, **148**, 1503-1515.

[9] Powrie, F., Leach, M.W., Mauze, S., Caddie, L.B. and Coffman, R.L. (1993) Phenotypically Distinct Subsets of $CD4^+$ T Cells Induce or Protect FROM Chronic Intestinal Inflammation in C. B-17 Scid Mice. *International Immunology*, **5**, 1461-1471. http://dx.doi.org/10.1093/intimm/5.11.1461

[10] Powrie, F., Mauze, S. and Coffman, R.L. (1997) $CD4^+$ T Cells in the Regulation of Inflammatory Responses in the Intestine. *Research in Immunology*, **148**, 576-581. http://dx.doi.org/10.1016/S0923-2494(98)80152-1

[11] Ennis, F.A., Verbonitz, M., Reichelderfer, P. and Daniel, S. (1976) Recombination of Influenza A Virus Strains: Effect on Pathogenicity. *Developments in Biological Standardization*, **33**, 220-225.

[12] Lin, G.H., Sedgmen, B.J., Moraes, T.J., Snell, L.M., Topham, D.J. and Watts, T.H. (2009) Endogenous 4-1BB Ligand Plays a Critical Role in Protection from Influenza-Induced Disease. *Journal of immunology*, **182**, 934-947. http://dx.doi.org/10.4049/jimmunol.182.2.934

[13] Wan, Y.Y., Leon, R.P., Marks, R., Cham, C.M., Schaack, J., Gejewski, T.F. and Degregori, J. (2000) Transgenic Expression of the Coxasackie/Adenovirus Receptor Enables Adenoviral-Mediated Gene Delivery in Naive T Cells. *Proceedings of the National Academy of Sciences of the United States of America*, **97**, 13784-13789. http://dx.doi.org/10.1073/pnas.250356297

[14] Cottey, R., Rowe, C.A. and Bender, B.S. (2001) Influenza Virus. In: Coico, R., Ed., *Current Protocols in Immunology*, John Wiley and Sons, Hoboken. http://dx.doi.org/10.1002/0471142735.im1911s42

[15] Poussier, P., Ning, T., Chen, J., Banerjee, D. and Julius, M. (2000) Intestinal Inflammation Observed in IL-2R/IL-2

Mutant Mice Is Associated with Impaired Intestinal T Lymphopoiesis. *Gastroenterology*, **118**, 880-891. http://dx.doi.org/10.1016/S0016-5085(00)70174-0

[16] Quah, B.J., Warren, H.S. and Parish, C.R. (2007) Monitoring Lymphocyte Proliferation *in Vitro* and *in Vivo* with the Intracellular Fluorescent Dye Carboxyfluorescein Diacetate Succinimidyl Ester. *Nature Protocols*, **2**, 2049-2056. http://dx.doi.org/10.1038/nprot.2007.296

[17] Marmour, M.D. and Julius, M. (2001) Role for Lipid Rafts in Regulating Interleukin-2 Receptor Signaling. *Blood*, **98**, 1489-1497. http://dx.doi.org/10.1182/blood.V98.5.1489

[18] Filby, A., Seddon, B., Kleczkowska, J., Salmond, R., Tomlinson, P., Smida, M., Lindquist, J.A., Schraven, B. and Zamoyska, R. (2007) Fyn Regulates the Duration of TCR Engagement Needed for Commitment to Effector Function. *Journal of Immunology*, **179**, 4635-4644. http://dx.doi.org/10.4049/jimmunol.179.7.4635

[19] Sugie, K., Jeon, M. and Grey, H.M. (2004) Activation of Naive CD4 T Cells by Anti-CD3 Reveals an Important Role for Fyn in Lck-Mediated Signaling. *Proceedings of the National Academy of Sciences of the United States of America*, **101**, 14859-14864. http://dx.doi.org/10.1073/pnas.0406168101

[20] da Silva, A., Rosenfield, J., Mueller, I., Bouton, A., Hirai, H. and Rudd, C. (1997) Biochemical Analysis of p120/130: A Protein-Tyrosine Kinase Substrate Restricted to T and Myeloid Cells. *The Journal of Immunology*, **158**, 2007-2016.

[21] Bettelli, E., Carrier, Y., Gao, W., Korn, T., Strom, T.B., Oukka, M., Weiner, H.L. and Kuchroo, V.K. (2006) Reciprocal Developmental Pathways for the Generation of Pathogenic Effector TH17 and Regulatory T Cells. *Nature*, **441**, 235-238. http://dx.doi.org/10.1038/nature04753

[22] Veldhoen, M., Hocking, R.J., Atkins, C.J., Locksley, R.M. and Stockinger, B. (2006) TGF$\beta$ in the Context of an Inflammatory Cytokine Milieu Supports de Novo Differentiation of IL-17-Producing T Cells. *Immunity*, **24**, 179-189. http://dx.doi.org/10.1016/j.immuni.2006.01.001

[23] Khanolkar, A., Fuller, M.J. and Zajac, A.J. (2004) CD4 T Cell-Dependent CD8 T Cell Maturation. *Journal of Immunology*, **172**, 2834-2844. http://dx.doi.org/10.4049/jimmunol.172.5.2834

[24] Williams, M.A., Tyznik, A.J. and Bevan, M.J. (2006) Interleukin-2 Signals during Priming Are Required for Secondary Expansion of $CD8^+$ Memory T Cells. *Nature*, **441**, 890-893. http://dx.doi.org/10.1038/nature04790

[25] Wilson, E.B. and Livingstone, A.M. (2008) Cutting Edge: $CD4^+$ T Cell-Derived IL-2 Is Essential for Help-Dependent Primary $CD8^+$ T Cell Responses. *Journal of Immunology*, **181**, 7445-7448. http://dx.doi.org/10.4049/jimmunol.181.11.7445

[26] Thomas, P.G., Keating, R., Hulse-Post, D.J. and Doherty, P.C. (2006) Cell-Mediated Protection in Influenza Infection. *Emerging Infectious Diseases*, **12**, 48-54. http://dx.doi.org/10.3201/eid1201.051237

[27] Gillis, S., Ferm, M.M., Ou, W. and Smith, K.A. (1978) T Cell Growth Factor: Parameters of Production and a Quantitative Microassay for Activity. *Journal of Immunology*, **120**, 2027-2032.

[28] Robb, R.J. and Smith, K.A. (1981) Heterogeneity of Human T-Cell Growth Factor(s) Due to Variable Glycosylation. *Molecular Immunology*, **18**, 1087-1094. http://dx.doi.org/10.1016/0161-5890(81)90024-9

[29] Smith, K.A. (1988) Interleukin-2: Inception, Impact, and Implications. *Science*, **240**, 1169-1176. http://dx.doi.org/10.1126/science.3131876

[30] Sojka, D.K., Bruniquel, D., Schwartz, R.H. and Singh, N.J. (2004) IL-2 Secretion by $CD4^+$ T Cells *in Vivo* Is Rapid, Transient, and Influenced by TCR-Specific Competition. *Journal of Immunology*, **172**, 6136-6143. http://dx.doi.org/10.4049/jimmunol.172.10.6136

[31] Sadlack, B., Merz, H., Schorle, H., Schimpl, A., Feller, A.C. and Horak, I. (1993) Ulcerative Colitis-Like Disease in Mice with a Disrupted Interleukin-2 Gene. *Cell*, **75**, 253-261. http://dx.doi.org/10.1016/0092-8674(93)80067-O

[32] Willerford, D.M., Chen, J., Ferry, J.A., Davidson, L., Ma, A. and Alt, F.W. (1995) Interleukin-2 Receptor Alpha Chain Regulates the Size and Content of the Peripheral Lymphoid Compartment. *Immunity*, **3**, 521-530. http://dx.doi.org/10.1016/1074-7613(95)90180-9

[33] Schorle, H., Holtschke, T., Hunig, T., Schimpl, A. and Horak, I. (1991) Development and Function of T Cells in Mice Rendered Interleukin-2 Deficient by Gene Targeting. *Nature*, **352**, 621-624. http://dx.doi.org/10.1038/352621a0

[34] Poussier, P., Ning, T., Banerjee, D. and Julius, M. (2002) A Unique Subset of Self-Specific Intraintestinal T Cells Maintains Gut Integrity. *Journal of Experimental Medicine*, **195**, 1491-1497. http://dx.doi.org/10.1084/jem.20011793

[35] Papiernik, M., de Moraes, M.L., Pontoux, C., Vasseur, F. and Penit, C. (1998) Regulatory CD4 T Cells: Expression of IL-2R Alpha Chain, Resistance to Clonal Deletion and IL-2 Dependency. *International Immunology*, **10**, 371-378. http://dx.doi.org/10.1093/intimm/10.4.371

[36] Kameyama, K., Nemoto, Y., Kanai, T., Shinohara, T., Okamoto, R., Tsuchiya, K., Nakamura, T., Sakamoto, N., Totsuka, T., Hibi, T. and Watanabe, M. (2010) IL-2 Is Positively Involved in the Development of Colitogenic $CD4^+$ IL-7R Alpha High Memory T Cells in Chronic Colitis. *European Journal of Immunology*, **40**, 2423-2436.

http://dx.doi.org/10.1002/eji.200939764

[37] Latour, S., Roncagalli, R., Chen, R., Bakinowski, M., Shi, X., Schwartzberg, P.L., Davidson, D. and Veillette, A. (2003) Binding of SAP SH2 Domain to FynT SH3 Domain Reveals a Novel Mechanism of Receptor Signalling in Immune Regulation. *Nature Cell Biology*, **5**, 149-154. http://dx.doi.org/10.1038/ncb919

[38] Qian, D., Lev, S., van Oers, N.S., Dikic, I., Schlessinger, J. and Weiss, A. (1997) Tyrosine Phosphorylation of Pyk2 Is Selectively Regulated by Fyn during TCR Signaling. *Journal of Experimental Medicine*, **185**, 1253-1260. http://dx.doi.org/10.1084/jem.185.7.1253

[39] Davidson, D., Shi, X., Zhang, S., Wang, H., Nemer, M., Ono, N., Ohno, S., Yanagi, Y. and Veillette, A. (2004) Genetic Evidence Linking SAP, the X-Linked Lymphoproliferative Gene Product, to Src-Related Kinase FynT in $T_H2$ Cytokine Regulation. *Immunity*, **21**, 707-717. http://dx.doi.org/10.1016/j.immuni.2004.10.005

[40] Beinke, S.R., Phee, H., Clingan, J.M., Schlessinger, J., Matloubian, M. and Weiss, A. (2010) Proline-Rich Tyrosine Kinase-2 Is Critical for CD8 T-Cell Short-Lived Effector Fate. *Proceedings of the National Academy of Sciences of the United States of America*, **107**, 16234-16239. http://dx.doi.org/10.1073/pnas.1011556107

[41] Veale, M., Raab, M., Li, Z., da Silva, A.J., Kraeft, S.K., Weremowicz, S., Morton, C.C. and Rudd, C.E. (1999) Novel Isoform of Lymphoid Adaptor FYN-T-Binding Protein (FYB-130) Interacts with SLP-76 and Up-Regulates Interleukin 2 Production. *Journal of Biological Chemistry*, **274**, 28427-28435. http://dx.doi.org/10.1074/jbc.274.40.28427

[42] Griffiths, E.K., Krawczyk, C., Kong, Y.-Y., Raab, M., Hyduk, S.J., Bouchard, D., Chan, V.S., Kozieradzki, I., Oliveira-dos-Santos, A.J., Wakeham, A., *et al.* (2001) Positive Regulation of T Cell Activation and Integrin Adhesion by the Adapter Fyb/Slap. *Science*, **293**, 2260-2263. http://dx.doi.org/10.1126/science.1063397

[43] Yablonski, D., Kadlecek, T. and Almeida, A.R. (2001) Identification of a Phospholipase C-$\gamma$1 (PLC-$\gamma$1) SH3 Domain-Binding Site in SLP-76 Required for T-Cell Receptor-Mediated Activation of PLC-$\gamma$1 and NFAT. *Molecular and Cellular Biology*, **21**, 4208-4218. http://dx.doi.org/10.1128/MCB.21.13.4208-4218.2001

[44] Meldrum, E., Parker, P.J. and Carozzi, A. (1991) The PtdIns-PLC Superfamily and Signal Transduction. *Biochimica et Biophysica Acta*, **1092**, 49-71. http://dx.doi.org/10.1016/0167-4889(91)90177-Y

[45] Hogan, P.G., Chen, L., Nardone, J. and Rao, A. (2003) Transcriptional Regulation by Calcium, Calcineurin, and NFAT. *Genes & Development*, **17**, 2205-2232. http://dx.doi.org/10.1101/gad.1102703

# Deleterious Nonsynonymous SNP Found within *HLA-DRB*1 Gene Involved in Allograft Rejection in Sudanese Family: Using DNA Sequencing and Bioinformatics Methods

**Mohamed M. Hassan[1,2*], Sofia B. Mohamed[3], Mohamed A. Hussain[4], Amar A. Dowd[1]**

[1]Faculty of Medical Laboratory Sciences, University of Medical Science and Technology, Khartoum, Sudan
[2]Faculty of Medical Laboratory Sciences, Al Zaiem Al Azhari University, Khartoum, Sudan
[3]Tropical Medicine Research Institute, Khartoum, Sudan
[4]Department of Pharmaceutical Microbiology, International University of Africa, Khartoum, Sudan
Email: [*]mhassan0210@gmail.com

## Abstract

**Renal transplantation provides the best long-term treatment for chronic renal failure. Single-nucleotide polymorphisms (SNPs) play a major role in the understanding of the genetic basis of many complex human diseases. Also, the genetics of human phenotype variation could be understood by knowing the functions of these SNPs. It is still a major challenge to identify the functional SNPs in a disease-related gene. This work explored how SNPs mutations in *HLA-DRB*1 gene could affect renal transplantation rejection. This study was carried out in Ahmed Gasim Hospital, Renal Dialysis Center during the period, from September 2012 to November 2013. Blood samples from five Sudanese patients (different families) with known renal transplantation rejection were collected before hemodialysis, furthermore one blood sample for control. DNA sequences results and detected SNPs were analyzed using bioinformatics tools (BLAST, SIFT, nsSNP Analyzer, PolyPhen, I-mutant, BioEdit, CPH, Chimera, Box shade and Project Hope). In addition, international databases were used for datasets [NCBI, Uniprot]. Results showed that, three SNPs were detected; two of three SNPs were predicted as tolerant or benign (rs1059575, novel) and one was deleterious (rs17885437). This study concluded that the identification of pathological SNPs could be an answer to unknown causes for a lot of organ transplantation rejection cases.**

[*]Corresponding author.

## Keywords

**Renal Transplantation Rejection, Single Nucleotide Polymorphisms (SNPs), Nonsynonymous Variant, *HLA-DRB*1 Gene, Sudanese Families**

## 1. Introduction

Around the world in 2002 there were over 1.1 million patients estimated to have end stage renal disease (ESRD) with addition of 7% annually [1]. In the same token and according to world health organization in 2011 Sudan was ranking number nine in kidney disease mortality (2.3%) [2]. In USA the incidence and prevalence of ESRD are expected to increase by 44% - 85% gradually between 2000 and 2015 [3]; in other side the incidence rate in Sudan is expected to be around 70 - 140/million inhabitants/year [4]. In conclusion we can say that chronic renal disease (CRD) is becoming a real major public health problem worldwide [5].

Human leukocyte antigen (HLA) system is the name of human major histocompatibilty complex (MHC). A group of cell-surface antigen-presenting proteins are encoded by a region on the short arm of chromosome: 6 in the distal portion of the 21.3 band; several different types of gene are arranged in the form of three regions: class I, II and III. Most of these genes are polymorphic, arranged close together and are generally inherited as a haplotype [6]. Class II MHC antigens are encoded by genes *HLA* (*DP*, *DM*, *DOA*, *DOB*, *DQ*, and *DR*) loci, and involved in list of the immunoglobulin supergene family [7].

*HLA-DRB*1 belongs to the HLA class II beta chain paralogs. The class II molecule is a heterodimer consisting of an alpha (DRA) and a beta chain (DRB), both anchored in the membrane. It plays a central role in the immune system by presenting peptides derived from extracellular proteins. Class II molecules are expressed in antigen presenting cells (APC: B lymphocytes, dendritic cells, macrophages). The beta chain is approximately 26 - 28 kilo Dalton (kDa). It is encoded by 6 exons. Exon one encodes the commander peptide; exons two and three encode the two extracellular domains; exon four encodes the transmembrane domain; and exon five encodes the cytoplasmic tail. Within the DR molecule the beta chain contains all the polymorphisms specifying the peptide binding specificities. DRB1 is expressed at a level five times higher than its paralogs DRB3, DRB4 and DRB5; also DRB1 is present in all individuals and the Allelic variants of DRB1 are linked with either none or one of the genes DRB3, DRB4 and DRB5. In addition, there are five related pseudogenes: DRB2, DRB6, DRB7, DRB8 and DRB9 [8].

Single nucleotide polymorphisms (SNPs) are variations of a single base, either between two homologous chromosomes within a single individual, or between two individuals [9]. Genetic polymorphisms are well-recognized sources of individual differences in disease risk and treatment response [10]. While the majority of SNPs have no biological consequences, a fraction of gene substitutions have functional significance and provide the basis for the diversity found among humans [10]. However, during the last decade, single nucleotide polymorphisms (SNPs) have become increasingly used because of their abundance in the genome, ease of replication in different laboratories and simplicity of analysis [11]. Recent studies have shown that single-nucleotide polymorphisms (SNPs) are associated with allograft rejection in kidney transplantation recipients [12].

## 2. Material & Methods

### 2.1. Patient Recruitment

This study was a hospital-based case control study, in Ahmed Gasim hospital in the period from September 2012 to November 2013. Five individuals from different families, had undergone renal transplantation whether they develop (acute/hyper acute/chronic) rejection. Sample size include five patients and one control, convenience sampling technique was choose which is based on elements selected from a population on the basis of what elements are easy to obtain. Sometimes a convenience sample is called a grab sample as we essentially grab members from the population for our sample. This is a type of sampling technique that does not rely upon a random process, such as we see in a simple random sample, to generate a sample. Committee of ministry of health, Khartoum state approved the protocol and a written informed consent was obtained from all participants prior to study participation.

## 2.2. Mutational Detection Using Automated DNA Sequencer

Genomic DNA (gDNA) were extracted from the patient's peripheral blood leukocytes using CinnaPure DNA extractions kits. Sequencing done for the area within *HLA-DRB*1 gene (301 base pairs), region location of chromosome 6: 32584100, 32584400. Using Roche/454 Genome Sequencer FLX + Titanium, Deep sequencing up to 1000 bp read length and up to 1.1 Gb/run.

## 2.3. Data Prediction and Analysis Using Bioinformatics Tools

Firstly; DNA sequences were compared with the NCBI human reference genome (www.ncbi.nlm.nih.gov) to check DNA sequencing quality and specificity by using BLAST (basic local alignment search tool), it's a fast sequence similarity searching (http://blast.ncbi.nlm.nih.gov/Blast.cgi) (**Figure 1**). Secondly; sequences were submitted—in sequence alignment form—to BoxShade (online tool) and BioEdit (software package) for multiple sequence alignment results, **Figure 2** and **Figure 3**. BoxShade available at: http://www.ch.embnet.org/software/BOX_form.html. Thirdly; three identified SNPs were submitted to NCBI human reference genome for the second time to check if the identified SNPs are known or novel, then protein sequence of SNPs were get from UniProt database (**Table 1**) (http://www.uniprot.org/) and submitted respectively to SIFT-Sorting Intolerant From Tolerant—(An online server was used to rate intolerant from tolerant nonsynonymous single-base nucleotide polymorphism (nsSNP), and alignments between an order sequence with a large number of homologous sequences to predict if an amino acid substitution will have a phenotypic effect, score result of each new residual ranges from zero to one, when score is below or equal to 0.05 the amino acid substitution is predicted to be intolerant, and tolerated if the score is greater than 0.05 [13]. Poly Phen (Polymorphism Phenotyping) is a server which predicts possible impact of an amino acid substitution on the structure and function of a human protein by analysis of multiple sequence alignment and protein 3D structure, using eight sequence and three structural based which selected automatically by masterful interactive algorithm, in addition that calculates position-specific independent count scores (PSIC) for each of two variants, and then computes the PSIC scores difference between two variants, where the higher a PSIC score difference, the higher functional impact a particular amino acid substitution is likely to have. Prediction outcome can be one of probably/possibly damaging or benign [14]. nsSNP Analyzer is a tool used to predict whether a nsSNP has a phenotypic effect. Its predict results contains information at functional and structural level, provides additional information about the

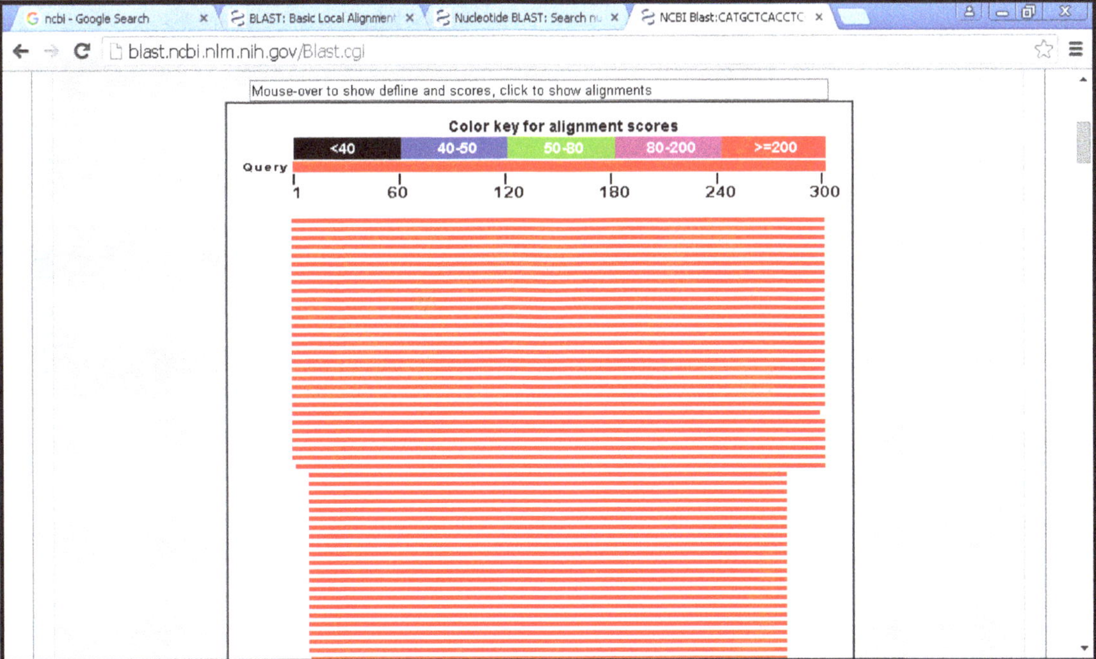


**Figure 1.** BLAST results. The score of each alignment is indicated by one of five different colors, which divides the range of scores into five groups, where red color shows the highly similar (≥200).

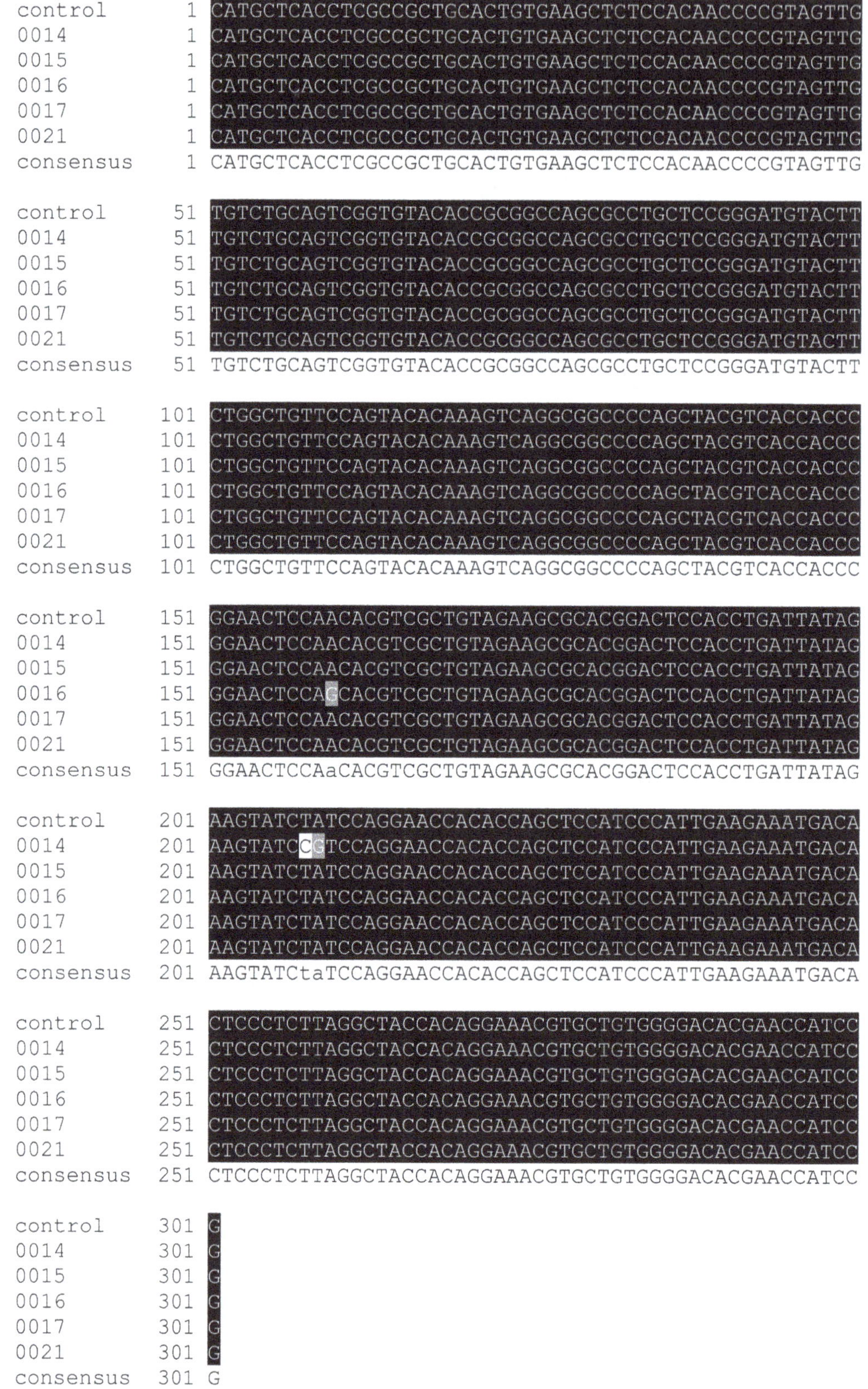

control 1 CATGCTCACCTCGCCGCTGCACTGTGAAGCTCTCCACAACCCCGTAGTTG
0014 1 CATGCTCACCTCGCCGCTGCACTGTGAAGCTCTCCACAACCCCGTAGTTG
0015 1 CATGCTCACCTCGCCGCTGCACTGTGAAGCTCTCCACAACCCCGTAGTTG
0016 1 CATGCTCACCTCGCCGCTGCACTGTGAAGCTCTCCACAACCCCGTAGTTG
0017 1 CATGCTCACCTCGCCGCTGCACTGTGAAGCTCTCCACAACCCCGTAGTTG
0021 1 CATGCTCACCTCGCCGCTGCACTGTGAAGCTCTCCACAACCCCGTAGTTG
consensus 1 CATGCTCACCTCGCCGCTGCACTGTGAAGCTCTCCACAACCCCGTAGTTG
control 51 TGTCTGCAGTCGGTGTACACCGCGGCCAGCGCCTGCTCCGGGATGTACTT
0014 51 TGTCTGCAGTCGGTGTACACCGCGGCCAGCGCCTGCTCCGGGATGTACTT
0015 51 TGTCTGCAGTCGGTGTACACCGCGGCCAGCGCCTGCTCCGGGATGTACTT
0016 51 TGTCTGCAGTCGGTGTACACCGCGGCCAGCGCCTGCTCCGGGATGTACTT
0017 51 TGTCTGCAGTCGGTGTACACCGCGGCCAGCGCCTGCTCCGGGATGTACTT
0021 51 TGTCTGCAGTCGGTGTACACCGCGGCCAGCGCCTGCTCCGGGATGTACTT
consensus 51 TGTCTGCAGTCGGTGTACACCGCGGCCAGCGCCTGCTCCGGGATGTACTT
control 101 CTGGCTGTTCCAGTACACAAAGTCAGGCGGCCCCAGCTACGTCACCACCC
0014 101 CTGGCTGTTCCAGTACACAAAGTCAGGCGGCCCCAGCTACGTCACCACCC
0015 101 CTGGCTGTTCCAGTACACAAAGTCAGGCGGCCCCAGCTACGTCACCACCC
0016 101 CTGGCTGTTCCAGTACACAAAGTCAGGCGGCCCCAGCTACGTCACCACCC
0017 101 CTGGCTGTTCCAGTACACAAAGTCAGGCGGCCCCAGCTACGTCACCACCC
0021 101 CTGGCTGTTCCAGTACACAAAGTCAGGCGGCCCCAGCTACGTCACCACCC
consensus 101 CTGGCTGTTCCAGTACACAAAGTCAGGCGGCCCCAGCTACGTCACCACCC
control 151 GGAACTCCAACACGTCGCTGTAGAAGCGCACGGACTCCACCTGATTATAG
0014 151 GGAACTCCAACACGTCGCTGTAGAAGCGCACGGACTCCACCTGATTATAG
0015 151 GGAACTCCAACACGTCGCTGTAGAAGCGCACGGACTCCACCTGATTATAG
0016 151 GGAACTCCAGCACGTCGCTGTAGAAGCGCACGGACTCCACCTGATTATAG
0017 151 GGAACTCCAACACGTCGCTGTAGAAGCGCACGGACTCCACCTGATTATAG
0021 151 GGAACTCCAACACGTCGCTGTAGAAGCGCACGGACTCCACCTGATTATAG
consensus 151 GGAACTCCAaCACGTCGCTGTAGAAGCGCACGGACTCCACCTGATTATAG
control 201 AAGTATCTATCCAGGAACCACACCAGCTCCATCCCATTGAAGAAATGACA
0014 201 AAGTATCCGTCCAGGAACCACACCAGCTCCATCCCATTGAAGAAATGACA
0015 201 AAGTATCTATCCAGGAACCACACCAGCTCCATCCCATTGAAGAAATGACA
0016 201 AAGTATCTATCCAGGAACCACACCAGCTCCATCCCATTGAAGAAATGACA
0017 201 AAGTATCTATCCAGGAACCACACCAGCTCCATCCCATTGAAGAAATGACA
0021 201 AAGTATCTATCCAGGAACCACACCAGCTCCATCCCATTGAAGAAATGACA
consensus 201 AAGTATCtaTCCAGGAACCACACCAGCTCCATCCCATTGAAGAAATGACA
control 251 CTCCCTCTTAGGCTACCACAGGAAACGTGCTGTGGGGACACGAACCATCC
0014 251 CTCCCTCTTAGGCTACCACAGGAAACGTGCTGTGGGGACACGAACCATCC
0015 251 CTCCCTCTTAGGCTACCACAGGAAACGTGCTGTGGGGACACGAACCATCC
0016 251 CTCCCTCTTAGGCTACCACAGGAAACGTGCTGTGGGGACACGAACCATCC
0017 251 CTCCCTCTTAGGCTACCACAGGAAACGTGCTGTGGGGACACGAACCATCC
0021 251 CTCCCTCTTAGGCTACCACAGGAAACGTGCTGTGGGGACACGAACCATCC
consensus 251 CTCCCTCTTAGGCTACCACAGGAAACGTGCTGTGGGGACACGAACCATCC
control 301 G
0014 301 G
0015 301 G
0016 301 G
0017 301 G
0021 301 G
consensus 301 G


**Figure 2.** Multiple sequence alignment using BoxShade software. Black colour shows conserved regions, gray and white colour shows the mutants regions.

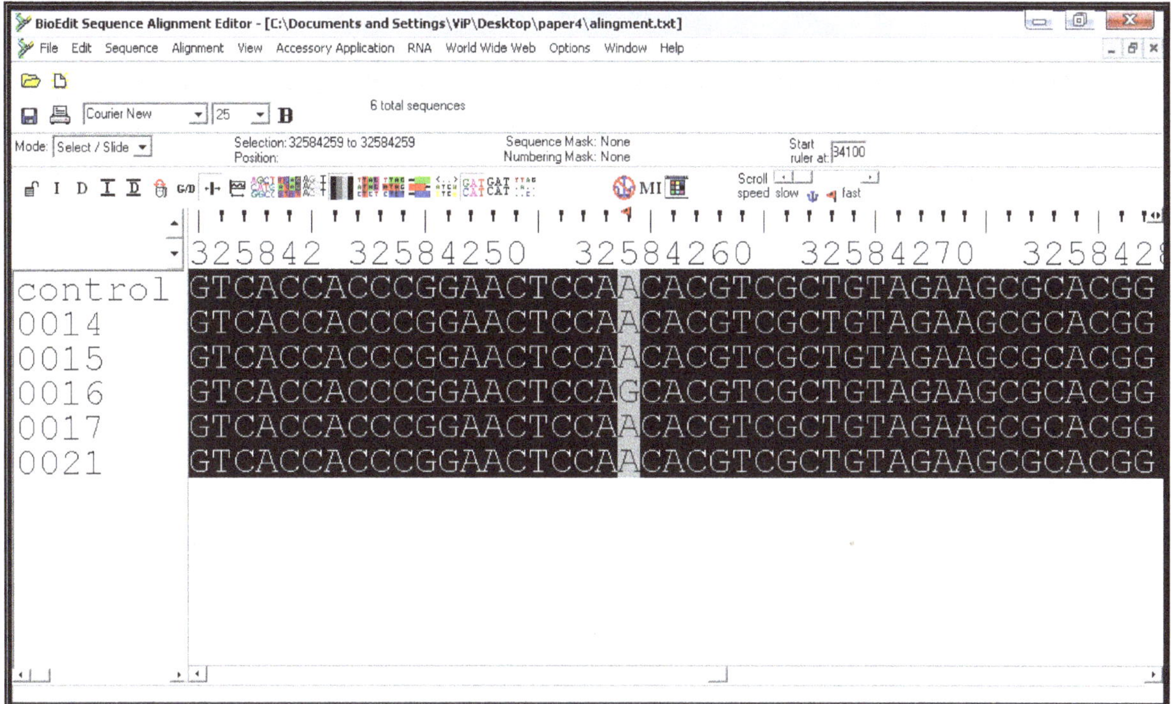

**Figure 3.** Multiple sequence alignment using BioEdit (software package), the upper rule numbers show the chromosome location, gray colour shows the pathological SNP (rs17885437) location (chr:6, 32584259).

**Table 1.** Gene and protein information of identified SNPs obtained from (NCBI & UniProt) databases. (www.ncbi.nlm.nih.gov, http://www.uniprot.org/)

| Sample code No. | Gene | SNP ID | Chromosome location | New nucleotide base pair (bp) | Protein ID | Amino acid change |
|---|---|---|---|---|---|---|
| Pt 0.0014 | *HLA-DRB*1 Gene bank ID: 3123 | rs1059575 | Chr6: 32584308 | G | NP_002115 | D57E |
| | | Novel | Chr6: 32584307 | C | - | S56S |
| Pt 0.0016 | | rs17885437 | chr6: 32584259 | G | NP_002115 | G74R |

SNP to facilitate the interpretation of results, e.g., structural environment and multiple sequence alignment [15]. Results summarized in **Table 2** and **Table 3**. Previous servers available at: SIFT (http://sift.bii.a-star.edu.sg/), nsSNP Analyzer (http://snpanalyzer.utmem.edu/), PolyPhen-2 (http://genetics.bwh.harvard.edu/pph2/). After that protein sequence of pathological or damaging predicted SNP was submitted to I-mutant and Project Hope servers to predict the stability index and some physiochemical properties change due to SNP variant [16] [17], **Table 4** and **Table 5**. I-mutant (version 3.0) available at: (http://gpcr2.biocomp.unibo.it/cgi/predictors/I-Mutant3.0/I-Mutant3.0.cgi), Project Hope (http://www.cmbi.ru.nl/hope/home). Fourthly; protein sequence of deleterious SNP placed to get protein secondary structure using GOR IV tool (secondary structure prediction tool) and result shown in **Figure 4**, (https://npsa-prabi.ibcp.fr/cgibin/npsa_automat.pl?page=npsa_gor4.html), then for the same sequence, homology modeling (3D structure) was predicted using CPH-models 3.2 server, after that for visualization of protein 3D structure and identification of native/new residues types, chimera software was used **Figure 5** and **Figure 6**. CPH server available at: http://www.cbs.dtu.dk/services/CPHmodels/. Lastly; protein sequence of deleterious SNP placed in ProtParam tool (a tool which allows the computation of various physical and chemical parameters for a user entered sequence. The computed parameters include the molecular weight, theoretical pI, amino acid composition, atomic composition, extinction coefficient, estimated half-life, instability index, aliphatic index and grand average of hydropathicity-GRAVY-) [18] (**Table 6**). http://web.expasy.org/protparam/.

**Table 2.** Predicted results of SIFT and nsSNP analyzer servers.

| SNP ID | Amino acid variant | Phenotype prediction | Environment | Area buried | Frac polar | Secondary structure | SIFT prediction | Prediction score |
|---|---|---|---|---|---|---|---|---|
| rs1059575 | D57E | Neutral | P1S | 0.445 | 0.406 | S | TOLERATED | 1 |
| Novel | S56S | - | - | - | - | - | TOLERATED | 0.05 |
| rs17885437 | G74R | Disease | EC | 0.126 | 0.552 | C | DAMAGING | 0.01 |

Environment: The structural environment of the SNP calculated by the environment program, Area buried: Solvent accessibility score, Frac polar: Environmental polarity score, SIFT and Score: Ranges from 0 to 1, the amino acid substitution is predicted damaging if the score is ≤0.05, and tolerated if the score is >0.05.

**Table 3.** Output for PolyPhen-2 server.

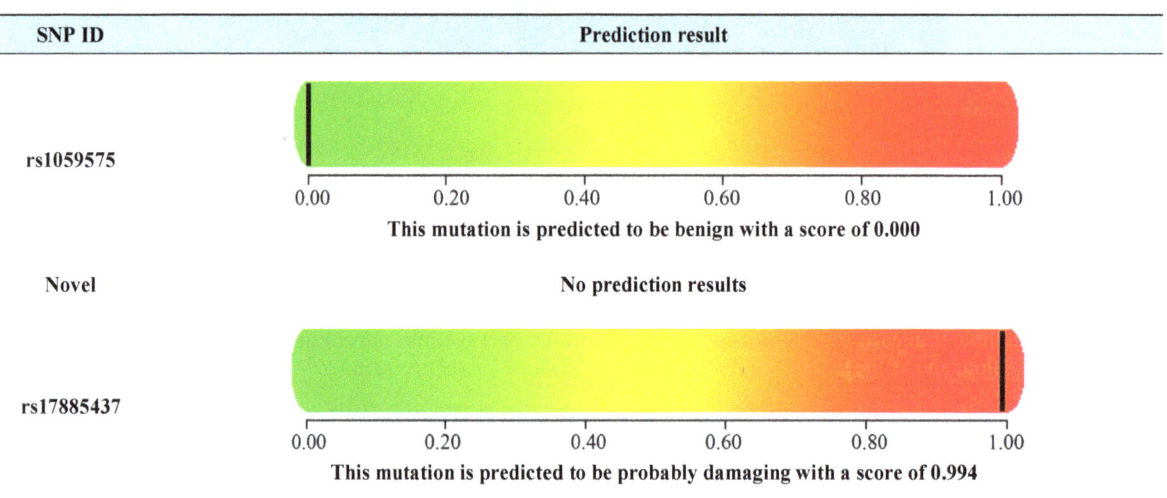

| SNP ID | Prediction result |
|---|---|
| rs1059575 | 0.00 0.20 0.40 0.60 0.80 1.00<br>**This mutation is predicted to be benign with a score of 0.000** |
| Novel | **No prediction results** |
| rs17885437 | 0.00 0.20 0.40 0.60 0.80 1.00<br>**This mutation is predicted to be probably damaging with a score of 0.994** |

PolyPhen-2 score (range from 0 to 1): Probably damaging (~ >0.80), possibly damaging (~ >0.60 to 0.80) and benign (~ ≤0.60).

**Table 4.** Protein stability based on standard free energy change using I-mutant 3.0.

| SNP ID | Amino acid position | WT | MT | PH | Temp (˚C) | Stability | DDG value prediction Kcal/mol |
|---|---|---|---|---|---|---|---|
| rs1059575 | 57 | D | E | 7.0 | 25 | Decrease | −0.54 |
| Novel | 56 | S | S | 7.0 | 25 | - | - |
| rs17885437 | 74 | G | R | 7.0 | 25 | Decrease | −1 |

WT: Wild type amino acid, MT Mutant type amino acid, DDG: DG (New Protein)-DG (Wild Type) in Kcal/mol (DDG < 0: Decrease stability, DDG > 0: Increase stability), RI: Reliability index.

## 3. Results

### 3.1. Check the Sequencing Results

BLAST results showed high similarity to Homo sapiens *HLA-DRB*1 gene for all sequences (samples and control), with identical percentage between 92% - 93%, and these results showed great sequencing results (**Figure 1**).

### 3.2. Multiple Sequence Alignment

Alignment showed the highly conserved target sequencing region for all sequences. Three SNPs were detected, first SNP was in sample (0016) and other two SNPs were within sample (0014) (**Figure 2** and **Figure 3**).

**Table 5.** Physicochemical properties of deleterious nsSNP (G74R) using Project Hope server.

| Differences | Glycine (native amino acid) | Arginine (mutant amino acid) |
|---|---|---|
| Schematic structure | $H_2N$ OH O | $H_2N$ NH NH $H_2N$ OH O |
| Size | Small in size | Bigger in size |
| Charge | Natural in charge | Positively charge and it could make repulsion between the mutant residue and neighboring residues |
| Flexibility | Most flexible of all residues | Can abolish this function which it might be necessary for the protein's function |
| Conservation | Highly conserved | Not observed at all, this mean in just some rare cases the mutation might occur without damaging the protein |

**Table 6.** Computation of some physical and chemical parameters of protein (ID: NP_002115) using Prot Param tool.

| Properties | Calculates |
|---|---|
| - Molecular weight: | 30030.1 |
| - Theoretical pI | 7.64 |
| - Amino acid composition | Ala (A) 11 4.1%<br>Arg (R) 19 7.1%<br>Asn (N) 8 3.0%<br>Asp (D) 9 3.4%<br>Cys (C) 6 2.3%<br>Gln (Q) 14 5.3%<br>Glu (E) 17 6.4%<br>Gly (G) 24 9.0%<br>His (H) 6 2.3%<br>Ile (I) 3 1.1%<br>Leu (L) 27 10.2%<br>Lys (K) 8 3.0%<br>Met (M) 6 2.3%<br>Phe (F) 16 6.0%<br>Pro (P) 13 4.9%<br>Ser (S) 21 7.9%<br>Thr (T) 18 6.8%<br>Trp (W) 5 1.9%<br>Tyr (Y) 10 3.8%<br>Val (V) 25 9.4%<br>Pyl (O) 0 0.0%<br>Sec (U) 0 0.0% |
| - Total number of negatively charged residues (Asp + Glu) | 26 |
| - Total number of positively charged residues (Arg + Lys) | 27 |
| - Formula: | $C_{1344}H_{2064}N_{370}O_{390}S_{12}$ |
| - Total number of atoms: | 4180 |
| - Extinction coefficients: (extinction coefficients are in units of $M^{-1}\cdot cm^{-1}$, at 280 nm measured in water). | 42,775 |
| - Estimated half-life | 30 hours |
| - Aliphatic index | 75.38 |
| - Grand average of hydropathicity (GRAVY) | −0.260 |

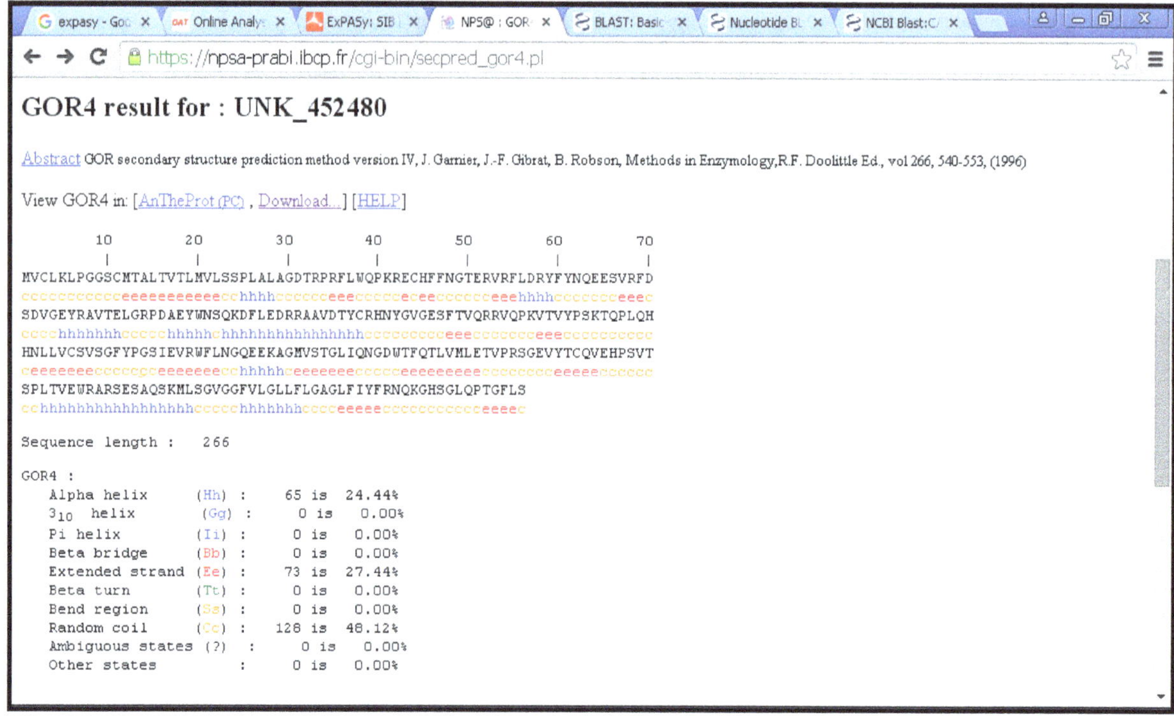


**Figure 4.** Shows primary and secondary structure of deleterious nsSNP related protein (NP_002115) using GOR IV tool, small box within the figure refers to mutant amino acid position of (rs17885437).

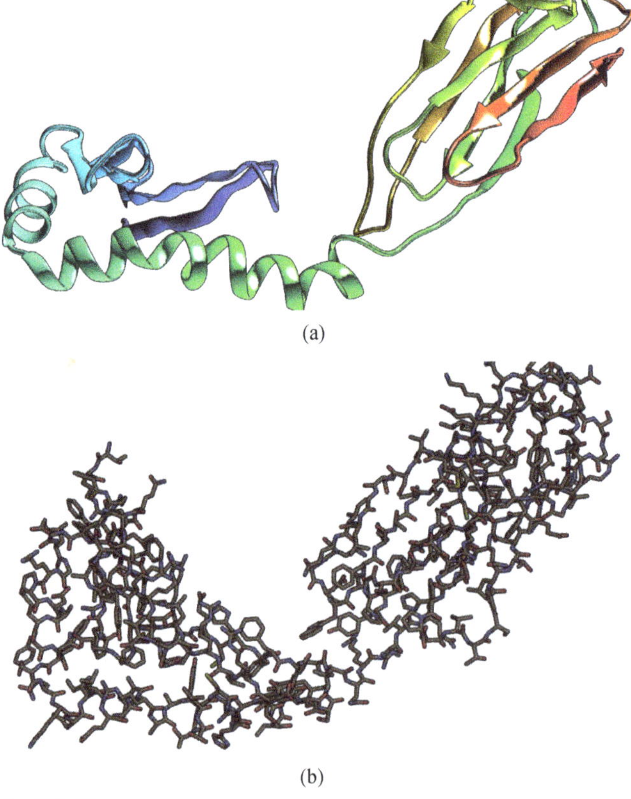

(a)

(b)

**Figure 5.** Shows protein tertiary structure (homology modeling) of deleterious nsSNP related protein (NP_002115). (a) Overview of the protein in ribbon-presentation; (b) Overview of all protein atoms.

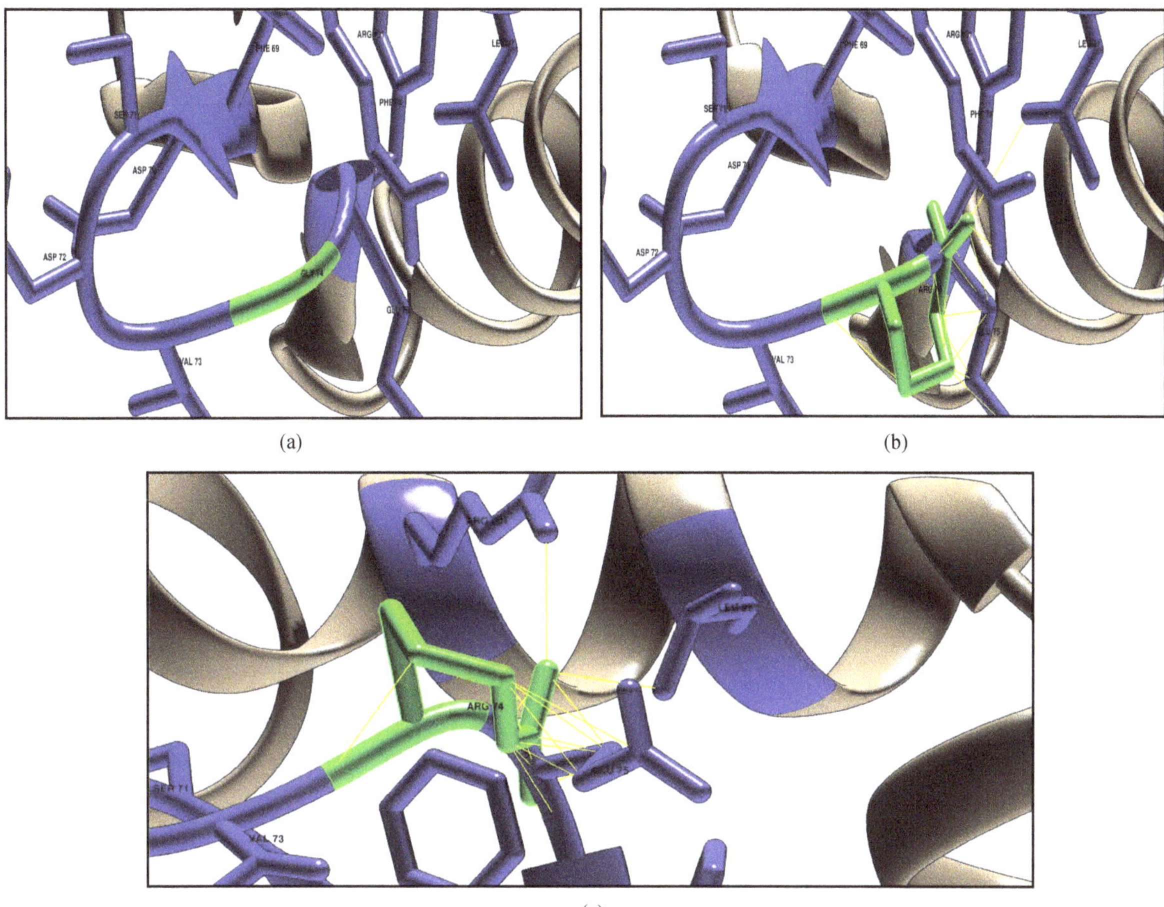


**Figure 6.** Shows *HLA-DRB1* protein structure (ID: NP_002115) using Chimera software (v 1.8). The target residue colored green and the surrounding closest residues colored blue, where (a) represent the native structure with Glycine in position 74; (b) represent the mutated structure with Arginine in position 74, mutant amino acid shows clashes (26 points contacts in fine yellow lines) with other neighbor residues; (c) Shows clashes from different side angle.

## 3.3. Differentiates between Deleterious and Tolerant (Non Damaging) SNPs

Three tools were used to predict the functionality of three detected SNPs, results showed that two of three SNPs were predicted as tolerated and third one as damaging (**Table 2** and **Table 3**).

### Prediction of Change in Stability Due to SNPs Used I-Mutant 3.0 Server

Protein sequence of target SNPs was submitted, results show stability change (decrease) for two SNPs (rs1059575, rs17885437) with deferments DDG values (**Table 4**).

## 3.4. Predicted Physical and Chemical Properties Change Due to SNP

Protein sequence of just a predicted pathological SNP was submitted to Project Hope server, results show that there were wide physiochemical changes due to single variant from wide type (Glycine) to new type (Arginine) (**Table 5**).

## 3.5. Visualized the Protein Homology Modeling

Homology modeling of target pathological SNP did used CPH model 3.2 server, and then model was visualized used chimera software, results shown the structural difference between wide and new amino acid in position 74 with 26 point contact (clash contact) of the mutant residue with neighbor atom, this contact point will increase the severity of damaging (**Figure 6**).

## 4. Discussion

The study involved a group of five renal transplant known rejection patients on hemodialysis (plus one control), patients were dialyzing two to three times per week, and they were at different duration of renal transplant rejection from two to ten years when samples had been collected. Our main objective was to detect presence of SNPs through Sudanese genome of 23 pathological nsSNPs which identified located worldwide in this chromosome location through *in silico* study done by Hassan (2014).

Three SNPs were detected in this study using DNA sequencing technology, two of the three were known SNPs in dbSNPs (SNPs database) (rs1059575, rs17885437), and the third SNP was a novel SNP (not found in dbSNP). Then bioinformatics tools were used to determine the effect of three detected SNPs on the protein structure and function, we found that two were tolerant and one is damaging. The damaging SNP in HLA complex genes may affect renal transplantation rejection. From the above, the results are similar to Hassan's results [8]. Novel SNP located in chromosome 6: 32584307, where nucleotide changed from thiamine to cytosine (T/C) and the codon had been changed from TCT to TCC, both codon encoded by the same amino acid Serine (degeneracy of genetic code), which means that SNP has no effect on protein level (tolerant SNP).

## 5. Conclusion

HLA typing using SNPs analysis is a suitable, accurate and cheap way to cover all types of HLA genes and could be used whole over the world. Damaging SNPs detections also could be an answer for unknown causes of many organ transplantation rejection cases. Results showed the power and impact of *in silico* tools on biomedical research and their ability to uncover the cause of genetic variations in different genetic diseases.

## Disclosure Statement

The authors declare that they have no conflicts of interest related to this work.

## References

[1] Lysaght, M.J. (2002) Maintenance Dialysis Population Dynamics: Current Trends and Long-Term Implications. *Journal of the American Society of Nephrology*, **13**, 37-40. http://jasn.asnjournals.org/content/13/suppl_1/S37.long

[2] (WHR) World Health Rankings. http://www.worldlifeexpectancy.com/world-health-rankings

[3] Gilbertson, D.T., Liu, J., Xue, J.L., Louis, T.A., Solid, C.A., Ebben, J.P. and Collins, A.J. (2005) Projecting the Number of Patients with End-Stage Renal Disease in the United States to the Year 2015. *Journal of the American Society of Nephrology*, **16**, 3736-3741. http://jasn.asnjournals.org/content/16/12/3736.long http://dx.doi.org/10.1681/ASN.2005010112

[4] Elsharif, M.E. and Elsharif, E.G. (2011) Causes of End-Stage Renal Disease in Sudan: A Single-Center Experience. *Saudi Journal of Kidney Diseases and Transplantation*, **22**, 373-376. http://www.sjkdt.org/article.asp?issn=13192442;year=2011;volume=22;issue=2;spage=373;epage=376;aulast=Elsharif

[5] Barsoum, R.S. (2006) Chronic Kidney Disease in the Developing World. *New England Journal of Medicine*, **354**, 997-999. http://www.nejm.org/doi/full/10.1056/NEJMp058318 http://dx.doi.org/10.1056/nejmp058318

[6] Mehra, N.K. (2001) Histocompatibility Antigens. Encyclopedia of Life Sciences. Nature Publishing Group. http://web.udl.es/usuaris/e4650869/docencia/segoncicle/genclin98/recursos_classe_%28pdf%29/revisionsPDF/HLA.pdf

[7] Bodmer, W.F. (1987) The HLA System: Structure and Function. *Journal of Clinical Pathology*, **40**, 948-958. http://jcp.bmj.com/content/40/9/948.full.pdf http://dx.doi.org/10.1136/jcp.40.9.948

[8] Hassan, M.M., Dowd, A.A., Mohamed, A.H., Mahalah, S.M.O.S., *et al.* (2014) Computational Analysis of Deleterious nsSNPs within HLA-DRB1 and HLA-DQB1 Genes Responsible for Allograft Rejection. *International Journal of Computational Bioinformatics and In-Silico Modeling*, **3**, 562-577. http://bioinfo.aizeonpublishers.net/content/2014/6/562-577.html

[9] Uricaru, R., Rizk, G., Lacroix, V., Quillery, E., *et al.* (2015) Reference-Free Detection of Isolated SNPs. *Nucleic Acids Research*, **43**, e11. http://www.ncbi.nlm.nih.gov/pmc/articles/PMC4333369/pdf/gku1187.pdf http://dx.doi.org/10.1093/nar/gku1187

[10] Berno, G., Zaccarelli, M., Goril, C., Tempestilli, M., *et al.* (2014) Analysis of Single-Nucleotide Polymorphisms (SNPs) in Human CYP3A4 and CYP3A5 Genes: Potential Implications for the Metabolism of HIV Drugs. *BMC Medical Ge-*

*netics*, **15**, 76. http://www.biomedcentral.com/content/pdf/1471-2350-15-76.pdf
http://dx.doi.org/10.1186/1471-2350-15-76

[11] Zhan, X., Dixon, A., Batbayar, N., Bragin, E., *et al.* (2015) Exonic versus Intronic SNPs: Contrasting Roles in Revealing the Population Genetic Differentiation of a Widespread Bird Species. *Heredity* (*Edinb*), **114**, 1-9. http://www.nature.com/hdy/journal/v114/n1/pdf/hdy201459a.pdf
http://dx.doi.org/10.1038/hdy.2014.59

[12] Kim, S.K., Park, H.J., Seok, H., Jeon, H.S., *et al.* (2014) Association Studies of Cytochrome P450, Family 2, Subfamily E, Polypeptide 1 (CYP2E1) Gene Polymorphisms with Acute Rejection in Kidney Transplantation Recipients. *Clinical Transplantation*, **28**, 707-712. http://onlinelibrary.wiley.com/doi/10.1111/ctr.12369/pdf
http://dx.doi.org/10.1111/ctr.12369

[13] Ng, P.C. and Henikoff, S. (2001) Predicting Deleterious Amino Acid Substitutions. *Genome Research*, **11**, 863-874. http://genome.cshlp.org/content/11/5/863
http://dx.doi.org/10.1101/gr.176601

[14] Ramensky, V., Bork, P. and Sunyaev, S. (2002) Human Nonsynonymous SNPs: Server and Survey. *Nucleic Acids Research*, **30**, 3894-3900. http://nar.oxfordjournals.org/content/30/17/3894.long
http://dx.doi.org/10.1093/nar/gkf493

[15] Bao, L., Zhou, M. and Cui, Y. (2005) nsSNP Analyzer: Identifying Disease-Associated Nonsynonymous Single Nucleotide Polymorphisms. *Nucleic Acids Research*, **33**, W480-W482.
http://nar.oxfordjournals.org/content/33/suppl_2/W480.abstract
http://dx.doi.org/10.1093/nar/gki372

[16] Capriotti, E., Fariselli, P., Calabrese and Casadio, R. (2005) Predicting Protein Stability Changes from Sequences Using Support Vector Machines. *Bioinformatics*, **2**, 54-58.
http://bioinformatics.oxfordjournals.org/content/21/suppl_2/ii54.abstract
http://dx.doi.org/10.1093/bioinformatics/bti1109

[17] Venselaar, H., Beek, T., Kuipers, R.K., Hekkelma, M.L. and Vriend, G. (2010) Protein Structure Analysis of Mutations Causing Inheritable Diseases. An e-Science Approach with Life Scientist Friendly Interfaces. *BMC Bioinformatics*, **11**, 548. http://www.biomedcentral.com/1471-2105/11/548
http://dx.doi.org/10.1186/1471-2105-11-548

[18] Gasteiger, E., Hoogland, C., Gattiker, A., Duvaud, S., *et al.* (2005) Protein Identification and Analysis Tools on the ExPASy Server. In: Walker, J.M., Ed., The Proteomics Protocols Handbook, Humana Press, 571-607.
http://link.springer.com/protocol/10.1385%2F1-59259-890-0%3A571
http://dx.doi.org/10.1385/1-59259-890-0:571

20

# IL-4, IL-10 and TNF-$\alpha$ Polymorphisms in Idiopathic Membranous Nephropathy (IMN)

**Mauro Giacomelli[1,2*], Rajesh Kumar[1,2], Giacomo Tampella[1,2], Simona Ceffa[3], Mario Bontempelli[3]**

[1]Institute of Molecular Medicine "Angelo Nocivelli", University of Brescia, Brescia, Italy
[2]Scuola di Dottorato in Scienze della Riproduzione e dello Sviluppo, University of Trieste, Trieste, Italy
[3]Immunology Laboratory, Ospedali Riuniti of Bergamo, Bergamo, Italy
Email: *mauro.giacomelli@unibs.it

## Abstract

**Idiopathic membranous nephropathy (IMN) is a Th2 nephritogenic immune disorder. It is caused by the accumulation of immune complexes, mainly IgG4, at the basal glomerular membrane that leads to the damage of the glomerular barrier and subsequent injury of podocytes. Our aim was to evaluate the relationship between cytokine polymorphisms and IMN. We investigated the cytokine polymorphisms in forty-five patients and one hundred twenty-four healthy individuals, using polymerase chain reaction-sequence specific primers (PCR-SSP). We showed a significant increase in allelic frequencies of the alleles -590T and -33T of IL-4 gene and -308A of TNF-$\alpha$ gene, in IMN patients. In addition, we observed an increased frequency of allele -1082G in IL-10 gene in a subgroup of patients with CD4/CD8 ratio major than 2, when compared either to control subjects or the subgroup of patients with CD4/CD8 ratio minor than 2. Moreover, analyzing the Th1/Th2 cytokines in serum and urine, we found increased levels of IL-4 in serum and IL-5 in urine of patients. We deduce that the alleles -590T and -33T of IL-4 and -308A of TNF-$\alpha$ may be associated with IMN. In addition, in patients with increased T helper lymphocytes, IL-10 -1082G polymorphism can also play a role in the pathogenesis of the disease. These findings remark the role of Th2 immune response and suggest the association between polymorphic variants of IL-4, IL-10 and TNF-$\alpha$ genes with the development of IMN and therefore giving a better insight in pathogenesis of this disease.**

## Keywords

**Interleukin-Four, Tumor Necrosis Factor-$\alpha$, Interleukin-Ten, Idiopathic Membranous Nephropathy, Immunoglobulin G Sub-Class 4**

*Corresponding author.

# 1. Introduction

Idiopathic membranous nephropathy (IMN) is a rare immune disease and also the most common cause of nephrotic syndrome in adults. It is caused by the accumulation of immune complexes in the basal glomerular membrane, which in turn damages the podocytes through complement-dependent processes. The major role of podocytes is to synthesize the components of glomerular filtration barrier [1]. The damaged podocytes cause a decrease in the filtration capacity of the glomerulus, resulting in marked proteinuria. The immune complexes deposited in the subepithelial glomerulus in IMN patients are mainly IgG4 [2]-[4].

IgG4 is a subclass of antibodies that is produced in response to prolonged and recurrent antigenic stimulations [5], or to helminthic infections [6]. These antibodies are monovalent and have low avidity. IgG4 antibodies are unable to bind the complement, but they form small non-precipitating complexes [7] [8]. The serum levels of these antibodies are often increased in subjects affected by IMN [2] [3].

IMN is a Th2 nephritogenic immune disorder. T helper lymphocytes, which are often increased in these patients, produce significantly more IL-4 [9], whereas B lymphocytes generate more IgG4, than healthy individuals, when cultured in presence of IL-4 [10]. IL-4 is a major Th2 cytokine that induces the isotype switching towards IgG4 and IgE, this induction is potentiated by IL-10, another Th2 cytokine [11]-[13].

The polymorphisms of IL-4 and IL-13 are already associated to the minimal change nephrotic syndrome (MCNS), a disorder of pediatric age characterized by an increase in IgE levels [14]. Moreover, genetic variants of STAT6, which transduces the signal through the IL-4 receptor alpha (IL-4Ralpha), are also linked to MCNS's clinical course [15]. Nevertheless, a direct correlation between IL-4 polymorphisms and IMN was never established.

Some authors indicated that the impaired immune response in IMN could be also related to the B cell compartment. In fact, there are also large infiltrates of B CD20 positive lymphocytes in tubule-interstitial compartment [16]. The role of these B cells in pathogenesis of the IMN is still unknown. B cells probably act as antigen presenting cells (APCs) rather than antibody producing cells. In fact Rituximab, an anti-CD20 antibody, is currently used in the treatment of the Membranous Nephropathy [17] [18].

The cytokines are key factors in modulating the immune response and class switching of antibodies. Cytokines modulate the activity of T and B lymphocytes, regulate cellular activities and the response to pathogens. The polymorphisms in promoter regions of cytokine genes can influence the transcriptional and expression levels of these cytokines [19]-[23].

Many research groups have established the link between these polymorphisms and various pathologies. For instance, the variant -572C of IL-6 gene and the polymorphism -308A of TNF-*α* and TNF d2 allele were associated to IMN in different ethnic groups [24] [25]. Moreover, it is demonstrated that TNF-*α*-308A can also cause Non Idiopathic Membranous Nephropathy [26].

In this study we evaluated the association between polymorphisms in cytokine genes and IMN. We also evaluated the amount of Th1/Th2 cytokines in the serum and the urine collected before the therapeutic treatment. Finally, on the basis of the ratio of CD4/CD8 T lymphocytes, we analyzed whether there were differences in the frequencies of polymorphisms between patients and control group.

# 2. Materials and Methods

## 2.1. Subjects

For this study, one hundred twenty-four controls (Bone marrow donors), aged between 27 and 52 years (mean age 43.5; 70 male and 54 female) [27] and forty-five IMN patients, aged between 21 and 77 years (mean age 51.3; 26 male and 19 female) were enrolled.

Samples were collected at the Department of Nephrology and Immunology of Ospedali Riuniti of Bergamo, between October 2002 and May 2008. Physical examination, hematochemical and urine analysis, 24 h urinary collection, albumin, creatinine and cholesterol levels, 24 h creatinine clearance and daily urinary protein excretion have defined the diagnosis of membranous nephropathy (MN). The diagnosis was confirmed on renal biopsies with microscopic and immunofluorescence techniques. Clinical examination and laboratory data excluded the presence of other alterations that could define secondary membranous nephropathies. In fact these patients were negative for tumors, systemic lupus, viral hepatitis infections or other causes of MN like rheumatoid arthritis. These patients were negative for ANA (antinucleus antibodies), RF (Rheumatoid factor), Hepatitis B and Hepatitis C markers (HBsAg and anti-HCV).

Twenty-four healthy subjects were analyzed for cytokines levels evaluation in serum and urine. Informed consent was obtained from each participant, and the local ethics committee approved the present study.

### 2.2. Single Nucleotide Polymorphism Analysis by PCR-SSP (Sequence Specific Primers)

DNA was extracted from 300 μl of peripheral blood by automatic extractor GenoM$^{TM}$-6 Robotic Workstation (Qiagen). The polymorphism typing was defined by Heidelberg cytokine gene polymorphisms SSP kit (Protrans medizinische diagnotiche produkte, Hockenheim, Germany).

The following polymorphisms were analysed: IL-1$\alpha$ (T/C −889), IL-1$\beta$ (C/T −511, T/C +3962), IL-12 (C/A −1188), IFN-$\gamma$ (A/T UTR 5644), TGF-$\beta$ (C/T codon 10, G/C codon 25), TNF-$\alpha$ (G/A −308, G/A −238), IL-2 (T/G −330, G/T +166), IL-4 (T/G −1098, T/C −590, T/C −33), IL-6 (G/C −174, G/A nt 565), IL-10 (G/A −1082, C/T −819, C/A −592), IL-1R (C/T pst 11,970), IL-1RA (T/C mspa 111,100) and IL-4R$\alpha$ (G/A +1902).

PCR reaction was performed using Ampli Taq DNA polymerase 5 U/μl, (Applied Biosystems) in GeneAmp PCR System 9700 thermal cycler (Perkin Elmer) using following protocol: initial denaturation at 94˚C for 2 minutes; denaturation at 94˚C for 15 seconds; annealing and extension at 65˚C for 1 minute (10 cycles), denaturation at 94˚C for 15 seconds; annealing at 61˚C for 50 seconds; extension at 72˚C for 30 seconds (20 cycles).

Amplicons were visualized by electrophoresis on 2% agarose gel containing ethidium bromide 0.625 mg/ml.

### 2.3. Measurement of Cytokine Levels in Serum and Urine.

The levels of IL-4, IL-5, IL-10, TNF-$\alpha$ and IFN-$\gamma$ were evaluated by ELISA (Bender MedSystems) with detection limit of 1, <2, 1, 2.5 and 1 pg/ml respectively. All samples were read in triplicate with an ELISA plate reader, Gralis-Microplate-Reader (Spa Laboratory Bouty). Serum and urine samples were collected before diagnosis and frozen at −80˚C until the analysis.

### 2.4. Flow Cytometry Analysis of Lymphocyte Subpopulations

Blood samples from patients were collected at the time of diagnosis and lymphocyte subpopulations were evaluated using FACSCalibur$^{TM}$ cytometer (Becton Dickinson). Whole blood was stained with the following antibodies: anti-CD3/CD4/CD8/CD45 and anti-CD3/CD19/CD16 + 56/CD45 (Becton Dickinson). All flow cytometric data were analyzed by FlowJo software 7.5. (TreeStar Inc.).

### 2.5. Statistical Analysis

The association between allelic or genotype frequencies and IMN was calculated through contingency tables 2 × 2 and 2 × 3 respectively, calculating $\chi^2$ test. Cytokine levels, CD4/CD8 ratio comparison and protein daily excretion were analyzed by variance analysis and subsequent execution of the Bonferroni test. A $p$-value less than 0.05 was considered statistically significant.

## 3. Results

### 3.1. Allelic and Genotype Frequency of IL-4, IL-10 and TNF-$\alpha$ in IMN Patients

1) Allele frequency:

The allele frequencies for IL-4 -590T and -33T, were increased in patients when compared to healthy controls ($p < 1 \times 10^{-6}$, $p < 1 \times 10^{-6}$ respectively). The distribution of TNF-$\alpha$ -308A allele was also statistically different between the two groups ($p = 0.0001$), (**Table 1**). Whereas, for IL-10, the allele -1082G didn't show any differences in the two groups analyzed ($p = 0.14$), while the allele -819C was slightly increased in patients ($p = 0.046$), (**Table 1**).

Other analyzed polymorphisms didn't show any significant differences in the two groups (data not shown).

2) Genotype frequency

The genotype distribution was significantly different for IL-4 T-590C, IL-4 T-33C, TNF-$\alpha$ G-308A and IL-10 G-1082A (**Table 2**) among the two groups. For IL-4 T-590C, genotypes TT, TC and CC were respectively 13.3%, 60% and 26.7% in patients vs. 2.4%, 9.6% and 88% in control subjects ($p < 1 \times 10^{-6}$). For IL-4 T-33C the genotypes TT, TC, and CC were respectively 4.4%, 57.8% and 37.8% in patients vs. 2.5%, 15.3% and 82.2% in control subjects ($p < 1 \times 10^{-6}$).

**Table 1.** The allele frequencies for cytokine polymorphisms in IMN patients respect to healthy controls.

| | | Ctrls (n = 248) | IMN Pts (n = 90) | IMN Pts vs Ctrls | |
|---|---|---|---|---|---|
| | | % (n) | % (n) | $\chi^2$ | *p* Value |
| -590T | IL-4 | 7.3 (18) | 42.2 (38) | $\chi^2 = 55.899$ | $p < 1 \times 10^{-6}$ |
| -590C | | 92.7 (230) | 57.8 (52) | | |
| -33T | IL-4 | 10 (25) | 33.3 (30) | $\chi^2 = 24.528$ | $p < 1 \times 10^{-6}$ |
| -33C | | 90 (223) | 66.7 (60) | | |
| -1082G | IL-10 | 39 (97) | 49 (44) | $\chi^2 = 2.209$ | $p = 0.1371$ |
| -1082A | | 61 (151) | 51 (46) | | |
| -819C | IL-10 | 68 (169) | 80 (72) | $\chi^2 = 3.975$ | $p = 0.0461$ |
| -819T | | 32 (79) | 20 (18) | | |
| -308A | TNF-*α* | 8 (20) | 24.4 (22) | $\chi^2 = 14.811$ | $p = 0.0001$ |
| -308G | | 92 (228) | 75.6 (68) | | |

**Table 2.** The genotype frequencies for cytokine polymorphisms in IMN patients respect to healthy controls.

| | | Ctrls (n = 124) | IMN Pts (n = 45) | IMN Pts vs Ctrls | |
|---|---|---|---|---|---|
| | | % (n) | % (n) | $\chi^2$ | *p* Value |
| IL-4 T-590C | TT | 2.4 (3) | 13.3 (6) | $\chi^2 = 60.910$ | $p < 1 \times 10^{-6}$ |
| | TC | 9.6 (12) | 60 (27) | | |
| | CC | 88 (109) | 26.7 (12) | | |
| IL-4 T-33C | TT | 2.5 (3) | 4.4 (2) | $\chi^2 = 32.085$ | $p < 1 \times 10^{-6}$ |
| | TC | 15.3 (19) | 57.8 (26) | | |
| | CC | 82.2 (102) | 37.8 (17) | | |
| IL-10 G-1082A | GG | 9.7 (12) | 31.1 (14) | $\chi^2 = 13.304$ | $p = 0.0013$ |
| | GA | 58.8 (73) | 35.6 (16) | | |
| | AA | 31.5 (39) | 33.3 (15) | | |
| IL-10 C-819T | CC | 48.5 (60) | 64.5 (29) | $\chi^2 = 5.350$ | $p = 0.069$ |
| | CT | 39.5 (49) | 33.3 (15) | | |
| | TT | 12 (15) | 2.2 (1) | | |
| TNF-*α* G-308A | AA | 3.3 (4) | 6.7 (3) | $\chi^2 = 17.869$ | $p = 0.0001$ |
| | GA | 9.7 (12) | 35.5 (16) | | |
| | GG | 87 (108) | 57.8 (26) | | |

Furthermore, for TNF-*α* G-308A, the genotypes AA, GA, and GG were present respectively in 6.7%, 35.5% and 57.8% of patients, compared to 3.3%, 9.7% and 87% of healthy subjects, ($p = 0.0001$). Finally, for IL-10, the genotypes GG, GA, and AA of G-1082A were respectively found in 31.1%, 35.6% and 33.6% of patients vs. 9.7%, 58.8% and 31.5% of healthy controls ($p = 0.001$). We did not find any significant differences in genotypes CC, CT, and TT for IL-10 C-819T, (**Table 2**).

## 3.2. CD4/CD8 Ratio in IMN Patients

The CD4/CD8 ratio is often increased in IMN, which likely represents a distinctive tract of the altered immune response associated to the pathogenesis of the disease [10] [28]-[31]. Hence, we calculated the CD4/CD8 ratio in 25 control subjects and 45 IMN patients. In control group the ratio was 1.54 +/− 0.23 whereas in IMN patients we identified two different subgroups, one with CD4/CD8 ratio greater than two (2.87 +/− 0.83, n = 24) and another subgroup with ratio less than two (1.51 +/− 0.3, n = 21). We did not find healthy controls with CD4/CD8 ratio greater than two. The differences between the subgroup of patients with CD4/CD8 ratio > 2 was statistically significant when compared either to control subjects (1.54 +/− 0.23 vs. 2.87 +/− 0.83, $p < 0.001$) or the subgroup of patients with CD4/CD8 ratio < 2 (2.87 +/− 0.83 vs. 1.51 +/− 0.3, $p < 0.001$). On the other hand there was no statistical difference observed when the subgroup of patients with CD4/CD8 ratio < 2 was matched to control subjects (1.54 +/− 0.23 vs. 1.51 +/− 0.3, $p = 0.15$).

### 3.3. Allelic and Genotype Frequency of IL-10 in IMN Patients with Increased CD4/CD8 Ratio

In order to better investigate the meaning of CD4/CD8 ratio in IMN patients, we assessed it in relationship with cytokine polymorphism frequencies.

Our results showed that the variants G-1082A and C-819T for IL-10 is statistically increased in patients with CD4/CD8 ratio > 2 respect to healthy subjects ($p = 0.005$ and $p = 0.011$, respectively), (**Table 3**).

We also compared the group of patients with ratio CD4/CD8 > 2 to the group of patients with CD4/CD8 ratio < 2, for the same alleles.

The allele frequency for IL-10 -1082G was increased in group with CD4/CD8 >2 ($p = 0.011$), while there were no differences for −819C allele in the two subgroups of patients ($p = 0.102$), (**Table 3**).

The genotype frequency was also different between the subgroup of patients with CD4/CD8 ratio > 2 and healthy controls group. For IL-10 G-1082A, the genotype frequency of GG, GA, and AA was 37.5%, 50% and 12.5% in patients, while the frequency was 9.7%, 58.8% and 31.5% in healthy controls ($p = 0.001$). For IL-10 C-819T, the genotype frequency of CC, CT, and TT was 75%, 25% and 0% in patients, while the frequency was 48.5%, 39.5% and 12% in healthy controls ($p = 0.034$), (**Table 4**).

Finally, we also compared the genotypes among the two subgroups of patients according to the CD4/CD8 ratio. The genotype frequency of GG, GA, and AA for IL-10 G-1082A was significantly different in two groups; 37.5%, 50% and 12.5% in CD4/CD8 > 2 subgroup and 23.8%, 19%, and 57.2% in CD4/CD8 < 2 subgroup, respectively ($p = 0.006$), (**Table 4**).

### 3.4. Cytokines Levels in Serum and Urine

We investigated cytokine levels in serum of both patients and healthy controls. The results showed only one significantly altered cytokine, *i.e.* IL-4. Its levels were 55.40 +/− 72.41 pg/ml in patients vs. 0.20 +/− 0.98 pg/ml in healthy controls ($p = 0.001$), (**Table 5**).

Furthermore, cytokine levels in urine were altered for two cytokines. For IL-5 were 5.59 +/− 7.51 pg/ml vs. 0.00 +/− 0.00 pg/ml ($p = 0.001$); while IL-10 levels were 1.22 +/− 1.66 pg/ml vs. 0.00 +/− 0.00 pg/ml ($p = 0.001$), in patients and healthy control subjects, respectively, (**Table 6**).

Finally, the comparison between the subgroup of patients with ratio CD4/CD8 > 2 vs. CD4/CD8 < 2 subgroup, showed a significant difference for IL-10, in urine. Ten patients with ratio CD4/CD8 > 2, compared to eight pa-

**Table 3.** The allele frequencies for cytokine polymorphisms in IMN patients with ratio CD4/CD8 > 2 respect to healthy controls and respect to IMN patients with ratio CD4/CD8 < 2.

| | | Ctrls (n = 248) | IMN Pts (CD4/CD8 > 2) (n = 48) | IMN Pts (CD4/CD8 < 2) (n = 42) | IMN Pts (CD4/CD8 > 2) vs Ctrls | | IMN Pts (CD4/CD8 > 2) vs IMN Pts (CD4/CD8 < 2) | |
|---|---|---|---|---|---|---|---|---|
| | | % (n) | % (n) | % (n) | $\chi^2$ | *P* value | $\chi^2$ | *p* Value |
| **-590T**<br>**-590C** | IL-4 | 7.3 (18)<br>92.7 (230) | 43.8 (21)<br>56.2 (27) | 42.8 (18)<br>57.2 (24) | $\chi^2 = 43.678$ | $p < 1 \times 10^{-6}$ | $\chi^2 = 0.0163$ | $p = 0.898$ |
| **-33T**<br>**-33C** | IL-4 | 10 (25)<br>90 (223) | 35.4 (17)<br>64.6 (31) | 31 (13)<br>69 (29) | $\chi^2 = 19.172$ | $p = 1.18 \times 10^{-5}$ | $\chi^2 = 0.0502$ | $p = 0.822$ |
| **-1082G**<br>**-1082A** | IL-10 | 39 (97)<br>61 (151) | 62.5 (30)<br>37.5 (18) | 33.3 (14)<br>66.7 (28) | $\chi^2 = 8.050$ | $p = 0.0045$ | $\chi^2 = 6.503$ | $p = 0.011$ |
| **-819C**<br>**-819T** | IL-10 | 68 (169)<br>32 (79) | 87.5 (42)<br>12.5 (6) | 71.4 (30)<br>28.6 (12) | $\chi^2 = 6.445$ | $p = 0.0111$ | $\chi^2 = 2.681$ | $p = 0.102$ |
| **-308A**<br>**-308G** | TNF-α | 8 (20)<br>92 (228) | 29 (14)<br>71 (34) | 19 (8)<br>81 (34) | $\chi^2 = 15.599$ | $p = 7.79 \times 10^{-5}$ | $\chi^2 = 0.754$ | $p = 0.385$ |

**Table 4.** The genotype frequencies for cytokine polymorphisms in IMN patients with ratio CD4/CD8 > 2 respect to healthy controls and respect to IMN patients with ratio CD4/CD8 < 2.

| | | Ctrls (n = 124) | IMN Pts (CD4/CD8 > 2) (n = 24) | IMN Pts (CD4/CD8 < 2) (n = 21) | IMN Pts (CD4/CD8 > 2) vs Ctrls | | IMN Pts (CD4/CD8 > 2) vs IMN Pts (CD4/CD8 < 2) | |
|---|---|---|---|---|---|---|---|---|
| | | % (n) | % (n) | % (n) | $\chi^2$ | *P* value | $\chi^2$ | *P* Value |
| **IL4 T-590C** | **TT** | 2.4 (3) | 16.7 (4) | 9.5 (2) | $\chi^2 = 41.042$ | $p < 1 \times 10^{-6}$ | $\chi^2 = 0.840$ | $p = 0.656$ |
| | **TC** | 9.6 (12) | 54.2 (13) | 66.7 (14) | | | | |
| | **CC** | 88 (109) | 29.1 (7) | 23.8 (5) | | | | |
| **IL4 T-33C** | **TT** | 2.5 (3) | 4.2 (1) | 4.8 (1) | $\chi^2 = 26.184$ | $p = 2.1 \times 10^{-6}$ | $\chi^2 = 0.476$ | $p = 0.788$ |
| | **TC** | 15.3 (19) | 62.5 (15) | 52.4 (11) | | | | |
| | **CC** | 82.2(102) | 33.3 (8) | 42.8 (9) | | | | |
| **IL-10 G-1082A** | **GG** | 9.7 (12) | 37.5 (9) | 23.8 (5) | $\chi^2 = 13.790$ | $p = 0.0010$ | $\chi^2 = 10.389$ | $p = 0.006$ |
| | **GA** | 58.8 (73) | 50 (12) | 19 (4) | | | | |
| | **AA** | 31.5 (39) | 12.5 (3) | 57.2 (12) | | | | |
| **IL-10 C-819T** | **CC** | 48.5 (60) | 75 (18) | 52.4 (11) | $\chi^2 = 6.746$ | $p = 0.0343$ | $\chi^2 = 3.103$ | $p = 0.212$ |
| | **CT** | 39.5 (49) | 25 (6) | 42.8 (9) | | | | |
| | **TT** | 12 (15) | 0 (0) | 4.8 (1) | | | | |
| **TNF-*α* G-308A** | **AA** | 3.3 (4) | 4.2 (1) | 9.5 (2) | $\chi^2 = 24.472$ | $p = 5.1 \times 10^{-6}$ | $\chi^2 = 4.769$ | $p = 0.092$ |
| | **GA** | 9.7 (12) | 50 (12) | 19 (4) | | | | |
| | **GG** | 87 (108) | 45.8 (11) | 71.5 (15) | | | | |

**Table 5.** Th1/Th2 cytokine levels in serum.

| | Serum | | | |
|---|---|---|---|---|
| | **Ctrls (n = 24) (Mean +/− sd) pg/ml** | **IMN Pts (n = 24) (Mean +/− sd) pg/ml** | ***p* Value** | **Detection Limit pg/ml** |
| **IL-4** | 0.20 +/− 0.98 | 55.40 +/− 72.41 | $p = 0.001$ | 1 |
| **IL-5** | 0.00 +/− 0.00 | 0.94 +/− 3.01 | $p = 0.142$ | < 2 |
| **IL-10** | 0.00 +/− 0.00 | 1.95 +/− 5.86 | $p = 0.116$ | 1 |
| **TNF-*α*** | 0.00+/−0.00 | 1.06 +/− 3.13 | $p = 0.109$ | 2.5 |
| **IFN-*γ*** | 0.05 +/− 0.16 | 0.52 +/− 0.65 | $p = 0.001$ | 1 |

**Table 6.** Th1/Th2 cytokine levels in urine.

| | Urine | | | |
|---|---|---|---|---|
| | **Ctrls (n = 22) (Mean +/− sd) pg/ml** | **IMN Pts (n = 18) (Mean +/− sd) pg/ml** | ***p* Value** | **Detection Limit pg/ml** |
| **IL-4** | 0.00 +/− 0.00 | 9.63 +/− 40.55 | $p = 0.271$ | 1 |
| **IL-5** | 0.00 +/− 0.00 | 5.59 +/− 7.51 | $p = 0.001$ | < 2 |
| **IL-10** | 0.00 +/− 0.00 | 1.22 +/− 1.66 | $p = 0.001$ | 1 |
| **TNF-*α*** | 0.00 +/− 0.00 | 0.79 +/− 1.29 | $p = 0.006$ | 2.5 |
| **IFN-*γ*** | 0.00 +/− 0.00 | 0.10 +/− 0.23M | $p = 0.037$ | 1 |

tients with ratio CD4/CD8 < 2, had the levels of IL-10 to 1.87 +/− 1.62 pg/ml and 0.47 +/− 0.42 pg/ml, respectively, ($p = 0.031$). All the other cytokines evaluated were either normal when compared to control group, or under the detection limits of relative ELISA kit.

### 3.5. Association between Cytokine Polymorphisms and Clinical Data

The analysis of allele and genotype frequencies did not show significant differences when clinical data such as gender, age at onset, or other clinical complications collected during follow-up, were considered (data not shown).

Instead, the analysis of the clinical parameters collected before treatment, showed a significant correlation, but only between proteinuria and the polymorphism T-590C of IL-4. Indeed, the genotypes TT, CT and CC had levels of proteinuria to 4.92 +/− 2.09, 3.74 +/− 1.31 and 3.0 +/− 0.81 g/day, respectively, ($p = 0.022$), (**Figure 1(a)**).

For IL-4 T-33C, the proteinuria levels in TT, TC and CC were 4.75 +/− 0.63, 3.88 +/− 1.62 and 3.19 +/− 1.10 g/day, respectively, ($p$ = not significant), (**Figure 1(b)**).

However, we did not observe other correlations between polymorphisms investigated and other parameters such as albumin levels, cholesterol levels or creatinine clearance (data not shown).

## 4. Discussion

In this study, we revealed the association between polymorphisms in IL-4 (T-590C, T-33C) and in TNF-$\alpha$ (G-308A) and the development of IMN syndrome. In addition, in a subgroup of patients with increased T-helper lymphocytes, an association is shown between IL-10 polymorphisms G-1082A and C-819T and the disease. Furthermore, we showed that the cytokine levels of IL-4 in serum and IL-5 and IL-10 in urine are often increased in IMN patients.

These data are in agreement with the hypothesis that IMN is a Th2 type immune-mediated pathology. Some authors already described that T-helper lymphocytes of patients affected by IMN have increased production of IL-4 [9] and B lymphocytes, stimulated with IL-4, generate more IgG4 compared to healthy individuals [10]. In the latter study, the authors showed the increased expression of IL-10 and IL-13 in PBMCs, as well as an increase in CD4/CD8 ratio in patients.

The increased CD4/CD8 ratio in IMN represents the altered immune response associated to the pathogenesis of the disease [10], [28]-[31]. We found that CD4/CD8 ratio was greater than two only in twenty four patients out of forty five. Nevertheless, in this subgroup, we observed the presence of two predominant polymorphisms of IL-10. IL-10 is one of the major Th2 cytokines, which acts on B lymphocytes stimulating the production of antibodies. In particular, this effect is further enhanced on B lymphocytes that are already IgG4 committed. In fact, in PBMCs stimulated with anti CD40 and IL-4, the addition of IL-10 increases IL-4 induced $\gamma$4 transcription and IgG4 production [11]-[13]. The most frequent allele of IL-10 in group of patients with CD4/CD8 ratio more than two was -1082G, which is associated to the increased production of IL-10 [20] [32], in fact in this subgroup of patients the levels of IL-10, in the urine, were higher compared to patients with CD4/CD8 ratio less than two.

Therefore, in the group of patients with increased CD4/CD8 ratio, IL-10 can be related to the pathogenesis of IMN and it might represent a new insight in the pathogenesis of this disease, as well as its role has been shown in other kidney diseases [33].

Moreover, IL-10 is a strong anti-inflammatory cytokine, which down regulates the production of TNF-$\alpha$ and the activity of APCs [34]-[36]. IL-10, as for TNF-$\alpha$, is not only produced by Th2 lymphocytes but also by mo-

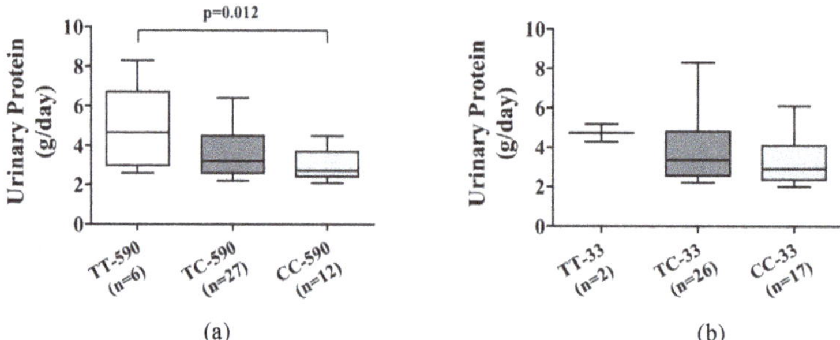


**Figure 1.** Boxplots of proteinuria levels by -590 and -33 IL-4 genotypes, in IMN patients.

nocytes and macrophages. It has been observed that inflammatory cells recruited to glomerulus and the visceral epithelial cells produce TNF-*α* in IMN [37]. In a similar way, IL-10 can also be produced in loco by the inflammatory cells recruited to the damaged glomerulus. Therefore, the presence of IL-10 in urine, but not in serum, can be partly explained as an effect of inflammatory response triggered by the presence of TNF-*α*. In agreement with this observation some authors described the presence of IL-10 in glomerular lesions, in patients affected with glomerulonephritis [38].

Likewise, IL-4 and IL-5 are both produced by Th2 lymphocytes. IL-4 is up regulated by peripheral T-helper cells in IMN [9], demonstrating its' systemic origin rather than produced in loco after glomerular damage. However in some cases, it has been demonstrated that there are increased mRNA levels of IL-4 and IL-5 in renal biopsies from MN patients, giving an evidence of local origin of these cytokines at the site of inflammation [39]. So, our results for the presence of IL-4 in serum are in agreement with Masutani *et al.* [9], while the presence of IL-5 in urine can be related to the immunological phenomena in glomerulus, as partly stated by Ifuku *et al.* [39] Nevertheless, these results confirm an injurious immune response due to T lymphocytes dysregulation in IMN pathogenesis.

The association between polymorphisms G-308A in TNF-*α* and IMN has already been described [25] [26]. Bantis C *et al.* [26] showed that the allele −308A was more frequent in patients affected by membranous glomerulonephritis. Likewise, the genotype distribution for genotypes GG, GA, and AA were also different. Similar results were shown by Tibaudin *et al.* [25] in IMN, where frequency of -308A allele was increased in patients. Nevertheless they did not suggest any significant and independent influence of different genotypes on diseases' progression. The increased levels of TNF-*α* in urine [40]-[42] and its expression in kidney cells [37] [40]-[42] of IMN affected patients, suggest a role of TNF-*α* in this syndrome. Hence, the presence of TNF-*α* together with IL-10 in urine emphasizes the significance of inflammatory processes and the role of TNF-*α* in the pathogenesis of IMN.

This role is more evident considering that the allele -308A of TNF-*α* is associated with a high expression of this cytokine [22]-[23]. TNF-*α* plays a role in the pathogenesis by contributing to the alterations of glomerular filtration barrier [43]. Besides, -308A allele of TNF-*α* is in linkage with HLA-B8/DR3 haplotype [44], which is also associated to the development of IMN [45]. Recent studies have further shown that TNF-*α* polymorphisms increase susceptibility to develop other forms of kidney disease [46].

The relevance of IL-4 (which is not in linkage disequilibrium with the MHC complex genes) and other Th2 cytokines is already described in the context of Minimal Change Nephrotic Syndrome, where the polymorphism T-590C of IL-4 [14] were more frequent in patients. Additionally, in some cases, the polymorphism T-590C of IL-4 is linked to the up regulation of this cytokine [19]. The potential role of this "high producer" genotype is also described in other Th2 mediated pathologies like atopic dermatitis, allergies and asthma. For example, our group described the association of T-590C polymorphism with asthma in the Italian population [27] and Kawashima *et al.* associated the same polymorphism with atopic dermatitis in the Japanese population [19].

Furthermore, we found an increase in two polymorphisms of IL-4 in our cohort of patients, namely T-590C and T-33C, moreover, we showed that T-590 allele is also associated with a proteinuria increment.

Moreover, we observed increased levels of IL-4 in serum of patients with IMN. This observation was in agreement with Masutani *et al.* [9] who described an increase of Th2 lymphocytes in peripheral blood of IMN patients. The key role of IL-4 might be the induction of isotype switching towards IgG4 [10], which is the main antibody subtype to accumulate in glomerular epithelium, causing the alterations and pathogenesis of this disease. The relevance of IL-4 has also been shown in other nephropathies. For example, Acharya B *et al.* described the association between minimal change nephrotic syndrome (MCNS) and C-590T polymorphism of IL-4 [14]. MCNS is the most common nephrotic syndrome in children and it is associated with proteinuria, hypogammaglobinemia, hypercholesterolemia and increased levels of IgE in serum. MCNS is also characterized by an aberrant immune response of T lymphocytes. Furthermore, factors derived from T cells are responsible for the alterations at glomerular barrier observed in this syndrome [47]-[50]. So, the same mechanisms can also be considered in the pathogenesis of IMN.

However, the association between the allele T-590 and the production of IL-4 remains questionable.

Li *et al.* have recently confirmed, through a study of meta-analysis, that the genotype -590TT is associated with an increase in the risk of developing allergic rhinitis. However, they have not shown a correlation between the serum level of IL-4 and allergic rhinitis [51]. While, Amirzargar *et al.* have shown that T-590 allele is associated with increased levels of IgE in vivo, as well as to the predisposition to asthma development [52]. The same correlation was observed in the cohort of asthmatic subjects by Smolnikova *et al.* In addition, here, the author shows that the T-590 allele of IL-4 is responsible for an increase in serum levels of IL-4 [53], confirming what we have observed in our group of patients.

## 5. Conclusion

In conclusion, our results suggest that polymorphisms in cytokine genes, mainly IL-4, IL-10 and TNF-$\alpha$ can be associated to IMN, suggesting that this pathology can be considered as a complex disease and that multiple mechanisms might be involved in its pathogenesis. Moreover, to our knowledge, this is the first study to associate IL-4 polymorphisms in Italian population to the Idiopathic Membranous Nephropathy.

## Acknowledgements

We are grateful to the unit of Nephrology of Ospedali Riuniti of Bergamo for their contribution to this work.

## References

[1] Nangaku, M., Shankland, S.J. and Couser, W.G. (2005) Cellular Response to Injury in Membranous Nephropathy. *Journal of the American Society of Nephrology*, **16**, 1-9. http://dx.doi.org/10.1681/ASN.2004121098

[2] Imai, H., Hamai, K., Komatsuda, A., Ohtani, H. and Miura, A.B. (1997) IgG Subclasses in Patients with Membranoproliferative Glomerulonephritis, Membranous Nephrophaty, and Lupus Nephritis. *Kidney International*, **51**, 270-276. http://dx.doi.org/10.1038/ki.1997.32

[3] Kuroki, A., Shibata, T., Honda, H., Totsuka, D., Kobayashi, K. and Sugisaki, T. (2002) Glomerular and Serum IgG Subclasses in Diffuse Proliferative Lupus Nephritis, Membranous Lupus Nephritis, and Idiophatic Membranous Nephrophaty. *Internal Medicine*, **41**, 936-942. http://dx.doi.org/10.2169/internalmedicine.41.936

[4] Ohtani, H., Wakui, H., Komatsuda, A., Okuyama, S., Masai, R., Maki, N., Kigawa, A., Sawada, K. and Imai, H. (2004) Distribution of Glomerular IgG Sublcass Deposits in Malignancy-Associated Membranous Nephropathy. *Nephrology Dialysis Transplantation*, **19**, 574-579. http://dx.doi.org/10.1093/ndt/gfg616

[5] Aalberse, R.C., Van der Gaag, R. and Van Leeuwen, J. (1983) Serologic Aspects of IgG4 Antibodies. I. Prolonged Immunization Results in an IgG4 Restricted Response. *The Journal of Immunology*, **130**, 722-726.

[6] Iskander, R., Das, P.K. and Aalberse, R.C. (1981) IgG4 Antibodies in Egyptian Patients with Schistosomiasis. *'International Archives of Allergy and Immunology*, **66**, 200-207. http://dx.doi.org/10.1159/000232819

[7] Doi, T., Kanatsu, K., Mayumi, M., Hamashima, Y. and Yoshida, H. (1991) Analysis of IgG Immune Complexes in Sera from Patients with Membranous Nephropathy: Role of IgG4 Subclass and Low-Avidity Antibodies. *Nephron*, **57**, 131-136. http://dx.doi.org/10.1159/000186239

[8] van de Zee, J.S., van Swieten, P. and Aalberse, R.C. (1986) Serologic Aspects of IgG4 Antibodies. II. IgG4 Antibodies Form Small, Nonprecipitating Immune Complexes Due to Functional Monovalency. *The Journal of Immunology*, **137**, 3566-3571.

[9] Masutani, K., Taniguchi, M., Nakashima, H., Yotsueda, H., Kudoh, Y., Tsuruya, K., Tokumoto, M., Fukuda, K., Kanai, H., Hirakata, H. and Iida, M. (2004) Up-Regulated Interleukin-4 Production by Peripheral T-Helper Cells in Idiopathic Membranous Nephrophaty. *Nephrology Dialysis Transplantation*, **19**, 580-586. http://dx.doi.org/10.1093/ndt/gfg572

[10] Kuroki, A., Iyoda, M., Shibata, T. and Sugisaki, T. (2005) Th2 Cytokines Increase and Stimulate B Cells to Produce IgG4 in Idiopathic Membranous Nephropathy. *Kidney International*, **68**, 302-310. http://dx.doi.org/10.1111/j.1523-1755.2005.00415.x

[11] Jeannin, P., Lecoanet, S., Delneste, Y., Gauchat, J.F. and Bonnefoy, J.Y. (1998) IgE versus IgG4 Production Can Be Differentially Regulated by IL-10. *Journal of Immunology*, **160**, 3555-3561.

[12] de Vries, J.E., Punnonen, J., Cocks, B.G. and Aversa, G. (1993) The Role of T/B Cell Interactions and Cytokines in the Regulation of Human IgE Synthesis. *Seminars in Immunology*, **5**, 431-439. http://dx.doi.org/10.1006/smim.1993.1049

[13] Lecart, S., Morel, F., Noraz, N., Pène, J., Garcia, M., Boniface, K., Lecron, J.C. and Yssel, H. (2002) IL-22, in Contrast to IL-10, Does Not Induce Ig Production, Due to Absence of a Functional IL-22 Receptor on Activated Human B Cells. *International Immunology*, **14**, 1351-1356. http://dx.doi.org/10.1093/intimm/dxf096

[14] Acharya, B., Shirakawa, T. and Gotoh, A. (2005) Polymorphism of the Interleukin-4, Interleukin-13, and Signal Trasducer and Activator of Transcription 6 Genes in Indonesian Children with Minimal Change Nephrotic Syndrome. *American Journal of Nephrology*, **25**, 30-35. http://dx.doi.org/10.1159/000083729

[15] Ikeuchi, Y., Kobayashi, Y., Arakawa, H., Suzuki, M., Tamra, K. and Morikawa, A. (2009) Polymorphisms in Interleu-

kin-4-Related Genes in Patients with Minimal Change Nephrotic Syndrome. *Pediatric Nephrology*, **24**, 489-495. http://dx.doi.org/10.1007/s00467-008-1003-y

[16] Cohen, C.D., Calvaresi, N. and Kretzler, M. (2005) CD20-Positive Infiltrates in Human Membranous Glomerulonephritis. *Journal of Nephrology*, **18**, 328-333.

[17] Ruggenenti, P., Chiurchiu, C., Abbate, M., Perna, A., Cravedi, P., Bontempelli, M. and Remuzzi, G. (2006) Rituximab for Idiopathic Membranous Nephropathy: Who Can Benefit? *Clinical Journal of the American Society of Nephrology*, **1**, 738-748. http://dx.doi.org/10.2215/CJN.01080905

[18] Remuzzi, G., Chiurchiu, C., Abbate, M., Brusegan, V., Bontempelli, M. and Ruggenenti, P. (2002) Rituximab for Idiopathic Membranous Nephropathy. *The Lancet*, **360**, 923-924. http://dx.doi.org/10.1016/S0140-6736(02)11042-7

[19] Kawashima, T., Noguchi, E., Arinami, T., Yamakawa-Kobayashi, K., Nakagawa, H., Otsuka, F. and Hamaguchi, H. (1998) Linkage and Association of an Interleukin-4 Gene Polymorphism with Atopic Dermatitis in Japanese Families. *Journal of Medical Genetics*, **35**, 502-504. http://dx.doi.org/10.1136/jmg.35.6.502

[20] Turner, D.M., Williams, D.M., Sankaran, D., Lazarus, M., Sinnott, P.J. and Hutchinson, I.V. (1997) An Investigation of Polymorphism in the Interleukin-10 Gene Promoter. *European Journal of Immunogenetics*, **24**, 1-8. http://dx.doi.org/10.1111/j.1365-2370.1997.tb00001.x

[21] Kim, J.M., Brannan, C.I., Copeland, N.G., Jenkins, N.A., Khan, T.A. and Moore, K.W. (1992) Structure of the Mouse IL-10 Gene and Chromosomal Localization of the Mouse and Human Genes. *Journal of Immunology*, **148**, 3618-3623.

[22] Louis, E., Franchimont, D., Piron, A., Gevaert, Y., Schaaf-Lafontaine, N., Roland, S., Mahieu, P., Malaise, M., De Groote, D., Louis, R. and Belaiche, J. (1998) Tumour Necrosis Factor (TNF) Gene Polymorphism Influences TNF-α Production in Lipopolysaccharide (LPS)-Stimulated Whole Blood Cell Culture in Healthy Humans. *Clinical and Experimental Immunology*, **113**, 401-406. http://dx.doi.org/10.1046/j.1365-2249.1998.00662.x

[23] Wilson, A.G., Symons, J.A., McDowell, T.L., McDevitt, H.O. and Duff, G.W. (1997) Effects of a Polymorphisms in the Human Tumour Necrosis Factor α Promoter on Transcriptional Activation. *Proceedings of the National Academy of Sciences of the United States of America*, **94**, 3195-3199. http://dx.doi.org/10.1073/pnas.94.7.3195

[24] Chen, S.Y., Chen, C.H., Huang, Y.C., Chuang, H.M., Lo, M.M. and Tsai, F.J. (2010) Effect of IL-6 C-572G Polymorphism on Idiopathic Membranous Nephropathy Risk in a Han Chinese Population. *Renal Failure*, **32**, 1172-1176. http://dx.doi.org/10.3109/0886022X.2010.516857

[25] Thibaudin, D., Thibaudin, L., Berthoux, P., Mariat, C., Filippis, J.P., Laurent, B., Alamartine, E. and Berthoux, F. (2007) TNFA2 and D2 Alleles of the Tumor Necrosis Factor Alpha Gene Polymorphism Are Associated with Onset/Occurrence of Idiopathic Membranous Nephropathy. *Kidney International*, **71**, 431-437. http://dx.doi.org/10.1038/sj.ki.5002054

[26] Bantis, C., Heering, P.J., Aker, S., Siekierka, M., Kuhr, N., Grabensee, B. and Ivens, K. (2006) Tumor Necrosis Factor-α Gene G-308A Polymorphism Is a Risk Factor for the Development of Membranous Glomerulonephritis. *American Journal of Nephrology*, **26**, 12-15. http://dx.doi.org/10.1159/000090706

[27] Ricciardolo, F.L., Sorbello, V., Silvestri, M., Giacomelli, M., Debenedetti, V.M., Malerba, M., Ciprandi, G., Rossi, G.A., Rossi, A. and Bontempelli, M. (2013) TNF-α, IL-4R-α and IL-4 Polymorphisms in Mild to Severe Asthma from Italian Caucasians. *International Journal of Immunopathology and Pharmacology*, **26**, 75-84.

[28] Ozaki, T., Tomino, Y., Nakayama, S. and Koide, H. (1992) Two-Color Analysis of Lymphocyte Subpopulations in Patients with Nephrotic Syndrome Due to Membranous Nephropathy. *Clinical Nephrology*, **38**, 75-80.

[29] Zucchelli, P., Ponticelli, C., Cagnoli, L., Aroldi, A. and Beltrandi, E. (1988) Prognostic Value of T Lymphocyte Subset Ratio in Idiopathic Membranous Nephropathy. *American Journal of Nephrology*, **8**, 15-20. http://dx.doi.org/10.1159/000167547

[30] Cagnoli, L., Tabacchi, P., Pasquali, S., Cenci, M., Sasdelli, M. and Zucchelli, P. (1982) T Cell Subset Alterations in Idiopathic Glomerulonephritis. *Clinical & Experimental Immunology*, **50**, 70-76.

[31] Bannister, K.M., Drew, P.A., Clarkson, A.R. and Woodroffe, A.J. (1983) Immunoregulation in Glomerulonephritis, Henoch—Schonlein Purpura and Lupus Nephritis. *Clinical & Experimental Immunology*, **53**, 384-390.

[32] Castro-Santos, P., Suarez, A., López-Rivas, L., Mozo, L. and Gutierrez, C. (2006) TNFα and IL-10 Gene Poly-morphisms in Inflammatory Bowel Disease. Association of −1082 AA Low Producer IL-10 Genotype with Steroid Dependency TNFα and IL-10 Gene Polymorphisms in IBD. *American Journal of Gastroenterology*, **101**, 1039-1047. http://dx.doi.org/10.1111/j.1572-0241.2006.00501.x

[33] Rianthavorn, P., Chokedeemeeboon, C., Deekajorndech, T. and Suphapeetiporn, K. (2013) Interleukin-10 Promoter Polymorphisms and Expression in Thai Children with Juvenile Systemic Lupus Erythematosus. *Lupus*, **22**, 721-726. http://dx.doi.org/10.1177/0961203313486192

[34] Fiorentino, D.F., Zlotnik, A., Mosmann, T.R., Howard, M. and O'Garra, A. (1991) IL-10 Inhibits Cytokine Production by Activated Macrophages. *Journal of Immunology*, **147**, 3815-3822.

[35] de Waal Malefyt, R., Abrams, J., Bennett, B., Figdor, C.G. and de Vries, J.E. (1991) Interleukin 10 (IL-10) Inhibits Cytokine Synthesis by Human Monocytes: An Autoregulatory Role of IL-10 Produced by Monocytes. *Journal of Experimental Medicine*, **174**, 1209-1220. http://dx.doi.org/10.1084/jem.174.5.1209

[36] de Waal Malefyt, R., Haanen, J., Spits, H., Roncarolo, M.G., te Velde, A., Figdor, C., Johnson, K., Kastelein, R., Yssel, H. and de Vries, J.E. (1991) Interleukin 10 (IL-10) and Viral IL-10 Strongly Reduce Antigen-Specific Human T Cell Proliferation by Diminishing the Antigen-Presenting Capacity of Monocytes via Downregulation of Class II Major Histocompatibility Complex Expression. *Journal of Experimental Medicine*, **174**, 915-924. http://dx.doi.org/10.1084/jem.174.4.915

[37] Neale, T.J., Rüger, B.M., Macaulay, H., Dunbar, P.R., Hasan, Q., Bourke, A., Murray-McIntosh, R.P. and Kitching, A.R. (1995) Tumor Necrosis Factor-*α* Is Expressed by Glomerular Visceral Epithelial Cells in Human Membranous Nephropathy. *American Journal of Pathology*, **146**, 1444-1454.

[38] Niemir, Z.I., Ondracek, M., Dworacki, G., Stein, H., Waldherr, R., Ritz, E. and Otto, H.F. (1998) *In Situ* Upregulation of IL-10 Reflects the Activity of Human Glomerulonephritides. *American Journal of Kidney Diseases*, **32**, 80-92. http://dx.doi.org/10.1053/ajkd.1998.v32.pm9669428

[39] Ifuku, M., Miyake, K., Watanebe, M., Ito, K., Abe, Y., Sasatomi, Y., Ogahara, S., Hisano, S., Sato, H., Saito, T. and Nakashima, H. (2013) Various Roles of Th Cytokine mRNA Expression in Different Forms of Glomerulonephritis. *American Journal of Nephrology*, **38**, 115-123. http://dx.doi.org/10.1159/000353102

[40] Honkanen, E., von Willebrand, E., Teppo, A.M., Törnroth, T. and Grönhagen-Riska, C. (1998) Adhesion Molecules and Urinary Tumor Necrosis Factor-*α* in Idiopathic Membranous Glomerulonephritis. *Kidney International*, **53**, 909-917. http://dx.doi.org/10.1111/j.1523-1755.1998.00833.x

[41] Kshirsagar, A.V., Nachman, P.H. and Falk, R.J. (2003) Alternative Therapies and Future Intervention for Treatment of Membranous Nephropathy. *Seminars in Nephrology*, **23**, 362-372. http://dx.doi.org/10.1016/S0270-9295(03)00047-0

[42] Wu, T.H., Tsai, C.Y. and Yang, W.C. (1998) Excessive Expression of the Tumor Necrosis Factor-*α* Gene in the Kidneys of Patients with Membranous Glomerulonephritis. *Chinese Medical Journal* (*Taipei*), **61**, 524-530.

[43] Tabibzadeh, S., Kong, Q.F., Kapur, S., Leffers, H., Ridley, A., Aktories, K. and Celis, J.E. (1995) TNF-*α* Induces Dyscohesion of Epithelial Cells. Association with Disassembly of Actin Filaments. *Endocrine*, **3**, 549-556. http://dx.doi.org/10.1007/BF02953018

[44] Wilson, A.G., de Vries, N., Pociot, F., di Giovine, F.S., van der Putte, L.B. and Duff, G.W. (1993) An Allelic Polymorphism within the Human Tumor Necrosis Factor Alpha Promoter Region Is Strongly Associated with HLA A1, B8, and DR3 Alleles. *Journal of Experimental Medicine*, **177**, 557-560. http://dx.doi.org/10.1084/jem.177.2.557

[45] Reichert, L.J., Koene, R.A. and Wetzels, J.F. (1998) Prognostic Factors in Idiopathic Membranous Nephropathy. *American Journal of Kidney Diseases*, **31**, 1-11. http://dx.doi.org/10.1053/ajkd.1998.v31.pm9428445

[46] Farid, T.M., Abd El Baky, A.M., Khalefa, E.S., Talaat, A.A., Mohamed, A.A., Gheita, T.A. and Abdel-Salam, R.F. (2011) Association of Tumor Necrosis Factor-*α* Gene Polymorphisms with Juvenile Systemic Lupus Erythematosus Nephritis in a Cohort of Egyptian Patients. *Iranian Journal of Kidney Diseases*, **5**, 392-397.

[47] Tomizawa, S., Maruyama, K., Nagasawa, N., Suzuki, S. and Kuroume, T. (1985) Studies on Vascular Permeability Factor Derived from T Lymphocytes and Inhibitory Effect of Plasma on Its Production in Minimal Change Nephrotic Syndrome. *Nephron*, **41**, 157-160. http://dx.doi.org/10.1159/000183572

[48] Cho, B.S., Yoon, S.R., Jang, J.Y., Pyun, K.H. and Lee, C.E. (1999) Up-Regulation of Interleukin-4 and CD23/ FcepsilonRII in Minimal Change Nephrotic Syndrome. *Pediatric Nephrology*, **13**, 199-204. http://dx.doi.org/10.1007/s004670050592

[49] Neuhaus, T.J., Shah, V., Callard, R.E. and Barratt, T.M. (1995) T-Lymphocyte Activation in Steroid-Sensitive Nephrotic Syndrome in Childhood. *Nephrology Dialysis Transplantation*, **10**, 1348-1352.

[50] Neuhaus, T.J., Wadhwa, M., Callard, R. and Barratt, T.M. (1995) Increased IL-2, IL-4 and Interferon-Gamma (IFN-Gamma) in Steroid-Sensitive Nephrotic Syndrome. *Clinical & Experimental Immunology*, **100**, 475-479. http://dx.doi.org/10.1111/j.1365-2249.1995.tb03725.x

[51] Li, Z.P., Yin, L.L., Wang, H. and Liu, L.S. (2014) Association between Promoter Polymorphisms of Interleukin-4 Gene and Allergic Rhinitis Risk: A Meta-Analysis. *Journal of Huazhong University of Science and Technology* (*Medical Sciences*), **34**, 306-313. http://dx.doi.org/10.1007/s11596-014-1275-3

[52] Amirzargar, A.A., Movahedi, M., Rezaei, N., Moradi, B., Dorkhosh, S., Mahloji, M. and Mahdaviani, S.A. (2009) Polymorphisms in IL4 and iLARA Confer Susceptibility to Asthma. *Journal of Investigational Allergology and Clinical Immunology*, **19**, 433-438.

[53] Smolnikova, M.V., Smirnova, S.V., Freidin, M.B. and Tyutina, O.S. (2013) Immunological Parameters and Gene Polymorphisms (*C*-590*T IL4*, *C*-597*A IL*10) in Severe Bronchial Asthma in Children from the Krasnoyarsk Region, West Siberia. *International Journal of Circumpolar Health*, **72**. http://dx.doi.org/10.3402/ijch.v72i0.21159

21

# Pregnancy Specific Beta-1 Glycoprotein in Women with Eclampsia, Kaduna State, Nigeria

**Jim M. Banda[1*], Geoffrey C. Onyemelukwe[2], Bolanle O. P. Musa[2], Oladapo S. Shittu[3], Zulai A. Sarkin-Pawa[3], Aliyu A. Babadoko[4], Aisha I. Mamman[4], Adamu G. Bakari[5], Suraj Junaid[6]**

[1]Pathology Department, Faculty of Medicine, Kaduna State University, Kaduna, Nigeria
[2]Immunology Unit, Department of Medicine, Ahmadu Bello University Teaching Hospital, Zaria, Nigeria
[3]Department of Obstetrics and Gynaecology, Ahmadu Bello University Teaching Hospital, Zaria, Nigeria
[4]Department of Haematology and Blood Transfusion, Ahmadu Bello University Teaching Hospital, Zaria, Nigeria
[5]Department of Medicine, Ahmadu Bello University Teaching Hospital, Zaria, Nigeria
[6]Federal College of Veternary and Medical Laboratory, National Veterinary and Research Institute, Vom, Nigeria
Email: [*]jimbanda31@yahoo.com

## Abstract

**This was a comparative cross-sectional study of eclamptic and normal healthy pregnant women conducted in kaduna State, Nigeria to determine Pregnancy Specific beta-1 Glycoprotein (PSG-1) levels in the peripheral blood of third trimester women with eclampsia (EC; n = 38), normal healthy pregnant and non pregnant women controls (PC; n = 25 and NPC; n = 25 respectively), age and parity matched, attending labour rooms/wards and Antenatal Clinics (ANC) of Ahmadu Bello University Teaching Hospital Shika, Zaria and four other Hospitals in Kaduna state, Nigeria. Participants with smear positive malaria, seropositive for human immunodeficiency virus (HIV) or any other known clinical infection were excluded from this study. Pregnancy specific beta-1 glycoprotein levels were estimated using Quantikine ELISA kits. Data obtained were analyzed using SPSS version 20.0 (Chicago, USA) and Graph pad Prism 6.0. Results were expressed as mean ± standard deviation while Kruskal Wallis test was used to determine the significant differences. A p-value of less than 0.05 was considered to be significant. The mean serum level of PSG-1 in EC was 2.53 ± 0.11 pg/ml, PC; 2.56 ± 0.03 pg/ml) and NPC; 0.62 ± 0.20 pg/ml. There was no significant difference between EC and PC ($P > 0.05$). Pregnant women (with and without EC) had significantly higher mean serum values compared to NPC $p < 0.05$. While pregnancy was associated with high levels of PSG-1, the study did not support the hypothesis of low PSG-1 level in EC. A longitudinal study to capture changes in PSG-I levels in the course of pregnancy as they manifest is recommended.**

[*]Corresponding author.

## Keywords

**Eclampsia, Pregnancy Specific Beta-1 Glycoprotein**

## 1. Introduction

Eclampsia has remained a significant public health threat in both developed and developing countries, contributing to maternal and perinatal morbidity and mortality globally [1] [2]. However, the impact of the disease is felt more severely in developing countries including Nigeria [3]-[5]. Report show that in Nigeria, 37,000 women die annually due to PE and EC related complications and it accounts for up to 40% of maternal death in Northern Nigeria [6].

Eclampsia, the occurrence of generalized convulsion (s) in association with signs of preeclampsia (hypertension and proteinuria) in pregnancy and not caused by epilepsy or other convulsive disorders in pregnancy. While pre-eclamppsia (PE) and EC are not distinct disorders but the manifestation of the clinical features of the same condition [7], some features suggest that EC may have an immune pathology [8]. Also susceptibility to EC varies from one woman to another, indicating genetic and immune factors [9].

Pregnancy-specific glycoproteins (PSGs) are expressed throughout human pregnancy and are the most abundant fetal proteins secreted by the placental syncytiotrophoblast into the maternal bloodstream in mid to late pregnancy (~200 - 400 μg/ml) [10]. Pregnancy specific glycoproteins are produced by ten *PSG* genes (*PSG*1-P*SG*9, *PSG*11) and belong to the carcinoembryonic antigen (CEA) family, part of the immunoglobulin (Ig) super family [11].

Studies of PSG function have largely focussed on their role in modulating the maternal immune system. Pregnancy specific glycoproteins isolated from the human placenta have an inhibitory effect on phytohaemagglutinin or allogeneically stimulated lymphocytes [12]. Subsequently, it was shown that recombinant mouse and human PSGs induce production of anti-inflammatory cytokines such as interleukin-10 (IL-10) and transforming growth factor beta-1 (TGF$\beta$1) by monocytic, macrophage and dendritic lineages in vitro and in vivo [13] [14]. In the human, elevated PSG levels are associated with improved symptoms of rheumatoid arthritis during pregnancy [15]. These findings are consistent with PSGs contributing to modulation of maternal immune responses during pregnancy. More recently, PSGs were shown to be pro-angiogenic in *in vitro* assays, an activity mediated by interactions with cell surface glycosaminoglycans and the induction of TGF$\beta$1 and vascular endothelial growth factor A (VEGF-A) [16]. Pregnancy specific glycoproteins are expressed from the preimplantation blastocyst stage of development [17] and therefore may have a role in promoting angiogenesis in the placental bed in the early pregnancy, or perhaps in vascular endothelial protection and repair in the maternal circulation in later pregnancy. Consistent with the proposed immunoregulatory and angiogenic functions of PSGs, deregulation of PSG expression has been reported in disorders of pregnancy associated with pro-inflammatory and anti-angiogenic phenotypes. For example, low levels of PSGs have been reported in maternal circulation of first and second trimester pregnancies complicated by intrauterine growth retardation and preeclampsia [18], [19]. What are the alterations or changes that may occur in PSG-1 levels women with established EC? This question therefore, forms the basis of this study. The objective of this study was to measure PSG-1 levels in the peripheral blood of women with EC and to compare the data obtained with values in normal pregnant women and normal healthy non-pregnant controls with the hope of understanding the role of PSG-1 in the pathogenesis of EC.

## 2. Materials and Methods

### 2.1. Study Area

This was a comparative cross sectional study, conducted in Gynaecology and Obstetrics Departments of Ahmadu Bello University Teaching Hospital (ABUTH) Shika, Zaria, Hajiya Gambo Sawaba General Hospital (HGSGH), Zaria, Barau Dikko Specialist Hospital (BDSH) Kaduna, Yusufu Dantsoho Memorial Hospital (YDMH) Kaduna and General Hospital (GH) Kafanchan. Patients and controls were enrolled as they present. Ethical clearance was obtained from the Scientific and Health Research Ethics Committee of the Ahmadu Bello University teaching hospital Shika-Zaria and the Kaduna State Ministry of Health (KSMOH) before commencing the study. Patients retained the right to deny consent for or opt out of the study at any stage. Patient confidentiality was maintained throughout the study.

For the women with EC: third trimester women with identifying features of high blood pressure (≥140/90), proteinuria (2+ dip stick testing of random urine) and tonic-clinic convulsion, who were previously normotensive and nonproteinuric after 20 weeks of gestation [20]. For the controls: third trimester healthy pregnant women (normotensive and nonproteinuric) age and parity matched with EC above and non-pregnant healthy (normotensive and nonproteinuric) age matched with EC and PC [21]. Participants that refused consent or opt out, tested sero-positive for human immunodeficiency virus (HIV), blood smear positive for malaria test, or any known clinical disorder were excluded from the study.

### 2.2. Clinical Evaluation and Selection of Participants

All the participants were briefed about the nature of the study and written informed consent was taken from all the recruits. Blood pressure was measured using a simple mercury sphygmomanometer on right hand arm in a supine position after 10 min. rest by the collaborating clinician at the antenatal clinic (ANC)s of the Obstetrics and Gynaecology Department of the respective hospitals. To perform dipstick urine analysis, combi-2 Medi-test strips were used. Clients who fulfilled the entry criteria were enrolled for the study. Participant's personal data such as age and parity, etc. were sourced from each participant in addition to the data resulting from the clinical and laboratory examination and entered into the study.

### 2.3. Blood Sample Collection.

A total of 5mls of blood were drawn from each research participants, after confirmation of diagnosis and before the administration of any drugs into plain tubes. Serum were extracted and stored in pre-labelled serum vials containing drops of trasylol (aprotonin)-Sigma USA and stored at −20˚C to inhibit degradation of PSGs.

### 2.4. PSG-1 Assay

Pregnancy specific beta-1 glycoprotein was assayed on batched serum samples by quantikine ELISA kits following the outlined protocol by pathare *et al.* [22]. Frozen (−20˚C) serum samples were thawed once and brought to room temperature at the time of assay. Serum samples (EC; n = 38, PC; n = 25, NPC; n = 25) were dispensed along side with dilutions of standards (recombinant PSG-1) into wells of the micro titre ELISA plates pre-coated with monoclonal antibodies against the human PSG-1 to be assayed and incubated at room temperature for 2 hours. The plates were washed four times with buffer (phosphate buffer saline-0.05% and Tween 20). Conjugates (polyclonal antibody against PSG-1 to horseradish peroxidase-HRP) were added and incubated for 2 hours at room temperature. Unbound enzymes were washed out while the bound enzymes were then detected by incubation in the dark with substrate solutions (stabilized hydrogen peroxides and tetramethylbenzidine-TMB). The plates were scanned using a microplate reader (Bio-Rad, USA) set at 450 nm with wave length correction set at 570nm. A standard curve was then generated from the known standards. Concentrations of PSG-1 in the specimen were determined by comparing sample optical density with the values on the standard curve.

### 2.5. Statistical Analysis

The data obtained were analysed using the SPSS version 20.0 (Chicago, USA) and Graph Pad Prism 6.0. Results were expressed as mean ± standard deviation. Kruskal Wallis was used to determine significant differences. Comparisons were made between EC, PC and NPC. Test was carried out at 0.05 level of significant and $p < 0.05$ was considered significant.

## 3. Results

### 3.1. The Demographic and Clinical Characteristics of Women with EC, PC and NPC

The mean age and standard deviation of the groups were similar: EC (25.0 ± 5.9 years), PC (24.9 ± 5.7 years) and NPC (25.1 ± 5.9 years). The mean gestational age and parity for patients and controls were also similar: EC (37.2 ± 2.2 weeks and 1.4 ± 2.4) and PC; (37.1 ± 2.0weeks and 1.5 ± 2.5) respectively. Similarly, the mean BMI and standard deviation recorded was: EC (26.4 ± 4.3 $Kg/m^{2)}$, PC (25.8 ± 3.7 $Kg/m^{2)}$ and NPC (25.2 ± 4.3 $Kg/m^{2)}$. There was no statistical difference between EC, PC and NPC ($P > 0.5$) (**Table 1**). However, the mean values of blood pressures (systolic; diastolic) and standard deviation were noted to be higher in EC (171.6 ± 25.2 mmHg; 110.0 ± 10.7 mmHg) compared with PC, (111.6 ± 7.1 mmHg; 79.5 ± 11.3 mmHg) and NPC, (109.6 ± 6.6 mmHg; 84.2 ± 6.4 mmHg). There were significant differences between EC, PC and NPC ($p < 0.05$) (**Table 1**). Most of the eclamptic women (55.3%) were not booked in the facility at the time of study. While 100% of the pregnant women control had been booked who served as controls (**Table 1**). Urinary proteins (albumin), ≥2+ were recorded in all eclamptic women and non in PC and NPC. Similarly, tonic-clonic convulsions that occurred antepartum (16; 42.1%) and intrapatum (22; 57.9%) were recorded in the eclamptic women and non in the pregnant and non pregnant controls (**Table 1**).

**Table 1.** The demographic and clinical characteristics of women with EC, PC and NPC (Mean and ± SD).

| Characteristics | EC (n = 38) | PC (n = 38) | NPC (n = 38) |
|---|---|---|---|
| Age (years) | 25.0 ± 5.9 | 24.9 ± 5.7 | 25.1 ± 5.9 |
| Gestational age (wks) | 37.2 ± 2.2 | 37.1 ± 2.0 | - |
| BMI (Kg/m$^2$) | 26.4 ± 4.3 | 25.8 ± 3.7 | 25.2 ± 4.3 |
| Systolic BP (mmHg) | 171.6 ± 25.2* | 111.6 ± 7.1 | 109.6 ± 6.6 |
| Diastolic BP (mmHg) | 110.0 ± 10.7* | 79.5 ± 11.3 | 84.2 ± 6.4 |
| Proteinuria | ≥2+ | Not detected | Not detected |
| Antenatal booking | 55.3% | 100.0% | - |
| Antepartum convulsion | 16 (42.1%) | - | - |
| Intrapartum convulsion | 22 (57.9%) | - | - |

EC = Eclampsia, PC = Healthy Pregnant Control, NPC = Healthy Non Pregnant Control, BMI=Body Mass Index, BP= Blood Pressure *Eclampsia is significantly different from both controls at $p < 0.05$.

## 3.2. Pregnancy Specific Beta-1 Glycoprotein Levels in Eclampsia, Pregnant and Non-Pregnant Controls

In **Table 2**, the mean serum (log value) of PSG-1 in EC was 2.53 ± 0.11 pg/ml, while for the PC and NPC; it was 2.56 ± 0.03 pg/ml and 0.62 ± 0.20 pg/ml respectively.

While there was no significant difference between EC and PC ($P > 0.05$), women with EC had significantly higher mean serum values compared to NPC $p < 0.05$.

**Table 2.** Pregnancy specific beta-1 glycoprotein levels in eclampsia pregnant and non-pregnant controls.

| Parameter | EC (n = 38) (mean ± SD) | PC (n = 25) (mean ± SD) | NPC (n = 25) (mean ± SD) | P-value |
|---|---|---|---|---|
| Log PSG-1 (pg/mL) | 2.53 ± 0.11 | 2.56 ± 0.03 | 0.62 ± 0.20 | |
| Kruskal-Wallis | 56.46 | 57.82 | 13.00 | <0.001* |

PSG-I = Pregnancy Specific beta-1 glycoprotein, EC = Eclampsia, PC= Healthy Pregnant Control, NPC = Healthy Non-Pregnant Control. *PSG-1 in EC and PC are significantly different from NPC $P < 0.05$.

# 4. Discussion.

## Pregnancy Specific Beta-1 Glycoprotein (PSG-1)

The result of this study showed that women with EC and normal healthy pregnant women had higher mean serum levels of PSG-1($P < 0.05$) compared to concentration recorded in healthy non pregnant controls. Although, there was a decrease in the mean serum PSG-1 levels among the eclamptic women compared to the normal healthy pregnant group, the difference was not significant ($P > 0.05$).

This result agrees with findings of Onyemelukwe *et al.* [23] who studied 71 normal healthy pregnant women in northern Nigeria. They documented a low rise in PSG-1 up to 24 weeks, then a steep rise up to 36 wks followed by a gradual fall near term. The result of this study whoever, did not support the findings of Silver *et al.* [24] who reported significant low PSG levels in PE, the precursor of EC.

Pregnancy specific beta-1 glycoprotein, the major placental glycoproteins are a group of highly similar proteins synthesized in large amounts by the placenta trophoblast that together with the carcinoembryonic antigens comprise a subfamily within the immunoglobulin (Ig) super family [25]. During normal pregnancy, PSG molecules are released into the maternal circulation reaching 200 - 400 μg/ml in the serum at the end of gestation [26] and are thought to play a crucial role in supporting gestation and foetus protection against the maternal immune system [27]. Sacks *et al.* [28] proposed that pregnancy-specific factors induce the suppression of a specific arm of the maternal response and assumes the central role in maternal immunological adaptation. PSG modulates the immune response by inducing the secretion of anti-inflammatory cytokines such as IL-10, IL-6 and TGF-$\beta$ by human and murine cells ([29] [30]). PSG also suppress mixed lymphocyte reaction and T cell activation by mitogens [12].

In this study, the slight decreased mean PSG-1 value in the eclamptic women compared to normal healthy pregnant women control might in part be associated with the pathogenesis of EC. Lower levels of PSG-1 have been associated with certain human, pathological conditions such as autoimmune disease, spontaneous abortion, fetal retardation, low birth weight and hypoxia [27] [31]-[33].

Sacks *et al.* [28] have proposed that soluble placental products released directly into maternal circulation can generate specific pregnancy signals through interaction with innate immune system. Thus the innate immunity might be able to distinguish pregnant from non-pregnant states, producing unique signals that promote or prevent the lymphocytes response to alloantigen stimulation. While pregnancy is generally associated with high levels of PSG-1, the study did not support the hypothesis of low PSG-1 level in EC. There is a need for a longitudinal study to capture changes in PSG-1 levels as they occur for better understanding of pathophysiology of eclampsia as it surfaces.

## References


[1] Ghulmiyyah, L. and Sibai, B. (2012) Maternal Mortality from Preeclampsia and Eclampsia. *Seminars in Perinatology*, **36**, 56-59. http://dx.doi.org/10.1053/j.semperi.2011.09.011

[2] WHO (2011) Recommendations for Prevention and Treatment of Preeclampsia and Eclampsia. WHO Department of Maternal and Child Health, Geneva.

[3] Acquaah-Arhin, R. and Kwakwukume, E.Y. (2003) Trends in Eclampsia in Ghana at Korle-Bu Teaching Hospital, Accra, Ghana. *Nigerian Journal of Clinical Practice*, **6**, 1-4

[4] Adamu, Y.M., Salihu, H.M., Sathiakumar, N. and Alexander, G.R. (2003) Maternal Mortality in Northern Nigeria: A Population-Based Study. *European Journal of Obstetrics Gynecology and Reproductive Biology*, **109**, 153-159. http://dx.doi.org/10.1016/S0301-2115(03)00009-5

[5] Igberase, G. and Ebeigbe, P. (2006) Eclampsia: Ten-Years of Experience in a Rural Tertiary Hospital in the Niger Delta, Nigeria. *Journal of Obstetrics and Gynaecology*, **26**, 414-417. http://dx.doi.org/10.1080/01443610600720113

[6] WHO (2004) Coverage of Maternity Care: A Listing of Available Information. World Health Organization, Geneva.

[7] Shah, A.K. (2009) Preeclampsia/Eclampsia. http://emedicine.medscape.com/article/118427%200-overview

[8] Saito, S., Nakashima, A., Sakai M. and Sakai, Y. (2007) The Role of Immune System in Preeclampsia. *Molecular Aspect of Medicine*, **28**, 192-209. http://dx.doi.org/10.1016/j.mam.2007.02.006

[9] Duley, L. (2009) The Global Impact of Preeclampsia and Eclampisa. *Seminars in Perinatology*, **33**, 130-137. http://dx.doi.org/10.1053/j.semperi.2009.02.010

[10] Zhou, G.Q., Baranov, V., Zimmermann, W., Grunert, F., Erhard, B., *et al.* (1997) Highly Specific Monoclonal Antibody Demonstrates That Pregnancy-Specific Glycoprotein (PSG) Is Limited to Syncytiotrophoblast in Human Early and Term Placenta. *Placenta*, **18**, 491-501. http://dx.doi.org/10.1016/0143-4004(77)90002-9

[11] Kammerer, R. and Zimmermann, W. (2010) Coevolution of Activating and Inhibitory Receptors within Mammalian Carcinoembryonic Antigen Families. *BMC Biology*, **8**, 12. http://dx.doi.org/10.1186/1741-7007-8-12

[12] Harris, S.J., Anthony, F.W., Jones, D.B. and Masson, G.M. (1984) Pregnancy-Specific Beta 1-Glycoprotein: Effect on Lymphocyte Proliferation *in Vitro*. *Journal of Reproductive Immunology*, **6**, 267-270. http://dx.doi.org/10.1016/0165-0378(84)90015-9

[13] Ha, C.T., Waterhouse, R., Warren, J., Zimmermann, W. and Dveksler, G.S. (2005) N-Glycosylation Is Required for Binding of Murine Pregnancy-Specific Glycoproteins 17 and 19 to the Receptor CD9. *American Journal of Reproductive Immunology*, **59**, 251-258. http://dx.doi.org/10.1111/j.1600-0897.2007.00573.x

[14] Martínez, F.F., Knubel, C.P., Sánchez, M.C., Cervi, L. and Motrán, C.C. (2012) Pregnancy-Specific Glycoprotein 1a Activates Dendritic Cells to Provide Signals for Th17-, Th2-, and Treg-Cell Polarization. *European Journal of Immunology*, **42**, 1573-1584. http://dx.doi.org/10.1002/eji.201142140

[15] Fialova, L., Kohoutova, B., Pelísková, Z., Malbohan, I. and Mikulíková, L. (1991) Serum Levels of Trophoblast-Specific

Beta-1-Globulin (SP1) and Alpha-1-Fetoprotein (AFP) in Pregnant Women with Rheumatoid Arthritis. *Ceská Gynekologie*, **56**, 166-170.

[16] Ha, C.T., Wu, J.A., Irmak, S., Lisboa, F.A. and Dizon, A.M.L. (2010) Human Pregnancy Specific Beta-1-Glycoprotein 1 (PSG1) Has a Potential Role in Placental Vascular Morphogenesis. *Biology of Reproduction*, **83**, 27-35. http://dx.doi.org/10.1095/biolreprod.109.082412

[17] Jurisicova, A., Antenos, M., Kapasi, K., Meriano, J. and Casper, R.F. (1999) Variability in the Expression of Trophectodermal Markers Beta-Human Chorionic Gonadotrophin, Human Leukocyte Antigen-G and Pregnancy Specific Beta-1 Glycoprotein by the Human Blastocyst. *Human Reproduction*, **14**, 1852-1858. http://dx.doi.org/10.1093/humrep/14.7.1852

[18] Bersinger, N.A. and Odegard, R.A. (2004) Second and Third-Trimester Serum Levels of Placental Proteins in Preeclampsia and Small-for-Gestational Age Pregnancies. *Acta Obstetrics and Gynecology of Scandavania*, **83**, 37-45. http://dx.doi.org/10.1111/j.1600-0412.2004.00277.x

[19] Pihl, K., Larsen, T., Laursen, I., Krebs, L. and Christiansen, M. (2009) First Trimester Maternal Serum Pregnancy-Specific Beta-1-Glycoprotein (SP1) as a Marker of Adverse Pregnancy Outcome. *Prenatal Diagnosis*, **29**, 1256-1261. http://dx.doi.org/10.1002/pd.2408

[20] Chesley, L.C. (1985) Diagnosis of Preeclampsia. *Obstetrics and Gynecology*, **65**, 423-425.

[21] Teran, E., Escudero, C., Moya, W., Flores, M., Vallance, P. and Lopez-Jaramillo, P. (2001) Elevated C-Reactive Protein and Pro-Inflammatory Cytokines in Andean Women with Preeclampsia. *International Journal of Obstetrics and Gynecology*, **75**, 243-249. http://dx.doi.org/10.1016/S0020-7292(01)00499-4

[22] Pathare, A., Al Kindi, S., Alnaqdy, A., Daar, S., Knox-Macauly, H. and Dennison, D. (2004) Cytokine Profile of Sickle Cell Disease in Oman. *American Journal of Hematology*, **77**, 323-328. http://dx.doi.org/10.1002/ajh.20196

[23] Onyemelukwe, G.C., Ekwempu, C.C. and Alexander, L.C. (1985) Pregnancy Specific Glycoprotein (PSG1) in Normal Pregnancy in Nigeria. *Internal Journal of Obstetrics and Gynaecology*, **23**, 347-349. http://dx.doi.org/10.1016/0020-7292(85)90032-3

[24] Silver, R.M., Heyborne, K.D. and Leslie, K.K. (1993) Pregnancy Specific Beta 1 Glycoprotein (SP-1) in Maternal Serum and Ammiotic Fluid; Pre-Eclampsia, Small for Gestational Age Fetus and Fetal Distress. *Placenta*, **14**, 583-589. http://dx.doi.org/10.1016/S0143-4004(05)80211-5

[25] Horne, C.H., Towler, C.M., Pugh-Humphreys, R.G., Thomson, A.W. and Bohn, H. (1976) Pregnancy Specific Beta-1-Glycoprotein: A Product of the Syncytiotrophoblast. *Experientia*, **32**, 1197-1199. http://dx.doi.org/10.1007/BF01927624

[26] Lin, T.M., Halbert, S.P. and Kiefer, D. (1976) Quantitative Analysis of Pregnancy-Associated Plasma Proteins in Human Placenta. *Journal of Clinical Investigations*, **57**, 466-472. http://dx.doi.org/10.1172/JCI108298

[27] Lisboa, F.A., Warren, J., Sulkowski, G., Aparicio, M., David, G., *et al.* (2011) Pregnancy-Specific Glycoprotein 1 Induces Endothelial Tubulogenesis through Interaction with Cell Surface Proteoglycans. *Journal of Biological Chemistry*, **286**, 7577-7586. http://dx.doi.org/10.1074/jbc.M110.161810

[28] Sacks, G., Sargent, I. and Redman, C. (1999) An Innate View of Human Pregnancy. *Immunology Today*, **20**, 114-118. http://dx.doi.org/10.1016/S0167-5699(98)01393-0

[29] Snyder, S.K., Wessner, D.H. Wessells, J.L., Waterhouse, R.M., Zimmermann, W. and Dveksler, G.S. (2001) Pregnancy-Specific-Beta1 Glycoprotein Function as Immunomodulators by Inducing Secretion of IL-10, IL6 and TGF by Human Monocytes. *American Journal of Immunology*, **45**, 205-216. http://dx.doi.org/10.1111/j.8755-8920.2001.450403.x

[30] Blois, S.M., Sulkowski, M., Tirado-Gonzalez, I., Warren, J., Freitag, N., Klabb, B.F., Rifkin, D., Fuss, I., Strober, W. and Dveksler, G.S. (2014) Pregnancy Specific Beta-1 Activates Transformation Growth Factor Beta-1 and Prevent Dextran Sodium Sulfate-Induced Colitis in Mice. *Mucosal Immunology*, **7**, 348-358. http://dx.doi.org/10.1038/mi.2013.53

[31] Masson, G.M., Anthony, F. and Wilson, M. (1983) Value of Schwangerschftsprotein 1 (SP1) and Pregnancy-Associated Plasma Protein A (PAPP-A) in the Clinical Management of Threatened Abortion. *British Journal of Obstetrics and Gynaecology*, **90**, 146-149. http://dx.doi.org/10.1111/j.1471-0528.1983.tb08899.x

[32] Tamsen, L., Johansson, S.G. and Axelsson, O. (1983) Pregnancy-Specific Beta 1-Glycoprotein (SP1) in Serum from Women with Pregnancies Complicated by Intrauterine Growth Retardation. *Journal of Perinatal Medicine*, **11**, 19-25. http://dx.doi.org/10.1515/jpme.1983.11.1.19

[33] Arnold, L.L., Doherty, T.M., Flor, A.W., Simon, J.A., Chou, J.Y., Chan, W.Y. and Mansfield, B.C. (1999) Pregnancy-Specific Glycoprotein Gene Expression in Recurrent Aborters: A Potential Correlation to Interleukin-10 Expression. *American Journal of Reproductive Immunology*, **41**, 174-182. http://dx.doi.org/10.1111/j.1600-0897.1999.tb00530.x

# Permissions

All chapters in this book were first published in OJI, by Scientific Research Publishing; hereby published with permission under the Creative Commons Attribution License or equivalent. Every chapter published in this book has been scrutinized by our experts. Their significance has been extensively debated. The topics covered herein carry significant findings which will fuel the growth of the discipline. They may even be implemented as practical applications or may be referred to as a beginning point for another development.

The contributors of this book come from diverse backgrounds, making this book a truly international effort. This book will bring forth new frontiers with its revolutionizing research information and detailed analysis of the nascent developments around the world.

We would like to thank all the contributing authors for lending their expertise to make the book truly unique. They have played a crucial role in the development of this book. Without their invaluable contributions this book wouldn't have been possible. They have made vital efforts to compile up to date information on the varied aspects of this subject to make this book a valuable addition to the collection of many professionals and students.

This book was conceptualized with the vision of imparting up-to-date information and advanced data in this field. To ensure the same, a matchless editorial board was set up. Every individual on the board went through rigorous rounds of assessment to prove their worth. After which they invested a large part of their time researching and compiling the most relevant data for our readers.

The editorial board has been involved in producing this book since its inception. They have spent rigorous hours researching and exploring the diverse topics which have resulted in the successful publishing of this book. They have passed on their knowledge of decades through this book. To expedite this challenging task, the publisher supported the team at every step. A small team of assistant editors was also appointed to further simplify the editing procedure and attain best results for the readers.

Apart from the editorial board, the designing team has also invested a significant amount of their time in understanding the subject and creating the most relevant covers. They scrutinized every image to scout for the most suitable representation of the subject and create an appropriate cover for the book.

The publishing team has been an ardent support to the editorial, designing and production team. Their endless efforts to recruit the best for this project, has resulted in the accomplishment of this book. They are a veteran in the field of academics and their pool of knowledge is as vast as their experience in printing. Their expertise and guidance has proved useful at every step. Their uncompromising quality standards have made this book an exceptional effort. Their encouragement from time to time has been an inspiration for everyone.

The publisher and the editorial board hope that this book will prove to be a valuable piece of knowledge for researchers, students, practitioners and scholars across the globe.

# List of Contributors

**Mei Lin**
Department of Immunology and Infectious Diseases, The Forsyth Institute, Cambridge, USA
Department of Stomatology, Beijing Chao-Yang Hospital, Capital Medical University, Beijing, China

**Jiang Lin**
Department of Immunology and Infectious Diseases, The Forsyth Institute, Cambridge, USA
Department of Stomatology, Fourth Hospital of Harbin Medical University, Harbin, China

**Yuhua Wang**
Department of Immunology and Infectious Diseases, The Forsyth Institute, Cambridge, USA
Department of Stomatology, Shanghai 9th People's Hospital, Shanghai, China

**Nathalie Bonheur, Toshihisa Kawai and Xiaozhe Han**
Department of Immunology and Infectious Diseases, The Forsyth Institute, Cambridge, USA

**Zuomin Wang**
Department of Stomatology, Beijing Chao-Yang Hospital, Capital Medical University, Beijing, China

**Kohji Ohtubo**
Ishikawa Natural Medicinal Products Research Center, Ishikawa, Japan

**Nobuo Yamaguchi**
Ishikawa Natural Medicinal Products Research Center, Ishikawa, Japan
Department of Fundament Research for CAM, Kanazawa Medical University, Ishikawa, Japan

**Nurmuhamamt Amat and Dilxat Yimit**
Traditional Uighur Medicine Department, Xinjiang Medical University, Urumqi, China

**Parida Hoxur**
Traditional Chinese Medicine Hospital, Xinjiang Medical University, Urumqi, China

**Hiroshi Ushijima and Yousuke Watanabe**
Department of Fundament Research for CAM, Kanazawa Medical University, Ishikawa, Japan

**Heping Zhou**
Department of Biological Sciences, Seton Hall University, New Jersey, USA

**Kenji Kawakita**
Department of Physiology, Meiji University of Integrative Medicine, Kyoto, Japan

**Yong-Suk Kim**
Department of Acupuncture & Moxibustion, (Brain & Neurological Disorders and Pain), Kangnam Korean Hospital, Kyung Hee University, Seoul, Korea

**Nobuo Yamaguchi**
Kanazawa Medical University, Ishikawa, Japan

**Xiao-Pin Lin, Matsuo Arai and Naomi Takazawa**
Ishikawa Natural Medicinal Products Research Center, Kanazawa, Japan

**Shan-Yu Su**
School of Post-Baccalaureate Chinese Medicine, College of Chinese Medicine, China Medical University, Taichung, Taiwan

**Hitoshi Kubota and Nobuo Yamaguchi**
Ishikawa Natural Medicinal Products Research Center, Ishikawa, Japan
Department of Fundament Research for CAM, Kanazawa Medical University, Ishikawa, Japan

**Nurmuhamamt Amat and Dilxat Yimit**
Traditional Uighur Medicine Department, Xinjiang Medical University, Urumqi, China

**Parida Hoxur**
Traditional Chinese Medicine Hospital, Xinjiang Medical University, Urumqi, China

**Nobuo Yamaguchi**
Department of Fundamental Research for CAM, Kanazawa Medical University, Uchinada, Japan
Ishikawa Natural Medicinal Products Research Center, Kanazawa, Japan

**Takanao Ueyama**
Department of Medicine II, Kansai Medical University, Osaka, Japan

**Nurmuhamamt Amat and Dilxat Yimit**
Traditional Uighur Medicine Department, Xinjiang Medical University, Urumqi, China

**Parida Hoxur**
Traditional Chinese Medicine Hospital, Xinjiang Medical University, Urumqi, China

**Daisuke Sakamoto**
Department of Chest Surgery, Kanazawa Medical University, Himi Citizen Hospital, Himi, Japan

**Yuma Katoh**
Ishikawa Natural Medicinal Products Research Center, Kanazawa, Japan
Department of Respiratory Medicine, Tohkai Central Hospital, Gifu, Japan

**Ikkan Watanabe**
Ishikawa Natural Medicinal Products Research Center, Kanazawa, Japan

**Shan-Yu Su**
Department of Chinese Medicine, China Medical University Hospital, Taichung City, Taiwan
School of Post-Baccalaureate Chinese Medicine, College of Chinese Medicine, China Medical University, Taichung City, Taiwan

**Nobuo Yamaguchi**
Department of Fundamental Research for CAM, Kanazawa Medical University, Ishikawa, Japan
Ishikawa Natural Medicinal Products Research Center, Ishikawa, Japan

**Matsuo Arai**
Ishikawa Natural Medicinal Products Research Center, Ishikawa, Japan

**Tsugiya Murayama**
Ishikawa Natural Medicinal Products Research Center, Ishikawa, Japan
Faculty of Pharmaceutical Sciences, Department of Microbiology and Immunology, Hokuriku University, Ishikawa, Japan

**Hyo-Jung Kwon and Yong-Suk Kim**
Department of Acupuncture & Moxibustion, (Brain & Neurological Disorders and Pain), Kangnam Korean Hospital, Kyung Hee University, Seoul, Korea

**Yousuke Watanabe**
Ishikawa Natural Medicinal Products Research Center, Ishikawa, Japan

**Nobuo Yamaguchi**
Ishikawa Natural Medicinal Products Research Center, Ishikawa, Japan
Department of Fundament Research for CAM, Kanazawa Medical University, Ishikawa, Japan

**Isao Horiuch**
Traditional Uighur Medicine Department, Xinjiang Medical University, Urumchi, China
Traditional Chinese Medicine Hospital, Xinjiang Medical University, Urumchi, China

**Tsugia Murayama**
Faculty of Pharmaceutical Sciences, Department of Microbiology and Immunology, Hokuriku University, Ishikawa, Japan

**Pellegrino Mazzone, Ivan Scudiero, Angela Ferravante, Luca E. D'Andrea, Maddalena Pizzulo and Carla Reale**
Laboratory of Immunogenetics, Biogem, Via Camporeale, Ariano Irpino, Italy

**Marina Paolucci and Ettore Varricchio**
Dipartimento di Scienze e Tecnologie, Università del Sannio, Benevento, Italy

**Gianluca Telesio**
Laboratory of Immunogenetics, Biogem, Via Camporeale, Ariano Irpino, Italy
Dipartimento di Medicina molecolare Biotecnologie mediche, Università di Napoli "Federico II", Napoli, Italy

**Tiziana Zotti, Pasquale Vito and Romania Stilo**
Laboratory of Immunogenetics, Biogem, Via Camporeale, Ariano Irpino, Italy
Dipartimento di Scienze e Tecnologie, Università del Sannio, Benevento, Italy

**Mei Lin**
Department of Immunology and Infectious Diseases, The Forsyth Institute, Cambridge, USA
Department of Stomatology, Beijing Chao-Yang Hospital, Capital Medical University, Beijing, China

**Zuomin Wang**
Department of Stomatology, Beijing Chao-Yang Hospital, Capital Medical University, Beijing, China

**Xiaozhe Han**
Department of Immunology and Infectious Diseases, The Forsyth Institute, Cambridge, USA

**Nobuo Yamaguchi**
Department of Fundamental Research for CAM, Kanazawa Medical University, Ishikawa, Japan
Ishikawa Natural Medicinal Products Research Center, Ishikawa, Japan

**Wataru Hiruma and Kohei Suruga**
International Operation Department (FM Center for R & D), Kibun Foods Inc., Tokyo, Japan

**Nurmuhamamt Amat and Dilxat Yimit**
Traditional Uighur Medicine Department, Xinjiang Medical University, Urumchi, China

**Parida Hoxur**
Traditional Uighur Medicine Department, Xinjiang Medical University, Urumchi, China
Traditional Chinese Medicine Hospital, Xinjiang Medical University, Urumchi, China

**Daisuke Sakamoto**
Traditional Chinese Medicine Hospital, Xinjiang Medical University, Urumchi, China

**Kazuhiro Okamoto**
Department of Otolaryngology, Kanazawa Medical University, Ishikawa, Japan

**Shan-Yu Su**
Department of Chinese Medicine, China Medical University Hospital, Taiwan
School of Post-Baccalaureate Chinese Medicine, College of Chinese Medicine, China Medicinal University, Taiwan

**Ghousunnissa Sheikh, Venkata Sanjeev Kumar Neela, Satya Sudheer Pydi and Naveen Chandra Suryadevara,**
LEPRA-India, Blue Peter Public Health & Research Centre, Hyderabad, India

**Ramulu Gaddam and Sai Kumar Auzumeedi**
Government Chest & General Hospital, Hyderabad, India

**Suman Latha Gaddam**
Bhagwan Mahavir Medical Research Centre, Hyderabad, India
Osmania University, Hyderabad, India

**Vijaya Lakshmi Valluri**
LEPRA-India, Blue Peter Public Health & Research Centre, Hyderabad, India
Bhagwan Mahavir Medical Research Centre, Hyderabad, India

**Mohammad Ehlayel**
Weill Cornell Medical College, Doha, Qatar
Section of Pediatric Allergy-Immunology, Department of Pediatrics, Hamad Medical Corporation, Doha, Qatar

**Mahmoud F. Elsaid**
Weill Cornell Medical College, Doha, Qatar
Section of Pediatric Neurology, Department of Pediatrics, Hamad Medical Corporation, Doha, Qatar

**Rana Shami**
Section of Pediatric Neurology, Department of Pediatrics, Hamad Medical Corporation, Doha, Qatar

**Khalid Salem**
Department of Radiology, Hamad Medical Corporation, Doha, Qatar

**Abdulbari Bener**
Deptartment of Biostatistics & Medical Informatics, Cerrahpaşa Faculty of Medicine, Istanbul University, Istanbul, Turkey
Department Evidence for Population Health Unit, School of Epidemiology and Health Sciences, The University of Manchester, Manchester, UK

**Yasuteru Eguchi and Kei Yokokawa**
Ishikawa Natural Medicinal Products Research Center, Ishikawa, Japan

**Nobuo Yamaguchi**
Ishikawa Natural Medicinal Products Research Center, Ishikawa, Japan
Department of Fundament Research for CAM, Kanazawa Medical University, Ishikawa, Japan

**Nurmuhamamt Amat and Dilxat Yimit**
Traditional Uighur Medicine Department, Xinjiang Medical University, Urumqi, China

**Parida Hoxur**
Traditional Chinese Medicine Hospital, Xinjiang Medical University, Urumqi, China

**Wataru Hiruma**
International Operation Department (FM Center for R & D), Kibun Foods Inc., Tokyo, Japan
Faculty of Pharmaceutical Sciences, Fukuoka University, Fukuoka, Japan

**Kohei Suruga, Kazunari Kadokura, Tsuyoshi Tomita, Ayaka Miyata and Yoshihiro Sekino**
International Operation Department (FM Center for R & D), Kibun Foods Inc., Tokyo, Japan

**Masahiko Kimura and Nobufumi Ono**
Faculty of Pharmaceutical Sciences, Fukuoka University, Fukuoka, Japan

**Nobuo Yamaguchi**
Ishikawa Natural Medicinal Products Research Center, Ishikawa, Japan
Department of Fundamental Research for CAM, Kanazawa Medical University, Ishikawa, Japan

**Yasuhiro Komatsu**
Kitasato Institution for Life Science, Kitasato University, Tokyo, Japan
Sun R & D Institute for Natural Medicines Co. Inc., Tokyo, Japan

**C. A. Tony Buffington**
Department of Veterinary Clinical Sciences, The Ohio State University College of Veterinary Medicine, Columbus, USA

**Sarah Moodad, Nayla Al-Akl and Alexander M. Abdelnoor**
Department of Experimental Pathology, Immunology and Microbiology, Faculty of Medicine, American University of Beirut, Beirut, Lebanon

**Joseph Simaan**
Department of Pharmacology and Toxicology, Faculty of Medicine, American University of Beirut, Beirut, Lebanon

**Behrouz Moemeni and Michael Julius**
Sunnybrook Research Institute, Toronto, Canada
Department of Immunology, University of Toronto, Toronto, Canada

**Nathalie Vacaresse and Marina Vainder**
Sunnybrook Research Institute, Toronto, Canada

**Michael E. Wortzman and Tania H. Watts**
Department of Immunology, University of Toronto, Toronto, Canada

**André Veillette**
Laboratory of Molecular Oncology, Clinical Research Institute of Montreal, Montreal, Canada

**Thomas F. Gajewski**
Department of Pathology, University of Chicago, Chicago, IL, USA

**Mohamed M. Hassan**
Faculty of Medical Laboratory Sciences, University of Medical Science and Technology, Khartoum, Sudan
Faculty of Medical Laboratory Sciences, Al Zaiem Al Azhari University, Khartoum, Sudan

**Sofia B. Mohamed**
Tropical Medicine Research Institute, Khartoum, Sudan

**Mohamed A. Hussain**
Department of Pharmaceutical Microbiology, International University of Africa, Khartoum, Sudan

**Amar A. Dowd**
Faculty of Medical Laboratory Sciences, University of Medical Science and Technology, Khartoum, Sudan

**Mauro Giacomelli, Rajesh Kumar and Giacomo Tampella**
Institute of Molecular Medicine "Angelo Nocivelli", University of Brescia, Brescia, Italy
Scuola di Dottorato in Scienze della Riproduzione e dello Sviluppo, University of Trieste, Trieste, Italy

**Mario Bontempelli and Simona Ceffa**
Immunology Laboratory, Ospedali Riuniti of Bergamo, Bergamo, Italy

**Jim M. Banda**
Pathology Department, Faculty of Medicine, Kaduna State University, Kaduna, Nigeria

**Geoffrey C. Onyemelukwe and Bolanle O. P. Musa**
Immunology Unit, Department of Medicine, Ahmadu Bello University Teaching Hospital, Zaria, Nigeria

**Oladapo S. Shittu and Zulai A. Sarkin-Pawa**
Department of Obstetrics and Gynaecology, Ahmadu Bello University Teaching Hospital, Zaria, Nigeria

**Aliyu A. Babadoko and Aisha I. Mamman**
Department of Haematology and Blood Transfusion, Ahmadu Bello University Teaching Hospital, Zaria, Nigeria

**Adamu G. Bakari**
Department of Medicine, Ahmadu Bello University Teaching Hospital, Zaria, Nigeria

**Suraj Junaid**
Federal College of Veternary and Medical Laboratory, National Veterinary and Research Institute, Vom, Nigeria

www.ingramcontent.com/pod-product-compliance
Lightning Source LLC
Chambersburg PA
CBHW080246230326
41458CB00097B/3992

* 9 7 8 1 6 3 2 4 2 4 5 7 0 *